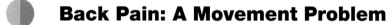

Back Pain: A Movement Problem

A clinical approach incorporating relevant research and practice

Dedication

In memory of my mother and for Ian

both who have always been there for me

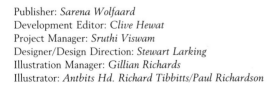

Publisher: *Sarena Wolfaard*
Development Editor: *Clive Hewat*
Project Manager: *Sruthi Viswam*
Designer/Design Direction: *Stewart Larking*
Illustration Manager: *Gillian Richards*
Illustrator: *Antbits Hd. Richard Tibbitts/Paul Richardson*

Back Pain: A Movement Problem

A clinical approach incorporating relevant research and practice

Josephine Key Dip Phys, PGD Manip. Ther.
APA Musculoskeletal Physiotherapist,
Edgecliff Physiotherapy Sports and Spinal Centre,
Edgecliff, New South Wales, Australia

Foreword by

Leon Chaitow ND DO
Registered Osteopathic Practitioner and Honorary Fellow,
University of Westminster, London, UK

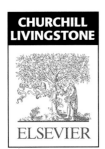

CHURCHILL LIVINGSTONE

ELSEVIER

Edinburgh London New York Oxford Philadelphia St Louis Sydney Toronto 2010

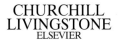

CHURCHILL
LIVINGSTONE
ELSEVIER

First published 2010, © Elsevier Limited. All rights reserved.

ISBN 978-0-7020-3079-6

British Library Cataloguing in Publication Data
A catalogue record for this book is available from the British Library

Library of Congress Cataloging in Publication Data
A catalog record for this book is available from the Library of Congress

your source for books,
journals and multimedia
in the health sciences

www.elsevierhealth.com

Working together to grow
libraries in developing countries

www.elsevier.com | www.bookaid.org | www.sabre.org

ELSEVIER   BOOK AID
             International   Sabre Foundation

The
Publisher's
policy is to use
**paper manufactured
from sustainable forests**

Printed in China

Contents

Foreword

An outside observer might consider – what with the plethora of professions focusing on the topic, and the ceaseless flow of research reports about it – that back pain might now be pretty well understood. However, those of us who labour at the coal-face, confronted daily by myriad versions of 'back pain', realise that the truth is somewhat different, with aetiologies almost as varied as the individuals with the symptoms.

Congresses and conferences devoted to different aspects of back pain come and go, almost always generating contrasting viewpoints, sometimes diplomatically managed, and sometimes not. However – by small incremental degrees – we appear to be inching forwards towards a realisation that it is actually possible, in many instances, to identify coherent patterns of dysfunction that relate to the reported pain, and that a degree of categorisation is often possible. As a result therapeutic choices can frequently be based on what the author of this fascinating book has described as 'a balance between practice-based evidence and evidence-based practice'. This book encourages that process by offering a deeper understanding of some of the processes of compensatory change that may at times be neglected when confronted by a pain-afflicted patient.

It was in the early 1980s that I first became aware of the work of the great Czech physician, Vladimir Janda. Along with many thousands of others, his landmark work has continued to inform my understanding of the human body. Of particular value were his explanations of patterns of dysfunction – for example – Upper and Lower Crossed Patterns ('syndromes'). These describe the veritable chain reactions that emerge when overused, hypertonic, muscle groups alternate with inhibited antagonists to form sequences of dysfunction that commonly translate into pain and other symptoms. (see Chapter 9)

The classical example Crossed Syndrome Pattern is exemplified by the individual whose head and neck are forward of their normal centre of gravity, chin poked anteriorly, with a combination of hypertonic shortened neck extensors/inhibited – possibly lengthened deep neck flexors; short-tight upper fixators of the shoulder (upper trapezius, levator scapula) as well as shortened shoulder protractors/alternating with weak inhibited lower shoulder fixators – including middle and lower trapezius ... and so on, down the body; with shortened lumbar erector spinae – inhibited core abdominal muscles – shortened hip flexors – inhibited gluteal muscles, and so on, involving a complex and compound series of adaptations and compensations, extending the full length of the body. What emerges are not just biomechanical stresses and strains and, inevitably, pain and dysfunction of affected muscles and joints. Additional pathophysiological changes impact on breathing function, and internal pelvic function – with major implications for the individual's health and wellbeing.

Janda not only described and codified such patterns, but via many years of research was able to offer cogent clinical guidelines as to how to begin the process of understanding and 'reading' them – using functional assessments such as the scapulo-humeral rhythm test, and hip abduction test – as examples.

Keen observation and analysis, over a long period, has allowed Josephine Key to accurately describe further elaborations on the theme of Crossed Syndromes, that have immense clinical value. Important insights emerge from Key's expansion of – for example – Janda's original Lower Crossed Syndrome – (where the pelvis translates posteriorly in relation to the trunk - see p. 219). Importantly she also recognised the obverse pattern - one in which the pelvis virtually translates anteriorly (see p.224). My own first reaction to seeing and reading about these expanded descriptions of Janda's work was to say – 'Of course, that's obvious!'. But what was not immediately obvious was that the physiological adaptations that flowed from one such Crossed Pattern would be so different from those flowing from another – with clear implications for subsequent clinical choices. Details of these changes are a small part of what remains for the reader to explore during the reading of this book.

Once the global scale of postural imbalances, and the habitual patterns of use with which these are associated, can be more effectively understood, rehabilitation and normalisation are more readily achievable. What has become clear in this greater understanding is the relative pointlessness – apart from offering symptomatic relief – of excessive therapeutic attention being paid to where pain is being experienced. Low back pain, for example, can well be the end-result of adaptive changes resulting from a primary lower limb imbalance, or a head/neck imbalance – and treating the area of pain without attention to the origin is – to paraphrase an old osteopathic term - no more than 'engine wiping'.

What Josephine Key and her collaborators have achieved in this book is to build on Janda's foundational body of work. If Janda was able to demonstrate *'what'* happens when posture goes wrong,

Key has taken the focus further towards the 'why?' adaptation failure culminates in pain, dysfunction and other symptoms.

Key, with ample reference to the research of others, has mined and collated the evidence of her many years of clinical practice, to effectively demonstrate the need for us to understand the ways in which overuse, misuse, abuse and disuse lead inevitably to altered posturo-movement control, and commonly to pain. How to read such changes more effectively, and how to integrate appropriate treatment and rehabilitation strategies, are the tools that are on offer from this excellent work.

All those working in manual/physical medicine – practitioners and therapists of all schools - can benefit from its' practical insights.

Leon Chaitow, ND DO
University of Westminster, London

In common parlance the spinal column is often referred to as the 'backbone'.

'Back pain' has generally come to mean that of the low back but can infer pain occurring anywhere between the shoulders and the bottom. This book about back pain and movement considers that the whole spine functions as an integrated system. Extending from the head to the tail bone, changed function in one region of the spinal column will be reflected in adaptations in other regions as their functioning is interdependent. Local spinal pain and related syndromes may not necessarily be the result of changed local function but result from a more widespread dysfunction.

Back pain science is becoming an enormous body of work, in particular that pertaining to the low back. More recently, cervical spine disorders are also attracting much more research interest. Increasingly, because of the exciting advances being made in motor control and pain research, there is a diagnosis and management shift from considering that certain pathological anatomical structures are responsible for 'back pain' to a more dynamic systems approach which sees that it is a variable *pathophysiology* in the interdependent functioning of the neuro musculoskeletal systems which is implicated in most spinal pain disorders. That changes in the underlying 'functional mechanisms' such as the control of movement drive the pain disorder which will in turn, influence the bio-psycho-social health of the individual.

This book chooses to focus more upon the aspect of back pain and movement. It attempts to explore and enhance the understanding of healthy movement control of the spine in Chapters 3, 4, 5 & 6; and in the subsequent chapters, the related changes in movement function that are evident in those with spinal pain disorders. Philosophically, an enhanced understanding enables the clinician and movement therapist to better identify the abnormal features and posturomovement defects presenting in that particular patient, laying the foundation for better differential diagnosis and rehabilitation.

This book examines many of the accepted contemporary models of thinking and approach and questions the veracity of some. The ideas proposed in this book have emanated from a clinician attempting a balance between practice based evidence and evidence based practice. In some instances, adjusted or alternate models are offered as a basis for thought and discussion that will hopefully stimulate debate. For some, the work will represent a certain paradigm shift: one which argues for a 'functional approach' – quality in the control of the functional kinematic patterns involved in our 'ordinary movements'. A motor control perspective is offered which argues that developmental and adaptive changes in movement underlie most 'back pain' syndromes.

I have attempted to marry the contemporary evidence available with clinically apparent altered patterns of motor response. In general terms these can be simply teased out to a case of too little control in some regions of the spine and too much in others, with certain predictable consequences.

I envisage that this book will provide helpful information and guidance for all those practitioners involved with managing people with back pain – physiotherapists, osteopaths, chiropractors and doctors of orthopedics, rheumatology, rehabilitation and manual medicine. Likewise for students of movement and those who are involved in re-educating movement – exercise physiologists, Pilates and yoga teachers and so on. In particular it is my hope that those working in the fitness industry such as personal trainers will look beyond advocating 'strength and toning' – and the resultant inevitable need for 'stretching', and begin to offer more responsible, physiological and functionally useful programmes for their many 'at risk' clients, so that in time they do not become a 'patient'.

Josephine Key

Acknowledgements

There are many I would like to acknowledge in my quest for a better understanding of back pain such as it is. At the outset, I am indebted to the many patients who trusted in my care, particularly in the earlier years when I knew so relatively little and who have over time tested my abilities yet taught me so much. It has been and still is a constant learning curve.

My early involvement 'with spines' was as a paediatric neurodevelopmental physiotherapist managing adolescents with adolescent idiopathic scoliosis of the spine. My conceptual understanding of 'functional movement control' was limited and there was little in the way of actual movement science to assist the clinician in determining 'what's wrong with the posturomovement control that this scoliosis happens?' and 'how do I help fix it?' After completing a Post Graduate Diploma in Manipulative Therapy at the University of Sydney, I later set up in private musculoskeletal practice. In 1984, this course was then very Maitland based and 'joint dominant'. While endeavouring to 'improve my manual skills' towards better patient outcomes I was still questioning 'why does back pain occur and what is appropriate exercise therapy?'

In the subsequent journey involved in attempting to answer these questions I am enormously indebted to the early influence of Professor Vladimir Janda and his notion of the interdependent dysfunction of the neuromyo-articular systems which helped make sense of the patient, where often multiple problems often coexist. While his work I consider largely did not receive the degree of accolade and respect it deserved during his lifetime, the direction of current research, diagnosis and clinical practice is very much in line with Janda's tenets that disturbed function is the 'underlying mechanism' which contributes to the development of pathological changes and otherwise underlies most musculoskeletal pain syndromes.

I would like to acknowledge the significant contribution of the growing body of important and more clinically relevant motor control research, a great proportion of which has emanated from fellow colleagues in Australia: Hodges, Richardson, Jull, O'Sullivan, Mosely and their associates to name a few.

I would also like to acknowledge the important insights gleaned from examining and exploring the work of certain pioneers in the realm of movement appreciation both healthy and otherwise. In particular:

- Berta and Karel Bobath for their work on the altered qualities of movement found in the delayed and abnormal development of movement in infancy; and much later:
- Bonnie Bainbridge Cohen for her further insights into the developmental process and quality of movement
- Moshe Feldenkrais whose work facilitated my appreciation of certain fundamental aspects of healthy movement. I am forever grateful for his notion and the title of one of his books, *The Elusive Obvious* – which 'deals with simple, fundamental notions of our daily life that through habit become elusive'
- Ida Rolf for her insights into 'structure' and aberrant patterns of imbalance in myofascial relationships
- Mabel Todd who understood 'bodily economy' and organic posturomovement reactions to the problem of resisting gravity as expressed in her book *The Thinking Body* published way back in 1937
- Irmgard Bartenieff, physiotherapist and movement educator who also influenced by Rudolph Laban, provided further insights into aspects and qualities of healthy movement.

I would also like to acknowledge my various teachers of Iyengar yoga over the years and for some time the Feldenkrais Method, and thank them for their guidance and the subjective insights and improved understanding they helped provide.

In particular I would like to acknowledge my colleagues at Edgecliff Physiotherapy Sports and Spinal Centre without whose support and valuable contribution towards the exploration and evolvement of the work culminating in this book would not have been possible. Especially the Senior Associates, Andrea Clift, Fiona Condie and Caroline Harley who have in particular constructively questioned and explored with me various aspects of the work as it evolved while also 'keeping me in line'. I am also indebted to Andrea for being the catalyst for the inception of the Therapeutic Exercise and Movement Classes which we commenced eight years ago. These classes have taught us much and as our understanding of the real problems of the movement difficulties experienced in people with spinal pain has been better appreciated, likewise the rationale behind the classes and content has continued to evolve. I would also like to thank the Associates within the practice, Micky Yim and Ajantha Suppiah for their valuable contribution and support. All teams depend upon a 'good organizer' and we are all grateful to have had our 'marvellous Nicole' (Crompton) run the practice in such a professional and responsible way such that the therapists can get on with their task. Thank you also Nicole for grappling with all the complexities of permissions and figure schedules – seemingly 'the last straw' when trying to honour a publishing deadline!

Perhaps most importantly, I would like to give special thanks to the real 'godfather' of this book – Leon Chaitow ND DO, esteemed practitioner and teacher, prolific author and editor of the internationally peer reviewed Journal of Bodywork and Movement Therapies. It was his suggestion that the understanding and application of our 'clinical detective work' and the ideas expressed in our published paper might be more fully realized in a book aimed towards practitioners. This work may otherwise well have remained 'a sleeper' – thank you Leon for your discernment and faith in its veracity.

Finally, I would like to honour my dear husband Ian for his love and patient understanding and support in general and particularly during the time of writing this book when, of needs be, I was often 'not there'.

Chapter One

Introduction

Back pain is usually a *symptom of dysfunction* in the musculoskeletal system.

Janda[1] suggests that pain, however undesirable, serves an important biological function acting as a warning signal that all is not well in the movement system. It may be functioning in a harmful way and rather like the warning light on your dashboard reminding you the car needs a service, pain heralds the 'tipping point' in a continuum of dysfunction. Addressing the dysfunction will generally ameliorate the pain. However, classical Western medicine has by and large tended to view pain within a 'disease model', hunting for 'the pathological' structure in order to arrive at diagnosis and 'fix it'. As we all know, the results have been less than promising and there is now a shift towards the possibility that disturbed function may be more important than structural damage as the physical basis of back pain.[1] When the dysfunction and pain continue unabated, secondary factors such as disability and psychosocial factors begin to create a complex picture of interlocking dysfunctions. The 'biopsychosocial model of dysfunction'[2] acknowledges the multifactorial nature of the 'problem of back pain' and contemporary treatment approaches generally embrace addressing each aspect as indicated.

Back pain is fundamentally a physical problem and the focus of this book is to primarily address the 'bio' aspect – the physical perspective of back pain.

Gracovetsky[3] has said 'restoring the function of the injured patient implies knowing what the normal function is, something which is still the subject of speculation'. In similar vein, Van Dieën[4] states 'the relationship between low-back pain and motor behavior is poorly understood. Consequently the (para) medical disciplines involved lack a theoretical basis for treatment and outcome evaluation'. Moseley[5] asks 'what is it about pain that changes the way people move?' Conversely, one could ask: 'what is it about the way people move that causes pain?'

The aim in this work is an attempt to assist the understanding of normal movement function and the *nature* of movement dysfunction seen in spinal pain patients. Understanding *how* and *why* movement is altered goes a long way towards effectively redressing it.

An integrative model of neuromusculoskeletal dysfunction is offered as both a theoretical and a practical framework to aid the understanding of dysfunction and enhance current clinical practice skill. It describes the consistently observed, more common altered patterns of postural and movement control seen clinically in patients with spinal pain and related disorders. While each person with back pain presents individually, we can observe the tendency for common features which can be collated into a general paradigm of dysfunction. In general, the kinematic patterns of movement adopted during the simple repetitive activities of daily living are altered as a result of changed posturomovement control, and contribute to repetitive microtrauma and 'injury'. Most back pain is a developmental movement disorder – a simple event often called an 'injury' can end up being a major problem. This helps explain the development and perpetuation of pain and related symptoms.

The model is somewhat of a paradigm shift – one of functional adaptation and maladaptation of posturomovement control as a common underlying genesis of most spinal pain disorders. It also provides a clinical classification system based upon posturomovement dysfunction providing a framework guiding assessment and management. Without a conceptual practical framework, there is a risk that 'evidence based research' is often misinterpreted and inappropriately applied to all patients regardless of that patient's presenting dysfunction. The aim of treatment interventions, both manual and therapeutic exercise, is to restore function. Manual treatment is necessary initially to alleviate pain and help normalize the local neuromuscular dysfunction. Retraining control of movement protects the spine against reoccurrence and helps restore function.

An appreciation of these more common changed responses in motor control helps to formulate the choices and enhance the quality of teaching therapeutic exercise in the rehabilitation of spinal musculoskeletal pain syndromes. We are seeing a larger group of patients presenting with symptoms resulting from, or exacerbated by, inappropriate exercise therapy. Hopefully an improved understanding of the problem can help rescue and refine the art of exercise therapy.

The work has emanated from the fruits of over 40 years of extensive clinical practice, scientific 'evidence' to hand and the diverse influences of inspired thinkers within the realms of therapeutic practice and somatic movement education. The clinical practice combination of manual therapist and movement educator has helped in seeing and understanding the relationships between joint and myofascial dysfunction and movement disorders. Conducting therapeutic exercise and movement classes has provided more opportunity for observing and recognizing certain 'patterns' of response which appear to be somewhat common in people with a history of spinal pain disorders.

Significantly however, by our observation, it appears that the boundary between 'normal' and abnormal movement function is often quite blurred and dysfunction may represent subtle variations from normal.[6] Similar patterns are often evident, albeit less marked, when observing the general public: students in a yoga class or similar exercise forum perhaps reflect common underlying tendencies in us all and which, when more pronounced, contribute to the development of pain syndromes. The presence of pain further compounds the dysfunction. Janda noted 'the high incidence of functional impairment makes it extremely difficult to estimate the borders between the norm and evident pathology'. The prevalence of low back pain appears to be on the rise in affluent urbanized countries.[7]

This book is addressed to the clinician to practically assist in the physical aspect of the management of patients with spinal pain disorders. It attempts to examine and provide an overview of ideal normal movement function of the torso and the functional interrelationship of its parts. This includes the significant aspects of normal motor development and the important qualities in normal movement control. It also describes the commonly observed inefficient patterns of axial muscle control and the close relationship between these and the development of changed articular function and pain syndromes.

References

[1] Janda V. Introduction to functional pathology of the motor system. Proc: VII Commonwealth and International Conference on Sport, Physical Education, Recreation and Dance, vol. 3. 1982.

[2] Waddell G. The Back Pain Revolution. Edinburgh: Churchill Livingstone; 2004.

[3] Gracovetsky S. Stability or controlled instability. In: Vleeming A, Mooney V, Stoeckart R, editors. Movement, stability & Lumbopelvic Pain: Integration of research and therapy. Edinburgh: Churchill Livingstone Elsevier; 2007.

[4] Van Dieën JH. Low back pain and motor behavior: contingent adaptations, a common goal. Proc. 6th Interdisciplinary World Congress on Low Back and Pelvic Pain. Barcelona; 2007.

[5] Moseley GL. Psychosocial factors and altered motor control. Proc. 5th Interdisciplinary World Congress on Low Back and Pelvic Pain. Melbourne; 2004.

[6] DonTigny RL. A detailed and critical biomechanical analysis of the sacroiliac joints and relevant kinesiology: the implications for lumbopelvic function and dysfunction. In: Vleeming A, Mooney V, Stoeckart R, editors. Movement, stability & Lumbopelvic Pain: Integration of research and therapy. Edinburgh: Churchill Livingstone Elsevier; 2007.

[7] Volinn E. The epidemiology of low back pain in the rest of the world: a review of surveys in low and middle income countries. Spine 1997; 22(15).

The problem of back pain

Just about any book or paper you read on low back pain (LBP) introduces the subject by restating the fact of the increasing 'epidemic' of low back pain and its enormous cost to society. We can fly man to the moon yet despite the advances of modern science the effective diagnosis and treatment of back pain remains somewhat of an elusive dilemma. Is it perhaps a case of losing sight of basic principles? To utilize Feldenkrais'[1] term, is it missing 'the elusive obvious'?

According to Janda,[2] excluding insidious pathology, most musculoskeletal pain is the result of impaired function in the motor system. Pain serves an important biological function,

It might even be said that the motor system suffers from our whims and thus has no other way of protecting itself than by producing pain'.[2]

The Eastern medical paradigm would tend to view pain as a valuable sign signalling harmful overstress in the system. Western medicine has had a vested interest in treating pain as a disease and back pain has certainly become this.

The diagnosis dilemma

Waddell[3] says: 'only with the introduction of western medicine does chronic back disability become common'. The approach of contemporary medicine is to search for a 'pathological' diagnosis, the cornerstone for instituting appropriate treatment. However, definite structural pathology is only evident in about 15% of patients with back pain.[3-5] The relationship between imaging and symptoms is weak.[4,6] There are inherent limitations to the accuracy of diagnostic tests and imaging studies have their greatest value in the exclusion of other conditions.[7] There is often relatively weak agreement between the results of medical 'physical examination' and the subjective reporting of pain and disability.[8] As Waddell[3] suggests the problem of back pain exists 'because we cannot diagnose any definite disease or offer any real cure' – 'if back pain becomes chronic patients soon realize that we do not know what is wrong'; and 'so when treatment for back pain fails, the professional may look for psychological reasons or other excuses'; 'the patient is likely to become defensive and both patient and professional may become angry and hostile'. Litigation and the potential 'reward' for back pain further muddy the waters. However, Hendler et al.[9] point out that the psychiatric abnormalities that are the normal response to chronic pain coupled with litigation tend to bias many physicians resulting in less extensive evaluation. They reported finding an organic origin for the pain, which had been overlooked in 98% of their sample group, who had been variously diagnosed as 'chronic pain', psychogenic pain' or lumbar strain'. No wonder the 'biopsychosocial model'[10] has evolved.

To aid diagnosis, Waddell[3] suggests a simple 'diagnostic triage' approach to determine management. As part of this framework, screening for 'red flags' indicating possible insidious pathology and 'yellow flags' indicating psychosocial risk factors are considered. Most patients will fall into either of three categories:

- Ordinary backache – 'the common or garden non-specific low back pain'
- Nerve root pain
- Serious spinal pathology which accounts for less than 1% of cases.

Most back pain is 'ordinary backache' which is 'non-specific'.[3] The remainder of patients have a 'specific' factor to account for their pain. Zusman[11] suggests that the term 'non specific' means essentially the inability of orthodox medicine to arrive at a definitive diagnosis for pain largely on the basis of structure, anatomy and biomechanics (SAB). However the patient has come to expect a SAB basis for his pain and may well prefer any reasonable diagnosis to uncertainty. The 'disc' provided a very handy hook on which the patient could hang his hat. Concerned people immediately 'understood the problem'. Unfortunately, as a result of these SAB beliefs and 'failure for various reasons, to obtain acceptable levels and/or duration of pain relief usually in association with the unproductive sequence of providers and treatments, effectively renders these patients chronic, partial or complete activity intolerant cripples'.[11] The patient's belief that the pain may signify 'serious damage', and provoking it might cause disablement, contributes towards the fear of moving, known as 'fear avoidance beliefs'[3]. The recognition of the negative impact of fear avoidance beliefs and deconditioning behavior led to the establishment of various task force groups that suggested the 'de-medicalization' of back pain and the avoidance of inactivity.[12] This was further reinforced by the Paris Task Force on Back Pain[13] which recommended the early resumption of 'activity of any form – rather than any specific activity'. Whilst these recommendations are understandable in helping to stem secondary factors contributing to the magnitude of the problem it is not a specific therapeutic solution to the underlying problem. In fact for many, the 'keep them moving' advice has contributed to the further entrenchment of already dysfunctional movement patterns, serving to perpetuate their 'non specific chronic pain' problem. If 'activity' and therapeutic exercise are to be effective they must specifically redress the *actual impairments*.

Classification systems for chronic low back pain

Chronic non specific low back pain (CNLBP) or 'ordinary' backache accounts for approximately 85% of back pain. The lack of a specific diagnosis has resulted in the lack of specific treatment interventions and poor outcomes. Various clinical classification systems have been proposed in attempt to improve intervention outcomes, some with dubious veracity.[14] In a review of the literature, Riddle[15] notes some classification systems are designed to determine the most appropriate treatment, some to aid in prognosis, and others to identify pathology. Still others place patients into homogenous groups based upon selected variables. Examining these is inclined to give one a headache, so laborious can they be. Riddle highlighted the limitations of the four most commonly cited systems, found those in current use did not meet many of the measurement standards and clinical utility was unclear.

The biopsychosocial paradigm acknowledges that CNLBP is a multifactorial problem.[3] Treatment interventions will only show positive outcomes when they appropriately address the patient's *actual prime impairments*. O'Sullivan[16] stringently argues for a classification system based upon the *specific mechanism underlying and driving the pain disorder*. He provides an excellent overview of the current operant classification/ diagnosis models which are summarized below.

- *Patho-anatomical model.* The traditional medical approach where abnormal structural findings such as 'disc prolapse' are assumed to be the cause of pain and treatment interventions provided on the basis of this assumption. (Extraordinarily, it appears that 'function affects structure' is rarely considered.)
- *Peripheral pain generator model.* Identification of the painful structure based upon history, clinical examination and diagnostic blocks. Treatment such as blocks and denervation procedures address the pain symptom without consideration for the underlying mechanism.
- *Neurophysiological model.* Central sensitization of pain secondary to sustained peripheral nociceptive input and changes in cortical mapping. Medical interventions inhibit both central and peripheral processing of pain.
- *Psychosocial model.* The impact of psychological and social factors upon the modulation of pain and in particular their capacity to increase the CNS mediated drive of pain. Poor coping strategies, anxiety, catastrophizing, hyper-vigilance tend to increase pain levels, disability and muscle guarding. Cognitive behavioral interventions can be effective. There is only

a small subgroup where these factors are primary. The danger, however, is that due to lack of an alternate diagnosis, physiotherapists are tending to classify most patients with CNLBP as primarily psychosocial driven. This is significant!

• *Mechanical loading model.* Both high and low levels of physical activity are reported risk factors for LBP; sustained end range loading; sudden and repeated loading, and related mechanical exposures are also influenced by ergonomic and environmental factors and have the potential for ongoing peripheral nociception and need to be addressed as part of management.

• *Signs and symptoms model.* Impairments in spinal movements and function, changes in segmental mobility, pain provocation tests; the effect of repeated movement on pain. The approaches of Maitland[17] and McKenzie[18–21] fall into this model which is based upon biomechanical and patho-anatomical models and have led to the treatment of signs and symptoms associated with CNLBP. Limited evidence of efficacy may reflect research designs and neglecting the biopsychosocial dimensions.

• *Motor control model.* This model includes the approaches of Richardson and Jull[22], Sahrmann[23] and O'Sullivan.[24,25] Movement and control impairments are highly variable and their presence does not establish cause and effect. Altered motor behavior is either protective or maladaptive which results in ongoing abnormal tissue loading and mechanically provoked pain. This group are amenable to tailored physiotherapy interventions directed at their specific physical and cognitive impairments with demonstrated positive outcomes.

• *Biopsychosocial model* – the multidimensional approach to dealing with CNLBP. The relative contributions of the different dimensions and their dominance will differ for each patient. Clinical reasoning allows determination as to which factors are dominant. Consideration of all factors allows for a diagnosis and mechanism based classification guiding management.

The subject of this book makes the case for adding another category to those summarized by O'Sullivan.

• *Functional movement model.* This encompasses the biopsychosocial paradigm with the major focus upon improving the understanding and skill of the physical therapist in better dealing with the problem of movement dysfunction in spinal pain disorders. It sees that altered function in the posturomovement system is the primary problem largely responsible for the development and perpetuation of most pain syndromes. A simple clinical classification system based upon altered posturomovement function guides assessment *functional diagnosis* and management. Specific, appropriate treatment interventions directed to both the 'peripheral pain generator' and the altered posturomovement function improves pain and ability and helps counter the development of secondary psychosocial problems. Restoring neurmyoarticular function helps restore the person.

The model is cognisant of all the above models but mainly rests within models 5–8 described above.

The need for clinical classification of chronic LBP for diagnosis and directing appropriate physical therapy

The classification of chronic low back pain (CLBP) into subgroups based upon movement impairments has been advocated by Sahrmann,[23,26] O'Sullivan[16,27] and colleagues.[28,29] Classification enables more appropriate, specific and effective interventions. Interventions adopting this approach have shown more positive outcomes.[30]

With regard to the motor control impairments found in patients with chronic low back pain, O'Sullivan[16,27] considers there are three main groups:

• The underlying pathology drives the pain and the movement impairment is secondary and adaptive.

• Those with dominant psychological and/or social problems and maladaptive coping strategies.

• The largest group where movement impairments are a maladaptive response to pain resulting in chronic abnormal tissue loading and ongoing pain and distress. Presentation is in either of two manners:

 • Movement impairment characterized by avoidant pain behavior, guarding and cocontraction and fear of movement. Management is based upon a cognitive behavioral model to reduce fear of movement and relax muscle tone by education and facilitating graduated movement exposure.

 • Control impairment characterized by no impairment in mobility but adopts provocative postures and movements and show defective motor control. Motor learning interventions based upon a cognitive behavior treatment model with the aim of changing faulty movement

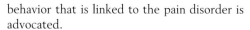

behavior that is linked to the pain disorder is advocated.

These two different strategies create either excessive or deficient spinal stability, [16] represent the primary physical problem and, with secondary cognitive problems, drive the pain disorder.

This book argues from a clinical perspective informed by research that motor control changes lead to the development of back pain and when pain arrives it further influences motor control as O'Sullivan, [16,27] Van Dieën [31] and others [32,33] describe. The 'functional movement model' sees that movement and control impairments often coexist in the one patient (see Ch. 8). The extent of each will be dependent upon the patient's functional classification and stage of the disorder.

The case for a functional classification system based upon posturomovement impairments

When function is disturbed it can be overwhelming for the therapist 'to see' and make sense of the patient in front of her. *Why* and *how* is he dysfunctional?

Assessing patterns of torso muscle recruitment, Nussbaum and Chaffin [34] noted that when they did not average experimental myoelectric data, but adopted a 'competitive neural network model', subjects formed consistent and finite clusters and could be categorized as either 'majority' or 'minority' type responders based on their individual muscle response patterns. They speculated that interindividual muscle recruitment differences may be important for assessing individual musculoskeletal risk.

Similarly, observant clinical practice delineates certain 'clusters' of response in the patterns of posturomovement control adopted by patients with spinal pain disorders. These appear to fall into two primary groups which can be readily discerned because of the typically altered standing posture and the position of the pelvis. This is associated with certain other typical changed responses. There are common features across both groups (Ch.8) and within each group (Ch. 9). Janda stressed the importance of faulty posture and its association with muscle imbalance and chronic pain syndromes. [35]

These two primary groups can be conveniently utilized as the basis for a therapeutic functional classification system based upon altered posturomovement control. While the 'pure' form of each primary

dysfunction picture is not necessarily prevalent, patients generally display 'majority' or 'minority' features of the primary picture. Other pictures of dysfunction emanate from these primary groups (Ch. 10).

The functional classification of patients helps provide a framework for guiding assessment, formulating a *dysfunctional diagnosis* and instituting appropriate treatment. This is in concordance with O'Sullivan [16] who suggested 'for a classification system to be clinically useful it should be based upon identifying the underlying mechanism(s) driving the disorder, in order to guide targeted interventions which in turn should predict the outcome of the disorder'.

The biopsychosocial model

First described by Engel in the 1970s, [36] one of the strengths of this model is that it encouraged broader thinking within medicine. It is now well accepted that chronic musculoskeletal pain is a multifaceted problem. The biopsychosocial model appreciates the functional interrelationships between the psyche and the soma and the consequent potential social effects that can occur in chronic pain states. The key clinical elements of this model described by Waddell [3] are:

- Physical dysfunction which leads to pain. How the patient reacts to the pain will affect and be affected by the other elements
- Beliefs and coping
- Distress
- Illness behavior
- Social interactions.

This is a most welcome departure from the conventional western biomedical disease model and research is even beginning to 'prove' aspects such as the deleterious effect of mental stress upon motor performance [37] and the reduction of psychological stress when pain is relieved. [38] Similarly the works of Linton, [39] Vlaeyen [40,41] and others have done much to enlarge the understanding of maladaptive behavioral responses to chronic pain. This has resulted in an increasing cognitive-behavioral approach as part of therapeutic management. Manual therapists need to understand and manage both the psychosocial and biomedical aspects of their patients and conceptual models have been proposed to help this integration. [42]

But what about the bio?

Getting the balance right between the various components can be a problem and the emphasis appears to have swung too far towards the psychosocial issues to the detriment of the physical aspects.[3,43] Is this partly because physiotherapists have not been doing their job? The research certainly points to this.[44,45] Poor research design and *inappropriate exercises* appear the major culprits, lending weight to O'Sullivan's call[16] for clinical classification systems in order to direct more effective interventions. Receiving 'physiotherapy' has been associated with a poorer prognosis and longer duration of back pain.[46] 'Physiotherapy' was defined as 'combinations of exercise therapy and modalities such as heat cold and massage and advice on daily behavior'. Here lies another problem. Something has to change! McGill states, 'No clinician will be effective if the cause of the patient's troubles is not removed'.[47] O'Sullivan[16] notes the increasing trend for physiotherapists to classify most patients with CLBP as primarily psychosocial driven due to lack of an alternative diagnosis. This is a real worry! If physical therapists do not adequately address the 'physical issues' and the patient is left with his pain yet told what is tantamount to 'it's all in your mind', it is no wonder he becomes behaviorally changed. For anyone who has had pain, it *is* depressing. Removing it is liberating.[38]

It should be mentioned that the 'somatic therapies' have always implicitly embodied an integrated biopsychosocial approach seeing that 'function' involves the whole person and whose personality is expressed in the way he moves. The work of Feldenkrais,[1,48] Hanna,[49,50] Bartenieff,[51] Hackney,[52] Bainbridge Cohen,[53] Hartley[54] and others has much to teach the 'biomedical' camp about movement and the whole person.

Evidence based practice

This has become the modern mantra. All evidence is not necessarily good evidence. Charlton and Miles[55] suggest, 'evidence based medicine is ripe for evaluation'. We are told we have a responsibility to deliver evidence-based treatment techniques yet what constitutes evidence? The two cornerstones of evidence based medicine are the randomized clinical trial (RCT) and meta-analysis and systematic reviews.[56] RCTs clearly have their strengths and weaknesses.

Berger[57] points out that equally valid yet less widely understood or used are qualitative and phenomenological methodologies that allow for detailed description and analysis and the whole person can be considered. Neither model is better than the other and each has inherent problems.

In the management of LBP, Delitto[58] notes the dichotomy between clinicians and researchers with a widening of the gap and discord in the debate, each accusing the other of being 'out of touch'. Caution should be exercised in the prescriptive use of 'clinical practice guidelines' where recommendations should be predicated upon three assumptions: science cannot define optimal care; the process of analysing evidence and opinion is imperfect; and patients are not uniform. While there are mountains of research studies, to date relatively few directly assist clinical practice.

Experimental design is often flawed in that it is 'unfunctional'. Numerous back pain research studies [59–63] have the subject seated with the pelvis restrained as they determine the responses of the back muscles. The pelvis is the platform and functional base of support for the spine directing much of its posturomovement control hence these outcomes should be viewed with some scepticism. With more interest in trunk muscle recruitment patterns research design is beginning to allow freedom of the hips and pelvis.[64]

Does evidenced based practice benefit patients? While there is emerging evidence that when evidence based management is practiced, patients benefit[65] at present there is simply not enough research on which to base clinical practice. As Berger[57] suggests, if we wait until everything we do is proven by research we will never practice. Rather we should think of *'evidence informed practice'*. Therapists have the responsibility to correlate the established scientific evidence and provide the queries and stimulus for further investigation. Some of the most exciting and clinically relevant research into the management of back pain is emanating from Australian researchers who are also clinicians and from centres where there is a healthy cross pollination between the researchers and clinicians. The brilliant insights of Janda resulted from clinical practice and his related research rendering him a key figure in the 20th century rehabilitation movement.[35]

Research can be misused in what Moore and Petty[66] describe as the 'Evidence-based practice technique syndrome' where every patient with a certain diagnostic label e.g. low back pain, is examined and regardless of what the findings are is placed in a stabilizing muscle re-education group or an aerobic activity group simply because they have back pain. Improved treatment outcomes will occur when *function is assessed* and *specific interventions* are *directed to the found dysfunction.*

Lastly, we should not forget that creative and intuitive clinicians have forged new directions. Without the intuitive insights of Bobath, Knott Maitland and others, many patients would not have been helped. The task for therapists becomes treating responsibly and systematically and collecting data as best we can using many methods, while 'Above all do no harm'.[57]

References

[1] Feldenkrais M. The Elusive Obvious or Basic Feldenkrais. Cupertino Ca: Meta Publications; 1981.

[2] Janda V. Introduction to functional pathology of the motor system, In: Proc. Vol 3. V11 Commonwealth and International Conference on Sport, Physical Education, Recreation and Dance; 1982.

[3] Waddell G. The back pain revolution. Edinburgh: Churchill Livingstone; 2004.

[4] Deyo RA, Weinstein JN. Low back pain. N Engl J Med 2001;344(5):363-70.

[5] Roy SH, Oddsson LIE. Classification of paraspinal muscle impairments by surface electromyography. Phys Ther 1998;78(8):838-51.

[6] Kleinstück F, Dvorak J, Mannion A. Are "structural abnormalities" on magnetic resonance imaging a contraindication to the successful conservative treatment of chronic nonspecific low back pain? Spine 2006;31(19):2250-7.

[7] Saal JS. General principles of diagnostic testing as related to painful lumbar spine disorders: a critical appraisal of current diagnostic techniques. Spine 2002;27(22):2538-45.

[8] Michel A, Kohlmann T, Raspe H. The association between clinical findings on physical examination and self reported severity in back pain: results of a population based study. Spine 1997;22(3): 296-303.

[9] Hendler N, Bergson C, Morrison C. Overlooked physical diagnoses in chronic pain patients involved in litigation, Part 2. Psychosomatics 1996;37(6): 509-17.

[10] Waddell G. Volvo award in clinical sciences: a new clinical model for the treatment of low back pain. Spine 1987;12(7): 632-44.

[11] Zusman M. Instigators of activity intolerance. Man Ther 1997; 2(2): 75-86.

[12] Fordyce WE, editor. Task force on Pain in the Workplace of the International Association for the Study of Pain. Seattle: IASP Press; 1995.

[13] Abenhaim L, et al. The role of activity in the therapeutic management of back pain: report of the International Paris Task Force on Back Pain. Spine 2000;25(4S):1S-33S.

[14] Fritz JM, George S. The use of a classification approach to identify subgroups of patients with acute low back pain: interrater reliability and short-term treatment outcomes. Spine 2000;25(1):106.

[15] Riddle DL. Classification and low back pain: a review of the literature and critical analysis of selected systems. Phys Ther 1998;78(7):708-37.

[16] O'Sullivan P. Diagnosis and classification of chronic low back pain disorders: maladaptive movement and motor control impairments as an underlying mechanism. Man Ther 2005;10:242-55.

[17] Maitland J. Vertebral Manipulation. London: Butterworths; 1986.

[18] McKenzie R. The lumbar spine: Mechanical diagnosis and treatment. Waikanae New Zealand: Spinal Publications; 1981.

[19] Werneke M, Hart D, Cook DA. Descriptive study of the centralization phenomenon: a prospective analysis. Spine 1999;24(7):676-83.

[20] Werneke M, Hart D. Discriminant validity and relative precision for classifying patients with nonspecific neck and back pain by anatomic pain patterns. Spine 2003;28(2):161-6.

[21] Wilson L, et al. Intertester reliability of a low back pain classification system. Spine 1999;24(3):248-54.

[22] Richardson CA, Jull GA. Muscle control – pain control. What exercises should you prescribe. Man Ther 1995;1(1):2-10.

[23] Sahrmann SA. Diagnosis and Treatment of Movement Impairment Syndromes. St Louis: Mosby; 2002.

[24] O'Sullivan PB, Twomey LT, Allison GT. Evaluation of specific stabilising exercises in the treatment of chronic low back pain with radiologic diagnosis of spondylolysis or spondylolisthesis. Spine 1997; 22(24):2959-67.

[25] O'Sullivan PB. Lumbar segmental 'instability': clinical presentation and specific stabilising exercise management. Man Ther 2000; 5(1):2-12.

[26] Maluf KS, Sahrmann SA, Van Dillen LR. Use of a classification system to guide nonsurgical management of a patient with chronic low back pain. Phys Ther 2000;80(11):1097-111.

[27] O'Sullivan P. Classification of lumbopelvic pain disorders - Why is it essential for management. Man Ther 2006;11:169-70.

[28] Dankaerts W, et al. The inter-examiner reliability of a classification method for non-specific chronic low back pain patients with motor control

impairment. Man Ther 2006;11:28-39.

[29] Dankaerts W, et al. Differences in sitting postures are associated with nonspecific chronic low back pain disorders when patients are subclassified. Spine 2006;31 (6):698-704.

[30] Dankaerts W, et al. The use of a mechanism-based classification system to evaluate and direct management of a patient with non-specific chronic low back pain and motor control impairment – A case report. Man Ther 2007;12(2):181-91.

[31] Van Dieën JH. Low back pain and motor behaviour: contingent adaptations, a common goal. Proc. 6th Interdisciplinary World Congress on Low Back and Pelvic Pain. Barcelona; 2007.

[32] Van Dieën JH, Cholewicki J, Radebold A. Trunk muscle recruitment patterns in patients with low back pain enhance the stability of the lumbar spine. Spine 2003;28(8):834-41.

[33] Cholewicki J, van Dieën JH. Editorial: muscle function and dysfunction in the spine. J Electromyogr Kinesiol 2003;13:303-4.

[34] Nussbaum MA, Chaffin DB. Pattern classification reveals intersubject group differences in lumbar muscle recruitment during static loading. Clin Biomech 1997;12(2):97-106.

[35] Morris CE, et al. Vladimir Janda, MD, DSc: Tribute to a master of rehabilitation. Spine 2006;31 (9):1060-4.

[36] Engel GF. The need for a new medical model: a challenge for biomedicine. Science 1977;196:129-36.

[37] Davis K, et al. The impact of mental processing and pacing on spine loading: 2002 Volvo award in Biomechanics. Spine 2002;27 (23):2645-53.

[38] Wallis BJ, Lord SM, Bogduk N. Resolution of psychological distress of whiplash patients following treatment by radiofrequency neurotomy: a randomized double-blind, placebo controlled trial.

[39] Linton S. A review of psychological risk factors in back and neck pain. Spine 2000;25:1148-56.

[40] Vlaeyen JWS, Crombez G. Fear of movement/(re)injury, avoidance and pain disability in chronic low back pain patients. Man Ther 1999;4(4): 187-95.

[41] Vlaeyen JWS, Vancleef LMG. Behavioral analysis, fear of movement/(re)injury and cognitive-behavioral management of chronic low back pain. In: Vleeming A, Mooney V., Stoeckart R, editors. Movement, Stability & Lumbopelvic Pain: Integration of research and therapy. Edinburgh: Churchill Livingstone Elsevier; 2007.

[42] Jones M, Edwards I, Gifford L. Conceptual models for implementing biopsychosocial theory in clinical practice. Man Ther 2002;7(1):2-9.

[43] Alford L. Findings of interest from immunology and psychoneuroimmunology. Man Ther 2007;12(2):176-80.

[44] Van Tulder M, Koes BW, Bouter LM. Conservative treatment of acute and chronic nonspecific low back pain: a systematic review of randomized controlled trials o the most common interventions. Spine 1997; 22(18):2128-56.

[45] Van Tulder M, et al. Exercise therapy for low back pain: a systematic review within the framework of the Cochrane Collaboration Back Review Group. Spine 2000;25(21): 2784-96.

[46] Van den Hoogen HJM, et al. The prognosis of low back pain in general practice. Spine 1997; 22(13):1515-21.

[47] McGill S. Low Back Disorders: evidence based prevention and rehabilitation. Champaign, Il: Human Kinetics; 2002.

[48] Feldenkrais M. Body and Mature behaviour: a study of anxiety, sex, gravitation and learning. New York: International Universities Press; 1949.

[49] Hanna T. Somatics; Reawakening the mind's control of movement, flexibility and health. Cambridge Ma: Da Capo Press; 1988.

[50] Hanna T. The body of life: creating new pathways for sensory awareness and fluid movement. Rochester: Healing Arts Press; 1979.

[51] Bartenieff I. Body movement: coping with the environment. Australia: Gordon and Breach; 2002.

[52] Hackney P. Making connections; Total body integration through Bartenieff Fundamentals. New York: Routledge; 2002.

[53] Bainbridge Cohen B., Sensing, Feeling and Action: the experiential anatomy oif body-mind centering. Northampton Ma: Contact Editions; 1993.

[54] Hartley LH. Wisdom of the Body Moving: an introduction to body-mind centering. Berkeley Ca: North Atlantic Books; 1989.

[55] Charlton BG, Miles A. The rise and fall of EBM. Q J Med 1998;91:371-4.

[56] Koes BW, Hoving JL. The value of the randomized clinical trial in the field of physiotherapy. Man Ther 1998;3(4):179-86.

[57] Berger D, Davis C, Harris S. What constitutes evidence? Phys Ther 1996;76(9):1011-4.

[58] Delitto A. Clinicians and researchers who treat and study patients with low back pain: are you listening? Phys Ther 1998;78 (7):705-7.

[59] Marras WS, et al. Spine loading characteristics of patients with low back pain compared with asymptomatic individuals. Spine 2001;26(23):2566-74.

[60] Stokes IAF, et al. Decrease in Trunk Muscular Response to Perturbation with Preactivation of Lumbar Spinal Musculature. Spine 2000;25(15):1957-64.

[61] Cholewicki J, et al. Delayed Trunk Muscle Reflex Responses Increase the Risk of Low Back Injuries. Spine 2005;30 (23):2614-20.

[62] Radebold A, et al. Muscle response Pattern to Sudden Trunk Loading in healthy Individuals and in Patients with Chronic Low Back Pain. Spine 2000;25(8):947-54.

[63] Van Dien JH, Cholewicki J, Radebold A. Trunk Muscle

Recruitment Patterns in Patients with Low Back Pain Enhance the Stability of the Lumbar Spine. Spine 2003;28(8):834-41.

[64] Silfies SP, et al. Trunk muscle recruitment patterns in specific chronic low back pain populations. Clin Biomech 2005;20(5):465-73.

[65] Imrie R, Ramey DW. The evidence for the evidence based medicine. Complement Ther Med 2000;8:123-6.

[66] Moore A, Petty N. Evidence-based practice – getting a grip and finding a balance. Editorial Man Ther 2001;6(4):195-6.

Chapter Three

The development of posture and movement

3

All movement is dependent upon related supporting postures for its control. Posture and movement are interdependent and develop hand in hand.

When observing the posture and movement behavior of people with spinal pain and related disorders one can usually see altered qualities and patterns of response. To help understand and appreciate these patterns, an examination of salient aspects of early motor development is helpful. This is not intended as a comprehensive treatise on the multiple aspects of development, but rather the opportunity to particularly see how movement control of the spine develops. To analyze the important component parts and the patterns of posture and movement as they emerge and contribute to the repertoire of adult movement control – in particular as they pertain to the development of axial and proximal girdle control, and so, effective control of the spine.

Motor development theories

The development of our movement control is a journey with gravity. From birth, the process of development begins to establish the basic components and patterns of all our movements. The evolution of effective postural control underlies the development of a reasonably predictable sequence of movement events and behaviors. For instance we learn to turn over, sit, crawl, stand and walk and so on. Theories of early motor development encompass two principal schools of thought:[1]

• *Reflex hierarchy* has been the more traditional approach to child motor development. This places great importance on the reflex substrate for the emergence of mature human patterns. The development of postural and movement control is dependent on the appearance of these tonic reflexes controlled at lower levels within the central nervous system (CNS). With neural maturation and development of the higher levels in the CNS – the mid brain and cortex, these reflexes are subsequently integrated into more functional postural and voluntary motor responses (Fig. 3.1).

• *A 'dynamic systems control'* approach considers that postural and movement control develop from a complex interaction of musculoskeletal and neural systems including perceptual, cognitive and motor processes collectively called the postural control system. *How* the elements within the system are organized depends on interactions between the individual, the task and the environment. 'Systems theory does not deny the existence of the reflexes but considers them as only one of the many influences on the control of posture and movement.' Trew[2] further elaborates: we are 'observed to perform specific motor tasks in similar ways despite the opportunity to get to the endpoint by a variety of routes. This suggests that, for many movement tasks, there is likely to be an optimum way of moving that requires the least energy for that length and weight of limb as well as the sort of movement required' However, there is still the opportunity to choose differing qualities of muscle action and performance which allow us to do that particular movement in similar but slightly different individual ways. The amount of skill we develop through practice of a movement determines how

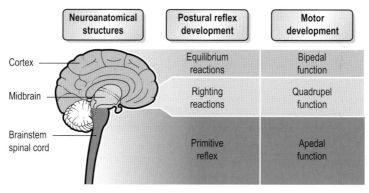

Fig 3.1 • Functional levels of the CNS in relation to neuromaturational theory.

flexibly we can accommodate to slightly different circumstances. Motor learning is a process of adjusting movement characteristics to a new task or challenge. This dynamic systems approach tends to link biomechanical and behavioral variables more than other models. Maturation, learning, perception practice and emotional factors all contribute to effective biopsychosocial development.[3]

Salient aspects of early sensorimotor development

According to Kolar[4,5] motor development is automatic and dependent upon sensory orientation, motivation and emotional need. It is characterized by the development of motor patterns which are genetically predetermined, overlap and allow for:

• the control of posture or position
• achievement of the vertical position
• purposeful phasic movements of the limbs.

Movement patterns occur through the development of muscle co-activation synergies which themselves are dependent on the body posture as a whole, and not that of a particular segment. Each stage of development is characterized by the development of specific partial motor patterns which, with the process of motor development, represent the basic elements of mature motor behavior.

Movement development in utero

Movement is life. It begins as that of cell division in the embryo and as the nervous system begins to mature, movements of the fetus begin to develop. Hartley[6] and Bainbridge Cohen[7] note the importance of

intrauterine movements in helping the nervous system develop. The first nerves to myelinate are, according to them, the vestibular nerves. As the fetus moves and is moved within the mother's body, sensory information from the vestibular nerves begins to be processed within its CNS. This perception of movement stimulates more movement or a change in movement which in turn elicits new sensory information – we are moved and then we receive sensory feedback about the movement. Sensorimotor learning thus begins in utero.

Neonatal period and change birth – 9 months

At birth, the CNS is still undeveloped. The lower centers of the CNS are more operant which is reflected in the infant's motor activity being largely influenced by neonatal reflexes, which are *automatic, stereotyped and predictable*. The baby's movements are crude with no component of voluntary control or meaningful direction. The body responds mechanically and automatically to a number of influences such as touch, sound, head or body position. This results in changes in muscle tone which then effects a posture and or movement response in a number of consistent patterns – termed 'the primitive reflexes'.[8]

Bobath[9] considers that normal motor development can be characterized by two sets of processes which are closely interwoven and dependent upon one another:

• The development of the normal postural reflex mechanism through the development of the righting, equilibrium and other adaptive and protective reactions. The development of these reactions is closely associated with normal postural tone which allows for maintenance of positions against gravity and the performance of normal movements.

• The inhibition of some of the reflex responses of the neonate such as primary standing and walking, and the startle reaction. Inhibition also shows itself in a change in the early total responses, such as the flexor withdrawal response from a total response which involves all segments of a limb to some only. This process of 'breaking up' the early total responses, makes possible a re-synthesis of parts of the total patterns in many and varied ways. This, in association with the development of the postural control mechanism mentioned above allows for the performance of selective movements and motor skill.

Primitive postural reflexes: early movement experiences of the neonate

In general, the neonate is flexed and symmetrical in all positions – in supine, prone, vertical or ventral suspension[9] due to dominant physiological flexor hypertonus. While he can turn his head he otherwise has poor head control and the only extension is reflex, via the Moro or startle reaction which bilaterally extends the arms. The emerging development of head control begins to initiate the development of extensor tonus. The symmetrical flexor activity starts to be broken up by the appearance of the asymmetrical tonic neck reflex at about 1 month old as the physiological extensor tone starts to appear. The legs are more mobile and show alternate incomplete flexion and extension via the reflex crossed extension kicking which also helps breaks up the symmetrical flexor tonus.

These various automatic reflex postural reactions which make up his early movement repertoire are stimulated by touch or pressure to particular areas of the body, passive movements of the head, torso or limbs, changes of position, changes in relation to gravity, or sudden unexpected sounds, movements, etc. The infant responds to the stimulus by moving toward it or drawing away; these responses support the potential for bonding or defending.[6] Importantly, these early responses help ensure survival and provide the infant with the experience of movement and support while he is in the process of developing his own higher level control. As this develops they either disappear or become integrated into higher order patterns of movement control. The timing of their appearance and disappearance, symmetry and intensity helps in the evaluation of early motor function. Their retention, under activity or over activity and asymmetry are indicative of potential motor problems.

It is not intended to comprehensively examine all the primitive reflexes but to look at the underlying influence of some towards important aspects of mature motor control.

Oral reflexes: beginning of head control

The rooting reflex is the first postural reflex that initiates movement of the head.[6] Mouth opening is associated with head extension while sucking or mouth closing is related to a sagittal flexion of the skull rocking on the first vertebra, the movement then transferring down the spine heralding the beginning of spinal movement control initiated from the head. Hartley[6] notes that if this pattern does not become fully integrated with the closing phase of this action not completely developed, habitual mouth opening and related hyperextended head postures ensue. This very common pattern underlies many neck shoulder and back problems in adulthood.

Other reflexes such as the Babkin and Grasp reflex provide additional stimulus to neck righting (rotation), to neck flexion and the initiation of head righting in supine. They also underlie the pattern for mouth–hand coordination[7] and establish midline focus for the mouth and hands.

Anal rooting reflex initiates movements from the tail

When the area around the anus is stimulated the infant will move its tail towards the touch. This reflex underlies the development of spinal movements which are *initiated from* the tail[7] (Fig. 3.2). 'Going long' from the tailbone also helps achieve a 'neutral spine'. These important functional actions are invariably difficult in people with back pain.

Galant's reaction:precursor to lateral movements

Stroking the back on one side elicits a side bending movement. This contributes towards initiating

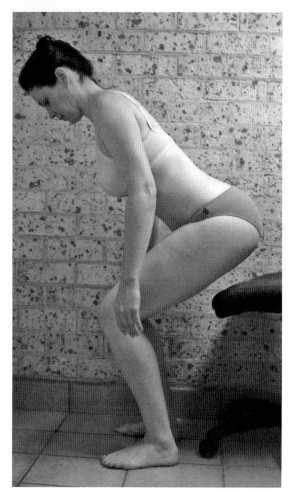

Fig 3.2 • Leading movements from the tailbone is basic to many daily activities.

unilateral trunk movement; provides the initial movement for rotation; is the precursor to the initiation of amphibian movement necessary for crawling, creeping and walking; helps break up the symmetrical patterns of flexor and extensor movement and is the beginning of asymmetrical movements.[8] If both sides are stimulated together the infant will extend the lumbar spine.[7]

Abdominal reflex underlies trunk flexion

Stimulation on either side of the navel when supine results in the infant ipsilaterally flexing the lumbar spine. If both sides are simultaneously stroked, the infant will flex the lumbar spine.[7] This reflex balances the galant and both contribute to moving the chest and pelvis through space.

First vertical antigravity experiences

The primary standing, primary stepping and placing reactions of the legs contribute towards the first sense of vertical self support. At this time the support reaction is primitive and incomplete as extensor tone is only present to the knees,[8] but they assist the infant to overcome the dominant flexor tonus contributing to the development of flexor and extensor tone balance and reciprocal leg movement for future standing and walking.

First extensor experience

The Moro reflex or startle reaction is characterized by reflex extension and abduction of the arms, opening of the hands and crying. It is a response to 'stress'. The reflex has two phases following the first phase described above, the infant flexes his head, curls his body, flexes and draws his arms across his body and closes its hands as though embracing himself. The legs may extend during both phases, unless they are already extended, in which case they may flex.[7] It allows the infant to first symmetrically widen through his chest and upper limbs and then to recover with an embrace. It is then a protective action. The reflex helps develop extensor tone in the arms at a time when physiological flexor tonus is dominant and establishes a base for all opening and closing movements of the torso. As stress is a common contemporary phenomenon, it is common to observe people adopting habitual postures which relate to the second stage Moro (Fig. 3.3).

Early protective responses

The flexor withdrawal reflex and the extensor thrust reflex underlie our neuromuscular patterns of 'protection'.
• **Flexor withdrawal** is a defensive (flight) reflex. Upon stimulation of the feet or hands of the extended limb, the infant reacts with a total flexion pattern of withdrawal. It assists in the early balancing of muscle tone between the flexors and extensors.[8] It underlies all flexion movements of

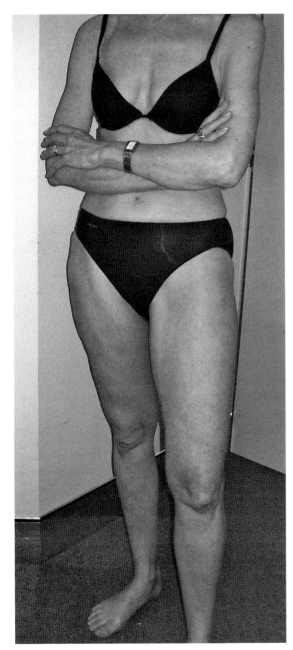

Fig 3.3 • Adults frequently adopt postures reflecting aspects of the second stage Moro reflex.

the leg or arm initiated from the feet or hands and leads into the negative supporting reflex of the lower limb, which prepares the hands and feet to release their contact with the ground in crawling, walking and jumping.[7]

• **Extensor thrust** reflex is elicited when the palm or sole of a flexed limb are stimulated leading to a total extension pattern of the limbs. This is defensive (fight) reflex and underlies all extension movements of the total arm or leg that are initiated from the hand or foot such as kicking, creeping, walking, climbing and equilibrium responses. This reflex leads into the positive supporting reflex of the upper and lower limbs.[7]

Reciprocal limb movements

Crossed extension kicking is a simple spinal reflex where if one leg is extended the other will flex. This is an integration of the flexor withdrawal on one side and the extensor thrust on the other side. It helps to develop alternating extensor tone in the lower extremities; break up symmetrical flexion and extension patterns, and is the precursor to amphibian movements in preparation for later reciprocal limb movements for crawling and walking patterns.

The amphibian reaction is an important appearance at 6 months of age and remains throughout life.[10] When the pelvis is lifted on one side, the arm and leg on the same side automatically flex (Fig. 3.4) This helps further break up the total flexor and extensor responses, produces weight shift and the experience of rotation through the trunk initiated from the pelvis. This is an important functional pattern and with further neuromuscular maturation, the infant develops his own selective control of this movement pattern. It is common that people with spinal pain have difficulty with this movement.

Positive supporting reactions underpin antigravity control

Establishment of the positive supporting reactions is an important aspect of developing antigravity control.

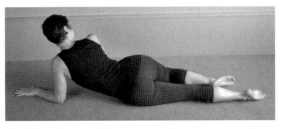

Fig 3.4 • The amphibian action provides important patterns of spinal movement.

• *Positive supporting reactions of the arms and legs.* This appears around the third month or so in both the legs and arms. The stimulus is initially exteroceptive from touch to the sole or palm, and then pressure adds a proprioceptive stimulus from stretch to the interosseous muscles. This stimulates the extensor muscles; however, the infant learns to co-contract the antagonist flexor muscles in a balanced and coordinated fashion to provide for dynamic stability of the joints[8] in weight bearing. Through this reflex, extensor tone begins to develop in the limbs from distal to proximal. It underlies all weight bearing on the upper and lower limbs and the spine. Through its action, forces pass from the support, through the limbs, proximal limb girdles and importantly *the baby's centre – the spine.*[7] This 'pushing away' is important in firing up the infants' antigravity responses. Bainbridge Cohen[7] notes that if this connection is not well established, the baby will substitute with the Propping Reaction.

• *Positive support from the head and tail.* Apart from Bainbridge Cohen's work,[7] these supporting reactions do not appear to be well appreciated in the literature. She and others[11] she has influenced who work in the area of improving movement performance, use the concept of the head and tail as 'limbs' from which to bear weight, initiate movement, and improve and refine control. The infants head pushes as it nuzzles. Support through the tail occurs in sitting and can be stimulated through play activities such as bouncing the infant's bottom on an adult's knee for '*Ride a cock horse*' and similar play. Both these early responses are important in establishing the initiation of movement control from the top and bottom of the spine as well as co-activation of antagonist muscles for dynamic control. Support from the tail is important in sitting. Commonly, in those people with back pain, there is difficulty initiating and controlling the spine from the head and tail bone.

Compensations can begin early

Attention parents and carers! According to Bainbridge Cohen (and others[14]), the Propping Response occurs when the infant is *placed in a position which is higher in relation to gravity than it could attain by 'pushing up' itself.* The baby responds by 'fixing' its limb(s) in 'total extension' and propping its body weight without connecting

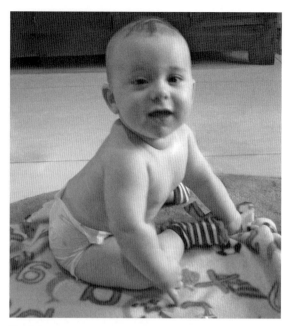

Fig 3.5 • Being placed in sitting too early encourages 'propping' and early axial imbalance.

the lines of force from the ground through its proximal limb girdles and through its centre – the spine. This occurs when the baby has not sorted out his own control and parents try to do it for him. There is excess influence from the Tonic Labyrinthine Reflex and under activity from the positive supporting reaction, which will then require excessive tone in the back muscles (Fig. 3.5). She maintains this is a common occurrence in adults with back problems and it is certainly a common finding in the clinical situation. Back pain research has also shown excess back muscle activity with a lack of the flexion relaxation phenomenon in people with back pain.[12,13]

Tonic attitudinal postural reflexes: produce changes in postural tone and body posture as a result of head position

These reflexes appear before or at birth and usually become integrated into more complex patterns of movement by 4–6 months of age. They are controlled at the spinal level and brain stem (the low brain). These tonic reflexes are not obligatory in normal development. They produce reliable changes in body posture as a result of a change in the head position.[1] They consist of:

Tonic labyrinthine prone and supine reflex (TLR)

This is apparent from birth to about 6 months after which it becomes integrated and 'disappears'. Changes in the position of the head and body in space affects the labyrinths which initiates the sensory input for the reflex arc. Increased postural/muscle tone develops on the *underside* of the body with respect to gravity. When the infant is supine this reflex produces an increase in extensor tone; when prone an increase in flexor tonus. If lying on the side, the tone in the underside body is facilitated. The subsequent development of more integrated control of flexion when supine and extension when prone modifies this reflex. This helps develop the patterns of flexor/extensor coactivation needed for spinal alignment and control. Bainbridge Cohen sees that the TLR, in increasing postural tone on the underside of the body, is the basis for 'grounding', drawing us down to the earth[7] – that from and through this, we can begin to move towards finding grounding in our verticality.

Asymmetrical tonic neck reflex (ATNR)

This is readily apparent at birth for two or more months. If the head is turned to the side, the arm and hand on the face side will extend reflexly, while the arm and leg on the skull side will flex. Its contribution in movement development is that it begins to break up the symmetrical flexion and extension patterns of movement; helps develop an alternation of these patterns; and enables each side of the body to be used separately. It also prepares the way for the integration of neck turning, visual fixation and reaching. As such it is fundamental to the establishment of visually directed reaching and eye hand coordination.[8]

Symmetrical tonic neck reflex (STNR)

This appears around the 5th to 6th month and begins to 'disappear' around the 9th month. Head flexion causes flexion of the upper extremities and extension of the lower limbs; head extension causes extension of the arms and flexion of the legs. As the prone TLR is being integrated and so becoming less obvious, the STNR develops. As the neck is developing dorsiflexion, stimulated by the labyrinthine and optical righting reflexes, the STNR facilitates the development of extensor tone concurrently in the upper limbs and flexor tone in the lower limbs. This alteration in flexor and extensor tone in the upper and lower body from changes in head flexion and extension facilitates the development of a balance between the flexors and extensors for stable positions against gravity. The infant gradually develops the ability to be prone on elbows and later to push up to extended elbows, to hands and knees and down again.

Integration and contribution of postural reflexes in the development of movement

In the developmental continuum, the postural reflexes supply the basic balance of muscle tone. This is a prerequisite to further control developing.

Bainbridge Cohen[7] also considers that the primitive reflexes establish the basic gross patterns of function that utilize and underlie all movements. She says:

> *They are the alphabet of movement and build and combine together to create more varied patterns of movement. If there is deficient development of these earliest and simplest reflexes, the more advanced patterns will be absent, weak or incomplete. The reflexes depend on each other for efficient functioning. For every reflex there is an opposite reflex which modulates it, each acting as a shadow to the other. In efficient movement, they interface and counter-support one another at all times, creating balanced postural tone and integrated movement.*

The primitive reflexes underlie the righting reactions and the equilibrium responses and so, support their development.

In early motor development, primitive reflexes are more obligatorily but not always triggered by specific stimuli. Bainbridge Cohen[7] sees that once that reflex has developed and then become appropriately integrated through higher central nervous control, that particular movement pattern will become part of one's automatic movement repertoire although *with or without the stimulus occurring, and in any plane in relation to gravity.* When looking at integrated movement in the adult we don't see the isolated reflexes but rather, *their underlying support and influence on the movement.*[7]

Importantly, if the reflexes do not develop in synchrony, they remain too static or fixated, and postural tone will be too low, too high or fluctuating and inconsistent. This problem is manifested in extremes in persons having overt brain dysfunction'. Minimal brain dysfunction is often described as 'clumsiness'.

Part of the thesis of this book is that in general people with spinal pain and related disorders demonstrate various, consistent and often subtle features of more primitive motor behavior. The continuing influence of the primitive and attitudinal reflexes can sometimes be observed in some aspects motor behavior in otherwise 'normal healthy adults'. For example, when on all fours and turning the head, the skull arm may flex indicating a lingering ATNR influence (Fig. 3.6). Likewise when on all fours the head may drop from the neutral position, the arms may flex somewhat and the patient will find good hip flexion difficult due to lingering STNR influence (Fig. 3.7).

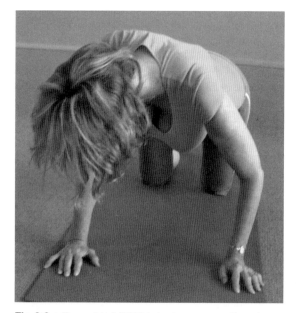

Fig 3.6 • Elements of ATNR behavior can sometimes be observed in the adult.

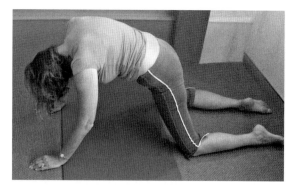

Fig 3.7 • Elements of STNR behavior is also sometimes observed.

Righting reactions: help develop more integrated control

Collectively these are a chain of actions that sequentially interact with each other to create a smooth transition from one developmental stage to the next and to maintain a proper relationship to the environment – nose vertical and eyes and mouth horizontal. These are more advanced patterns of movement than the primitive and attitudinal reflexes and are controlled by the midbrain. Some of them begin to develop at birth, are most dominant at 10–12 months of age and most of them remain active throughout life. There are five of these as follows:[1]

Three righting reactions: orient the head in space

These begin to make their appearance from birth onwards and bring the head into vertical orientation in space and in relationship to gravity.
- **Optical righting reaction (ORR)** which contributes to reflex orientation of the head using visual inputs – the eyes adjusting to the horizon
- **Labyrinthine righting reaction (LRR)** which orients the head to an upright vertical position in response to vestibular signals
- **Body on the head righting reaction (BOH)** which orients the head when the body is in the lateral position as a result of asymmetrical stimulation of proprioceptive and tactile signals as the body makes contact with a hard surface.

Orientation of the body with respect to the head and the ground

These righting reactions make their appearance around 6 months of age and persist through life. They bring the head and torso into mutual alignment in relationship to each other.

• **The neck on body righting reaction (NOB)**. This orients the body in response to cervical afferents, reporting changes in the position of the head and neck. There are two forms of this reflex: the immature form, resulting in log rolling which is present at birth and the mature form which subsequently develops producing segmental rotation of the body.[1]

• **The body on body righting reaction (BOB)**. This keeps the body oriented with respect to the ground or surface regardless of the position of the head. This is necessary for the development of the rotary components of movement and for developing higher skills for assuming the sitting and quadruped position.[8]

Landau reaction

This combines the effects of all three head righting reactions[1] and makes its appearance around 6 months of age. When the infant is supported under the chest in ventral suspension, he will first right his head followed by symmetrical extension which develops cephalocaudal down the spine to the thighs at the hips (Fig. 3.8). If the head is passively flexed the torso and thighs will follow suit and flex also.

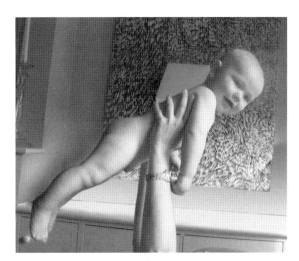

Fig 3.8 • The Landau reaction is important in the development of extension

This is an important reaction as it stimulates the development of extensor tone proximally to distally and so contributes greatly towards the infant developing sufficient extension tone to counteract the newborn's total body flexion. It also counterbalances the physiological extension which develops from the feet through the positive supporting reaction and so prepares the infant for effective antigravity postural and movement control and the development of upright posture.[3]

Significantly, it is a common clinical observation that many people with back pain demonstrate poor integration of this reflex – reflected in either too little or too much back extensor muscle activity.

Contribution of righting reactions to motor control

The labyrinths are the important contributors to the development of antigravity postures and balance at this stage of life. Movement of the head in any dimension stimulates some part of the labyrinths and appropriate postural responses develop. The increasing control of the head stimulates the development of extensor tone, particularly through the Landau reaction. The 'righting reactions underlie our ability to raise and maintain our heads and bodies upright against gravity in all postures and transitions from lying down to standing and to turning all positions in relationship to gravity and space. They are necessary for us to lift our heads, roll over, sit, crawl, creep, stand and walk'.[7]

In the developmental process the righting reactions are established before the equilibrium reactions and are a necessary component in their development.

Development overview: first 12 months

The automatic reactions for the maintenance of posture and equilibrium are developing – the postural reflexes are becoming integrated and the head righting reactions are active. The body righting reactions begin to appear. Head control improves and in prone initiates a process of general extension of the trunk and limbs against gravity which proceeds cephalocaudal to reach the hips and knees around the 6th month. Up until about the 5th or 6th month the baby moves with patterns of total flexion or extension against gravity.[8,9] Flexor and extensor musculature must develop until muscle tone between the two is balanced. While other muscle groups are developing, they are not as functional as the flexor and extensor groups – as rotation develops complete balance in all muscles will be acquired.[8] The total flexor and extensor patterns are gradually broken up so that the baby can crawl, kneel and sit with flexed hips and an extended spine and legs.

Important patterns of spinal stabilization: established 0–6 months

Kolar[4,5] considers that the first 6 months is a crucial stage in the development of the early patterns of spinal stability. He describes important stages as follows:

- **At 6 weeks** the infant shows coactivation between the cervical agonists and antagonists and active support through the arms begins. Breathing is abdominal.

- **At 3 months** the development of upper proximal girdle stability and control allows him to establish his first real support base through his elbows and symphysis pubis in prone. From this he is able to lift and hold up his head from his upper thoracic spine providing the first segmental movement (Fig. 3.9). This encourages further development of extensor tone and head rotation leads to side bending in his trunk. At the same time as he is developing support through the upper limb, he is also beginning to reach and grasp to the side in supine, the support base being his head, shoulder blades and buttocks.

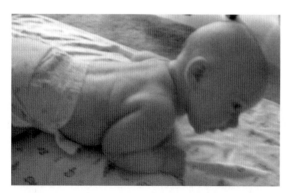

Fig 3.9 • At 3 months old head control and extension are beginning to develop.

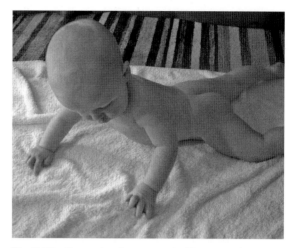

Fig 3.10 • Crossed pattern support with arm reach.

He develops balance between the upper and lower fixators of his shoulder girdle He develops the muscle synergies of coactivation responsible for regulating intra abdominal pressure (IAP).

- **By 4–5 months** in prone he can lift the head, shoulder and upper extremity against gravity as he is achieving crossed pattern support. The base of support is from the elbow and anterior superior iliac spine on one side and the medial condyle of the femur on the opposite side. His base of support shifts more caudally and the support pattern for the lower extremity is partially formed (Fig. 3.10). In supine he can lift his pelvis supporting himself on the thoracolumbar junction which is stabilized by muscular coactivation.

The lower shoulder blade also becomes the support for grasp in the midline and across the midline from 5–6 months. Stabilization in the sagittal plane is completed and this forms the basis for controlling all 'phasic' limb movements. He can now begin to develop the patterns for turning over. This is initiated in either the upper or lower limb girdle on the same side reaching or 'swinging' forward via two oblique muscle chains which appear at this time:[4]

- The first produces forward pelvic rotation in the direction of the supporting upper extremity. The contraction begins in the internal oblique of the 'upper' side, passing through the transversus abdominus to the external oblique on the opposite supporting 'lower' side. The dorsal muscles take part in the co-activation strategy including middle and lower trapezius of the 'lower' supporting shoulder girdle. The top leg comes forward (Fig. 3.11.)

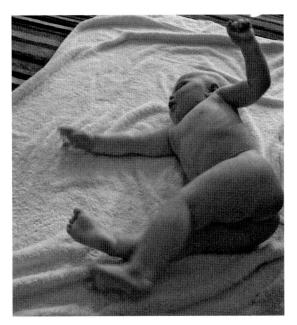

Fig 3.11 • First oblique chain leading with the pelvis.

• The second oblique chain taking part synergistically in rotation is formed by the abdominal muscles with pectoralis major and minor of both sides producing rotation of the upper part of the trunk and straightening the shoulder. The top arm leads the movement forward. (Fig. 3.12).

Kolar[4] makes an important point in noting the differentiation of muscle function which is established at this stage. The same muscles will have an opposite direction

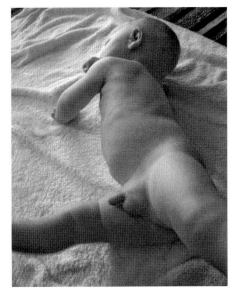

Fig 3.12 • Second oblique chain leading with the shoulder.

of pull depending upon whether the limb is supporting or 'swinging'. If the limb is supporting, the proximal limb girdle (scapula or pelvis) moves around a distal fixed humeral or femoral head. If the limb is 'swinging' the extremity muscles pull against a fixed or stabilized proximal point – the scapula or pelvis. The developing patterns of movement establish joint alignment or 'functional centration' for optimal load transfer.

Support or 'swinging' (reach) of the arm and leg is initially ipsilateral – both take place on the same side e.g. the arm and leg both reach forward.

• By six months stability in the sagittal plane is completed. His proximal limb girdles have developed increased control and stability of his thorax and abdominal development means his breathing pattern has moved from abdominal to lateral costal. Note in Fig. 3.13 how easily he supports both sets of limbs in flexion. Balance between the axial flexors and extensors renders his torso a functional 'cylinder' such that his whole spine is in contact in Fig. 3.14.

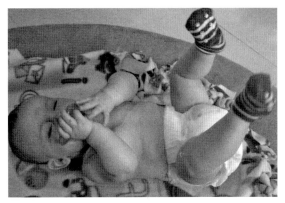

Fig 3.13 • Integration of the axial flexors and extensors allows for support of the limbs.

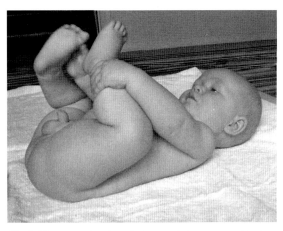

Fig 3.14 • Note that the whole torso is in contact with the support.

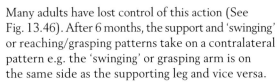

Many adults have lost control of this action (See Fig. 13.46). After 6 months, the support and 'swinging' or reaching/grasping patterns take on a contralateral pattern e.g. the 'swinging' or grasping arm is on the same side as the supporting leg and vice versa.

• If sagittal plane stability is not well established at this stage, he will substitute somewhere else in the system and will have to continue to do so.

Further development of motor control occurs through the emergence of the equilibrium reactions to create stability in balance needed for independent function no matter what position the body is in.

Equilibrium reactions: more highly integrated control

The development of the equilibrium reactions overlaps that of the righting reactions and is responsible for the modification and transformation of the righting reactions.[8] They begin to emerge around 6 months of age, take years to perfect and remain through life. These are highly integrated automatic patterns of reaction in response to disturbances of the centre of gravity, shifts of the centre of gravity over the base of support or into space. Their effective action depends upon adequate and continuous sensory information to integrate the necessary 'feed forward' and 'feedback' adaptive postural adjustments which occur in all activities. The response can vary from a subtle tonus shift to an overt movement depending on the situation.

In the child and adult equilibrium reactions will be elicited in varying ways:

• Through internal disturbance to balance through one's own movements such as breathing, moving the head and the limbs.

• Movement of the external supporting surface which threatens the base of support such as standing on an inclined surface; on a moving surface such as when standing up on the train. Conversely, slipping on a wet floor creates a similar response.

• Reacting to external forces such as lifting an awkward or heavy object or being pushed.

• Responding to stimuli which attract our interest in moving beyond our usual personal kinesphere such as moves in dance or simply, wanting that big red apple up there which is just out of reach.

In response to perturbation, Bainbridge Cohen[7] maps the development of the various equilibrium strategies as initially being through head righting,

followed by the gravity oriented protective equilibrium responses of the limbs which change the base of support. These are followed by the development of the higher level spatial reaching responses which serve to change the body's centre of gravity. She places them into five main categories and provides a very good account of them in well integrated mature motor behavior as follows.

Navel-yielding

Those responses which yield to gravity in which one curls the limbs around the navel and releases the body weight sequentially down to the ground thereby lowering the centre of gravity of the body.

Protective equilibrium reactions

• *Protective extension (parachute).* When the infant's centre of gravity is displaced too far such that he begins to fall, he will try to save himself by extending and reaching out his arm(s) and/or legs towards the ground in the direction of the fall and so he widens or changes his base of support. They first develop forwards, then sideways, backwards and diagonally. The high incidence of Colles' fractures in falls in the elderly attests to the reliability of the response throughout life.

• *Protective stepping.* When the supported standing infants' centre of gravity is displaced, he will step out with the leg in the direction of the fall – forwards, sideways, backwards and diagonally, and so extending or changing his base of support. This equilibrium response underlies walking.

• *Protective hopping.* When the older child is standing independently and one leg is lifted and gently displaced by someone else, the response will be to hop on the standing leg in the same direction, in order to move its base of support underneath its displaced centre of gravity.

As the protective equilibrium responses are integrated, the spatial-reaching equilibrium responses begin to emerge.

Spatial-reaching equilibrium reactions

When the infant begins to fall, he begins to curve his spine in the direction of the fall while reaching its

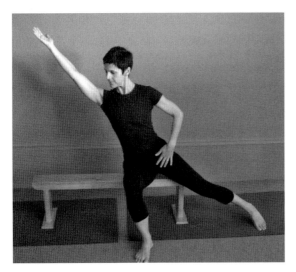

Fig 3.15 • Equilibrium reactions provide important patterns of axial control.

Outer-spatial equilibrium response

These are initiated distally from the head, tail, hands and/or feet and are the high level equilibrium reactions seen in the skilled mover whereby motivation draws the person beyond their personal kinesphere where the body moves far beyond the base of support and uses a combination of protective extension and spatial reaching to control the movement.

Most research into equilibrium responses has been conducted in the upright sitting and standing position. This is an easy position to better control the variables and has yielded important data. However, Bainbridge Cohen's description provides a better basis for understanding and therapeutically addressing alterations in functional movement control.

The next 5 years

Over the next 5 years in particular, the child energetically and endlessly explores and practices sensory and movement opportunities wherever possible. He constantly stimulates the further development of his postural equilibrium control, his movement repertoire and skills. He cannot stay still! The sensation of movement feeds the desire for more. There is evidence to suggest that in terms of motor memory, it is not the motor program that is remembered but the kinesthetic information generated during the movement.[3] The child's movements become increasingly controlled, smoother and faster as well as easier and more automatic in their execution. Movements also become more complex in their combinations and sequences. It is these combinations which provide the skills necessary to carry out particular sports activities.[3]

Kolar[4] maintains that the development of postural function is completed by age 4, when he can attain at each joint, the opposite position to that of the infant at birth. For example, at birth the predominant upper limb posture is one of flexion, protraction, internal rotation, and adduction. Upper limb patterns of movement are mature when he can extend and abduct the fingers, extend and radially deviate the wrist, the elbow in supination and extension, and the shoulder in depression, abduction and external rotation.

Motor skill development not only relies upon increasing control of balance, strength and coordination but also upon changing patterns of control. While he continues to develop a more consistent

head (head righting reactions) and its upper and lower limbs in the opposite direction of the fall. In so doing he changes the body's centre of gravity so that he maintains it over his base of support. Reaching on one side will often be coupled with spatial reaching of the opposite arm and leg (Fig. 3.15). This is an important movement pattern for the well being of spinal health and frequently there is an observed deficient response in people with back pain. The loss of competent axial control strategies and related spinal stiffness mean that when balance is threatened, he will have to compensate with protective extension or protective stepping to adjust his base of support. Responses such as grabbing with the arms are common also. Falls in the elderly become likely.

Spatial-turning equilibrium reactions

These are 'those responses where the head spine and limbs shape into a rounded form around a central body axis so that the body turns in space (in any plane) in order to:
• reorient the body's position in space as a last resort to keep from falling when a spatial-reaching response has been unsuccessful
• reorient the body's position in space as a transition from an unsuccessful spatial-reaching response to a gravity-oriented response, when the body is not in a position to reach the hands or feet to the earth.
• transfer the falling forces or momentum into circular forces e.g. rolling'.

and stable postural background, he also shows an increasing ability to select and isolate the sequence of movement most appropriate to the task without unnecessary movements or effort being used. As he improves his ability to refine modify or adapt his movements to changing needs, he develops multiple options for different movement strategies. He learns through movement and at the same time he develops his social cognitive behavioral abilities.

The advent of schooling and increasing sedentary leisure activities begin to limit the opportunities for the sensations and experiences necessary for fully realizing his sensorimotor potential. Generally, most of us do not develop this fully compared to someone dedicated to exploring and optimizing their movement abilities such as a dancer. We 'get by' with fairly modest posturomovement control as can be observed in many people in any public domain.

General comments about motor development

While normal motor development is generally a similar sequence of achievement in terms of the motor milestones, the stages overlap a lot and are variable. Each stage is supported by the previous and contributes to the next. Each person's development while similar is individual. It is the qualitative aspects which lead to the individual blueprint of our postural and movement responses. The baby learns control over the early reflexes mostly during the first 9 months, the time of moving around on the floor hence it is important has the opportunity to be there and work out his own motor progressions.[14] The early reflexes become integrated as part of his motor behavior yet their influence remains for an emergency e.g. flexor withdrawal on touching the hot plate!

Motivation is a strong driver of development – getting to what you want. However this determination can be deleterious as the infant can become frustrated e.g. tummy time is developmentally important yet the infant may not persevere, the parents responding by placing him in a sitting position (with a 'ready made' array of toys) or standing too early before he has developed his own means of getting there[14] (Fig. 3.16). This may well result in less ideal integration of the patterns of support and control in the preceding stages and the need for compensations which become necessary and habitual through life. It is important he finds his own way (Fig. 3.17). Any missed developmental stages are evident in the

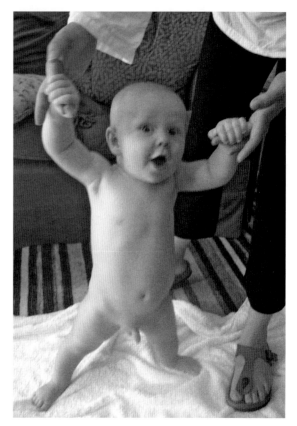

Fig 3.16 • Being stood too early before gaining ones own control risks missing important stages in motor development.

quality of one's posturomovement control.[15] In particular the development of the important components of weight shift and rotation may suffer where 'poor posture' and shades of 'clumsiness' result.

Motor learning outcomes are also influenced by the degree of practice, repetition and persistence in improving the motor act. Individual strategies for completion of a task will vary between people. The quality of the response will also be affected by variables such as opportunity; the context in which the action occurs; emotional state; cognitive learning; and the ability to effectively adapt to changed conditions.

Normal motor development: significant basic components overview

Fiorentino[8] cites four basic components in the developing patterns of movement which are necessary for the acquisition of motor skills, 'It is

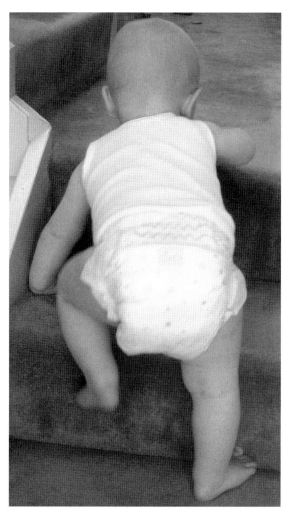

Fig 3.17 • In finding his own way he learns to master each important stage which underlie the development of further patterns.

necessary to have gross developmental patterns directed toward the stable position, especially against gravity'. These components are:

- head control
- development of extensor tone
- ability to rotate within the body axis
- development of equilibrium so that balance is possible, allowing freedom of the arms from their early role of support, so that they may develop as tools for skilled manipulative abilities.

These components are dependent upon 'normal muscle tone'. These are explored:

Muscle tone versus postural tone

The primitive postural reflexes play an important role in the development, regulation, degree, strength, balance and distribution of muscle tone through the body.[8] 'The regulation of muscle tone throughout the body for the maintenance of posture and movement is the function of the proprioceptive system'.[9] Postural tone is regulated by higher facilitatory and inhibitory influences from the brainstem, midbrain and cerebellum frontal and parietal lobes by a harmonious integration of exteroceptive and proprioceptive stimuli.[9]

Physiological flexion and extension: development of balanced muscle tone

At birth the infant's basic postural tone is predominantly flexor.[8,9] When the early primitive postural reflexes are elicited the antagonist muscle groups are inhibited. The reflexes provide the opportunity for experiencing both flexion and extension 'movements' and serve to modulate and balance one another's activity. If the reflexes don't develop in synchrony, or they remain too static or fixated, the developing postural tone will be too low, too high or fluctuating and inconsistent.[7]

If the *state* of muscle tone is altered it will affect the subsequent development of higher CNS controlled flexion and extension and the *balanced coactivation* between them, affecting the development of axial alignment and control and the coordination of posture and movement.[8]

Integration of early flexor and extensor response

The early predominantly reflex driven physiological flexion and extension responses are elicited more from the periphery – the hands or the feet 'up'. Initially these are primitive 'total patterns' with little differentiation between different body segments but are later modified. The development of *integrated control* of flexion and extension proceeds 'from the head down' to counterbalance and meet the physiological activity initiated from the periphery. The development of higher CNS control is characterized by the appearance of muscular *co-activation of antagonists*. The balanced activity and simultaneous activation of antagonists and their mutual reciprocal facilitation and inhibition allow the development of (peripheral) support bases through the limb girdles as well as the development of head control. Central development proceeds cephalocaudal and is met by control from the periphery which also has a cephalocaudal pattern, i.e. the first support base in prone is formed by the elbow and symphysis pubis[4] and facilitates the development of head control. In supine the infant learns to develop control of flexion of the body and so modifies the supine TLR and gains control against gravity. In prone he learns to develop control of extension of the body away from gravity and the effects of the prone TLR. In this process of development the infant becomes able in breaking up the earlier and more primitive total patterns of response. He re-synthesizes parts of each in various combinations so that he can flex and extend each body part independently e.g. flexion of his hips with extension of his spine. Through the integration of the reflexes and the emergence of the righting and equilibrium responses, physiological flexion and extension are integrated into the background of normal postural tone. Bainbridge Cohen[7] notes the importance of the infant having the opportunity to experience all positions in relation to gravity so that his postural tone will develop in a balanced and integrated manner on all body surfaces.

Normal postural tone does show variance – it is lower when we are calm and relaxed and higher when we are aroused and tense. Despite normal developmental achievements, depending upon our emotional, mental and physical activities, we may later influence our tone by adopting habitual patterns of response e.g. the stressed person who is always 'edgy,' 'uptight' and tense.

In clinical practice, one observes that the problem for some people with spinal pain is an alteration in their basic postural tone – either lower or higher. Associated with this is a proclivity for either respective flexor or extensor pattern dominance in posture and movement.

Importance of head control in movement

Apart from the important contribution that the peripheral somatosensory system provides, the head contains our primary organs of sense and perception – the eyes, nose, ears, labyrinths and the brain. All sensory experience is associated with movements of the head. The head initiates and largely influences our motor development. In the neonate, its movement

and position stimulate many of the early primitive reflexes which provide us with the first patterns of movement. Through emerging control of the head, the process of developing well organized movement begins to develop cephalocaudally in the extensor and flexor muscle systems. It is important that the stabilizing synergies of coactivation between the agonists and antagonist occur both in the neck itself (between the deep neck flexors and cervical extensors) to provide central alignment of the head on the neck as well as more caudally in the shoulder girdle/chest to provide adequate postural support for the movement. According to Kolar[5] this begins at 6 weeks of age and the pattern should be well established by 3 months of age. The righting reactions in response to visual, labyrinthine and spatial position of the head also begin to develop lateral and rotary movements. The equilibrium reactions are highly dependent on spinal adjustments, many of which are initiated from the head as well as the tail and through the spine.

In the adult, well developed and integrated control of the head on the neck allows options for preferentially moving and orienting the head for directing and focusing our sense organs and so optimizing wellbeing and survival. In functional terms, its position and control will affect the postural tone throughout the rest of the body given that some of the most essential afferent impulses for the static and dynamic regulation of body posture arise from the receptor systems in the connective tissues and muscles around the upper cervical joints.[16] In mechanical terms in the erect position, the head furnishes the cue for balance of the whole body.[17] Defective positioning and control of the head is a common observation in people presenting to the clinician. Frequently, the head is carried forward and largely controlled from 'extensor holding patterns' (Fig. 3.18) with consequent effects on the whole body and its systems, and the predictable emergence and presence of many clinical 'syndromes' and 'diagnoses'. Contrast this with the alignment in Figure 3.19.

Development of extension

The development of controlled extension is fundamental in establishing and maintaining vertical positions against gravity. However, it is important that as extension control develops, so does corresponding flexor control. The balanced coactivation of both antagonistic groups provides the

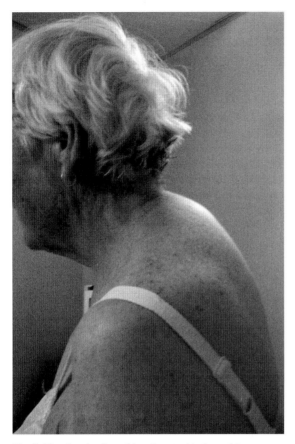

Fig 3.18 • Poorly aligned head control in the adult.

compensate for this deficiency the person will develop local and regional axial 'holding patterns' and show altered postural alignment.

Bainbridge Cohen[7] notes that if there are problems in the integration of the TLR, head righting reactions and the positive supporting reactions, two patterns will manifest:

• An overactive TLR and underactive positive supporting and head righting reactions will mean being 'drawn too much to the ground' e.g. this is well seen when on all fours. The person will 'prop' with their limbs and assume a flexed body posture with the head in flexion. Insufficient extension is apparent in the body and proximal limb girdles. There is deficient postural tone and coactivation of the spinal and proximal limb girdle muscles to support the spine and so alignment and control of the spine suffers. Their body postures and actions tend to reflect flexor predominance (Fig. 3.20) (see Ch. 9: 'APXS').

• An underactive TLR and overactive positive supporting and head righting reactions create a 'lack of bonding to the earth' where the person holds himself excessively away from the ground using too much muscle tension, e.g. when sitting with forward arm support or on all fours, the person will tend to overextend his neck and back (non uniform) and

appropriate patterns for axial and proximal girdle alignment, support and control in all planes in relation to gravity.

Initial extension as we have seen is reflex, 'total' and undifferentiated. The development of integrated or controlled extension through the body and limbs is initiated from head control, the three head righting reactions and through the Landau and positive support reactions. The positive support and Landau reactions also bring control into the proximal limb girdles. Flexion development is also influenced by head control, righting reactions and the need for flexor contribution for coactivation in the positive support reactions. As these develop, the infant develops the ability to selectively extend and control some body segments while he moves others into flexion. Both extension and flexion become differentiated, modulated and more refined. In all movements of extension there is support and control from the flexors and vice versa. Should this not happen, there is less strength and efficiency in the torso and to

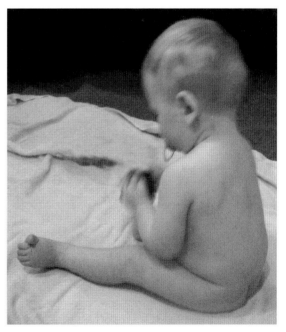

Fig 3.19 • Well aligned head control and developing spinal extension at around 7 months.

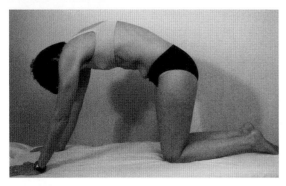

Fig 3.20 • Tendency towards propping and flexor dominance in all fours is seen in the adult.

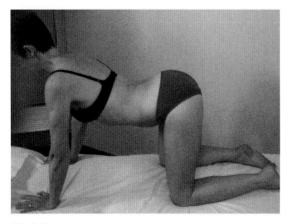

Fig 3.21 • A tendency to propping and extensor dominance in all fours can also be observed.

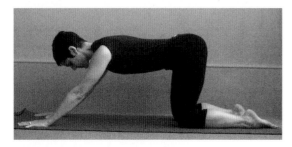

Fig 3.22 • Ideal alignment in all fours.

have poor flexor contribution to balanced activity of the torso muscles including the proximal limb girdles. There is poor balance in the postural tone and so poor support to provide for alignment and control of the torso and limbs. These people demonstrate a tendency for more extensor dominance in posture and movement (Fig. 3.21) (see Ch. 9: 'PPXS'). Compare Figs 3.20 and 3.21 with that in Fig. 3.22.

Development of rotation

Fiorentino[8] suggests that the development of rotation within the body axis is one of major consequence, as it underlies the development of the rotary components of the righting reactions and subsequent higher levels of normal sensorimotor achievement. In other words without adequate development of rotation, the further development of equilibrium responses and stable control in the axial skeleton will be compromised.

In the early stages of reflex flexor and extensor dominance, reflexes such as the galant and ATNR and the early righting reactions, provide the infant with his first experiences of lateral and rotary movement until he can develop his own control (Figs 3.11 & 3.12). Control of head rotation is important in the development of body rotation.

The initiation of controlled rotation within the body axis is dependent upon developing balance between the flexors and extensor muscle systems which allows for balanced muscle tone and good alignment of the body segments while it is rotating. Rotation allows the flexion and extension movements to have a more complex repertoire. Rotation and righting responses of the head and body when prone or supine involves a degree of weight shift which then necessitates the beginning of development of equilibrium responses for control. Lateral weight shift and rotation mutually interact. Stability and mobility elements begin to develop in each motor milestone as the infant gets up to sit, moves to hands and knees etc.

Poor flexor/extensor co-activation and balance means rotation does not develop well through the spine and proximal limb girdles. The rotation, if and when it occurs, tends to develop 'more in extension' or 'more in flexion' in certain regions of the torso. Fiorentino states that if the weight does not shift, rotation may not develop and we can infer that predictably if rotation does not develop, weight shift and stability will suffer.

Besides contributing largely towards stability, rotation within the body and between it and the proximal limb girdles also allows for the sequencing of movement through the spine and increased mobility and more effective use of the limbs e.g. rotating the trunk and shoulder girdle forward when upright allows the arm to reach further into space. Rotation also allows for crossing the midline of the body.

The development of rotation allows movement control to develop from its early principal sagittal orientation towards movements which encompass lateral and rotary components, and so enlargement of the personal kinesphere. Movement control begins to develop in three dimensions.

It is important to appreciate that all movements contain elements of rotation, however slight. In order to easily change positions or body levels up and down against gravity, rotary components need to be active. When rotary movement control is not well developed and integrated in the torso, the person will compensate with regional 'holding patterns' in the torso which serve to further limit his movements to a more sagittal orientation.

Development of weight shift

Weight shifts are a feature of all movements of the torso in some degree. The development of weight shift and rotation are closely associated. The initial weight shifts are passive in prone and supine where head turning tends to shift the weight to one side of the body. With the development of head control and the righting and later equilibrium reactions, weight shift over varying bases of support starts to become more controlled (Fig. 3.4). These initially occur more in the sagittal plane as the infant is establishing its flexor and extensor control. As it masters this and pushes up more against gravity, it begins to involve more lateral and diagonal shifts. Assisted by the positive supporting reactions, this lateral control is important as it provides for 'grounding' of one side of the body through the spine and proximal limb girdles and unloading of the contralateral side, facilitating unilateral limb mobility and control of the limbs. The increased use of asymmetrical limb movements afforded by effective weight shift further develops rotation and equilibrium development. The muscular tensions and countertensions set up in the torso form part of the matrix of postural control patterns providing for its mobility with stability.

The infant needs to develop control of weight shift in supine, prone, side lying sitting all fours, etc. In each new position he attains, the infant plays with and learns to shift his weight around in that position and to move in and out of it and from this position to another. Control thus allows him to be able to change the base of support and raise the centre of gravity. As his control develops, he is able to decrease the size of his base, e.g. from lying, to all fours, to sitting and standing with a wide base and then eventually to a narrow base.

When upright, weight shifts both subtle and overt, occur before and during all limb movements to adjust the centre of gravity within and over the base of support.

Further aspects of posturomovement development

Other important elements also contribute to our motor development.

Inhibition and the control of movement

Inhibition as well as excitation plays an important role in the control and differentiation of movement.[3]

As noted, motor development involves inhibition of some of the early reflex responses so that they disappear. In other of the primitive reflexes, inhibition serves to modulate or diminish the response such that the basic pattern of movement can be used but control over it improved e.g. the extensor thrust reflex is a pattern of total extension but this then develops into the positive supporting reaction which is a more evolved response to weight bearing.[7]

Inhibitory influences from higher levels of control in the CNS are involved in regulating all our movements. Inhibition allows us to modify and alter the response. As each new movement and posture is attained, the infant repetitively practices using it, and moves in and out of it. Inhibition helps her master and then improve the activity. Crude movements become more refined and economical as the unwanted and unnecessary aspects are reduced.

Clinical observation shows that in some respects, people with spinal pain tend to have some difficulty with this 'functional editing' of movement e.g. movements of the shoulder may involve unnecessary tension in the neck. Trunk flexion actions against gravity will often involve unnecessary tension and activity in the superficial neck and back muscles because of a corresponding deficiency in the patterns of axial stability. The ability to inhibit the habitual response and unwanted muscle activity is often much more difficult than activating certain muscle groups. As Sherrington noted, 'Inhibition is a motor act in itself – to not react is an action'.[18]

Movement develops in stages through three planes

Development is not a strictly linear process but occurs in overlapping waves with each stage containing elements of all the others – the previous stages underlie and support the successive stages. The infant learns to move around three axes and three planes. He first learns control of movements in the sagittal plane which in some respects can be seen as the primary movements. Here he develops symmetry around the transverse and longitudinal axes and when he has control of this he can develop movements around the two diagonal axes formed between the upper limb on one side and the contralateral lower limb.[14] Every limb movement requires stabilization in the sagittal plane as its first phase.[4]

The evolving rotary and oblique patterns underpin the reciprocal movement patterns between legs and arms. As the infant masters these, he can push up into more vertical postures and further develop the lateral and rotary components. Mastering these coronal and transverse plane movements allows control in three dimensions and the evolution of more complex movement patterns, better equilibrium and greater exploration of the personal kinesphere.

Observation of the habitual postures and movements in people with spinal pain and related disorders reveals certain common patterns of response. Most display some degree of incomplete stabilization in the sagittal plane. Accordingly, their movements are predominantly those in the sagittal plane. Muscle tonus and alignment suffer. Associated with this is an observed habitual under use or incompetent use of movements in the coronal and transverse planes – the lateral, diagonal and rotary components of movement. Tri-planar static and dynamic control of the spine and proximal limb girdles is deficient. This renders the spine more vulnerable to the effects of repetitive micro trauma as well as from more overt insults. The high incidence of back pain should not come as a surprise.

Posture is a reflection of the quality of neuromuscular status

Postural and movement control develop together and are interdependent. Normal postural control provides the proximal stability for the achievement of distal movement control and distal stability for proximal control. Control of movement precedes control of sustained postures. In this respect movement may be considered more primitive than sustained posture. Yet as motor behavior matures the stability of sustained posture is necessary for purposeful movement'.[19]

The term 'posture' is often used to describe both biomechanical alignment of the body, as well as the orientation of the body to the environment.[1] We have become used to thinking of 'posture' more in terms of upright posture. However each and any position adopted is 'a posture'. The posture adopted *in* any position is a reflection of the neuromuscular status of the person, and this is evident from birth through to adulthood. This is seen as changes in basic muscle tone or the unbalanced development of muscle response patterns which affect alignment of the body segments in any position. For example in side lying, the neonate's posture is one of 'total flexion' due to predominant physiological flexor tonus. The posture adopted by some adults with back pain can resemble the fetal position and tells a story about the quality of his neuromuscular status (Fig. 3.23). Altered alignment of the body segments will be a feature in all other positions.

Stability and mobility: constant relationship in movement

As each movement develops it is supported by the co-development of synergistic patterns of appropriate stabilization. This takes place automatically and unconsciously, programmed by the CNS.[4] Insufficient patterns of stabilization develop if each developmental stage is not well integrated. Kolar[5] stresses the importance of the patterns developed in the first 6 months in providing central/axial stability and control. Insufficient integration can be seen in the adult as altered alignment of the torso segments and poor coordination of breathing and postural and movement control.

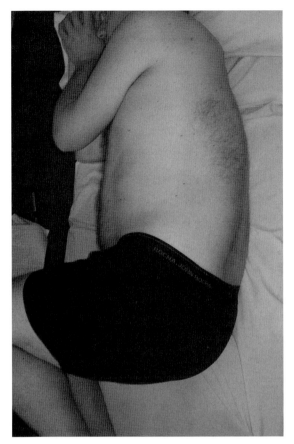

Fig 3.23 • Spontaneous postures adopted in lying reflect neuromotor activity.

In all movement, stability and mobility elements interact – there is a continual shifting and gradation from one through to the other. Problems arise when there is too much or too little of either.

Developmental patterns of movement: basic patterns of support and control for the spine

During the developmental process, certain primary patterns of movement emerge which commonly underlie all human movement. They have been described as the basic neurological patterns[20] but are also known as developmental patterns[6] and have been further elaborated as patterns of total body connectivity.[11] Bainbridge Cohen[7] describes them as follows:

Prevertebrate patterns

- **Cellular breathing** underlies all other patterns and postural tone. Breathing is internal movement and underlies movement of the body through external space. Movement in turn affects our breathing.
- **Navel radiation**. The relating and movement of all parts of the body via the navel. Movement should both *sequence through* the 'core' of the body and be *controlled from* the core.
- **Mouthing**. Movement of the body initiated by the mouth. This underlies movement of the head initiated from the ears and eyes.
- **Pre-spinal movement**. Soft sequential movements of the spine initiated via the interface between the spinal cord and the digestive tract.

Vertebrate patterns

Based upon four patterns of movement, these develop in the three planes of movement in prone supine and when upright:

- **Spinal movement**. Head to tail movement which correlates to the movement of fish – spinal flexion, extension, lateral flexion and rotation. Through this we develop rolling, discover the vertical axis of our bodies and establish the horizontal plane. We differentiate the front from the backs of our bodies. She sees that these patterns underlie the qualities of strength or lightness in our movements and are the ground from which we develop our inner and outer attention.
- It is important that all reflexes which underlie spinal movement are established in all their respective directions so that the development of spinal control is balanced in each direction. Bainbridge Cohen sees that spinal movement expresses our postural tone of attention. Movement of the extremities – homologous, homolateral and contralateral expresses our postural tone of intention.
- **Homologous movement**. Symmetrical flexion or extension movements of both arms or legs simultaneously. These movements underlie the quadruped position, movements such as push-ups and jumping with both legs. They utilize and establish the sagittal plane; differentiate the upper part of our bodies from the lower; and help us gain the ability to act (Fig. 3.24).

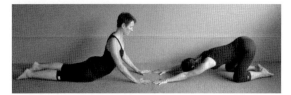

Fig 3.24 • 'Sphinx' and 'Allah' are homologous movements.

• **Homolateral movement**. Asymmetrical movement in which the arm and leg on the same side of the body flex or extend together which correlates to movement seen in reptiles. Movements such as crawling on our bellies; hopping on one leg; we establish the vertical plane; differentiate the right from the left side of our bodies and gain the ability to intend. These movements underlie mouth/eye/hand coordination and provide the foundation for reaching out into the world. They are involved in rolling over (Fig. 3.25).

• **Contralateral movement**. These movements emphasize the diagonal plane and are those in which the opposite arm and leg are flexing or extending together which correlates to movement of mammals. Movements such as creeping on our hands and knees, walking, running and leaping; we establish three dimensional movement; differentiate the diagonal quadrants of our bodies and gain the ability to integrate our attention, intention and action (Fig. 3.26).

The development of these patterns, according to Bainbridge Cohen, not only establishes the basic movement patterns but importantly the corresponding perceptual relationships including spatial orientation, body image and the basic elements of learning and communication.[20]

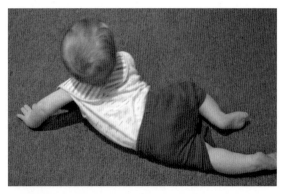

Fig 3.25 • Homolateral movements provide important components of motor patterns such as 'lengthening the side'.

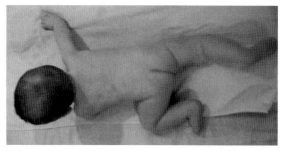

Fig 3.26 • Contralateral movements provide important diagonal cross support patterns between the proximal limb girdles and spine.

Push patterns

These first appear in the upper body – through the head and elbows and then hands and later in the tail knees and feet.[6] The infant pushes down into the ground or supporting surface, stimulating his internal receptor systems and his proprioceptive knowledge which help give him a sense of gravity, his own weight and support in movement. What is important to recognize is that *he pushes down through his base of support to 'get up'* through the vertical plane. These patterns underlie the basis of effective positive supporting responses. The push patterns occur through each stage: spinal, homologous, homolateral contralateral. Hackney[11] prefers the term yield and push patterns – the 'yield brings an aspect of bonding and contact with the support before separating with the push'. The push patterns precede and provide grounding for the reach and pull patterns – the infant pushes down through his base of support to reach up and so both are functionally related to the other as part of a movement phrase (see Ch.13, 'Grounding').

Reach and pull patterns

Developmentally these patterns develop after the yield and push patterns although development is never strictly linear. Hackney[11] coined this term as a refinement of the classic 'pull patterns'. A reach out from the base of support and body kinesphere towards an object of desire precedes a pulling towards the body, particularly when supported by a preceding yield and push. They also allow expressive use of space (Fig. 3.27).

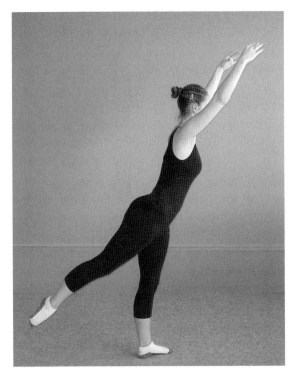

Fig 3.27 • Pushing up from the ground allows verticality and expressive reach.

Development of spinal support and control: overview

The two primary spinal curves are 'flexor' – the thoracic and pelvic are implicit in the spine at birth because of the design of the rib cage and pelvis which are attached to them.[17] The development of the compensatory cervical and lumbar curves is necessary in order that the spinal column can carry and control its own and all its superimposed weights. These secondary curves are formed as the infant develops extensor control of the head which then proceeds down the spine so he develops his lumbar curve. As he becomes more active throwing his arms and legs around and moving his head and the resultant deeper breathing, brings about a coordinated action of the whole spine. Todd[17] notes that this process is greatly aided by spells of crying and screaming since the diaphragm and lower lumbar and pelvic muscles are so closely associated. In the primary patterns of movement the breathing and locomotor apparatus interrelate aiding one another and so locomotion and breathing develop together.

The spine gets its initial support from the ground in passive form. The spinal patterns are the first to develop. They are initiated from the head through the oral rooting and sucking responses and the movement wave passes down the spine. In the early recumbent postures, the baby learns to wriggle up and down the bed. 'The Spinal Reach and Pull, patterns give the sense of elongation of the vertical axis and sequential movement travelling through the spine. Led by the head the spine begins to move in all directions creating the base for the development of body movement in three basic planes – vertical, sagittal and horizontal – and the diagonals which combine all three dimensions.'[6] Gracovetsky[21] says 'locomotion was first achieved by the motion of the spine. The limbs came after as an improvement not a substitute'.

In prone and supine the base of support with the ground is relatively enormous. The infant begins to shift his weight over this as he turns his head, reaches etc. This is the beginning of weight shift to support movement. There is a concept in physics, 'to every action there is an equal and opposite reaction' (Newton's 3rd law of motion).[2] As his weight shifts, the baby activates muscle pattern responses to control it. His muscles work as both stabilizers to support movement and to create a movement.[4] These get better as he develops the righting and equilibrium responses. He develops a dynamic interplay of the axial muscles in response to the ever changing conditions, depending upon his position in relationship to gravity, the goal of the movement and his stage of development.

What is particularly significant is that except for the very early stages of development, the infant never really moves in a pure plane movement. Extension develops with components of side bending and rotation and so on.

The head is the storehouse of sensory reception and perception. Increasing interest, emotional needs and interaction with his environment motivate the infant to orient and move his head. As control of flexion and extension proceeds down the spine from the head proximal to distal it is met by corresponding control developing from distal to proximal through the limbs and proximal limb girdles. Both the feet and hands have large fields of sensory receptors and pressure through these help fire up the normal postural reflex mechanism. Through the ipsilateral supporting and grasping patterns he develops turning over and then oblique sitting position develops. The points of support are the gluteus medius and the hand on the same side. When his grasping arm can be lifted 120°, crawling on all fours develops.[4] Patterns of axial control begin to further develop through the weight bearing push/pull patterns of the limbs. *Movement sequences from the limbs to the spine and from the spine to the limbs.* It is important to appreciate these rich sensory parts – the head, hands feet and tail, play a large role in the *initiation* of movement *from* them. In this way they promote the sequencing of movement through and between the limbs and spine. They are also involved in protecting equilibrium.

Spinal loading progressively occurs: neuromusculoskeletal system in the process of development

Gravity isn't the only force we need counter as we develop. 'In the physical universe, action and reaction are always equal and opposite'.[17] In the normal developmental process the various forces and stresses acting on the body facilitate the appropriate neuromuscular responses. The forces occur from within the body as a result of muscle activation as well as from the external environment. The spine is variously subjected to a number of loading influences:

• Lifting the weight of the head as well as positive support through the head and tail begin to load in compression and tension.

• The control of body weight shift as it develops in all positions creates lateral and rotary torques and appropriate coactivation responses of the 'body cylinder' muscle synergies. These include torsion shear and bending stresses.

• As the infant develops the push and reach patterns through all the limbs, it begins to develop spinal support through them and develop more strength against gravity. The torques through the proximal limb girdles are transferred through the spine which must be resolved by appropriate patterns of axial stability/mobility. Hartley[6] makes a very important observation that 'If the support of the limbs is lacking or incomplete, the spine will have to support itself once it is vertical. This is done through *holding* the body centrally, which creates a pattern of tension and rigidity in the spine and the surrounding tissues and organs'. This is explored further in Chapters 9 and 10.

• With the homologous push pull patterns, the child pushes itself forwards and backwards along

the floor and in so doing improves the developing balance between the flexors and extensors of the axial spine and proximal limb girdles. Forward and backwards weight shift control further develops.

• As it develops the homolateral push pull patterns, the infant learns to move with one side of the body stable while the other side is mobile. When on his belly, the arm and leg on one side of the body extend, elongating that side which also bears the body weight. The opposite side is unweighted and shortens, which frees the limbs to flex and reach and so on as he pushes himself forward and backwards. This is an important pattern for developing patterns of lateral weight shift with one side of the body lengthening and supporting. It is needed to push up onto his hands and knees, stand and walk. It is also important in upright lateral weight shift and equilibrium responses. Generally, it is a poorly integrated pattern of movement in the adult with back pain.

• As the contralateral patterns become established the diagonal and rotary torque and challenge increases and so he develops towards multiplanar control and equilibrium. Importantly a sequential rotation through the spine underlies the action of these patterns. Hartley[6] notes that either push or reach patterns may dominate the way he initiates his movements; either tendency can be, but is not necessarily a sign of incomplete development of the other phase. However if this is the case it will affect the quality and variety of the patterns axial support and control.

All these spinal patterns initially develop with the body in a horizontal relationship to the ground. As they become practiced, combined and further developed they *prepare and form the foundation of control of the torso* in the vertical upright postures and related patterns. The attainment of vertical upright control is further dependent upon the development of strength and control of the pelvic hip musculature as an organized base of support in order that the pelvis can perform its threefold function of weight bearing, transmission and movement. The axial patterns of control become further developed in the vertical postures over many years provided the environment is conducive.

Bainbridge Cohen[7] maintains that 'underneath ALL successful, effortless movement are integrated reflexes, righting reactions and equilibrium responses.' Inadequate integration during any stage of development creates the need for compensatory strategies which then become learned and a habitual part of the movement repertoire. In time they may become a patient.

References

[1] Shumway-Cook A, Woollacott MH. Motor Control: Theory and Practical Applications. Baltimore: Lippincott Williams & Wilkins; 2001.

[2] Trew M, Everett T. Human Movement: An introductory text. 5th ed. Edinburgh: Elsevier Churchill Livingstone; 2005.

[3] Burns YR, MacDonald J. Physiotherapy and the growing child. W B Saunders; 1996.

[4] Kolar P. Facilitation of Agonist-Antagonist Co-activation by reflex stimulation methods. In: Liebenson C, editor. Rehabilitation of the Spine: a Practitioner's Manual. Philadelphia: Lippincott Williams and Wilkins; 2007.

[5] Safarova M. Presenter - Course notes: Dynamic Neuromuscular stabilisation: according to Kolar. Sydney: Feb 2008.

[6] Hartley L. Wisdom of the body moving: an introduction to body mind centering. North Atlantic Books; 1989.

[7] Bainbridge Cohen B. The alphabet of movement: Primitive reflexes, righting reactions and equilibrium responses Part 1 and 2. In: Sensing, Feeling and Action. Northampton MA: Contact Editions; 1993.

[8] Fiorentino MR. A basis for sensorimotor development – normal and abnormal; The influence of Primitive Postural Reflexes on the Development and Distribution of Tone. Illinois: Charles C Thomas; 1981.

[9] Bobath K. The Motor Deficit in Patients with Cerebral Palsy Spastics. International Medical Publications in association with William Heinemann Medical Books; 1966.

[10] Fiorentino MR. Reflex Testing Methods for evaluating C.N.S. development. 2nd ed. Illinois: Charles C Thomas; 1973.

[11] Hackney P. Making Connections: Total Body Integration Through Bartenieff Fundamentals. New York: Routledge; 1998.

[12] Neblett R, et al. Quantifying the lumbar flexion relaxation phenomenon: theory, normative data, and clinical applications. Spine 2003;28(13):1435-46.

[13] Watson PJ, et al. Surface electromyography in the identification of chronic low back pain patients: the development of the flexion relaxation ratio. Clin Biomech 1997;12(3):165-71.

[14] Hermsen-van Wanroy M. Baby Moves; A step by step guide to enhancing your baby's development through his or her own natural movement. 2nd ed. New Zealand: Baby Moves Publications; 2006.

[15] Bartenieff I. Body Movement: Coping with the environment. Australia: Gordon and Breach; 2002.

[16] Grieve GP. Common Joint Problems. Churchill Livingstone; 1981.

[17] Todd ME. The Thinking Body. A Dance Horizons Book; 1937.

[18] Sherrington CS. Reflex inhibition as a factor in the co-ordination of movements and postures. Quart J Exp Physiol 1913;6:251.

[19] Knott M, Voss DE. Proprioceptive neuromuscular facilitation. Patterns and techniques. 2nd ed. New York: Harper and Rowe Publishers; 1968.

[20] Bainbridge Cohen B. Introduction to Body Mind Centering. In: Sensing, Feeling and Action. Northampton MA: Contact Editions; 1993.

[21] Gracovetsky S. An hypothesis for the role of the spine in human locomotion: a challenge to current thinking. J Biomed Eng 1985;7:205-16.

Chapter Four

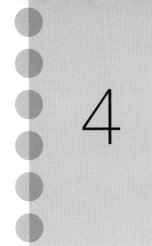

The analysis of movement

Movement analysis can be as daunting as it is complex, three-dimensional, always changing, and numerous aspects contribute towards functional control. Some basic underlying concepts are examined.

Basic concepts in posturomovement analysis

Kinematics

Kinematics describes motion in the body,[1] without regard for the forces or torques that may produce the motion.[2] Kinematic patterns of movement involve the alignment and relative contribution of various segments of the body in an action.

Kinetics

Kinetics describes the effect of forces upon the body.[2] Movement concerns the way we organize ourselves in relation to numerous forces, the most dominant and consistent of which is gravity. This deserves some consideration.

Line of gravity

The 'line of gravity' (LOG) refers to the vertical downward force that gravity constantly exerts upon the body whichever position it is in. Best visualized like a 'plumb line', it is an imaginary line to aid the conceptual understanding of 'gravity'. The development of posture and movement is a process of

learning to counteract this force so we can purposefully and safely move around. Ideally, we achieve a balanced response to gravity so that when vertical, the arrangement of the body segments is balanced around this 'force line' with minimum energy expenditure and easy equilibrium in the system. The further the body segments or body as a whole move away from this 'line', the greater is the demand for neuromuscular control.

Centre of gravity

The mass of a body in relation to gravity gives it weight. The centre of mass can be defined as the point about which the mass of an object is evenly distributed. While gravity acts upon all points of an object or segment of an object, its point of application is given as the centre of mass or centre of gravity (COG) of that object or segment.

The COG of the body in the anatomical upright position is considered to be at the level of the 2(nd) sacral vertebra, inside the pelvis.[1,3,4] However, the anatomical position does not necessarily equate to movement function because as soon as the configuration of the body segments changes so does the COG. Each segment of the body has its own COG. If two or more adjacent segments are going to move together as a single solid segment they can be represented by a single COG.[1] The COG can be raised for example when reaching up, or lowered if the legs or body bend, etc. Depending on the arrangement of the body segments it can be located at the edge of or outside the body. The LOG passes through the COG (Fig. 4.1).

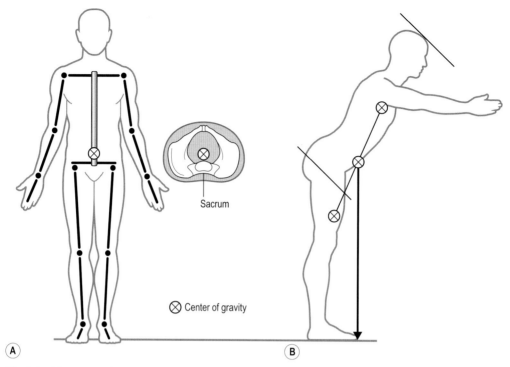

Sacrum

⊗ Center of gravity

(A)

(B)

Fig 4.1 • The centre of gravity is mainly located within the body (A) but can deviate outside the body (B).

The interaction between the LOG and the COG is in a constantly changing relationship in movement. In fact movement can be simply seen as shifting ones COG around with respect to the LOG. The body is most stable when segmental or global alignment is closer to the LOG and the COG is low and most vulnerable to instability when the body configuration moves outside the LOG and/or the COG is high. The neuromyofascial articular system anticipates and responds to the continual gravity induced sensory cues in order that we do not collapse or fall over.

Base of support

We bear our body weight through and within our support base. This is the surface area of that part of the body resting on the supporting surface. The size and shape of the base of support depends upon which posture the body has adopted e.g. lying, sitting, standing. In sitting the base is the two ischia and the feet. In standing the base is the area between the feet, which can be enlarged by standing with the feet apart. A larger base permits a wider excursion of the body without the LOG falling outside the base of support and so the more stable is

the position within which to move and express the self. The smaller the base of support, the less stable the position, particularly if the COG is high and the body configuration has moved outside the LOG.

Centre of pressure

This is the point of application of the ground reaction force through the base of support. This force reflects Newton's third law of action/reaction in that the force exerted by the body onto the ground is reflected back at the centre of pressure.[4] Pressure down into the ground stimulates a neuromuscular response of 'push up and lift'. This force is utilized a lot as we develop and maintain movement control against gravity. It may be exerted through any part of the body – the hands, feet, knees, ischia or even the head, as is the case when standing on the head! (See Ch.13).

Planes of motion

Posture and movement are generally analyzed and described in relation to the three cardinal planes. These planes of reference are derived from dimensions in space and are at right angles to each other. They are depicted in the context of the person standing in the anatomic position as illustrated and are carried over into other postures as the person moves (Fig. 4.2).

• The sagittal plane is vertical and divides the body into right and left halves. Movements primarily in the sagittal plane involve flexion and extension and forward – backward movements. It represents the 'side view'.

• The frontal or coronal plane is also vertical and divides the front and back body. Movements primarily in the frontal plane involve side bending, lateral motions, and abduction/adduction and inversion/eversion actions. It is the front/back view.

• The transverse or horizontal plane divides the body into upper (cephalad), and lower (caudal)

sections. Movements primarily in this plane involve rotation – within the body axis and in the limbs. It represents the 'bird's eye' view.

Posture

The term 'posture' is used to describe both biomechanical alignment of the segments of the body, as well as the orientation of the body to the environment.[5]

Commonly posture is thought of as alignment of the body in the upright sitting and standing positions. However, each and any position adopted is 'a posture'. The posture adopted *in any position* is a reflection of the neuromuscular status of the person, and this is evident from birth through to adulthood (see Ch. 3).

Postures are never static – there is *always a movement*, however slight, as in a subtle shift of muscle tonus. Postures underlie and support all movements. Posture is generated by movement and movement generated by posture. The two are inseparable and interdependent. However, static analysis aids conceptual understanding.

'Static' posture

Gracovetsky[6] describes posture as 'an average'– the steady erect stance is maintained by cycling through a sequence of different but closely related postures. This oscillation is necessary from a sensory perspective and to prevent continuous loading of the viscoelastic tissues.

The conventional view is the vertical alignment of the body segments with respect to the LOG. While more ideal than real, it is useful in helping detect deviations in the sagittal and frontal planes, the expected altered intrinsic forces and their possible biomechanical consequences.

Sagittal view

Optimum alignment of the segments and easy equilibrium is said to occur when the LOG passes through:

• the mastoid process of the skull
• slightly anterior to the shoulder joint
• through the bodies of the lumbar vertebrae[3]
• through centre of the pelvis anterior to the second sacral vertebra
• at or just behind the hip joint[3,4]
• just anterior to the knee and ankle joint (Fig. 4.3).

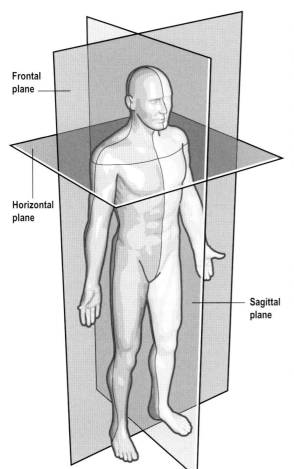

Frontal plane

Horizontal plane

Sagittal plane

Fig 4.2 • The three cardinal planes of motion.

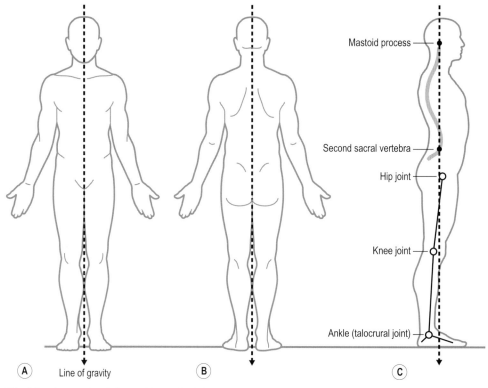

Fig 4.3 • Conventional views of frontal (A & B) and sagittal plane (C) postural alignment in relation to the 'line of gravity'.

Optimal alignment of the vertebral column is also said to occur when the LOG passes through the transitional or junctional regions of the spine.[7] Many consider that the T12/L1 articulation is quite central[8,9] being the point of inflection between the thoracic kyphosis and lumbar lordosis.[7] Ideal alignment is said to produce a torque that helps maintain the optimum shape of each spinal curve with the maximum torque at the convexity of each curve. When the line of gravity falls posterior there is an increased axial extensor torque; when it falls anterior there is an increased flexor torque.[2]

In the pelvis, 'ideally' the LOG passes through the greater trochanter yet posterior to the axis of the hip joint[1] but anterior to the sacroiliac joints.[9] This tends to nutate the sacrum while also creating an extensor moment at the hip and a tendency to passive posterior rotation of the pelvis.

Coronal view

The LOG passes directly through the centre of the head, trunk and pelvis and falls midway between the two feet. This conceptually divides the body into two symmetrical, equal halves (Fig. 4.3).

This view is useful for discerning lateral deviations and asymmetries in the body.

There is a constant though subtle postural sway in response to breathing[10] which provides continual sensory cues which keep refuelling the alignment of the segments and the antigravity response. Flexible and adaptable segmental control throughout the spine allows appropriate postural shifts and sets to balance and support movement.

Farhi[11] points to the observable close relationship between how we stand and breathe. Three patterns are generally apparent:

• Propping: we stand like a table on a floor 'holding ourselves up'. This is associated with hyperventilation and chest breathing.

• Collapsing: we drop to the earth without the necessary integrity through our structure to use gravity to our advantage. This results in a lethargic, laboured and shallow breathing pattern.

• Yielding: between the two patterns above, this represents the 'right' relationship where we give the weight of our body to the earth but at the same time we receive the rebound of gravity up through our bodies – an erect lightness which provides for an ease an effortless in breathing.

Dynamic posture

In functional terms posture is always dynamic as it is constantly changing and adapting to support movement. However, when walking, running, jumping, throwing and lifting[1] there is the increased challenge of adapting to further changed alignment of the segments, momentum and larger perturbations.

Quantitative and qualitative aspects of movement

Effective clinical practice relies upon the ability of the practitioner to analyze movement in the clinic in a relatively easy, practically relevant, and useful way. Trew[4] states 'it is relatively straight forward to measure some of the physical aspects of movement such as joint range or muscle strength in a non functional context but difficulty arises when the quality of the movement must also be considered'.

The skilled practitioner is one who has the ability to see the qualitative 'soft signs' as well as the 'hard signs' of objectively measurable movement. Janda considered that the quality of the motor performance was of greater importance than testing strength.[15]

The qualitative aspects of movement are observable

While the quantitative aspects of movement function are more derived from testing, the qualitative aspects are derived more through observation of the *patterns of motor response* in different situations. We are interested in the *quality* of a person's sensory–motor integration. Without any interference we note *how* he habitually chooses to stand, sit, bend over and perform some of the repetitive actions involved in daily living such as getting undressed or standing on one leg. Feldenkrais apparently coined the term '*acture*' – posture in action, to describe the observation of the person moving.[12] This can reveal a wealth of information such as the presence of organic or pathological movement patterns, discomfort during motion, the emotion behind the motion, the amount of sensory amnesia present, the range of motion, the quality of the breathing pattern and the quality of specific tasks

as in the transitions between lying, sitting standing and walking. We may decide to 'test' by observing *the manner in which* the patient spontaneously chooses to perform a requested task

These aspects of quality control in movement have probably received less attention because their interpretation is more subjective; they are usually the more subtle aspects of motor control and require an in depth understanding of the subject and considerable practical experience. The signs are relatively 'soft' and more difficult to objectively measure. These aspects are explored.

Doing it – but 'how' the movement happens: aspects of quality control in posturomovement

The following aspects are functionally interrelated in varying respects.

Observing the size, shape and symmetry of the superficial muscles tells a story

Janda[13] maintained that 'changes in muscle function play an important role in the pathogenesis of many painful conditions of the motor system and constitute an integral part of postural defects in general'. The muscles both cause and reflect altered function.[14]

Simply observing the appearance of the standing person's superficial muscles can provide insights about the patient's neuromuscular function.[15] The size shape and symmetry of a muscle provides clues to the level of its activity. Those muscles which are used a lot become bulkier and more prominent (Fig. 4.4) and those that aren't lose their definition or shape. The role of the deeper muscles in postural deviations may need to be confirmed or negated in later tests (Ch.13).

The ability to align the body segments in different functional acts

As infants we spent a deal of time down on the ground as we learned how to move along and get ourselves up against the force of gravity. As adults, we tend to spend most of our time upright in one

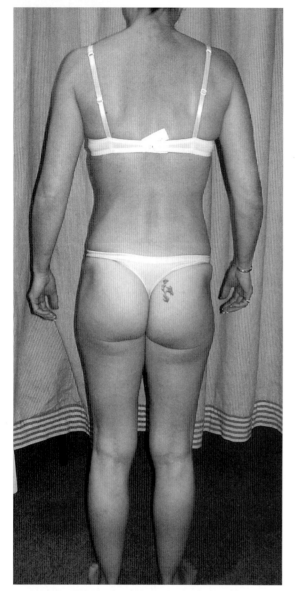

Fig 4.4 • Buttocks like these are an unusual clinical presentation – these are the result of weight training.

them, which the patient will repeatedly enact during the course of his day. Implicit is the way he does ordinary movements significantly contributes to his predicament.

The importance of this 'functional control' in everyday activities has also been recognized by McGill who has examined motion patterns of lifting[16] and O'Sullivan who has examined postural patterns of sitting in non back pain and back pain groups.[17,18]

The ability to generate appropriate patterns of axial stabilisation

Any muscle action requires adequate or fixation of one or both of its attachment points to have a firm origin from which to pull. Stability in the spine must ensure protection for the spine itself through movement as well as provide support counteracting the torques created by muscles attaching to the torso. Balanced co-activation between the flexors and extensors is basic to the complex patterns of axial stabilisation which provide three dimensional control.

All muscles contributing to the 'central stabilisation system' are interdependent in function. If one muscle is weak or overactive, this never remains isolated, but affects the static and dynamic function of the entire spine. Individual spinal segments will no longer be controlled in a balanced way. In particular, the diaphragm needs to become integrated into the patterns of central control.[19] Observing the quality of the breathing pattern and axial alignment at rest and during trunk and limb movements tells us a lot about the quality of axial control. Poor patterns of axial make balanced alignment difficult (Fig. 4.5).

Limb load tests e.g. the active straight leg raise test

The supine active straight leg raise test (ASLR) is a functional test which assesses the quality of the patterns of axial stabilization when the extended leg is lifted off the surface. First described by Mens et al.,[20] the extended leg should be able to effortlessly lift 5 cm. When control is optimal, three dimensional alignment of the pelvis[21] should be maintained as well as the alignment of the whole torso while breathing patterns are maintained.[22,23] The test as originally described, is positive if accompanied by a primary sensation of profound heaviness in the leg and /or pain[23] which is relieved by the application of bilateral compression through

way or another and our patterns of motor use represent a fairly constrained repertoire by comparison. Commonly, most of us use four basic spinopelvic posturomotor patterns and derivatives of them in the course of our daily living – standing, walking, sitting and bending/lifting/squatting.

Observing the person's habitual patterns of functional control in aligning the body segments or otherwise in these primary movement patterns is highly informative as it is these actions and derivatives of

Subjective complaints should not be the only decider of dysfunction as probably more important is the observed quality of the axial control patterns. Dysfunctional responses include loss of alignment, breath holding, central 'fixing' strategies and a functional 'disconnect' between the upper and lower torso. There are numerous other tests using either a short or long limb lever which can be applied in a similar manner in order to test and facilitate axial control strategies.

Sequence and degree of muscle activation in a movement

Movement stems from a starting point – a 'posture' developed on a base of support which is actively controlled before the actual movement happens. The work of Hodges[24,25] has shown that normally transversus abdominis is active *before* arm movement begins. Transversus is a member of the 'central stabilization system' – a coordinated trunk muscle synergy creating anticipatory postural adjustment to support limb movement.

Janda[15] maintained that examination of movement patterns provides a good indication of the quality of a person's motor control. In the presence of muscle imbalance or poor central nervous system regulation some typical abnormal patterns of muscle activation can be clinically observed. He described six basic movement patterns[15,26–28] which essentially test the quality of axial patterns of control.

- Head flexion in supine.
- Shoulder abduction in sitting.
- Push up from prone. This is a high level test and should be used with discretion.
- Hip extension prone.
- Hip abduction in side lying.
- Trunk curl in supine.

These are fully described elsewhere.[28] When changed, these usually show certain typical patterns of response. Appreciating the common features of dysfunction (Ch. 8) and clinical sub-classification helps predict the response (Chs 9 & 10).

Strength versus control

Janda was not interested in muscle strength but rather, the coordinated activity between different muscle groups in a synergy. He says this should be evaluated in at least three ways:[29]

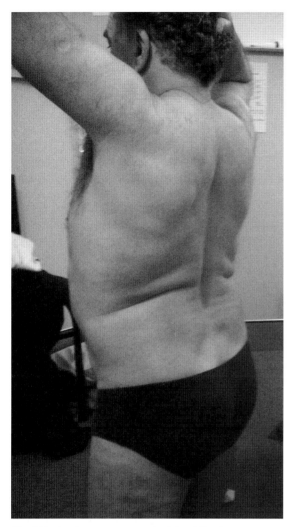

Fig 4.5 • Inadequate pattern of axial stabilization.

the ilia either just below the anterior superior iliac spines or at the level of the symphysis pubis[20] (above or below the hip joint). This compression is considered to enhance 'force closure' through the sacroiliac joint[21] by simulating muscle forces which would otherwise control the movement. The prone ASLR test similarly tests axial patterns of control including the breathing mechanism with hip extension in knee extension.

Because of the long lever arm of the leg, it represents a fairly high level challenge to the ability and quality of axial stability. While a positive test result has been shown to strongly correlate in people with pelvic ring instability,[20] a positive test does *not* necessarily confer sacroiliac joint instability. However, a positive test *is* indicative of suboptimal neuromuscular control in the torso and pelvic–hip complex.

• The sequence of activation of muscles in the synergy producing the movement i.e. an estimation of timing. Which muscles activate early and which come in later. Expecting appropriate patterns of anticipatory axial 'postural setting' and control to support limb movement or conversely the axial spine adjusting to movements initiated from the limbs. The 'onset' may be central or peripheral depending upon the movement. The point of initiation of a movement is important and the sequencing of the movement from it.

• Degree of activity of the main muscles or groups – which muscles dominate the movement and which are underactive.

• Estimation of activity of the so called 'parasitic muscles' – those which should not be activated in that particular movement

He is concerned with the quality of the response – *how* the task is performed and what, if any, substitutions and compensations occur.

There are a multitude of other functional movement pattern tests that can be looked at based on these and other principles. Choice will also depend upon which aspect of function needs examining, the age of the patient and the state of irritability of his tissues. The art in the practitioner is to be able to gauge what is an appropriate test for that person's stage of disorder. Liebenson[30] rightly says 'choosing the correct functional tests is an art not a science'.

It is interesting that current thinking and research is pointing more in this direction. Van Dieën et al[31] suggest that certain aspects such as altered timing of muscle activity and load sharing between muscles contribute towards the observed altered recruitment patterns seen in people with back pain. 'The changes involved are task dependent, related to the individual problem and hence highly variable between and probably within individuals'.

Motor skill involves various qualities of optimal motor control

Trew[4] states 'there is no consensus as to what constitutes quality of movement'. While this may be partly true in an academic sense, clinical practice assisted by the insights of Bartenieff[32] and others helps delineate certain qualities in skilled movement:

• Economy of effort: movement should be easy and pleasurable and not hard work

• Lightness of movement rather than heavy or 'bound'

• Efficiency: without superfluous movement or the use of unnecessary muscles which may interfere with or oppose the desired movement

• Modulation of the degree of force appropriate to demand: at times strength and power is required

• Sustained: a posture/movement should have endurance without hardening or 'holding'

• Selective: the ability to control the point of initiation of the movement, either from the centre or the periphery; the ability to perform precise discreet actions

• Smooth and free flow rather than jerky and uneven

• Speed: the ability to move both slowly and fast

• Flexibility and adaptability to changed environmental demands: the ability to suddenly and differently respond when needed

• Variety and variability: the availability of multiple movement strategies and the ability to select the appropriate strategy for the task and the environment[5]

• Relaxation: the ability to let go tension when the muscle(s) are not required to work.

Further aspects of movement function

Muscle states

Weakness vs inhibition

Specific weakness of certain muscles such as the lumbosacral multifidus has been objectively shown in people with back pain,[33,34] probably resulting from disturbed joint mechanics, pain and altered afference creating inhibitory phenomena.[35,36] Kendall[3] and Sahrmann[37] note 'over stretch weakness' can occur when a muscle is held in a lengthened position particularly during long periods of rest, certainly a common clinical finding in the lower scapula stabilizers due to principal arm use in front of the body and poor postural habits (Fig. 4.6).

However, Janda[27] maintained that often muscles that appeared weak were inhibited through changed central nervous motor regulation and performance

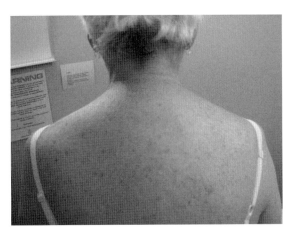

Fig 4.6 • Stretch weakness/underactivity of the interscapular and upper thoracic intrinsic muscles.

producing a systemic response in the muscular system with over activity in some muscles and underactivity in others.[13,15,27,29,36] Clinically the underactivity is observed as hypotonia, weakness and especially by a delayed sequence of activation in principal movement patterns. This underactivity in a muscle may also be due to direct inhibition because of hyper irritability of its antagonist in accordance with Sherrington's law of reciprocal innervation,[15] e.g. underactivity of the abdominals and related hyperactivity of the erector spinae. Janda says 'stretch or inhibition of a tight muscle can lead to spontaneous facilitation of an inhibited muscle leading to its inclusion in the movement chain and therefore improvement in key motor patterns'.[38] Importantly, when an inhibited or weakened muscle is resisted, its activity tends to decrease rather than increase.[15]

Kolar[19] notes that a muscle may appear weak when it is not, if there is inadequate stabilization of its attachment points, which itself is dependent upon a chain of muscles. Disturbed function of a muscle can therefore be caused by dysfunction of a far distant muscle. A good example is apparent weakness of the deep neck flexors because of inadequate stabilization of the thorax by the abdominals.

If back pain has been significant and longstanding and there is relative inactivity, general body de-conditioning 'weakness' can be expected and has been shown.[39] However, this is not the case in all patients by any means. Smeets and Wittink[40] question the deconditioning paradigm and point out that no convincing proof exists as studies have provided contradictory results. Clinically, many highly active sports people present with back pain.

Strength vs endurance

McGill[41] defines strength as 'the maximum force a muscle can produce during a single exertion to create joint torque; endurance is the ability to maintain a force for a period of time'. Studies have variously shown deficits in both in LBP subjects[31] Clinically, strength may be a problem for some; endurance appears to be a problem for all.

Both strength and endurance are dependent upon well coordinated *control* throughout the spine, and in particular from the support of the deep system (Ch. 5). Janda noted the tendency for dominant activity of certain 'postural muscles' in typical patterns.[38] Overactivity makes muscles stronger tending to inhibit their antagonist creating imbalance in patterns of movement. Clinically, muscles in some regions of the spine are found to be consistently overactive and 'strong' while others appear underactive and 'weak'. When too strong they often 'don't let go', evidenced by a commonly found lack of the flexion–relaxation response in studies of patients with back pain[42–45] (Fig. 4.7).

Van Dieën et al[31] suggest that this increased activation of the trunk muscles may be an adaptive response to pain aimed at limiting movement and so avoiding noxious tensile stresses on injured tissues. Clinically this response appears to be both the cause and the effect of pain. This is discussed more fully in Ch. 8.

Endurance however, or lack of it, particularly at low loads, is a common and significant clinical finding in patients with LBP and has been corroborated by

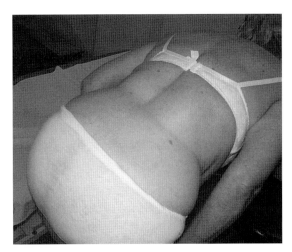

Fig 4.7 • Lack of flexion relaxation phenomenon in the thoracolumbar extensors.

studies.[31,41] Clinically, this is evident in most anti-gravity posturomovements and particularly in those which involve moving further away from the line of gravity. The provision of posturomovement 'staying power' appears to be one of the roles of the deep system (Ch.5). The Biering-Sorenson test [46,47] is a reasonably high level clinical test for trunk muscle strength and endurance. Modification in the Key Alignment and Control test (Ch.13) is a more functional alternative. The quality of the response is as informative as the measurable parameter of time.

Reduced endurance and fatigue are not necessarily the same; however, each will lead to the other. This is an interesting situation and will be dealt with more fully in Ch.7.

Muscle imbalance

Kendall[3] defined muscle imbalance as inequality in the strength of opposing muscles acting on a joint. Faulty alignment, inefficient movement and poor stabilization occur.

Janda[38] saw that impaired CNS motor regulation results in defective or uneconomical movement patterns. As a consequence, *imbalanced activity* between certain muscle groups develops. This includes altered timing, degree of activation and load sharing, altered concentric and eccentric control etc. As the spine is a system of multiple joints balanced activity between all muscles is important in its alignment and control, and particularly between the flexor and extensor systems.

Various forms of muscle activation and movement

Roles of muscles in movement

Many different muscles are involved in providing a movement but the forces generated by each vary considerably throughout a movement and each muscle can fulfil several roles in a pattern of movement:

• *An agonist or prime mover* is the muscle that plays the major role in initiating carrying out and maintaining a movement, e.g. ideally in hip flexion, iliopsoas is the prime mover assisted by the secondary superficial hip flexors acting as synergists.

• *An antagonist* is a muscle which works in the direction opposite to the agonist, e.g. if the agonist is a flexor, the antagonist is an extensor. The antagonists are often inhibited by a reflex

mechanism originating from the agonist known as reciprocal inhibition.[4] Otherwise, their eccentric contraction helps modulate movement.

• *Stabilizers or fixators* contract to control the position of the bone(s) to provide a stable base from which the agonist can contract, e.g. in the example of hip flexion, the lumbar spine and pelvic girdle must be appropriately controlled by the trunk muscles so that iliopsoas can act at the hip.

• *A synergist* is a muscle which helps or cooperates with other muscles in particular the prime mover, to perform a movement. It may help to stabilize a joint while an action is occurring. Janda[48] found synergistic activity in the hip adductors when testing hip flexion in sitting – particularly if resistance was applied. In reality, probably lots of synergists assist in a movement.

• *A synergy* is formed when a number of muscles cooperate and combine their activity to form a coordinated pattern of response – stability to support movement and or a movement sequence.

Concentric, isometric and eccentric muscle interplay

The nervous system stimulates a muscle to generate or resist force by utilizing various forms of action. The point of stabilization can either be proximal or distal.

• *A concentric muscle action* is a shortening muscle contraction. A simple example of concentric activity is flexing the hip. The point of stability is the pelvis.

• *An isometric contraction* occurs when there is no visible change in the length of the muscle, yet it maintains a constant level of tension[1] e.g. sustaining the hip in flexion.

• *An eccentric muscle action* is a lengthening muscle contraction which 'plays out' an action providing a braking or controlling action in a movement e.g. lowering the flexed hip.

A general simplification is that while the agonist is concentrically contracting the antagonists eccentrically contract in the modulation of movement. A nice example is the control of respiration and the IAP mechanism, where both the diaphragm and transversus abdominis are tonically coactivated – on inspiration, the diaphragm concentrically acts while transversus eccentrically lengthens and the converse pattern occurs during expiration.[49]

Eccentric muscle control deserves more attention

Clinically, patients with spinal pain disorders appear to have more difficulty with eccentric control particularly with lowering to gravity movements and those requiring more complex control hence further examination is warranted.

From a neurophysiological perspective, Enoka[57] says that there is accumulating evidence that control of eccentric contractions is different from that for concentric and isometric contractions. Eccentric contractions appear to be unique in several respects:

• Eccentric control strategies are *highly reliant upon afferent feedback* to provide information on the progress of the movement and achieve a desired trajectory. Eccentric contractions involve more sustained and often greater discharge by Group 1a afferents in the muscle spindles compared to concentric actions. Disruption to sensory feedback has been shown to disturb eccentric control and coordination. The predominant effect of feedback from Group 1a afferents is excitatory on motor neurons yet there is less EMG during an eccentric action. This is because:

• Fewer motor units are involved in an eccentric contraction compared with a shortening contraction. The reduced EMG is a consequence of the *greater force that muscles can exert* during these contractions. Compared with concentric, eccentric exercises may provide more effective stimulation for muscle hypertrophy.[57] The variability of motor unit discharge during eccentric actions can mean reduced steadiness in performance, particularly at 5% of MVC.[57]

• During eccentric contraction, the muscle stores elastic energy and some of this can be released during a concentric action. *When an eccentric contraction precedes a concentric one there is more power in the concentric action.*[57] This is also dependent upon the architectural properties of the muscle and the kinematic details of performance. A good example is the counter movement in a jump where the lowering to gravity precedes the spring giving it power. Another example is psoas in walking where it eccentrically lengthens during hip extension (increasing the stored elastic energy) before it contracts to flex the hip.[50] More subtle though important is its shuffling concentric/eccentric control of the column during lateral weight shift.

From a functional perspective, the interplay between the various modes of contraction is ever changing according to prevailing demands of posturomovement control. In order that the range and quality of movement is full there must be balanced activity between concentric/eccentric control.[51] Not all eccentric control is the same.[52,57] It can occur in response to:

• Lowering to gravity as when lowering a raised limb or moving down into a squat

• Controlling the momentum and lengthening of an outward swing such as kicking a ball

• To balance the concentric activity in antagonistic muscles as part of the coactivation patterns controlling a joint, and in resisting imposed loads during the give and take of posturomovement control.

Hartley[51] suggests that attempting to release muscle by forcefully stretching and pulling does not fundamentally change the muscle length and requires daily practice and tearing to keep the apparent length. Changing the 'mind' of the muscle in the way that it is used changes the unconscious neuromuscular patterns. By *focusing upon the eccentrically lengthening muscles in a movement*, and 'actively create (ing) the sensation of extending through the whole length of that muscle, we can in fact increase the contractility and natural resting length of the muscle and free it from a state of habitual contraction or tension'.[51] We have termed this 'active elongation' (see Ch.13). Bainbridge Cohen[52] notes dancers are more likely to injure themselves with 'pulls' and 'tears' during eccentric activity and the incidence of hamstring tears in football is legion.

The coordination and 'phrasing' of eccentric activity assists in balancing the forces in movement and in the sequencing and support of movement especially in the spine and other weight bearing structures.[52] Eccentric control thus plays an important role in posturomovement control. It is particularly involved in postural adjustment, weight shift and in 'yield and push' to provide 'grounding' through the base of support (Ch. 13) for antigravity control.

Co-activation or co-contraction of muscles

In practice when an agonist is called to perform a desired motion the agonist and antagonist contract simultaneously, and co-activation occurs.[1] While the agonist is concentrically contracting, the antagonist eccentrically contracts to balance its activity and help control the movement e.g. to bend your elbow, the extensors need to play out and lengthen. This co-activation provides stability for the joint; however it needs to be well modulated to allow for flexible adjustment of the joint, particularly important in weight bearing situations. If co-activation is excessive the joint becomes rigid or 'held'; if inadequate the joint(s) is not well controlled or 'unstable'. All skilled movement involves co-activation.

A certain level of muscular co-activation in the axial skeleton is always necessary in providing suitable stabilizing synergies for adaptable antigravity support and control in three dimensions. The application of external load such as carrying a bucket of water increases the response[53] and further so when preparing for short term unexpected and sudden loading or heavier loads. However, while protecting the spine, these greater responses are energetically and mechanically costly[54] if maintained beyond the time of their short term need. Problems arise when there is too much co-activation[55,56] or too little.[53] There is evidence that isometric strength training appears to involve a reduction in the coactivation of the antagonist.[57]

Clinical practice reveals common consistent patterns of reduced co-activation in some regions of the spine and excessive co-activation in others. The alignment, shape and function of the body change.

Open and closed kinetic chain movements

The performance of any task is achieved by a sequential activation of muscle synergies and movement of body segments referred to as a kinetic chain. Movement sequences from one limb girdle to the other through the spine. Movement control of the spine is further understood by considering the different roles the spine plays in the control of open and closed (kinetic) chain movements. Functional movement control includes mixed elements of both.

Open chain movements are those where the proximal parts are stabilized and the distal parts move, e.g. any free movement of a limb where *appropriate positioning and control of the axial spine and proximal girdles provide the stability* to support the limb movement. Here the femoral or humeral head move against the 'fixed' joint cavities of the proximal girdles (Fig. 4.8A). Free movements of the head and neck can also be seen as open chain movements; the point of stability provided by appropriate positioning and control of the thoracic spine and shoulder girdle etc. Open chain movements can be more ballistic in which case they may involve more activity of superficial muscles.

Closed chain movements are those where the more distal supporting part or limb provides the point of fixation or stability *and the more proximal parts are free to move.* The proximal axiogirdle

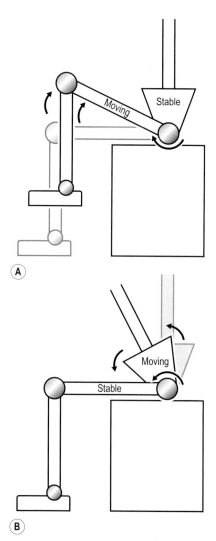

Fig 4.8 • Proximal stability with distal movement in (A) distal stability and proximal mobility in (B).

muscles now pull against a fixed more distal point and the joint cavities move around or against the femoral and/or humeral heads[19](Fig. 4.8B), e.g. sitting with the feet on the ground, the legs provide the point of stabilization allowing the pelvis to tilt on the femur enabling the torso to freely adjust and move (see Fig. 6.25). In all fours the limbs are the stable point and the proximal girdles and spine can move and adjust between them.

Studies on the pattern of quadriceps activation in open and closed chain movements of the knee have shown more balanced initial activation in closed chain movements.[58] The joint compression afforded in closed chain exercise facilitates more balanced co-contraction of the muscles around the joint rendering them a more superior form of exercise in providing optimal joint loading and stability.[59] The added proprioception afforded in closed chain movements more optimally recruits the deep Systemic Local Muscle System synergies (Ch. 5). They are a nice way to facilitate activation of this system in less gravitationally loaded postures so that reprogramming of the postural reflex responses can be experienced and learnt.

The head also initiates closed chain movements of the spine serving as the point of support, e.g. doing a head stand.

Anatomical vs functional actions of muscles

The brain knows about movement, not single muscles. No muscle works in isolation but as part of a synergy in varying manner of contraction required in that particular movement. Anatomists tend to describe the actions of single muscles according to a presumed shortening contraction occurring between the fixed proximal origin and the more distal insertion, i.e. principally in terms of open chain actions. Practically, muscles also work with a 'reversed origin and insertion' – where the distal attachment is stable and the proximal part moves as occurs in closed chain movements. A good example is serratus anterior providing stability for the ribs to move when weight bearing through the arm, and stabilizing the scapula when freely reaching the arm.

Understanding this principal is important in understanding functional movement control of the spine. Psoas demonstrates the principle well. Usually considered a hip flexor[60] yet in functional

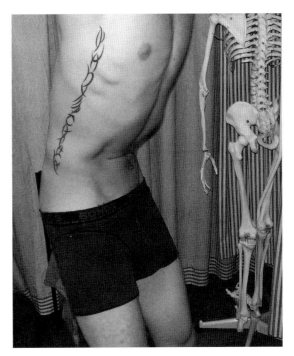

Fig 4.9 • Acute hamstring spasm changes the line of pull of psoas. Note the associated abdominal hyperactivity.

movement control it contributes to vertical stability and support of the spine, and controlling lateral flexion torques;[2,61] shows an oscillating concentric/eccentric action during walking;[61,62] helps control load transfer between the legs to the body; and it assists the functional pattern of flexing the pelvis on the femur[2] while helping to control the spine, as in the pattern of forward bending. In certain instances it could act as a hip extensor as Schleip[63] suggests, i.e. if in crook lying and performing a 'pelvic roll', psoas could contribute to synergies producing hip extension and lumbar flexion. Clinically, this is sometimes apparent in an acute trunk 'list' where hamstrings spasm posteriorly rotates the pelvis and psoas appears to flex the lumbar spine (Fig. 4.9).

McGill[64] found that loss of the lumbar lordosis changed the line of action of the largest extensor muscles, compromising their role to support anterior shear forces.

Mobilizing and stabilizing elements interact (see Ch.13)

Laban apparently taught: 'stability and mobility alternate ceaselessly'.[8,32] The role of muscles change during movement according to whether they are required to provide support or movement; work in closed or open chain movements; work eccentrically, concentrically etc. In addition, factors such as posture, the line of gravity, internal and external forces, weight shift etc., will all affect the timing and degree of muscle action and their shifting role between providing stability or mobility.

The two-joint muscles

A significant number of muscles span two joints. They are usually 'superficial' and generally known as 'global' muscles (see Ch. 5).

Enoka describes the two joint muscles as providing at least three advantages in control of the musculoskeletal system.[57]

- They allow coupled motion at the two joints they cross, e.g. the semimembranosus concurrently contributes to hip extension and knee flexion. This coupling can be achieved by a reduction in EMG in the one joint muscle (gluteus maximus) and an increased EMG in the two joint muscle (semimembranosus)
- The shortening velocity of a two joint muscle (e.g. rectus femoris) is less than half of its one joint synergist (vastus medialis oblique)and hence it is capable of exerting a force that is a greater proportion of the isometric maximum
- The two joint muscles can redistribute muscle torque, joint power and mechanical energy throughout a limb (Fig. 4.10).

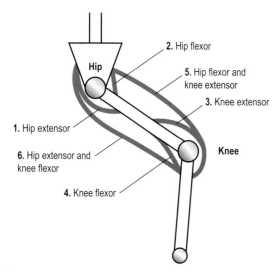

1. Hip extensor
2. Hip flexor
3. Knee extensor
4. Knee flexor
5. Hip flexor and knee extensor
6. Hip extensor and knee flexor

Fig 4.10 • Model of the hip and knee and the one and two joint flexor/extensor muscles.

- Muscles 1 and 3 are one joint hip and knee extensors
- Muscles 2 and 4 are one joint hip and knee flexors
- Muscles 5 and 6 are two joint muscles.

These muscles can be activated in various combinations to exert extensor torques about the hip and knee joints.

The role of the two joint muscles as described by Enoka is useful in understanding the 'extensor mechanism' and the myomechanics of the hips and knees in positioning and controlling the pelvis during the pattern of forward bending and lifting (see Ch. 6).

Balanced proximal girdle muscle force couples

Both proximal limb girdles house sockets to accommodate the big spheroidal heads of the long bones, allowing multiplanar movements at the shoulder and hip all of which are actually all rotations. This rotary action is controlled by means of coplanar muscle force couples formed when two or more muscles simultaneously produce forces in different linear directions, although the torques act in the same rotary direction[2] as in turning a steering wheel. This serves to either rotate the limb on the girdle or the girdle on the limb. In order that the joint remains centrated and the axis of rotation is 'pure' at the joint, the muscle force couples obviously need to be balanced. Problems arise when they are not.

Compensatory motion

Sahrmann[37] notes that the stabilizing action of muscles can either be excessive or insufficient. This will tend to create regions in the spine with reduced intersegmental movement and regions which are relatively flexible or even show excessive movement. When analyzing movement function in the spine, due regard should be paid for the occurrence of compensatory motion. Commonly this occurs in the cervical and lumbar spines as a result of insufficient movement in the thoracic spine, shoulders and hips and inadequate axiopelvic control (Fig. 4.11).

Motivation and motor performance

Parameters of functional evaluation have been strongly correlated with cognitive state.[65] Strength tests demand motivation and cooperation from the

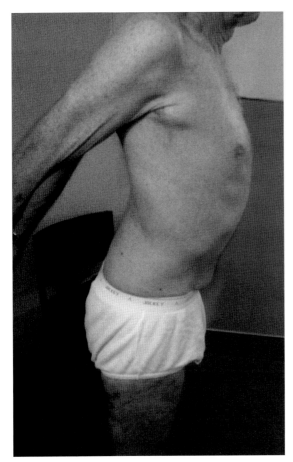

Fig 4.11 • Compensatory motion occurs in some regions of the spine when the thorax and shoulders are stiff.

patient which can confound objective assessment. Cox et al[65] suggest that complex spinal coordination is a better indicator of spinal dysfunction. Observing *how* the patient performs ordinary actions and tasking certain motor acts without the need for effort, reveals a lot about that person's *ability to organize* posture and movement control. Trying less hard does little to change the organization and so his ability to significantly influence the outcome. In fact, trying too hard invariably diminishes movement quality.

Continuum concept of dysfunction

In general terms pain doesn't 'just occur' but results from what Janda[66] termed a 'functional pathology of the motor system'. Neuromuscular dysfunction is evident before the onset of pain. He says:

The impairment is clinically recognizable even if symptoms are minimal. Depending upon the primary localization of the impairment, for example reflex changes in the corresponding segment may be deficient, or changes in movement patterns, early onset of fatigue and faster switch into more primitive movement patterns in fatigue of the motor system etc. The functional impairment will present itself, however by discomfort and pain if additional provoking factors come into play.

Pain results when one has run out of compensations. It may be considered as the major and most frequent sign of impaired function of the motor system.

Until recently the thinking has been that the motor control changes *occur as a result of pain*. In an excellent paper, Van Dieën et al[31] analyzed the literature to determine how LBP effects muscle recruitment in the trunk extensors. They found equivocal results – there is evidence for both increased and decreased muscle activity if you have back pain. They interpreted the altered activity as an adaptive functional response in order to mechanically stabilize the spine and limit noxious tensile stresses on painful tissues. Importantly they allowed that while disturbed motor control was not likely to be adaptive, *the loss of control leads to the adaptive changes* differs between patients and the developmental stage of the disorder.

There is some evidence emerging pointing towards pre-existing motor control changes.[67–69] When it is recognized that the dysfunction is pre-existing, and patients are sub-classified many of the outcomes reported in the literature can be better understood.

Janda's momentously important contribution towards the understanding of back pain is that altered control *precedes* the development of pain. When pain evolves, *further changes* in neuromuscular function occur. Patients presenting to the clinician display varying degrees of neuromusculoskeletal dysfunction at *varying stages of disorder*. Van Dieën et al.[31] importantly recognize that with respect to research studies, 'between-subject variation may occur to differences between patients in the developmental stage of their low back disorder'.

The clinician needs to gain some insight as to where in the continuum of dysfunction, the presenting patient lies (Fig. 4.12). An understanding of the expected patterns of normal and dysfunctional

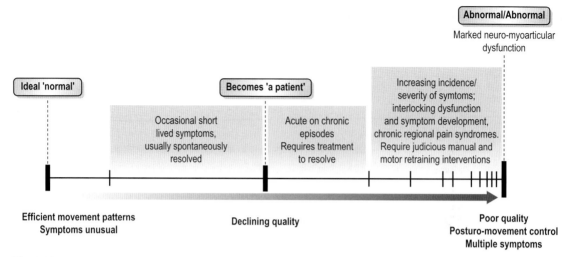

Fig 4.12 • Continuum concept of dysfunction.

control of movement allows the practitioner to choose to examine appropriate component parts of movement relevant to the stage of the patient's disorder and to be able to interpret the results.

The more common patterns of clinical presentation are presented in subsequent chapters to help the understanding of this and provide a framework for assisting assessment and intervention strategies.

References

[1] Norkin C, Levangie PK. Joint Structure and Function: a comprehensive analysis. 2nd ed. Philadelphia: F.A. Davis Company; 1992.

[2] Neumann DA. Kinesiology of the Musculoskeletal System: Foundations for Physical Rehabilitation. Missouri: Mosby; 2002.

[3] Kendall FP, McCreary EK, Provance PG. Muscles: Testing and Function – with Posture and Pain. 4th ed. Williams and Wilkins; 1993.

[4] Trew M, Everett T. Human Movement: an introductory text. 5th ed. Elsevier Churchill Livingstone; 2005.

[5] Shumway-Cook A, Woollacott MH. Motor Control: Theory and Practical Applications. 2nd ed. Maryland: Lippincott Williams and Wilkins; 2001.

[6] Gracovetsky S. Stability or controlled instability. In: Vleeming A, Mooney V, Stoeckart R, editors. Movement,

Stability & Lumbopelvic Pain. Edinburgh: Churchill Livingstone; 2007.

[7] Singer KP, Malmivarra A. Pathoanatomical characteristics of the thoracolumbar junctional region. In: Giles LGF, Singer KP, editors. Clinical anatomy and management of thoracic spine pain. Oxford: Butterworth Heinemann; 2000.

[8] Hackney P. Making Connections: total body integration through Bartenieff Fundamentals. New York: Routledge; 2002.

[9] Steindler A. Kinesiology of the Human Body under Normal and Pathological Conditions. Springfield, Illinois: Charles C Thomas; 1955.

[10] Hodges PW, et al. Coexistence of stability and mobility in postural control: evidence from postural compensation for respiration. Exp Brain Res 2002;144(3):293–302.

[11] Farhi D. The breathing book: Good health and vitality through essential breath work. New York: Henry Holt and Company; 1996.

[12] Mes S. Neurophysiology in Action. 5th Interdisciplinary World Congress on Low Back and Pelvic Pain. Melbourne; 2004 Post Congress Course proceedings.

[13] Janda V. Muscles, Central Nervous Regulation and Back Problems. In: Korr EM editor. Neurobiologic Mechanisms in Manipulative Therapy. New York: Plenum Press; 1978. p. 27–41.

[14] Tunnel PW. Protocol for Visual Assessment Postural Evaluation of the Muscular System through Visual Assessment. J Bodywork Movt Ther 1996;1(1):21–7.

[15] Janda V. Muscles and Motor Control in Back Pain: Assessment and Management. In: Twomey L, editor. Physical Therapy of the Low Back. New York: Churchill Livingstone; 1987. p. 253–78.

[16] McGill SM. Low Back Disorders: Evidence Based Prevention and Rehabilitation. USA: Human Kinetics; 2002.

[17] O'Sullivan PB, et al. Effect of Different Upright Sitting Postures on Spinal Pelvic Curvature and Trunk Muscle Activation in a Pain Free Population. Spine 2006;31(19): E707–12.

[18] Dankaerts W, et al. Altered patterns of Superficial Trunk Muscle Activation During Sitting in Non-specific Low Back Pain Patients: importance of sub classification. Spine 2006;31 (17):2017–23.

[19] Kolar P. Facilitation of Agonist-Antagonist Co-activation by Reflex Stimulation Methods. In: Liebenson C, editor. Rehabilitation of the Spine: A Practitioner's Manual. 2nd ed. Lippincott Williams and Wilkins; 2007.

[20] Mens JM, et al. The active straight leg raising test and mobility of the pelvic joints. Eur Spine J 1999;8:468–73.

[21] Lee D. The pelvic girdle: an approach to the examination and treatment of the lumbopelvic-hip region. 3rd ed. Edinburgh: Churchill Livingstone; 2004.

[22] O'Sullivan PB, et al. Altered motor control strategies in subjects with sacroiliac joint pain during active straight-leg-raise test. Spine 2002;27(1):E1–8.

[23] O'Sullivan PB, Beales DJ. Changes in pelvic floor and diaphragm kinematics and respiratory patterns in subjects with sacroiliac joint pain following a motor learning intervention: a case series. Man Ther 2007;12(3): 209–18.

[24] Hodges PW, Richardson CA. Inefficient Muscular Stabilisation of the Lumbar Spine Associated With Low Back Pain. A Motor Control Evaluation of Transversus Abdominis. Spine 1996;21(22): 2640–50.

[25] Hodges PW, Richardson CA. Altered Trunk Muscle Recruitment in People with Low Back Pain with Upper Limb Movement at Different Speeds. Arch Phys Med Rehab 1999;80 (9):1005–12.

[26] Janda V. Motor Learning Impairment and Back Pain. J Manual Medicine 1984;22:74–8.

[27] Janda V. Muscles and Cervicogenic Pain Syndromes. In: Grant R, editor. Physical Therapy of the Cervical and Thoracic Spine. New York: Churchill Livingstone; 1988. p. 153–66.

[28] Janda V, Frank C, Liebenson C. Evaluation of muscle imbalance. In: Liebenson C, editor. Rehabilitation of the spine: A practitioner's manual. 2nd ed. Philadelphia: Lippincott Williams and Wilkins; 2007.

[29] Janda V. Postural and Phasic Muscles in Low Back Pain. Proc. XIth Congress ISRD. Dublin; 1968. 553–4.

[30] Liebenson C. Integrated approach to the lumbar spine. In: Liebenson C, editor. Rehabilitation of the spine: A practitioner's manual. 2nd ed. Philadelphia: Lippincott Williams and Wilkins; 2007.

[31] Van Dieën JH, Selen LPJ, Cholewicki J. Trunk muscle activation in low-back pain patients, an analysis of the literature. J Electomyogr Kinesiol 2003;13:333–51.

[32] Bartenieff I. Body Movement: coping with the environment. New York: Routledge; 2002.

[33] Hides JA, et al. Evidence of Lumbar Multifidus Muscle Wasting Ipsilateral to Symptoms in Patients with Acute/Subacute Low Back Pain. Spine 1994;19(2 Suppl.):165–72.

[34] Hides JA, et al. Magnetic Resonance Imaging Assessment of Trunk Muscles During Prolonged Bed Rest. Spine 2007;32 (15):1687–92.

[35] Janda V. Muscle Weakness and inhibition (pseudoparesis) in back pain syndromes. Modern Manual Therapy of the Vertebral Column. Edinburgh: Churchill Livingstone; 1986. p. 197–201.

[36] Janda V. Muscles as a Pathogenic factor in Back Pain. Proc: I.F.O.M.T. New Zealand; 1980.

[37] Sahrmann SA. Diagnosis and treatment of Movement Impairment Syndromes. Missouri: Mosby; 2002.

[38] Janda V. Pain in the Locomotor System. Proc: Second Annual Interdisciplinary Symposium 'Rehabilitation in Chronic Low Back Disorders' LACC Post Grad. Division California; 1988.

[39] Mayer T, et al. Quantification of Lumbar Function: Part 2 Sagittal Plane Trunk Strength in Chronic Low Back Pain Patients. Spine 1985;10(8):765–72.

[40] Smeets R, Wittink H. The deconditioning paradigm for chronic low back pain unmasked? Pain 2007;130(3):201–2.

[41] McGill SM. Low back exercises: evidence for improving exercise regimens. Phys Ther 1998;78(7): 754–65.

[42] Ahern D, et al. Comparison of Lumbar Paravertebral EMG Patterns in Chronic Low Back Pain Patients and Non-patient Controls. Pain 1988;34(2): 153–60.

[43] Paquet N, Malouin F, Richards CL. Hip-Spine Movement Interaction and Muscle Activation Patterns During Sagittal Trunk Movements in Low Back Pain Patients. Spine 1994;19(5): 596–603.

[44] Watson PJ, et al. Surface Electromyography in the Identification of Chronic Low Back Pain Patients: the development of the flexion relaxation ratio. Clin Biomech 1997;12(3):165–71.

[45] Neblett R, et al. Quantifying the Lumbar Flexion-Relaxation Phenomenon: Theory, Normative Data, and Clinical Applications. Spine 2003;28(13): 1435–1446.

[46] Biering-Sorenson F. Physical measurements as risk indicators for low-back trouble over a one year period. Spine 1984;9:106–19.

[47] Liebenson C, Yeomans S. Quantification of Physical Performance Ability. In: Liebenson C, editor. Rehabilitation of the Spine: A Practitioner's Manual. Lippincott Williams and Wilkins; 2007. p. 244.

[48] Janda V. The Role of the Thigh Adductors in Movement Patterns of the Hip and Knee Joint. Brisbane Australia: Janda Compendium distributed by Body Control Systems.

[49] Hodges P. Abdominal mechanism and support of the lumbar spine and pelvis. In: Richardson C, Hodges P, Hides J, editors. Therapeutic exercise for lumbopelvic stabilisation: A motor control approach for the treatment and prevention of low back pain. 2nd ed. Churchill Livingstone Elsevier; 2004.

[50] Newton A. In: Gracovetsky on walking Structural integration Feb 2003.

[51] Hartley L. Wisdom of the Body Moving: An introduction to Body-Mind Centering. Berkeley: North Atlantic Books; 1989.

[52] Bainbridge Cohen B. The training problems of a dancer. In: Sensing, Feeling and Action: The experiential anatomy of Body-Mind Centering. Northampton: Contact Editions; 1993.

[53] Cholewicki J, Panjabi MM, Khachatryan A. Stabilising Function of Trunk Flexor-Extensor muscles Around a Neutral Spine Posture. Spine 1997;22(19):2207–12.

[54] Cholewicki J, McGill SM. Mechanical Stability of the in vivo Lumbar spine: implications for injury and chronic low back pain. Clin Biomech 1995;11(1):1–15.

[55] Marras W, et al. Spine Loading Characteristics of Patients with Low Back Pain Compared with Asymptomatic Individuals. Spine 2001;26(23):2566–74.

[56] Marras W, et al. Functional Impairment as a Predictor of Spine Loading. Spine 2005; 30(7):729–37.

[57] Enoka RM. Neuromechanics of human movement. 3rd ed. United States: Human Kinetics; 200.

[58] Stensdotter AK, et al. Quadriceps Activation in Closed and in Open Kinetic Chain Exercise. Medicine & Science in Sports and Exercise 2003;35(12):2043–7.

[59] Richardson CA, Jull G, Hodges P, Hides J. Therapeutic exercise for Spinal Segmental Stabilisation in Low Back Pain: Scientific basis and clinical approach. Edinburgh: Churchill Livingstone; 1999.

[60] Bogduk N, Twomey L. Clinical anatomy of the lumbar spine. Churchill Livingstone; 1987.

[61] Gracovetsky S. An hypothesis for the role of the spine in human locomotion: a challenge to current thinking. J Biomed Eng 1985;7:205–16.

[62] Todd ME. The thinking body. Hightstown NJ: Princeton Book; 1937.

[63] Schleip R. Lecture notes on psoas and adductors Sourced. www.somatics.de/Psoas&Adds.html

[64] McGill SM, Hughson RL, Parks K. Changes in lumbar lordosis modify the role of the extensor muscles. Clin Biomech 2000;15(10):777–80.

[65] Cox ME, et al. Relationship between functional evaluation measures and self assessment in nonacute low back pain. Spine 2000;25(14):1817–26.

[66] Janda V. Introduction to functional pathology of the motor systemProc: V11 Commonwealth and International Conference on Sport, Physical Education, Recreation and Dance, vol. 3. 1982.

[67] Moseley GL. Impaired trunk muscle function in subacute neck pain: etiologic in the subsequent development of low back pain? Man Ther 2004;9:157–63.

[68] Cholewicki, et al. Delayed trunk muscle reflex responses increase the risk of low back injuries. Spine 2005;30(23):2614–20.

[69] Gregory DE, Brown SHM, Callaghan JP. Trunk muscle responses to suddenly applied loads: Do individuals who develop discomfort during prolonged standing respond differently? J Electromyogr Kinesiol 2008;18(3):495–502.

5

Classification of muscles

General overview

Hannon[1] describes muscles as having a wide variety of functions serving as springs, engines, braces and brakes. Attempting to understand these versatile roles, scientists and clinicians have variously classified muscles according to certain characteristics such as morphology, actions or functional role. These are explored.

Individual muscle morphology

Morphology refers to the basic form or structure of a muscle. This involves two aspects:
• **The shape** of the muscle partly reflects its role. The direction of the muscle fibres are variously arranged into differing forms to generate differing ranges of force. In general, pennate muscles produce greater maximal force than fusiform muscles of similar size.[2]
• *Fibre type*. All skeletal muscles are composed of a spectrum of Type 1 and Type 11 fibres, the relative proportions of each within a single muscle will depend upon the principle role of that muscle as either a constant worker or as a producer of intermittent large range and or strong movements. As can be seen in Table 5.1, there are differences in histochemistry, contractile properties and metabolism of the different fibre types.

We see that the Type 1 fibres are more resistant to fatigue, are recruited early in low force muscle activity due to their small axon size. The number of muscle fibres in slow motor units is small and so motor unit recruitment can result in *fine*

gradations of force. These are also known as slow twitch fibres.

Type 11 fibres in contrast, are fast to contract and relax. They are recruited only during high force activity and fatigue rapidly. These are also known as fast twitch fibres. These also provide the rapid responses to perturbations of sudden and high loading.

According to Trew and Everett,[3] during low force contractions of a muscle, only Type 1 fibres may be recruited and so these are used mainly for normal everyday activities which do not require maximal or high force contractions. Their resistance to fatigue suits them well for this role. As the force generated by the muscle increases, the Type 11 fibres are progressively recruited and during maximal activity all motor units are involved. However maximal force rapidly declines due to the high fatigue rate of the force generating fibres. There is a wide variation in the proportion of the different fibre types between muscles and between people. Each person has a unique proportion of Type 1 to 11 fibres and the fibre type is largely determined genetically.[3] Each motor unit within a muscle contains fibres of only one type.[5]

Limb immobilization studies have demonstrated a conversion of fibre types with a decrease in slow twitch fibres and increase in the proportion of fast twitch.[6]

Classification of muscles according to functional role

In attempting to simplify and aid the conceptual understanding of the complex roles that muscles perform, various different functional classification

Table 5.1 Characteristic differences between skeletal muscle fibre types

Property	Type 1 fibre (slow twitch)	Type 11a fibre (fast twitch red)	Type 11b fibre (fast twitch white)
Muscle fibre type	Slow oxidative (SO)	Fast oxidative glycolytic (FOG)	Fast glycolytic (FG)
Fibre diameter	Small	Intermediate	Large
Muscle colour	Red	Red	white
Motor unit type	Slow (S)	Fast fatigue resistant (FR)	Fast fatigable (FF)
Motor unit size	Small	Medium	Large
Twitch tension	Low	Moderate	High
Mechanical speed	Slow	Fast	Fast
Rate of fatigue	Slow	Intermediate	Fast
Capillary density	High	Medium	Low
Myoglobin content	High	Medium	Low

Adapted from [3,4] (Trew & Everett 2005 and Norkin & Levangie 1992)

systems have been adopted. However, the different nomenclature used has to some extent confused the issue and there is a lack of general consensus on the subject. Each aspect is examined and a more holistic and inclusive classification system is subsequently proffered.

Movement actions

The simplest form of classification – muscles with equivalent or similar actions are grouped together, e.g. those muscles which externally rotate the hip are known as the external rotators of the hip. However, it is never so straight forward as the hip external rotators also play an important role in stabilizing and controlling the pelvis. In the torso we talk of the flexor and extensor systems of muscles which contribute to antigravity control as well as flexion extension and so on. Similarly we may talk of the upper limb flexors or the lower limb extensors.

Tonic and phasic muscles

Although a considerable amount of variability exists among muscles in regard to the number, size, arrangement and type of muscle fibres it has however, been common practice by some to classify the muscles themselves into two main groups as either predominantly tonic or phasic muscles.

Tonic muscles are those with a predominance of Type 1 fibres. These muscles work at a low grade of contraction in a sustained manner thus have a lot of endurance. They are often also termed stability or postural muscles as they help to maintain stability of the body,[4] e.g. the soleus is almost continually active in standing and owing to the high proportion of Type 1 fibres can make small adjustments in muscle tension required to maintain body balance and counteract gravity.

Phasic muscles are those muscles with a predominance of Type 11 fibres. These play a major role in large movements and those requiring more power and speed. They are either called mobility or phasic muscles. However, they fatigue more quickly and following intermittent bouts of high intensity exercise recover more slowly than the tonic muscles,[4] e.g. the gastrocnemius. Table 5.2 presents the more commonly used distinguishing features[4] of the tonic and phasic muscles.

Besides the differences in function and structure outlined above, Kolar[7] importantly draws attention to the differences in the neural control of the different muscle fibres – it is the type of the motor neuron which determines the type of muscle fibre, creating either tonic or phasic motor units. This difference becomes particularly striking in the light of our individual motor and phylogenetic or evolutionary

Table 5.2 Different characteristics of tonic and phasic muscles (after Norkin and Levangie[4])

	Tonic	Phasic
Fibre type	High proportion Type 1 fibres	High proportion Type 11 fibres
Fibre arrangement	Penniform	Parallel
Location	Deep and cross one joint	Superficial and cross more than one joint
Primary function	Stability	Mobility
Action	Extension, abduction and external rotation	Flexion adduction and internal rotation

development. At birth, the infant's posture is predominantly influenced by the phylogenetically older phasic (as described in Table 5.2) muscle system. (Kolar calls this the tonic system!) The tonic system (Table 5.2) is less evident, but *as the central nervous system (CNS) matures these muscles play an increasingly important part in the development of upright posture and its stabilization with movement* (Kolar calls this system the phasic system). This system is phylogenetically younger, more vulnerable and tends to become weak. Maturity of this system is not achieved until the child is 4 years old.

It is important to point out at this point that the nomenclature used by the Czech School of Manual Medicine can be confusing and appear contradictory as is evidenced by the paragraph above. This may account for a less wide understanding and acceptance of their valuable work. In addition it may contribute some of the current confusion on the subject. Their use of the terms tonic and phasic is different to that shown in Table 5.2, and further compounded when talking of postural and phasic muscles. This is further elaborated upon when examining Janda's classification, and the muscle classification debate (see p. 60).

Kolar[7] does clarify that tonic motor units have a more postural role and phasic motor units have a more kinetic role and that both motor units are present in differing proportions in every muscle. However, he also adopts the nomenclature used by Janda making his work more difficult to interpret.

Importantly, Kolar[7] questions which position is decisive in opposing gravity and I agree. He sees that in motor control, both types of muscles have dual functions participating in both posture and movement. The decisive difference between them consists of the timing of their development. Postural activity of the tonic system (his phasic) comes into play as central nervous control becomes more highly developed. The functioning between the two systems needs to become integrated and balanced.

Muscle classification according to Vladimir Janda

Professor Janda saw that the muscular system lies at a functional crossroad because it is influenced by stimuli from both the central nervous system and musculoskeletal system.[8] From the clinical point of view, Janda's significant contribution has been to show that dysfunction in the muscular system is usually a reflection of dysfunction in the peripheral or central neural system. Impaired central motor regulation results in defective or uneconomical movement patterns. As a consequence, imbalanced action between two structurally and functionally different muscle groups occurs in a systematic, regular and predictable manner.[9] He proposed a more general classification of muscles throughout the body into two groups based on characteristics of their structure and function and observed actions in the clinical situation. They are the 'postural muscles' which are prone to over-activity which in turn tends to create relative underactivity in the antagonistic 'phasic muscles'. These functional differences are further elaborated:

The '*postural muscles*' have a tendency to tightness, hypertonia, over-activity and shortening. They tend to be activated early and dominate in a given movement and in states of pain, fatigue, injury, stress and emotional states this tendency is increased. These muscles tend to be relatively 'strong'.

The '*phasic muscles*' are prone to inhibition, hypotonia, atrophy and weakening and are less readily activated in most movement patterns, particularly under conditions of injury fatigue and stress. He classified certain muscles into either functional group as shown in Table 5.3.

You will note that he was undecided about the role of the scalenes and the abdominals, classifying them differently at different times.

Janda defined the muscles which tend to become short and tight as those having an antigravity postural function, particularly those activated when standing on one leg. Janda[5] considered the postural

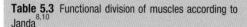

Table 5.3 Functional division of muscles according to Janda[8,10]

Postural: tightness prone muscles	Phasic: weakness prone muscles
Gastrosoleus	Peroneii[10]
Tibialis posterior	Tibialis anterior
Short hip adductors	Vasti particularly medialis
Hamstrings	Gluteus maximus, medius, and minimus
Rectus femoris	
Iliopsoas	Rectus abdominus[10]
Tensor fascia lata	Whole abdominal wall[8]
Piriformis	Serratus anterior
Erector spinae – especially lumbar, thoracolumbar and cervical potions	Rhomboids
	Lower and middle trapezius
	Short cervical flexors
Quadratus lumborum	Scalenes[8]
Pectorals	Extensors of the upper limb
Upper Trapezius /levator Scapulae	
Scalenes[10]	
Sternocleidomastoid	
Short deep cervical extensors	
Flexors of the upper limb	

muscles were approximately one-third stronger than those prone to inhibition. In subjects with altered or poor movement patterns their degree of activation increases. In addition, he notes that in certain structural lesions of the CNS, as seen in cases of cerebral vascular accident or cerebral palsy, the muscles which show evident spasticity are the same as those included in the postural group.

Janda himself said there were a lot of misconceptions and discrepancies about the use of the term 'postural muscles'.[11] However, examining his muscle system groupings it is apparent that they more closely resemble the phasic muscles as described in Table 5.2.

His nomenclature is confusing for our purposes as you will see (p. 60). However, conceptually and functionally his approach has been very helpful.

Local and global muscles acting on the lumbar spine

Bergmark[12] in examining the conditions for mechanical stability in the lumbar spine presented a concept of functional muscle classification into local and global muscles as they acted to control local stability in the lumbar spine including transfer of load between the thorax and pelvis (Fig. 5.1)

The *local system* includes 'all those muscles which have their origin or insertion (or both) at the lumbar vertebrae with the exception of psoas'. The muscles included are shown in Table 5.4. This system is involved in the posture of the lumbar spine and used to 'control the (lumbar) curvature and to give sagittal and lateral stiffness to maintain mechanical stability of the lumbar spine'.

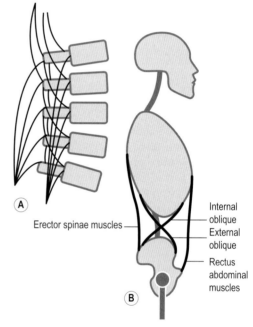

Erector spinae muscles

Internal oblique
External oblique
Rectus abdominal muscles

Fig 5.1 • The local (A) and global (B) muscles.

Table 5.4 Local and global muscles of the lumbar spine described by Bergmark[12]

Local muscles	Global muscles
Multifidus	Thoracic erector spinae which is about $2/3$ of the muscle area
Interspinales and intertransversarii	Internal and external obliques
Lumbar erector spinae – medial and lateral fibres	Rectus abdominus
	Lateral fibres of quadratus lumborum
Medial fibres quadratus lumborum	

The *global system* 'consists of the active components i.e. the muscles and IAP which transfer the load directly between the thoracic cage and pelvis'. The muscles have 'origin on the pelvis and insertions on the thoracic cage'. These include the global muscles shown in Table 5.4. The main role of this system 'appears to be to balance the outer load so that the resulting force transferred to the lumbar spine can be handled by the local system. Thus large variations of the distribution of the outer load should give rise to only small variations of the resulting load on the lumbar spine. The local system therefore is essentially dependent upon the magnitude (not the distribution) of the outer load and of the posture (curvature) of the lumbar spine'.

He says 'the global system can be said to respond to changes of the line of action of the outer load whereas the local system responds to changes in the posture of the lumbar spine. Both systems respond to changes in the magnitude of the outer load'. 'Generally speaking, smaller forces in the global system imply larger forces in the local system as could be expected'. He says intra abdominal pressure (IAP) theoretically has a local and global mechanical role. 'The global role is to act directly on the thoracic cage or on the curved global muscles. The local action consists of the transverse force in the posterior direction acting directly on the lumbar spine thus inducing a flexion moment'.

This paper has been very influential and is frequently quoted in the literature. This is interesting, as his is a study in mechanical engineering looking at forces and load transfer in the lumbar spine rather than functional control of movement. He admits that how the CNS controls loads is not sufficiently understood to allow detailed modeling; does not include iliopsoas in the local system or accord it any role in lumbar control; and treats the thoracic cage as a rigid body. While he thought psoas should be referred to the global system he excluded both it and latissimus dorsi from his analysis as he felt they do not have a substantial role in maintaining mechanical stability of the back system.

While his muscle classification principle is very useful, it needs to be applied to more than the lumbar spine and we need to appreciate that control of the lumbar spine will be dependent upon control through the entire axial skeleton including the pelvis.

The influence of Bergmark:stabilizers and mobilizers

Richardson et al[14]., collectively known as The Queensland Group, have produced some fine research and have been at the forefront of the motor control approach to effective lumbopelvic stabilization in the treatment of low back pain. They have been strongly influenced by Bergmark as seen in Table 5.5, choosing to include transversus abdominus and some of internal oblique into the local group.[14,42]

In addition, Richardson[13] also makes distinction between monoarticular, bi-articular and multijoint muscles. Their capacity to provide joint stabilization differs in each category. The monoarticular muscles could also be called local muscles. The multijoint muscles are phylogenetically the oldest and can be called the global muscles.[13]

Comerford and Mottram[15] have interlinked the concepts of local/global and stabilizer/mobilizer into what they see as a more clinically useful classification. This encompasses three different functional muscle roles: local stability muscles; global stability muscles; global mobility muscles. Some muscles stabilize and some mobilize.

However, there are inherent problems for understanding functional control in seeing some muscles as stabilizers and others as mobilizers. As we have seen in Chapter 3 in the process of motor development, movement and stability develop together and

Table 5.5 Categorization of the lumbar and abdominal muscles based on their role in stabilisation according to Richardson et al.[14]

Local stabilizing system	Global stabilizing system
Intertransversarii	Longissimus thoracis pars thoracis
Interspinales	
Multifidus	Iliocostalis lumborum pars thoracis
Longissimus thoracis pars lumborum	
Iliocostalis lumborum pars lumborum	Quadratus lumborum lateral fibres
Quadratus lumborum - medial fibres	Rectus abdominus
Transversus abdominus	Obliquus externus abdominus
Obliquus internus abdominus (fibre insertion into thoracolumbar fascia)	Obliquus internus abdominis

are always in constant interaction in mature motor behavior. Kolar[7] points out that any muscle may be required to work in a stabilizing role one moment and then as a movement producer the next. While some muscles may appear to have a predominantly stabilizing role e.g. the local muscles in the lumbar spine as described by Bergmark, importantly, they also sub serve a postural role and are also producers of fine subtle movements as well as being controllers and discrete adjusters. Danneels et al.[16] found increased multifidus action in concentric lifting which could indicate that it participates in torque production. It is an oversimplification of function and erroneous to consider that they do not produce any appreciable movement and 'just stabilize'.

Cholewicki and VanVliet[17] refute the classification of muscles into local and global as a means for discriminating between muscles responsible for intersegmental stability and spine motion. All trunk muscles contribute to spine stability and their contribution depends upon many variables including posture and loading conditions. McGill[18] and Kavcic et al.[19] express similar sentiments. The patterns of muscle activation change as the form and magnitude of spine loading patterns change (See 'spinal stability' p. 86).

Muscle classification debate

Is muscle classification relevant and if so, which of the above muscle classifications is most clinically useful? As can be seen, muscle classification has depended in part upon which aspects of function have been appreciated.

In 2000, the *Journal of Bodywork and Movement Therapies* published a paper entitled 'The muscle designation debate: the experts respond'.[20] The paper was a response to readers who had communicated their confusion over the apparent contradictions in the way that different researchers and clinicians refer to muscle categorizations. The editor says 'When words postural/phasic or stabilizer/mobilizer are applied to particular muscles practical as well as linguistic difficulties become apparent'.[20] The preceding classification summary highlights the problem.

The principal confusion probably stems from Janda's use of the terms postural and phasic muscles (see page 57). Comparing Table 5.2 – tonic and phasic muscles with Table 5.4 – postural and phasic muscles of Janda – we see that frequently his

'postural muscles' equate more to the muscles with a high Type 11 fibre content which are actually phasic muscles as defined in Table 5.2. Janda later tended to describe the postural muscles more in terms of 'tightness prone' while still maintaining that they were the ones predominantly activated when standing on one leg – the primary posture, according to him. The confusion becomes further compounded when both he[8] and Kolar[7] at times use the term 'tonic muscle system' referring to those muscles as described in his 'postural group' when in fact they are describing phasic muscle activity. Kolar[7] however, does also allow that tonic motor units have a postural role.

Most of the respondents in the above mentioned paper appeared to be in agreement that phasic muscles (as defined in Table 5.2) equate to global muscles, mobilizer muscles, kinetic muscles, and, by inference, Janda's postural muscles. Muscles with a more postural function have a greater proportion of Type 1 fibres and tonic motor units and have tended to be called local or stabilizer muscles. They behave with some similarity to Janda's phasic muscles as he described them.

Most respondents agreed that the principal issue was altered motor control rather than strength and endurance. All incorporate various aspects of muscle classification into clinical practice.

The case for a new and inclusive muscle classification system based upon posturomovement control

'Muscle impairment classifications should describe categories and provide a basis for treatment'.[21] Although any classification of muscles is likely to be an oversimplification, appreciating the nature of posturomovement function as it develops helps inform a clinically useful muscle classification system which encompasses the structural and functional properties of muscles in a functional movement context.

Normal postural reflex mechanism (NPRM)

Good movement control requires good postural control which is dependent upon normal functioning of this system. As we have seen, this is not present at birth but with the motor development of the infant, this will become highly complex and varied and allow the development of motor skill in a gravity based environment.

Functions ascribed to the postural reflex mechanism

In the 'ideal' state, the functions mediated by the normal postural reflex mechanism can be essentially distilled as providing:

- *'Uprightness'* against gravity with the axial skeleton and the proximal limb girdles optimally aligned and controlled with respect to the line of gravity and the current requisite activity, with minimal muscular effort. This includes axial spinal segmental control in the normal spinal curves, particularly the lumbar lordosis and the generation of intra abdominal pressure (IAP) for spinal support. The proprioceptive system probably provides the predominant graviceptive information.[22] Feldenkrais[23] considered that people with a fine kinesthetic sense maintain tonic muscular activity with less effort. Effort disables the ability to detect small differences.

- *Breathing* in an energy efficient manner i.e. principally via the diaphragm with related function of the axial skeleton providing optimal alignment and control to allow effective movement of the ribs and adjustments within the thoracic cage to shifts in the centre of gravity; to allow diaphragmatic breathing to continue despite strong actions of many of the large muscles attaching to the thoracic cage e.g. abdominals, serratus anterior/posterior, pectorals. Breathing is the most fundamental motor act.

- *Maintenance of equilibrium* in both 'low' and 'high' load antigravity situations by the provision of:

  - Anticipatory 'feed-forward' postural presetting and 'stability' of the axial skeleton to support limb movement. Studies conducted by Cresswell[24] and Hodges[25] demonstrate the role of transversus abdominus as part of a feed-forward postural synergy.

  - Compensatory 'feed-back' adjustments and postural reactions activated by sensory events following loss of desirable alignment and control resulting from intrinsic and extrinsic perturbations to the body while stationary or moving.

- Equilibrium in the low load state is accomplished by small segmental rotary shifts and adjustments of the axial skeleton and proximal limb girdles to perturbations in the centre of gravity caused by, e.g. breathing, head turning, limb use, unstable base of support, torque produced by large superficial muscle action etc.

- Equilibrium control in high load states is accomplished by more forceful coactivation of the whole muscle system to control the relationship of individual spinal segments as well as that between the various body parts while accommodating the forces imposed by gravity or otherwise.

- *Appropriate postural sets to support limb movement* – involve prepositioning and adaptive movements of the axial skeleton and proximal limb girdles in appropriate spatial relationships for effective limb activity. This includes control of weight shift.

The NPRM essentially controls forces – gravity and the intrinsic/extrinsic forces related to it, to provide a stable platform of control on which to superimpose movements. Without this, the person has to 'hold himself up' and is not free to adjust and selectively move his spine and proximal limb girdles. Many with spinal pain and related disorders can move, but cannot adequately posture themselves prior to and during movement. The postural system is dependent upon gravity, suitable demand and adequate proprioceptive and other afferent information for its wellbeing.

Ideally, we demonstrate a 'central intelligence' in the torso – balancing upright control, movement and breathing in an energy efficient manner.

Proposed functional classification of muscles

When the aspects of function provided by the NPRM are appreciated in movement control, holistic muscle designation becomes more apparent and clinically useful.

The proposed model applies to the body as a whole, particularly the torso. Its genesis results from the integration of clinically observed changed muscle behavior, contemporary thought and available research to date. It includes a similar polarity of spatially defined muscle function as proposed by Bergmark, as well as structural and functional differences according to convention and also that proposed by Janda.

The concept of a local and global muscle system acting on the lumbar spine has gained acceptance as a result of Bergmark's influence. However, clinically, lumbar spine problems are also functionally linked to problems elsewhere in the spine. Hence it makes sense to try to understand spinal control in a more universal way. Anatomical and empirical knowledge suggests that different functions are sub served by the deep and superficial muscles. Accordingly, the muscular system in particular that pertaining to function of the torso, is essentially seen in terms of a *systemic deep system* and a *systemic superficial system*. In health, optimal motor control involves systemic local function with balanced systemic global activity. The whole dynamically functions to permit grace, economy of effort in fruitful and refined action appropriate to the situation or task.

This classification is functionally related and of course conceptual, as no muscle or system works in isolation but as part of a coordinated synergy within and between the systems related to need.

The work of Richardson et al.[14] and in particular Hodges,[14,26] has largely been about examining aspects of deep system function. The manner of response noted in those muscles which have been studied in this system implicates separate CNS control.

Moseley et al.[27] also showed different activation behaviors between muscles in the deep and superficial muscle systems of the lumbar spine and Lee has shown that this also occurs in the thoracic spine.[28,29]

Systemic local muscle system (SLMS)

It is proposed that the role of the SLMS is more closely linked to the underlying functions provided by the NPRM: antigravity support; the more 'intrinsic' movements – spinal segmental control, small postural shifts and adjustments and discrete movements; and the fundamental motor act – respiration. This is in line with Richardson et al.[26] who proposed that 'the local muscles form part of a larger antigravity muscle system which links the joints of the entire functional kinetic chain including both the upper and lower limbs'.

They function to provide inner support and control of the axial skeleton as a whole and particularly around the body's centre of gravity. They provide the foundation for movement (Fig. 5.2).

The more general features of this system are explored and summarized in Table 5.6.

• The torso muscles in this system are generally *deep*, often small and may be uni- or poly segmental. Being close to the joint they control and many containing a large number of muscle spindles, it is likely that they have a large role in kinesthetic sense and postural control. The small deep intersegmental muscles of the spine contain a very high density of muscle spindles and more than likely act as large proprioceptive transducers[30] or vertebral position sensors at every segmental level.[31] Optimal spinal movement control depends on adequate sensory input into and from this system. Normal studies involving reduced mechanical loading or microgravity and related reduced proprioceptive input have demonstrated atrophy[32] and conversion of these deep muscles from slow tonic firing to more phasic function.[33]

• Their form and function produces *more continuous but varying tonic motor activity at low levels of contraction*[34] which provides endurance and staying power, particularly useful in counteracting gravity and maintaining the breathing cycle. Tonic low level activation of transversus in standing has been reported.[35,36] Saunders et al.[37] found tonic activation of transversus during walking which continued into running up to speeds of $3ms^{-1}$. Clinically they are best recruited during slow, sustained and non effortful movements.

• Rather than generators of force, their principal role is more one of *antigravity postural control including stability*. This entails movement which is subtle and finely modulated! Activity oscillates between concentric and eccentric control as required. The adoption of upright postures with the spine aligned close to the normal spinal curves and the line of gravity have been shown to readily activate various muscles in this system.[38–40] The deep abdominal muscles have also been shown to automatically respond to postural changes evoked through decreasing the base of support while sitting.[41]

• Their *early activation prior to a movement occurring*[25,27,42,43] renders the torso as an adjustable, yet stable base of support to allow for more effective and even forceful actions of the large more superficial global muscles as required. Their early action is also necessary to create appropriate axial 'postural sets' for effective control of the head and weight shift for limb movements.

• The muscles work *synergistically in patterns of co-activation as part of a coordinated system*

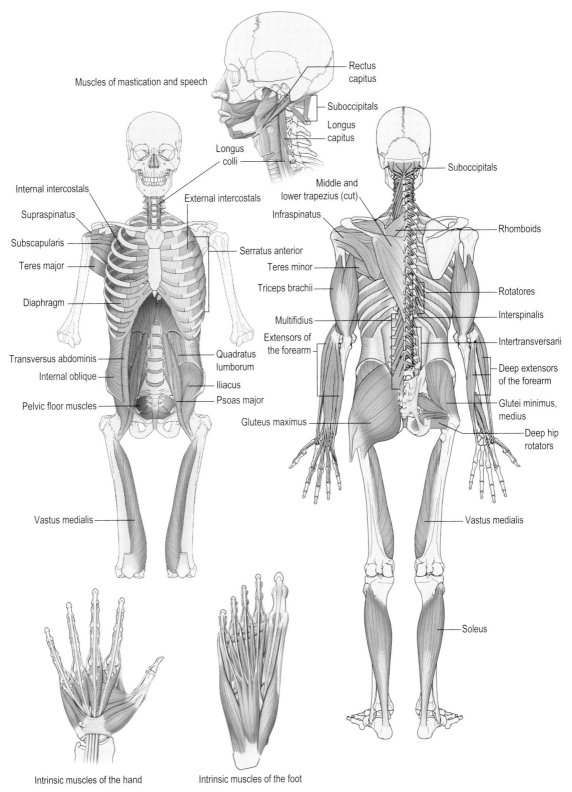

Fig 5.2 • Graphic depiction of the conceptual systemic local muscle system (SLMS) as a continuous innermost sleeve of myofascial support.

Muscles of mastication and speech

Rectus capitus

Suboccipitals

Longus capitus

Longus colli

Internal intercostals

Supraspinatus

Subscapularis

Teres major

Diaphragm

External intercostals

Serratus anterior

Transversus abdominis

Internal oblique

Pelvic floor muscles

Quadratus lumborum

Iliacus

Psoas major

Vastus medialis

Middle and lower trapezius (cut)

Infraspinatus

Suboccipitals

Rhomboids

Teres minor

Triceps brachii

Multifidius

Extensors of the forearm

Gluteus maximus

Rotatores

Interspinalis

Intertransversarii

Deep extensors of the forearm

Glutei minimus, medius

Deep hip rotators

Vastus medialis

Soleus

Intrinsic muscles of the hand

Intrinsic muscles of the foot

Table 5.6 Different structural and behavioral characteristics between the SLMS and the SGMS

	Systemic local muscle system (SLMS) deep system	Systemic global muscle system (SGMS) superficial system
Architecture	1° small, deep, more pennate Uni and polysegmental	1° large, superficial, more fusiform Polysegmental
Fibre type/activity	Type I fibre/tonic motor unit dominant	Type II fibre/phasic motor unit dominant
Role	1° postural/stabilizing/control and small movements and shifts at low force generation.	1° larger movements; ballistic; higher force and faster speed 2° postural/stabilizing at higher magnitude loads
Loading	Work more so and optimally in closed chain movements	Work more so and optimally in open chain movements particularly fast/ballistic
Timing	Pre activate before SGMS in movement	Activate after SLMS in movement
Action	Work in synergies in patterns of coactivation	Work singly or as part of a synergy; co-activate in high load or perturbation situations
Directionality	Non direction dependent	Direction dependent
Activation	1° bilateral activation - may/not be symmetrical	1° unilateral activation; asymmetrical
Inherent behavioral tendency	Tend to: inhibition, hypotonia, atrophy weakness, delayed activity particularly in states of pain injury fatigue, stress emotion	Tendency to: over activity, strength tightness shortness and to dominate in movements particularly in states of pain injury fatigue stress and emotion or when working out new or complex movements[9]

response. Balanced co activation or co-contraction around a joint provides for stability of the joint[26] and centered joint control and load transmission. This is particularly important in the spine where the control of the segments against gravity including compressive and shear forces is particularly important. Coordinated coactivation not only ensures control around individual joints but also control of the orientation and alignment of the spine as a whole. Another example of synergistic coactivation is the generation of the intra abdominal pressure mechanism (IAP) which depends upon coactivation and modulation between the diaphragm, transversus abdominis and pelvic floor. Studies of some of the muscles which are active in deep system synergies have demonstrated early coactivation e.g. of the diaphragm with transversus abdominis;[44,45] pelvic floor muscles with abdominal muscle activity;[46] transversus with deep multifidus;[27] internal oblique with multifidus.[43]

• The *patterns of muscle activation may be independent of movement direction*. Perturbation studies of the spinal reaction forces engendered from limb movement have shown that transversus and multifidus continue to be active with repetitive movement of the arm in both directions[25,27] and similarly so with movements of the leg.[24,47] McCook et al.[48] have shown consistent transversus activity during both trunk flexion and extension. However, Allison et al.[49] measured transversus bilaterally and found its activity was specific to the direction of arm movement. Herrington[50] reported symmetrical action occurred in different positions, particularly in standing.

• Clinically it appears that this muscle system *response is more bilateral however this may not necessarily be symmetrical*[49] as it controls reaction forces or allows for movement adjustments during say weight shift. Danneels et al.[16] found bilateral coactivation of internal oblique and multifidus in asymmetric lifting tasks with differences in the symmetry of multifidus activity between lifting and lowering.

• The *inherent behavior* of the muscles in this system is more akin to Janda's 'phasic muscles'. He maintains they have a *tendency to hypotonia, atrophy weakness and inhibition and to be less readily activated in movement patterns particularly under conditions of pain,*[51] *injury, fatigue and stress and emotional states.*[10,52,53] Weight bearing appears to be a significant afferent factor in generating antigravity extensor muscle activity, particularly the one joint extensors. Selective atrophy of multifidus muscle has been shown to occur after 8 weeks of bed rest in otherwise healthy individuals.[32,54] Richardson[55] notes the 'weight bearing muscles' tend to more readily fatigue.

However, there appear to be some important differences between Janda's 'phasic muscle' group and the SLMS:

• The SLMS appears to have a greater role in basic postural control. Janda saw his 'postural muscle' (tonic) group as more important in postural control.[11,56]

• Janda was more concerned about the effects of the postural muscles and clearer about classifying them. Those classified as phasic were less numerous.[10] He stated that those muscles he had not classified 'can be described as neutral or not yet determined'[9] or 'doubtful'.[57] We have included more muscles in this system than Janda did in his phasic group.

• He did not necessarily see the 'phasic muscle' activity as a deep or systemic response.

• Clinical evidence points to iliacus and psoas as important inclusions in this deep system. Janda classified them in his 'postural muscle' group.

Effective activity of the SLMS promotes a 'supple uprightness' – 'buoyancy', elongation, opening, and flexibility of the torso. When the system is working well, the person has equipoise, grace and lightness in movement. And he breathes well.

Systemic global muscle system (SGMS)

There appears to be much less ambiguity and confusion about this system. The muscles in this system equate to those in Janda's Postural Muscle group;[9,10] Bergmark's Global muscles;[12] with subsequent adoption by Richardson et al.,[13,58] O'Sullivan,[59,60] Comerford and Mottram.[15] Many are two-joint muscles (see Ch. 4).

These more superficial muscles are generally polysegmental and provide for the more 'extrinsic' movements and are activated in situations of larger perturbations of the torso and limb movements, particularly if fast or large 'actions' using effort. They are short acting force producers. They show a direction dependent stabilizing role.[19] Smith et al.[61] demonstrated selective recruitment of the phasic ankle extensors in ballistic fast paw shake movements in cats. Wohlfahrt et al.[62] found that rapid abdominal exercises appear to recruit the prime moving (superficial) muscles with a simultaneous decrease in static (deep) abdominal function. Richardson[63] also notes that these muscles are more favorably activated in open chain ballistic or speed loading situations. Conversely, the deep one joint muscles are optimally recruited in closed chain longitudinal loading which provides joint compression and constant sensory input from the periphery guiding motor performance. Janda[64] suggested that there may be a correlation between these muscles with a tendency to tighten and those participating mainly in flexor reflexes and a correlation between muscles with a tendency to weakness and those participating in extensor reflexes.

The muscles in this system require a stable and adaptable base of support provided by good preceding systemic local muscle activation.

They have an *inherent tendency* to be *easily activated,*[65] *strengthened* and *dominate in posture and movement patterns* in low and high load situations and are *prone to tightness*[26] and *shortness.*[10] Janda maintained that their *action is increased in states* of *pain, fatigue,*[66] *injury,*[67] *stress and effort* or when *working out new or complex movement patterns.*[9] Tight muscles also act in an inhibitory way on their antagonists[64] *It is important that the therapist fully appreciates this inherent behavior.* This is certainly the case clinically and is observed in the fitness industry where overactivation of these muscles has largely given rise to the 'stretch industry'.

A generally overactive global system will manifest in diminishing our dimensions, making our bodies shorter, narrower flatter and effectively closing them.[68] The person moves in a loping, heavy and somewhat grounded and awkward manner. This system is dominant in states of action, stress, tension and effort – the 'flight and fight' response with related sympathetic dominance. The aggressive, fighting warrior postures are SGMS dominant.

The more general features of their behavior are summarized in Table 5.6.

Assignation of muscle/groups into each functional system

The assigning of muscles into either group as shown in Table 5.7 has been much influenced by Janda and serves as a guiding principle. It is based upon muscle architecture, their role in more ideal postural and movement control and their behavioral tendencies determined through research and observed in clinical practice. Obviously there is not a clear demarcation between systems as they both cooperate in a coordinated manner in posturomovement function. These tendencies appear to be inherent in us all – with or without back pain. The presence of back pain tends to compound the picture.

System switching behavior

Motor behavior is complex and variable. Depending upon the pattern of neuromuscular strategies a person adopts, some muscles belonging in one functional muscle system may begin to act as though in the other. This may only involve a part of the muscle. When the *behavior* of a muscle changes, so does its role in posturomotor control. The most notable clinical observations are:

- Abdominal imbalance. Some of the superficial muscles or part of a muscle exhibit SGMS behavior creating imbalance within the group:
  - Hyperactivity of the 'upper abdominals' and hypoactivity of the 'lower abdominals'. This clinical observation is also corroborated by Kendall [69] who saw it as the most common altered pattern.
  - O'Sullivan et al.[70] found altered motor control strategies during the active straight leg raise test in subjects with sacroiliac joint pain. This included underactivity of the deep transversus and lower internal oblique with related hyperactivity of the more superficial oblique abdominals, in particular external oblique.
- Psoas may become overactive and tight and act as a global muscle
- Serratus anterior acts in a global manner.
- Piriformis & the obturator group act in a global manner

Abdominal muscle group

Functionally these are a very interesting group of muscles. Hodges' work[25,36,42,47] has convincingly

---

Table 5.7 Suggested classification into SLMS and SGMS of those muscles deemed significant in torso and related function

Systemic local muscle system (SLMS)	Systemic global muscle system (SGMS)
Short intersegmental muscles of the entire axial spine: rotatores; interspinales; intertransversarii; suboccipitals (recti & obliques)	Erector spinae: 1° thoracolumbar and cervicothoracic
Multifidus of entire axial spine: 1° deep	Quadratus lumborum: 1° lateral fibres
Deep neck flexor group: longus capitis & colli	Sternocleidomastoid
Abdominal group in particular the deep muscles: transversus abdominus, internal oblique & 'lower abdominals'	Scalenes
Pelvic floor muscles	Upper trapezius; levator scapula
Diaphragm	Serratus posterior: sup & 1° inferior
Intercostals: internal and external; levators costarum	Pectorals
Psoas	Latissimus dorsi: 1° lateral fibres
Iliacus	Hamstrings
Quadratus lumborum: 1° medial fibres	Rectus femoris
Glutei: minimus, medius, maximus	Tensor fascia lata
Lower and medial scapular stabilizers: middle and lower trapezius; rhomboids	Short hip adductors
Serratus anterior	Gastrocnemius
Intrinsic foot and hand muscles	Flexors of the upper limb
Soleus	
Deep rotators of the hip and shoulder	
Jaw, masticatory and speech muscles	
Vasti: 1° medialis	
Extensors of the upper limb	

confirmed transversus abdominus as an important deep system synergist with probable separate CNS control to some or all of the others. Internal oblique has also been found to behave in a similar manner.[31,43] This early activity has led to its inclusion in the local system by some[13,16] such that in the literature the deep abdominals consist of the transversus and internal oblique. These can be viewed as the major stabilizers.[71] However, some count internal and certainly external oblique as a global muscle[13] and rectus abdominus always earns that title. Although clinically, parts of these muscles may be tight or overactive, other regions are underactive. The entire abdominal wall may be underactive. The obliques and rectus are also important for postural alignment and orientation and control of the thorax on the lumbar spine as well as the generation of IAP at higher magnitude loads, hence their inclusion into the SLMS.

Urquhart et al.[72–74] found regional variations in the structure and recruitment of transversus abdominis and internal oblique in a healthy population. More tonic activity was greatest in the lower and middle regions compared to the upper region which showed more phasic activity in line with its greater role here with respiration. They also showed the postural responses differed between body positions with recruitment delayed in sitting compared to standing.[74] This variation of structure and function within a muscle lends credence to the examination of patterns of movement in controlling certain actions rather than individual muscle function. While individual muscles have been grouped to aid conceptual understanding, it is the degree of their synergistic activity in a movement which is significant.

While clinically, underactivity of the deep abdominals is usual, both over activity and under activity in the superficial abdominals can occur. As significant, is the different activity level between 'upper' and 'lower' sections of the group.

Changed patterns of activity within and between the abdominal and the iliopsoas groups in concert with altered deep system control, largely gives rise to the two primary clinical classification systems for back pain (see Ch. 9).

The case for the inclusion of iliacus and psoas in the SLMS

It has been common practice to lump these two muscles together as one, despite the fact that they have separate nerve supplies and have been shown to have task dependent independent activation as well as synergistic coactivation between them.[38]

Janda classified the iliopsoas as a 'postural muscle' (global system in our context). Bergmark nominated psoas as a global muscle,[12] but chose to exclude it from his model. He ignored iliacus. However, their anatomical architecture and empirical evidence in functional control point to their inclusion as important members of the deep SLMS.

Apart from the work of Andersson et al.,[38] iliacus' important contribution to functional control of the spine has been largely overlooked. Review of the literature on psoas reveals conflicting views as to its primary role – spinal control or hip flexion. Functional control of movement involves both. As Andersson et al.[38] point out; activation of a muscle is not always predictable from its anatomical arrangement and mechanical advantage but involves a high degree of task specificity.[75] This will also involve its action in relationship to the line of gravity as well as synergistically counteracting both internal and external forces. The contribution of iliacus and psoas in lumbopelvic movement control will be dealt with more fully in Chapter 6.

Importantly an antigravity postural role has been ascribed to psoas by numerous authors. While McGill sees quadratus lumborum as the most important stabilizer of the lumbar spine[76] he does accord some stabilizing role to psoas in the presence of some hip flexor torque.[31] In a simulated model, he proposed that it has the potential to posturally stabilize the spine with compressive loading and with bilateral activation.[77] However, symmetrical activation (the analogy of guy wires stabilizing the mast), imposes large compressive forces to the spine.[78] EMG studies have further confirmed postural activity of psoas in standing,[79] sitting[38] and also in bending and lifting.[80,81] An antigravity postural stabilizing role for psoas has also been supported by Gracovetsky,[82] Gibbons,[83] Penning[84] and Travell and Simons.[85]

Overview

The architecture and functional behavior of the SLMS as described forms a reasonably continuous inner neuromyofascial sleeve of support which provides a primary platform of control for body postures and movements (Fig. 5.2). The muscular system can be conceptually viewed as comprising an 'inner tube' supporting the 'outer slings'. The deep muscles are the supporters; the superficial muscles are the tensioners. The deep muscles provide the foundation for control while the superficial are more akin to scaffolding. There is a lively interplay between 'inner connectivity' and 'outer expressivity'.[86,87]

Drawing attention to the myofascial continuity of the muscular system, Myers[88] notes that the deep 'locals' determine the postural 'set' more than the superficial 'expresses' and are 'too often ignored because they are out of sight out of mind'. The SLMS has some similarities with his 'Deep Front Line' and 'Lateral Line'. The SGMS has features in common with his 'Superficial Front and Backlines', the 'Functional Lines' and the 'Spiral Line'. He notes the influence of the early German anatomist Hoepke in him seeing the spiral and oblique muscular chains in the superficial muscle system (Fig. 5.3). Similarly, others have described anterior and posterior oblique muscle slings[89] and also local longitudinal and lateral slings[90] in the global muscle system, which are proposed to assist regional stabilization of the pelvis.

Interestingly, Beach[91–93] recently presented a 'new model of human movement' with an evolutionary and embryonic perspective. As the mesoderm splits it forms a trilaminar myofascial external body wall. The two superficial layers contain 'fields of contractility' which are whole organism in scope and produce core mammalian movement patterns such as flexing/extending, lateral flexing and twisting. If carried too far these archetypal movement patterns will shorten and buckle the body. The deepest layer provides a field of contractility whose prime function is squeezing and sucking the body wall to thus preserve longitudinal integrity. Included is the anterior scalenes, transversus, the diaphragm, the intercostals, quadratus lumborum and levator ani.

The recognition of the concept of intrinsic and extrinsic musculature and their differing roles has it seems always been in some respects culturally acknowledged. Analyzing Egyptian art, Brecklinghaus[94] notes that the people portrayed 'give the impression of having been well balanced with respect to the integrated use of their intrinsic and extrinsic musculature and rarely display the over developed armored extrinsic musculature typical in fighting and aggressive cultures'.

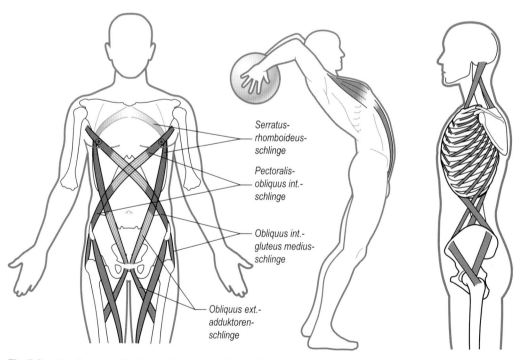

Serratus-
rhomboideus-
schlinge

Pectoralis-
obliquus int.-
schlinge

Obliquus int.-
gluteus medius-
schlinge

Obliquus ext.-
adduktoren-
schlinge

Fig 5.3 • Functional myofascial meridians according to Hoepke.

References

[1] Hannon JC. Wartenberg Part 3: Relaxation training, centration and skeletal opposition: a conceptual model. J Bodyw Mov Ther 2006;10:179–96.

[2] Neumann DA. Kinesiology of the musculoskeletal system: foundations for physical rehabilitation. St Louis: Mosby; 2002.

[3] Trew M, Everett T. Human movement: an introductory text. Edinburgh: Elsevier; 2005.

[4] Norkin CC, Levangie PK. Joint structure and function: a comprehensive analysis. Philadelphia: F.A. Davis; 1992.

[5] Tunnell PW. The muscle designation debate: the experts respond. J Bodywork & Movement Therapy 4(4):237–41.

[6] Enoka RM. Neuromechanics of human movement. 3rd ed. Champaign Il: Human Kinetics; 2002.

[7] Kolar P. Facilitation of agonist-antagonist co-activation by reflex stimulation methods. In: Liebenson C, editor. Rehabilitation of the spine: a practitioner's manual. 2nd ed. Baltimore: Lippincott Williams and Wilkins; 2007. p. 531–65.

[8] Janda V, Frank C, Liebenson C. Evaluation of muscle imbalance. In: Liebenson C, editor. Rehabilitation of the spine: a practitioner's manual. 2nd ed. Philadelphia: Lippincott Williams and Wilkins; 2007. p. 203–25.

[9] Janda V. Muscles as a pathogenic factor in back pain. In: Proc. I.F. O.M.T. New Zealand; 1980.

[10] Jull GA, Janda V. Muscles and motor control in low back pain: assessment and management. In: Twomey L, editor. Physical therapy of the low back. New York: Churchill Livingstone; 1987. p. 253–78.

[11] Janda V. On the concept of postural muscles and posture in man. Aust J Physiother 1983; 29(3):83–4.

[12] Bergmark A. Stability of the lumbar spine: a study in mechanical engineering. Acta Orthop Scand (Suppl. No. 230): 1989;60.

[13] Richardson CA. The muscle designation debate: the experts respond. J Bodyw Mov Ther 2000;4(4):235–6.

[14] Richardson C, Jull G, Hodges P, Hides J. Therapeutic exercise for segmental stabilisation in low back pain: Scientific basis and clinical approach. Edinburgh: Churchill Livingstone; 1999. p. 14.

[15] Comerford MJ, Mottram SL. Movement and stability dysfunction – contemporary developments. Man Ther 2001; 6(1):15–26.

[16] Danneels LA, et al. A functional subdivision of hip, abdominal and back muscles during asymmetric lifting. Spine 2001;26(6): E114–21.

[17] Cholewicki J, VanVliet J. Relative contribution of trunk muscles to the stability of the lumbar spine during isometric exertions. Clin Biomech 2002;17(2):99–105.

[18] McGill SM. Coordination of muscle activity to assure stability of the lumbar spine. J Electromyogr Kinesiol 2003; 13(4):353–9.

[19] Kavcic N, et al. Determining the stabilising role of individual torso muscles during rehabilitation exercises. Spine 2004;29(11): 1254–65.

[20] Chaitow L. The muscle designation debate: the experts respond. J Bodyw Mov Ther 2000;4(4):225–41.

[21] Roy SH, Oddsson LIE. Classification of paraspinal muscle impairments by surface electromyography. Phys Ther 1998;78(8):838–51.

[22] Vaugoyeau M, et al. Proprioceptive contribution of postural control as assessed from very slow oscillations of the support in healthy humans. Gait Posture 2008;27(2):294–302.

[23] Feldenkrais M. Body and mature behavior: a study of anxiety, sex, gravitation and learning. New York: International Universities Press Inc; 1949.

[24] Cresswell AG, Oddsson L, Thorstensson A. The influence of sudden perturbations on trunk muscle activity and intra-abdominal pressure while standing. Exp Brain Res 1994;98:336–41.

[25] Hodges PW, Richardson CA. Feed-forward contraction of transversus abdominis is not influenced by the direction of arm movement. Exp Brain Res 1997;114:362–70.

[26] Richardson C, Hodges P, Hides J. Therapeutic exercise for lumbopelvic stabilisation: a motor control approach for the treatment and prevention of low back pain. 2nd ed. Edinburgh: Churchill Livingstone; 2004.

[27] Moseley GL, Hodges PW, Gandevia SC. Deep and superficial fibres of lumbar multifidus muscle are differentially active during voluntary arm movements. Spine 2002;27(2):E29–36.

[28] Lee LJ, Coppieters MW, Hodges PW. Differential activation of the thoracic multifidus and Longissimus thoracis during trunk rotation. Spine 2005;30(8):870–6.

[29] Lee LJ, Coppieters MW, Hodges PW. Anticipatory postural adjustments to arm movement reveal complex control of paraspinal muscles in the thorax. J Electromyogr Kinesiol (IN PRESS).

[30] Bogduk N, Twomey LT. Clinical anatomy of the lumbar spine. Melbourne: Churchill Livingstone; 1987.

[31] McGill S. Low back disorders: evidenced based prevention and rehabilitation. USA: Human Kinetics; 2002.

[32] Hides JA, et al. Magnetic resonance imaging assessment of trunk muscles during prolonged bed rest. Spine 2007;32(15): 1687–92.

[33] Richardson CA. Prevention of musculoskeletal injury: integration of the past and present for the future. In: Proc.

69

1st International Conference on Movement Dysfunction. Edinburgh; 2001.

[34] O'Sullivan P. Motor control and pain disorders of the lumbo-pelvic region. In: Proc. 5th Interdisciplinary World Congress on Low Back and Pelvic Pain. Melbourne; 2004.

[35] De Troyer, et al. Transversus abdominus function in human. J Appl Physiol 1990;68:1010–6.

[36] Hodges PW, Gandevia SC, Richardson CA. Contractions of specific abdominal muscles in postural tasks are affected by respiratory manoeuvres. J Appl Physiol 1997;83:753–60.

[37] Saunders SW, Rath D, Hodges PW. Postural and respiratory activation of the trunk muscles changes with mode and speed of locomotion. Gait Posture 2004;20(3):280–90.

[38] Andersson E, et al. The role of the psoas and iliacus muscles for stability and movement of the lumbar spine, pelvis and hip. Scand J Med Sci Sports 1995;5:10–6.

[39] O'Sullivan, et al. Evaluation of the flexion relaxation phenomenon of the trunk muscles in sitting. Spine 2006; 31(17):2009–16.

[40] Sapsford R, Richardson CA, Stanton WR. Sitting posture affects pelvic floor muscle activity in parous women: an observational study. Aust J Physiother 2006;52:219–22.

[41] Ainscough-Potts AM, Morrissey MC, Critchley D. The response of the transverse abdominus and internal oblique muscles to different postures. Man Ther 2006;11:54–60.

[42] Hodges PW. Is there a role for transversus abdominus in lumbo-pelvic stability? Man Ther 1999; 4(2):74–86.

[43] Hungerford B, Gilleard W, Hodges P. Evidence of altered lumbo-pelvic muscle recruitment in the prescence of sacroiliac joint pain. Spine 2003;28(14): 1593–600.

[44] Hodges PW, Butler JE, McKenzie D, Gandevia SC. Contraction of the human diaphragm during postural adjustments. J Physiol 1997; 505(2):239–548.

[45] Allison G, et al. The role of the diaphragm during abdominal hollowing exercises. Aust J Physiother 1998;44:95–104.

[46] Sapsford R, Hodges PW. Contraction of the pelvic floor muscles during abdominal manoeuvres. Arch Phys Med Rehab 2001;82:1081–8.

[47] Hodges PW, Richardson CA. Contraction of the abdominal muscles associated with movement of the lower limb. Phys Ther 1997;77:132–42.

[48] McCook DT, Vicenzino B, Hodges PW. Activity of the deep abdominal muscles increases during sub maximal flexion and extension efforts but antagonistic co-contraction remains unchanged. J Electromyogr Kinesiol (IN PRESS).

[49] Allison GT, Morris SL, Lay B. Feedforward responses of transversus abdominus are directionally specific and act asymmetrically: implications for core stability theories. J Ortho Sports Phys Ther 2008;38(5): 228–37.

[50] Herrington L. Does transversus abdominis contract symmetrically in asymptomatic individuals in response to changes in position? In: Proc. 6th Interdisciplinary World Congress on Low Back and Pelvic Pain. Barcelona; 2007.

[51] Hodges PW, et al. Experimental muscle pain changes feedforward postural responses of the trunk muscles. Exp Brain Research 2003;151:262–71.

[52] Janda V. Postural and phasic muscles in the pathogenesis of low back pain. In: Proc. X1th Congress IRSD. Dublin; 1968. p. 553–54.

[53] Janda V. Sydney: Course notes; 1984; 1985; 1989; 1995.

[54] Belavy DL. (F)lying to mars: how spaceflight research helps healthcare. Australian Physiotherapy Association. MPA Intouch Magazine 2008;(Issue 2).

[55] Richardson C. The deload model of injury. In: Therapeutic exercise for lumbopelvic stabilisation: a motor control approach for the treatment and prevention of low back pain. 2nd ed. Edinburgh: Churchill Livingstone; 2004. p. 105–17.

[56] Janda V. Pain in the locomotor system- a broad approach. In: Aspects of manipulative therapy. Melbourne: Churchill Livingstone; 1984. p. 148–51.

[57] Janda V. Muscle weakness and inhibition (pseudoparesis) in back pain syndromes. In: Modern manual therapy of the vertebral column. Edinburgh: Churchill Livingstone; 1986. p. 197–201.

[58] Richardson CA, Jull GA, Hides J. A new clinical model of the muscle dysfunction linked to the disturbance of spinal stability: implications for treatment of low back pain. In: Twomey L, editor. Physical Therapy of the low back. 3rd ed. New York: Churchill Livingstone.

[59] O'Sullivan PB. Lumbar segmental 'instability': clinical presentation and specific stabilising exercise management. Man Ther 2000; 5(1):2–12.

[60] O'Sullivan PB. 'Clinical instability' of the lumbar spine: its pathological basis, diagnosis and conservative management. In: Boyling JD, Jull JA, editors. Modern manual therapy. Amsterdam: Elsevier; 2004. p. 311–22.

[61] Smith JL, Betts B, Edgerton VR, Zernicke RF. Rapid ankle extension during paw shakes: Selective recruitment of fast ankle extensors. J Neurophysiol 1980;43(3):612–20.

[62] Wohlfahrt D, Jull G, Richardson C. The relationship between the dynamic and static function of the abdominal muscles. Aust J Physiother 1993;39(1):9–13.

[63] Richardson C. The role of weightbearing and non-weight bearing muscles. In: Therapeutic exercise for lumbopelvic stabilisation: a motor control approach for the treatment and prevention of low back pain. 2nd ed. Edinburgh: Churchill Livingstone; 2004. p. 93–102.

[64] Janda V. Muscles, central nervous motor regulation and back problems. In: Korr IM, editor. Neurobiologic mechanisms in manipulative therapy. New York: Plenum Press; 1978.

[65] O'Sullivan PB, et al. Effect of different upright sitting postures on spinal-pelvic curvature and trunk muscle activation in a pain free population. Spine 2006; 31(19):E707–12.

[66] Potvin JR, O'Brien PR. Trunk muscle co-contraction increases during fatiguing isometric lateral bend exertions: possible implications for spine stability. Spine 1998;23(7):774–80.

[67] Sole G, et al. Altered muscle activation of hamstring muscles following posterior thigh injury. In: Proc. 6th Interdisciplinary World Congress on Low Back and Pelvic Pain. Barcelona; 2007.

[68] Bond M. The new rules of posture: how to sit, stand, and move in the modern world. Rochester: Healing Arts Press; 2007.

[69] Kendall FP, McCreary EK, Provance PG. Muscles: testing and function. 4th ed. Baltimore: Williams and Wilkins; 1993.

[70] O'Sullivan PB, et al. Altered motor control strategies in subjects with sacroiliac joint pain during the active straight leg raise test. Spine 2002;27(1):E1–8.

[71] Norris CM. Spinal stabilisation: stabilisation mechanisms in the spine. Physiotherapy 1995;81 (2):72–9.

[72] Urquhart DM, et al. Regional morphology of transversus abdominis and internal oblique. In: Proc. Musculoskeletal Physiotherapy Australia Twelfth Biennial conference. Adelaide; 2001.

[73] Urquhart DM, et al. Abdominal muscle recruitment during a range of voluntary exercises. Man Ther 2005;10(2):144–53.

[74] Urquhart DM, Hodges PW, Story IH. Postural activity of the abdominal muscles varies between regions of these muscles and between body positions. Gait Posture 2005;22(4):295–301.

[75] Andersson EA, et al. EMG activities of the quadratus lumborum and erector spinae muscles during flexion-relaxation and other motor tasks. Clin Biomech 1996;11(7): 392–400.

[76] McGill SM. Low back exercise: evidence for improving exercise regimens. Phys Ther 1998; 78(7):754–65.

[77] Santaguida PL, McGill SM. The psoas major muscle: a three dimensional geometric study. J of Biomechanics 1995;28(3): 339–45.

[78] Santaguida PL, McGill SM. A 3D mechanical study of the psoas major muscle with respect to the spine. J Biomech 1993;26(3):351.

[79] Basmajian JV. Electromyography of iliopsoas. Anat Rec 1958;132:127–32.

[80] Nachemson A. Electromyographic studies on the vertebral portion of the psoas muscle; with special reference to its stabilising function of the lumbar spine. Acta Orthop Scand 1966;2:177–90.

[81] Nachemson A. The possible importance of the psoas muscle for stabilisation of the lumbar spine. Acta Orthop. Scand 1968;1:47–57.

[82] Gracovetsky S. An hypothesis for the role of the spine in human locomotion: a challenge to current thinking. J Biomed Eng 1985;3:205–16.

[83] Gibbons SGT. The model of psoas major stability function. In: Proc. 1st International Conference on Movement Dysfunction. Edinburgh; 2001.

[84] Penning L. Psoas muscle and lumbar spine stability: a concept uniting existing controversies. Critical review and hypothesis. Eur Spine J 2000;9:577–85.

[85] Travell JG, Simons DG. Myofascial pain and dysfunction: the trigger point manual the lower extremities, vol. 2. Baltimore: Williams and Baltimore; 1992.

[86] Bartenieff I. Body movement: coping with the environment gordon and breach australia. 2002.

[87] Hackney P. Making connections: total body integration through bartenieff fundamentals. New York: Routledge; 2002.

[88] Myers TW. Anatomy trains: myofascial meridians for manual and movement therapists. Edinburgh: Churchill Livingstone; 2001.

[89] Vleeming A, et al. The posterior layer of the thoracolumbar fascia: its function in load transfer from spine to legs. Spine 1995;20:753.

[90] Lee D. The pelvic girdle: an approach to the examination and treatment of the lumbopelvic-hip region. 3rd ed. Edinburgh: Churchill Livingstone; 2004.

[91] Beach P. The contractile field: a new model of human movement. J Bodyw Mov Ther 2007; 11(4):308–17.

[92] Beach P. The contractile field: a new model of human movement. Part 2. J Bodyw Mov Ther 2008;12(1):76–85.

[93] Beach P. The contractile field: a new model of human movement. Part 3. J Bodyw Mov Ther 2008;12(2):158–65.

[94] Brecklinghaus HG. The rowing style in ancient Egypt. Found: http//www.Somatics.de/ BrecklinghausRowing.

Chapter Six

Salient aspects of normal function of the torso

6

The spine or 'backbone' is the segmented connecting rod of the body common to all vertebrates. However, man is unique, in being the only one to have evolved to a consistent upright posture on two legs upon which the spine is further required to function both vertically and horizontally in relation to the earth's surface while balancing its super incumbent load. More specialized function of the limbs has evolved more complex function in the proximal limb girdles and as we have seen their control is intimately related to control of the spine. Rolf[1] describes the spine as the 'vital core that integrates the human with his gravity environment poorly, well or adequately as the case may be'. Its function is complex and various aspects considered important in facilitating improvement in its control are explored. This is examined within four main functional components:

- The axial spine
- The pelvic girdle
- The upper pole of the 'body cylinder'
- Functional interrelationship between the upper and lower body cylinder.

Part A: The axial spine

Structural mechanical aspects

The axial spine functions as a system

No one part of the spine functions independently. The treatment of low back pain continues to provide poor outcomes. Perhaps the focus of much of the research and interventions has been too specific

to the lumbar spine, without understanding the functional interrelationships between all four regions of the spine. Control of the spine as a whole is also mutually dependent upon control of the rest of the axial skeleton – the occiput, thorax and proximal limb girdles – all function as part of an interrelated support and movement system.

The spine performs many roles

In the process of phylogenesis and ontogenesis the spine's structural architecture has evolved providing for its many roles. The process of our motor development ensures the necessary spectrum of patterns of neuromuscular control needed to serve its various functions. Much of the current spine research is involved with trying to dissemble and better understand these responses and how they are altered in people with spinal pain.

The spine is a remarkable piece of structural bio-engineering acting as the central support yet also capable of assuming different shapes in multiple planes. It has been described as an unstable structure stabilized by the nervous system.[2] Its roles can be essentially distilled as providing:

- A flexible yet stable central weight bearing column supporting and connecting the head and limbs and assisting load transfer between them.
- Acting as a scaffold or lattice supporting myofascial structures, it also helps distribute weight.[1]
- Movements which enlarge the scope of head and limb movements.

- Contribution to the support and function of the breathing mechanism.
- Contribution to locomotion. Gracovetsky states 'the spine does not stop at L5. It goes all the way to the acetabulum'[2] and acts as an 'engine' whereby the lordotic lumbar spine converts a lateral bending moment into an axial torque which drives pelvic rotation in walking.[3]
- Its geometry and structure of alternating viscoelastic and firm elements allow it to act as a spring loaded shock absorber, while its elastic recoil helps minimize the energy expenditure of locomotion and movement.
- It houses and protects the central nervous system and supports the autonomic nervous system. When spinal function is healthy so is the person. When spinal joints are 'out of kilter', altered afference can influence the function of the entire nervous system.

The requirement for both effective stability and mobility is achieved through the interdependent function between the nervous, myofascial and osseo-ligamentous systems as has been suggested by Janda[4] and White and Panjabi.[5]

The spine is more centrally located within the body than is generally appreciated. Its pyramidal shape and frontal plane symmetry means it can support, carry and control all its superimposed weights.[6] Maintaining control of the regions where the curves change, particularly the thoracolumbar and lumbosacral is important in balancing the structure of the lower spine. The natural state of the lumbar spine is *arched*. Gracovetsky[3] and Farfan[7] have long stressed the biomechanical advantage of the lumbar lordosis and hip extension for effective upright activity.

A neutral spine and the 'neutral zone'

While the spine can readily change its form, it is important that it is able to return to 'home base' or its neutral alignment. Here, the curves assume their physiologic position and act to balance one another; the head is balanced over the pelvis such that there is minimal displacement from the line of gravity, and minimal muscle work is needed to maintain the position. There is balance of all segments in all planes. The curves are characterized by a range defined by natural variability.[8] This can also be influenced by differing postural habits, body types and

training effect and so on. Clinically, those with spinal pain have altered perception of a neutral spine and difficulty achieving this throughout the spine.

The term 'neutral zone' was conceived by White and Panjabi[5] who defined control of the neutral zone as 'a low load response near or beyond the neutral position.... up to the beginning of significant resistance...due to the application of a small force'.[5] Movement further into range is into the 'elastic zone' up to the physiological limit, after which, 'failure' occurs. This is more likely with the adoption of end range postures with or without superimposed movements. White and Panjabi[5] state 'a significant amount of spinal motion takes place around the neutral position (which) is not accounted for'. In most usual everyday activities, a lot of the required spinal movement ideally oscillates in and around the neutral zone or 'mid position' of every spinal segment in the axial column under fairly low loads and is directionally balanced. This is important to recognize when facilitating functional neuromuscular control of the spine. The active control of these small low load movements is largely performed by the systemic local muscle system (SLMS). Larger loads and movements into the 'elastic zone' involve more activity from the SGMS (see Ch. 5).

The spine comprises multiple functional spinal units (FSU)

Otherwise known as the motion segment, the FSU is the smallest segment of the spine that exhibits the biomechanical characteristics similar to those of the whole spine.[5] It consists of two adjacent vertebrae, the articulating surfaces between them – the two facet joints, separated by an intervertebral disc, and the connecting ligamentous tissues. The behavior of the FSU is dependent upon the physical properties of each of these components. Generally speaking, motion at any FSU is extremely limited and consists of a small amount of gliding (translation) and rotation.[9] This occurs from a combination of rocking through the disc[30] and sliding of the facets which act to steer the movement. The total behavior of the spine results from the composite behaviors of the multiple FSUs connected in series which constitute its structure.

Significantly, between each intervertebral level, the spinal nerve exits through the intervertebral foramen (Fig. 6.1). Here it has important relations.

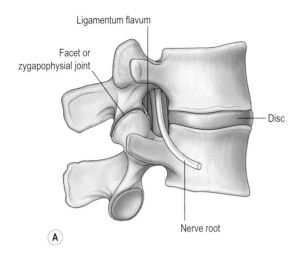

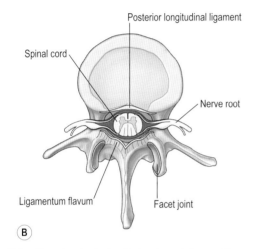

Fig 6.1 • Functional spinal unit showing relations of the disc and particularly the facet joint to the spinal nerve from the side (A) and above (B).

In the front is the intervertebral disc and adjacent regions of the vertebral body. Behind are the facet or zygapophysial joints.[10] Like any synovial joints, these can become inflamed and swollen when the vertebral mechanics change. This spinal joint inflammation not only disturbs local joint function but can also compromise the lumen of the foramen and directly impact upon the spinal nerve creating local and referred pain syndromes (Ch.12). The marked implications of facet inflammation are understood when injecting saline into the joints of pigs produced an immediate reduction in paraspinal muscle activity.[11] Clinically, most spinal pain and related disorders stem from dysfunction of one (or multiple) FSUs where, through altered loading, both the disc and the facet are implicated. When the disc loses height the facet mechanics change. Effective clinical interventions generally result from restoring the movement in the facet and through the segment which reduces the inflammation and so the pain.

Movements of the axial spine

The health of the spinal joints is largely dependent upon a variety of repeated small amplitude movements. Normal antigravity control is provided by a well integrated normal postural reflex system including balanced activity between the deep and superficial muscle systems. The fine modulation of flexor/extensor co-activity provides the appropriate sagittal alignment of the spine so that the occiput is balanced over the sacrum. This provides good foundations for movement.

Spinal movements result from the contribution of small movements in some or all of the FSUs. Spinal motion is generally described as flexion/ extension, lateral bending and rotation occurring in the sagittal, frontal and horizontal planes respectively. Lateral bending produces translation and rotation of the vertebrae in the frontal plane as well as axial rotation because of the inherent properties of the FSU.[5]

Functional movements are actually rarely pure plane, but variable combinations of these movements albeit within a primary movement direction, providing three-dimensional control. Axial movement is more one of adjustment and sequencing through the spinal segments. Big movements are provided by the large multi-axial ball and socket joints. Problems ensue if their movement is reduced so that some regions of the spine become the axis of movement.

In crude terms, all vertebrae consist of a body and a bony ring with processes containing the articulating surfaces. In each region there are differences in the size of the vertebral body and the orientation of the facet joints consistent with its load bearing role and which favors some movements over others.

Kinematic differences thus occur within each region of the spine and in depth analyses are provided by numerous authors.[5,9,12] Figure 6.2 shows the segmental and regional movement characteristics. Briefly:

- **Cervical.** The most mobile region of the spine with freedom of movement in all three planes.
- **Thoracic.** The facet shape affords more mobility in rotation and lateral flexion and least mobility in extension. Rotation freedom decreases in a cranio-to caudal direction.[12]

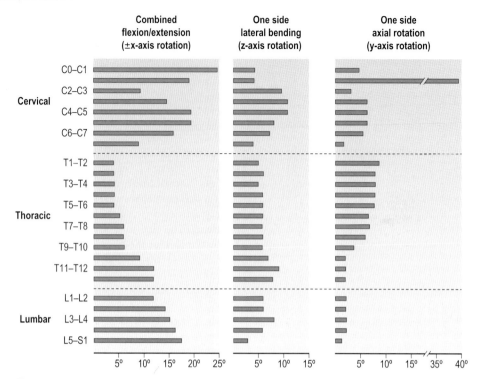

Fig 6.2 • Composite summary of segmental kinematics and regional variations. Reproduced from White AA and Panjabi MM. 1990 with permission JB. Lippincott & Co.

• *Lumbar.* Facet orientation favors movements in the sagittal plane – flexion and extension, with a cephalocaudal increase.[5] A recent study[13] has shown most segmental sagittal movement at L3/4 followed by L4/5. Side bending and particularly rotation are limited. Rotation has been shown to increase in flexed postures leaving all segmental structures more vulnerable.[14] However reduced rotation at the end of flexion and extension ranges compared with that in the neutral position has been shown.[15]

• *Sacrococcygeal.* The vertebral segments within the sacrum and coccyx are fused, but there is a fibrocartilaginous joint between them[10] which allows flexion and extension deemed by some to be largely passive[16] while others see it as the most mobile part of the pelvis[17] Lee[18] reported a MRI study which showed flexion of the coccyx with pelvic floor muscle contraction and extension during a Valsalva maneuver or straining. The sacrum is stabilized in the pelvic ring which limits its mobility and provides stability. Movements of the sacrum/coccyx principally involve those in the sagittal plane – nutation and counternutation with some

torsion and side bending. Ipso facto, these movements involve corresponding movements in both the spine and the pelvis.

A decrease in the range of all spinal movements with increasing age is apparent.[19]

Pelvic (sacral) spatial position affects spinal alignment

The sacrum/coccyx forms the base of the spine. The pelvis is partly formed by and in turn also supports them and so control of its spatial position will affect the alignment and control of the whole spine, the lumbar spine in particular. This is the case for all static and dynamic postures and movements in all planes both in relationship to the body and gravity. This is important to appreciate. While the static picture does not necessarily equate to functional reality, the principles provide for conceptual ease and can be extrapolated to all spinal movements.

In the frontal plane when the pelvis is in the neutral balanced position the spine is vertical, symmetrical and balanced. If the pelvis is oblique or laterally tilted, the pelvis will shift to the high side, the lumbar spine will side bend to that side. This in turn will then create compensatory adjustments throughout the spine – a pronounced case of which is seen in scoliosis.[23]

In the sagittal plane the lumbar spinal curvature is clearly dependent upon pelvic tilt.[23] A neutral lordosis is achieved with a corresponding neutral tilt of the pelvis. A neutral pelvis has been variously defined:

• When either the anterior iliac spines lie on a horizontal with the posterior iliac spines or the anterior superior iliac spine lies on a vertical with the symphysis pubis.[9]

• Rolf defines pelvic balance as a horizontal line between the coccyx and pubes and a vertical between the pubes and anterior iliac spine[1] (Fig. 6.3).

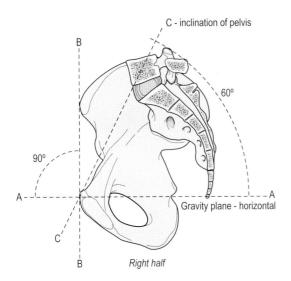

C - inclination of pelvis

60°

90°

A - A
Gravity plane - horizontal

Right half

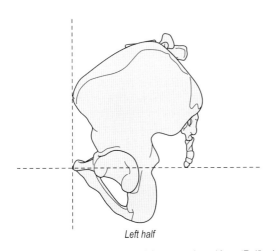

Left half

Fig 6.3 • A balanced 'neutral' pelvis – reproduced from 'Rolfing' with permission Harper and Rowe New York 1977.

• However, Rock[20] suggests that in optimal functional alignment, the anterior superior iliac spines move slightly in front of the symphysis which facilitates dynamic activity in the postural reflex mechanism. Here the shear forces imposed upon the sacro-iliac joint (SIJ) are offset as the sacrum is suspended between the two innominates in slight nutation.[18]

• When the pelvis tilts anteriorly the lordosis increases.[21]

• When the pelvis tilts posteriorly the lordosis reduces and the lumbar spine flexes.

Mutual behavior between the curves

A change in one curve will generally be reflected in the others. Try lying down on the floor with your knees bent. If you flatten your low back to the floor, invariably your chin will poke forward and your neck hyper extend. If you increase the lumbar lordosis the neck will lengthen and the chin retract. This has implications for clinical practice. Black et al.[22] showed this opposite relationship between lumbar and cervical posture in sitting – as the lumbar spine moved toward extension, the cervical spine flexed and vice versa. Marked stiffness in the thoracic spine will modify this response.

The junctional regions

According to Lewit,[23] not all vertebral segments have the same importance for the functioning of the spine. There are 'key segments or regions', mostly the transition areas where the anatomy and the function in the column changes between very mobile and relatively immobile regions. These 'junctional regions' marry the transitions between the three principal units of body weight – the head thorax and pelvis. They accommodate forces while transmitting movement through the spine. They occur at the top and bottom of the segmented spine and the top and bottom of the thorax. Ideally, the line of gravity passes through them.[24,25] Lewit maintains it is in these regions that the spinal column suffers first jeopardizing function of the spine as a whole, and causing secondary lesions.[23] They all share a common tendency to hypomobility or stiffness creating compensatory relative increased mobility in segments adjacent and/or far removed.

• *The craniocervical junction (C0/1/2).* These are the most anatomically and kinematically complex joints in the axial skeleton.[5] They allow triplanar mobility, rotation at C1/2 and sagittal nodding of the occiput on the condyles being most significant. In physiological terms the receptive field for the tonic neck reflexes which influence muscle tone throughout the postural trunk musculature lie mostly within the C0/1 and C1/2 joints.[26] Importantly, if function here is disturbed, there is frequently hypertonus of the 'postural muscles', disturbances of equilibrium and locomotor/movement deficit[23] which has to be compensated for elsewhere in the cervical spine.

• *The cervicothoracic junction (C7/T1/2)* where the most mobile region of the spine, the neck, joins the relatively immobile thoracic spine and where the powerful muscles of the upper limb and shoulder attach to the torso. Dysfunction over this junction contributes towards compensatory movements in the neck and is implicated in shoulder pain syndromes.

• *The thoracolumbar junction (T10/11/12/L1)* where the less mobile thorax joins the more mobile lumbar spine. Nature has attempted to soften the transition with the 11th and 12th ribs floating and bearing similarity to transverse processes. The upper facet joints of T12 retain the thoracic pattern while the lower joints have the lumbar pattern. According to White and Panjabi[5] and Bergmark,[27] the highest torsional stiffness is typically exhibited at this junction and the T12/L1 FSU is a site of high stress concentration. Clinically, it is a region which suffers badly from both postural collapse and regional muscular holding patterns. Disturbed function here causes intense spasm not only of the back muscles but also the psoas[23] in particular, as well as compromised diaphragm function. This is common and clinically important.

• *The lumbosacral junction (L5/sacrum)* where the relatively rigid sacrum joins the more mobile segmented lumbar spine. Disturbance of the hip–pelvis complex affects saccral kinematics which in turn affects the kinematics of L5/S1 segment as well as the alignment of the rest of the spine.

The head–tail bone relationship

The head and tail bone or coccyx represent the top and bottom of the spine and in a well balanced upright spine they are aligned. The head is balanced on the occipital condyles and the coccyx through the pelvis is balanced on the femoral condyles. Ideally this relationship is also maintained in numerous other postures whatever the base of support.

The head and the tail bone can be viewed as functional 'limbs'. Thus there are six 'limbs' *from which* spinal movement may be initiated. Additionally the spine transmits sequences and adjusts movements between the upper and lower body and between the various 'limbs'. Hackney[28] notes that in all movements both simple and complex, where the spine is a dynamic link between the limbs and the upper and lower body, the 'head and tail are in a constant and always changing interactive relationship'.

Unhealthy spinal control is characterized by a poor head/tail relationship, difficulty initiating movement from the six 'limbs' as well as controlling the 'centre'.

Spinal loading and the control of forces in movement

White and Panjabi[5] define load as 'a general term describing the application of a force and/or moment (torque) to a structure'. All structures including the body are subject to forces and in the physical universe action and reaction are always equal and opposite. Movement is loading. It can occur in response forces acting on the body which in turn creates other forces which further need to be controlled. While 'forces' and 'loads' may imply the idea of 'maximal', in the spine they can be minimal occasioning merely a tonus shift to counter them.

Interested in structural balance and the mechanical forces which affected this, Todd[6] says 'the direction in which any force acts upon an object in relation to its internal axis determines the nature of the stress endured by the object'. She lists 'axial and other stresses'.

• *Compression and tensile* stresses are called axial as both operate along the axis without changing it. In the skeleton the compression members are the uprights, the bones, and the direction of the forces is downward with gravity. 'The tensile members are the suspensory parts which direct weight to points on the upright

The role of the 'passive tissues'

These provide structural support and help counter the applied forces to the spine. Importantly, most exhibit viscoelastic behavior, in particular the disc. This means that when a constant load is applied to the tissues, over time they will deform or 'creep'. The tissues are variably sensitive to the rate that the load is applied. The load can be tensile or compressive. When the load is removed the tissue may not recover and return to its origin dimensions, known as 'hysteresis'. Both creep and hysteresis have been shown to increase with age.[29] These phenomena play a significant role in spinal pain syndromes. The adoption of habitual altered posturomovement strategies creates chronic aberrant loading of the tissues.

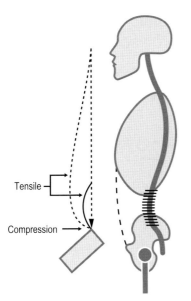

Fig 6.4 • Vertebral column as a spring. Balance of tensile and compression forces in the axial spine. Reproduced from "The Thinking Body" Mabel E Todd 1937 with permission from Princeton book company.

which may be received and transferred to the ground through the bones'. The direction of tensile forces is opposed to gravity (Fig. 6.4).

If these two forces are combined or directed in such a way as to interfere with the axis, three other stresses may occur as follows:

• *Torsion* where the tension or compression is so exerted as to cause the structure to twist about its axis which weakens the structure for support in the area affected

• *Shearing* occurs when the force is directed at an angle to its axis causing one part to slide over the other disrupting its axis

• *Bending* is a combination of tension and compression applied in such a way that the axis is curved so that the structure is weakened for support. It may be caused by an unevenly distributed load or a too top heavy load. It is the most serious of the stresses and the hardest to counter.

The effect that loading has on the spine will also depend on the duration and the magnitude of the force. These can be divided into two main categories:[5]

• Short duration–high amplitude as in a jerk lift

• Long duration–low magnitude as in postural collapse.

Loading can be static or dynamic. Dynamic loading with a repetitive pattern is called cyclic loading.

The vertebrae

The architecture of vertebrae makes them well designed to bear compressive loads, most of which is taken through the vertebral body although some occurs through the facet joints.[5,30] The vertebral bodies become progressively larger at the bottom of the spine and studies have shown these to be stronger in compressive loading as may be expected. Bone mineral content has been shown to increase in response to mechanical demand.[31] In general though, vertebral strength decreases with age.[5]

The facet joints or posterior intervertebral joints[30] contribute to load sharing. The amount of compressive load borne will depend upon the spinal posture and has been shown to vary between nil (becomes tension loading in marked flexion) and nearly half the load in extension.[5] Their geometry affords them a significant role in checking the tensile, torsional, shear and bending stresses that the spine is subject to.

The intervertebral disc

Its design provides for the combined roles of weight bearing and load transference while allowing multidirectional rocking movements between the vertebrae. Besides compression, the dense annular fibres act like strong ligaments and help resist tensile, torsional, bending and shear stresses. However, combined loads make it more vulnerable. Flexion bending and torsional loads are probably more harmful than compression,[5] although both cyclic and high compressive forces in hyperextension have demonstrated disc damage.[32] The disc also has the capacity to absorb and store energy, has elastic recoil and provides shock absorption[30] and damping through the spine. In its healthy state, acting as a tense pillow between the vertebrae, it assists the correct apposition of the facet joints and so helps ensure their function and stability. Intradiscal pressure within normal physiological ranges appears to provide an essential mechanical stimulus for maintenance of the proteoglycan matrix and the consequent load bearing capacity of the disc.[33] As we age, the disc degenerates. This can be apparent from the age of 20 and by the age of 50, 97% of all lumbar discs have been shown to be degenerated, in particular the lowest three levels.[5] When the disc degenerates, the facet joints tend to stiffen or can override, become sloppy and 'unstable'. Segmental dysfunction involves the whole FSU – problems with the disc involve the facets and vice versa. It is quite extraordinary how this one structure has been assumed to be the mainstay of most low back pain. Treatment directed at the movement impairment of the whole segment invariably ameliorates the pain while the radiological changes remain the same, being usual and age related.

Ligaments

Binding the vertebrae together, ligaments readily resist tensile forces in the direction in which the fibres run. As such they are also good at resisting torsion, shear and bending. With the muscles, they share the role of providing stability to the spine within its physiologic curves and ranges of motion including maintaining the relationship between each vertebra, protecting the spinal cord and nerve roots. They demonstrate adaptive changes in response to increasing demand or immobilization.[34] They are considered sensory organs and have significant input to sensation and reflexive/synergistic activation of muscles.[35] Solomonow et al.[36] demonstrated that mechanical overload of spinal ligaments recruits local muscles in a protective response which increases with the ligament stress. 'The functional complexity of ligaments is amplified when considering their inherent viscoelastic properties such as creep, tension–relaxation, hysteresis and time or frequency-dependent length-tension behavior'.[35] Dysfunctional ligaments thus result in various sensorimotor disorders.

The dynamic role of the neuromyofascial system

Fascial system

The thoracolumbar fascia has been ascribed a biomechanical role in the stability of the lumbar spine. In fact, Gracovetsky[37] considers it the most important structure insuring the integrity of the spinal machinery. Traditionally though, fascia has not been considered as a system and accorded little importance in musculoskeletal mechanics. However, there is growing interest in the potential major role that fascia may play in providing structural support, stability and contributing to movement coordination. It has been described as:

The soft tissue component of the connective tissue system that permeates the human body forms a whole body, continuous three-dimensional matrix of structural support. It interpenetrates and surrounds all organs, muscles, bones and nerve fibres, creating a unique environment for body systems functioning. It includes all fibrous connective tissues, including aponeuroses, ligaments, tendons, retinacula, joint capsules, organ and vessel tunics, the epineurium, the meninges, the periostia and all the endomysial and intermuscular fibres of the myofascia.[38]

According to Rolf,[1] there are different kinds of fascial sheaths. The superficial is a fibroareolar tissue that houses much of the body fats, can stretch in any direction and adjust quickly to strains of all kinds. The deep fascia is a denser layer, provides good resistance to tensile strain and its smooth coating permits neighbouring structures to slide over one another. She was particularly interested in the fascial envelope surrounding muscle. Rolf[1] and her disciples and those interested in biotensegrity[39] view the fascia as the prime organ of support and the bones, rather than providing support in the Newtonian sense, act as spacers serving to position and relate different areas of connective tissue. This may help explain how the 'human spine can accept loads from any direction with arms and legs cantilevered out in any direction'.[39] Muscles provide the source and direction of movement and as they are encased within it and attach to it, they can act as tensioners to the system. Variously described as the 'internet',[40] 'the endless web',[41] 'a spider's web reaching out to every nook and cranny',[42] being a continuous system – a force applied to one part or a local restriction – can have quite far reaching as well as local effects. The anatomical continuity of the myofascial and viscerofascial systems as well as the neuroanatomical relationship of somatic and visceral structures mean that recruitment patterns of spinal muscles may change due to dysfunction of structures outside the musculoskeletal system.[42]

Artificially increasing the tension in the lumbar fascia has been shown to alter lumbar segmental translation and rotation.[43] Fascia is also capable of remodeling in response to changing mechanical loads and muscle activity.[44] Recent research has demonstrated the presence of smooth muscle like contractile cells in fascia with higher densities found in the lumbar fascia indicating its ability to influence musculoskeletal mechanics.[45] Smith[46] provides a seductive view of its role: 'fascia is now seen as an antagonist to muscular action, and movement is seen less as the coordinated action of antagonistic muscles and more in terms of the elastic and oscillatory properties of the myofascial network as a whole'. As well as its static attributes, fascia 'has the potential for certain rhythmic or oscillatory movement patterns that arise from its elastic, hydraulic and tensegrity properties'. 'These inherent rhythmic movement patterns are independent of muscle activity. However, they may be either reinforced or inhibited by muscle action'. 'Muscular action works primarily to maintain the oscillatory patterns with an occasional and timely input of energy each movement cycle'. The whole body response seen in Craniosacral Therapy[47] is based upon the concept of a fascial continuity throughout the body. Gracovetsky[48] remarks 'it is the viscoelastic behavior of collagen that drives the stability of the spine... the integrity of the collagen structure is as important as that of the muscles'. The fascial system appears to serve as the structural and functional link between the frank passive and active tissues in movement.

Neuromuscular system

This interdependent system converts a structural body into a functional body.

In our relationship with gravity, the body is constantly adjusting to changing circumstances. We do this through information coming from our senses, from within (proprioception) and without (exteroception). Proprioception essentially provides position and movement sense. It allows us to sense the

position and movement of joints; to sense the force effort and heaviness associated with muscle contractions; and the ability to perceive the timing of muscle actions.[49] Exteroception comes through the senses with which we orient ourselves to the environment and the sense of space around us – vision labyrinths and touch.

Effective motor control is dependent upon adequate peripheral afference from receptors in the joints, ligaments, fascia muscles tendons etc so that the magnitude and timing of the muscle response is appropriate to the loading conditions. The various kinesthetic receptors are in tissues which are viscoelastic and the adoption of slouched postures has been shown to subsequently affect subjects' ability to reposition their spines.[50] Normally we can accurately spatially position our spine and this is independent of the magnitude of the range of movement.[51] Brumagne[52] has shown that precise muscle spindle input from multifidus is essential for accurate positioning of the pelvis and lumbosacral spine in sitting.

The neuromuscular system essentially deals with balancing the intrinsic and extrinsic forces imposed upon the body as a result of gravity, movement and loads. This system is fragile and its dysfunction, according to Janda,[53] is one of the first signs to be clinically recognizable and is responsible for the genesis of many spinal pain disorders. There are certain normal neuromuscular responses relating to spinal control which merit looking at.

Aspects of normal neuromuscular behavior around the spine

Muscle coactivation or cocontraction (see Ch. 4)

This is a normal muscle response from the trunk muscles in order that the spine may be controlled in a stable neutral posture[54] and ready to respond to the complex and unexpected loading patterns during our everyday activities. The column is supported and controlled from all sides. Activity at low load states is primarily in the deep SLMS and as the load increases so does the magnitude of the coactivation, as the superficial muscles become more involved. Antagonistic trunk muscle coactivation occurs during sudden loading of the torso, accelerations of the torso as in slipping, isometric trunk moments, axial torques and heavy exertions in order to provide the necessary stability.[54] Co-contraction is a normal response to fatigue as the spine attempts to protect itself.[55] However, Radebold et al.[56] showed that sudden perturbations to the trunk in normal people produced more flexible muscle recruitment responses in the superficial muscles and did not necessarily involve co-contraction. Their study did not access the deeper muscles.

At high loads, trunk muscle coactivation resembles muscle guarding or splinting and spinal motion is limited. Quint et al.[57] showed this can be reduced by as much as 20%. High levels of co-contraction have been shown to degrade postural control.[58] While stabilizing the spine to manage heavy loads, it imparts a high compressive loading on the spine. In the normal state this is not a problem, as they are generally short lived to say lift a box, or prevent a fall.

Flexion relaxation phenomenon

Studies have shown that when standing still and bending forward, the low back extensors eccentrically contract and then fall electrically silent, the load then being borne by the passive tissues – ligaments, disc, gut and some elastic recoil in the muscles,[59] and the fascial system.[60] The point in the flexion range where this occurs is variably reported as between two-thirds of maximum trunk flexion (and corresponding half-range hip flexion),[61] to near the end of trunk flexion.[59] The relaxation effect has also been reported to include the hamstrings and much of the thoracic erector spinae.[60] However, relaxation of the lumbar extensors associated with reciprocal thoracic erector spinae activation has also been found.[62] Bogduk et al.[63] estimate that the thoracic erector spinae contribute to 50% of the total extensor moment exerted on L4/5. Andersson et al.[64] found that quadratus lumborum did not relax with the lumbar extensors suggesting a postural stabilizing role for this muscle.[59]

Limiting the posterior shift of the pelvis and hip flexion has been shown to produce the response earlier in range.[65] While a lack of this response is a common finding in subjects with LBP suggesting an increased 'protective' role from the superficial extensors, it is not universal. The question needs to be asked as to the desirability of depending on

the passive tissues. In functional movement, is the flexion relaxation response different? Is it partly a consequence of decreased SLMS coactivation synergies affording poor adaptable support and control where limiting pelvic shift and locking the legs allows one to utilize the passive system more than is healthy?

O'Sullivan et al[66] have examined the response when moving from sitting upright to slumped sitting. They found that superficial multifidus and internal oblique – both important in segmental control, exhibited a consistent and significant decrease in activity at mid range spinal flexion. The thoracic erector spinae response was highly variable with several different patterns of activity demonstrating the variable and complex nature of motor control. They found that adopting a neutral lordosis in sitting, best facilitated activity in the deep system muscles.

The reflex muscular responses to arousal/stress

Arousal, a state of internal alertness, is a component of several emotional responses including fear and anxiety and is mediated by the neuroendocrine system and includes the limbic system.[67] The level of arousal can vary from deep sleep to the fight-or-flight response. The body and mind are inextricably linked, our emotions being reflected in our neuromuscular being. Stress is a natural phenomenon and necessary for our survival. There is a normal cyclic variation between periods of stress when we are aroused and periods of relaxation where depleted energy is restored. In times of stress or hyper arousal, the sympathetic system is activated initiating a 'fight or flight response'. This occasions an increase in the cardiac and respiratory rate and other bodily changes to get ready for action. Hyperventilation is part of this normal reaction to sudden danger or excitement. There is over activity of the general body musculature, particularly of the facial and jaw muscles, neck and shoulders. Activity in the SGMS predominates. The upper limbs are held in flexion, the trunk is generally held stiff and because of tension in the abdominal musculature, diaphragmatic breathing can be inhibited and replaced by upper chest breathing.[68] Classically adduction and flexion patterns are symptomatic of stress.[68,74] The higher levels of muscle activation found in states of increased arousal have been shown to decrease performance in highly anxious subjects yet improve it in those less anxious.[67]

Repeated exposure to stress creates a risk that stress changes from a natural transient reaction to a chronic pathological state. The person finds it difficult to relax. Symptoms such as hyperventilation syndrome become common and will have effects on the whole body including the neuromuscular system.[69,70,71] The line between normal and abnormal behavior becomes blurred.

The protective and defensive reactions

It is a basic instinct of all animals and humans to protect or defend themselves when threatened.

Hanna[72] was influenced by Selye's statement that stress is a response to good things as well as bad. He describes stress as being both positive and negative and creating a specific reflex response of the neuromuscular system in two basic ways:

• Positive or **'eustress'** is the action and perhaps effort response which primarily activates the extensor muscle system. It is assertive behavior and Hanna termed it the Green Light Reflex. Its specific effect is the habitual contraction of the back muscles – the extensor system. It contributes to a 'posture of defense'.

• Negative or **'distress'** creates a basic neuromuscular withdrawal response which primarily occurs on the front of the body. It is a primitive reflex of survival – a 'rapid motor act' that helps our survival by withdrawing from danger. Hanna termed it the Red Light Reflex – a protective response to negative events which threaten us such as fear and anxiety. It is associated with a reflex contraction of the abdominal muscles which pulls the trunk into more flexion, depresses the chest, inhibits activity of the diaphragm and so causes shallow breathing. It contributes to a 'posture of protection'. Trauma will invoke a protective response guarding against pain, e.g. trunk list. These are *unconscious, involuntary rapid reflex motor acts* which *primarily affect the muscles around the body's centre of gravity.*

Bond[40] suggests that the horizontal, crosswise muscles (the vocal, thoracic and pelvic diaphragms) are the sites of our most internal motions of protection as they constrict whenever we hunker down under pressure. Acting like valves through the vertical axis of the body, their closure blocks the adaptive responses to gravity through the body. Again, these reactions are characterized by associated over activity in the superficial systemic global muscle system (SGMS). When repeatedly triggered, which is indeed common in today's stress inducing society, these basic responses easily become habitual behavior. As Hanna says:

Habituation is the simplest form of learning. It occurs through the constant repetition of a response. When the same bodily response occurs over and over again, its pattern is gradually 'learned' at an unconscious level. Habituation is a slow relentless adaptive act which ingrains itself into the functional patterns of the central nervous system.[72]

And this occurs in 'normal' 'healthy' as yet 'pain free' people!

In states of acute pain, we are all familiar with the need to protect, guard, splint and 'hold against', particularly if we sense the pain 'is causing damage'. This is generally associated with reflex breath holding. If pain persists the risk is that the splinting and holding persist. These responses are important when working with patients both with manual treatment and therapeutic directed exercise. Accessing painful joints and stiff regions can provoke discomfort. The art of the therapist is to gauge the right degree of intervention so that these responses are not triggered. The patient's belief systems regarding pain being 'good' or 'bad' can further sensitize the response or otherwise. It is also common to see these reactions being triggered during many fitness endeavors such as gyms and some yoga studios where being pushed beyond one's capability engenders features of unconscious 'defending' and 'holding against' in the motor response patterns.

Effort response

Movement should on the whole be easy and effortless, achieved from well integrated activity between the SLMS and the SGMS. When performing a task that requires a high level of effort, there is a spread of activation to other muscles besides those principally responsible for the task. This enhances postural stability and enables the transfer of power across joints by the two-joint muscles.[67]

Laban[73] was interested in the economy of effort afforded by the use of appropriate motor skills. Efficiency is gauging the right proportionality of weight, space, timing and control of the flow of movement. The inherent rhythm in movement is important and is disturbed by the use of excess and unnecessary effort. 'Any inappropriate use of movement is just a waste of effort.'[73] The harder we work the more the SGMS is called into action, a feature of their innate behavior (see Ch.5). In times of higher loading they serve to provide the added stiffness the spine needs. However, the amount of effort expended needs to match the demand of the situation. People with a poorly integrated systemic local muscle system rely more on their SGMS and so tend to use more effort than necessary in low load activities and with unhealthy kinematic patterns. Importantly, those actions requiring increased effort, should involve the adoption of biomechanically sound movement patterns.

Often, when a person 'tries to please' and 'tries too hard' he invariably activates a neuromuscular response which is more effortful and SGMS dominant than is required by the situation. Excess effort in movement leads to grosser movement. This is a common response in people being directed in exercise, whether it is therapeutic or recreational.

Postural equilibrium

Feldenkrais noted: 'human upright posture is a dynamic equilibrium...our nervous system as well as our body works to restore equilibrium rather than to keep it.'[74] How we physically organize ourselves in relation to gravity is reflected in both our posture and our breathing. The primary breathing muscles are also postural muscles. The body constantly adjusts to the disturbance created by breathing and so even in the 'static' state there is always a degree of movement in the form of small oscillations of postural sway. In adulthood, for most functional tasks we maintain a vertical orientation of the body. In the process of establishing and maintaining this verticality we use multiple sensory references including gravity (the vestibular system), the support surface (the somatosensory system) and the relationship of our body to objects in the environment (visual system).[75]

Postural stability or balance is the ability to maintain the body in equilibrium in both 'static' and dynamic states and this will change as the body configuration changes. The smaller and the more unstable the base of support (see Ch.4) the greater is the demand from the control system. The central nervous system (CNS) automatically attempts to control the orientation of the head and trunk with respect to the gravity axis. The magnitude of the perturbation both intrinsic and extrinsic and its duration will determine the relative contribution from the deep and superficial systems. If SLMS activity is reduced, it is common to observe central 'holding patterns' in the torso which will compromise the equilibrium responses in the torso. Too much trunk muscle coactivation degrades postural control.[58] Habitual postures influence how muscles are recruited and coordinated for recovery of stability.

Todd[6] notes that upright equilibrium occurs when the pelvis can act as a mechanical de-coupler and freely swing between the spinal axis and the leg axis which are not in continuous but parallel planes. These axes result from the effects of gravity, bones muscles, ligaments and fascia. All are involved in maintaining a balance between the compression forces coming down through the spine at the back and the tensile forces being transmitted up the front. The two planes should be parallel to the line of gravity which bisects the body vertically through the three main centres of weight. Keeping them parallel and close together will bring all joints of the connecting parts into the best mechanical relationship and equilibrium (Fig. 6.5).

Ideal alignment of the body segments minimizes the effect of gravitational forces and reduces the amount of muscle activity needed to remain upright and for equilibrium.

Most of the postural stability control research has been conducted in standing. Functional equilibrium is necessary in all manner of 'postures'. Vertical equilibrium has been examined in the following ways:

• Changes in the amplitude of postural sway during quiet stance. Traditionally, small amplitude movements of the body reflected as the centre of pressure over the base of support (BOS) have been seen to reflect 'good' control of balance and larger amplitude movements to reflect 'poor' control.[75] When sensory inputs are decreased the centre of pressure motion tends to increase.

• Motor strategies as a response to perturbed stance. Characteristic patterns of synergistic muscle activity occur in response to perturbation.

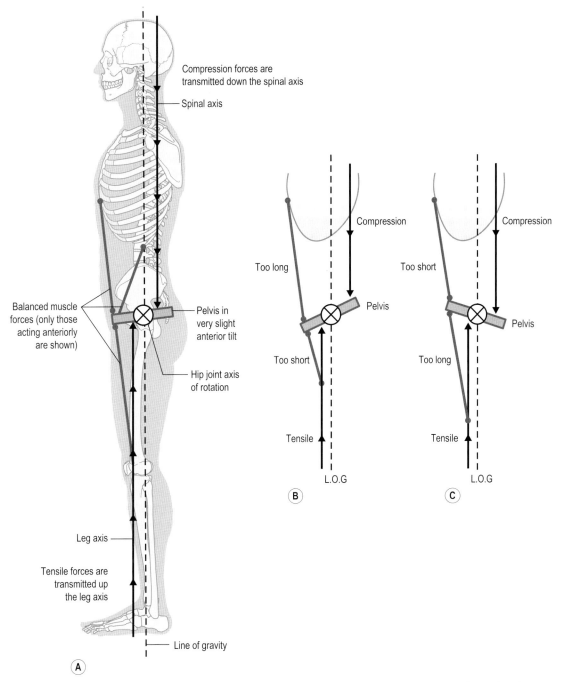

Fig 6.5 • The pelvic cantilever should swing freely between the spinal axis and the leg axis. (A) Imbalance in the tension elements disturbs equilibrium (B) and (C). Adapted from Todd 'The Thinking Body' with permission from Princeton Book Company.

Anteroposterior stability

The common patterns of response are:
• *The ankle strategy.* Here anteroposterior stability is regained by a sequential firing of the gastrosoleus, hamstrings, and finally the paraspinal muscles to return the body mass over the BOS. It is apparently most commonly used when perturbations to equilibrium are small and the support surface is firm.[75] Adequate

ankle mobility and strength is required for effective control.

• **The hip strategy.** This strategy controls motion of the centre of mass of the body by producing large and rapid motion at the hip joints with anti phase rotations at the ankles.[75] The hip strategy is used in response to larger faster perturbations, or when the support surface is compliant or smaller than the feet as when standing on a beam. Artificially increasing hip and trunk stiffness has shown reduced balance control and increased arm movements to regain stability.[76] Poorly integrated lumbopelvic–hip control including hip stiffness as well as hyperstability of the trunk through muscular 'holding' patterns will obviously jeopardize balance.[77]

• **The stepping strategy.** When the closed chain strategies are insufficient a step or a hop are used to return the BOS back under the centre of mass of the body. This may be a more common response in people with back pain – changing the BOS seems easier than resolving the perturbation through the body? (See Ch. 3.)

Researchers believe that in normal people, combinations of all three strategies are used in controlling sagittal displacements.[75] These anteroposterior responses are organized in a distal to proximal manner.

Mediolateral stability

Here control occurs primarily through the hip, pelvis and trunk as there is little mediolateral movement in the knee and ankle. Apparently these show a descending response organization, with head movements occurring first, followed by those in the hip and the ankle. Head movements occur in the opposite direction to those at the hip and ankle.[75] Of significance is the clinical observation that many with back pain have altered head control and ability to control lateral weight shift. Stability is therefore likely to be predictably compromised.

Spinal stability: examining proposed mechanisms which contribute control

It has been said that structures build their needs. However, the human spine is often seen to be a complex mechanical structure which is inherently unstable. This notion probably stems in part from early *in vitro* studies which found buckling occurred at fairly low forces. Related studies and Panjabi's influence,[78,79] has lead to the current concept of 'instability' and that the spine is 'not stiff enough'. In fact clinical practice and some of the recent research shows that parts of it at least, are 'too stiff'.

Gracovetsky[2] points out that 'it is not clear to what extent the hypotheses underlying these engineering 'stability' theories are appropriate for viscoelastic structures. Current concepts of musculoskeletal stability are developed without considering the advantages of being an unstable structure stabilized by a complex control system'. The process of our motor development ensures the necessary spectrum of patterns of neuromuscular control needed to serve its function.

Similarly, Todd[6] suggests that the living being maintains its stability because it is excitable and capable of modifying itself according to external stimuli and adjusting the response to the stimulation. Slight instability is the necessary condition for the true stability of the organism. Bond[40] suggests that if our perceptual orientation to our surroundings is insufficient, we compensate by stabilizing too much, the muscle contractions serving to diminish our dimensions making our bodies shorter, narrower flatter and effectively closing them. Movement has limited expression.

Various dynamic mechanisms are proposed to contribute to the spine's stability and function and are explored.

The intra-abdominal pressure mechanism (IAP)

This was first proposed by Bartelink[80] as a mechanism to protect the spine when lifting heavy loads. It is a 'high load' strategy. Utilizing a natural reflex response the Valsalva maneuver, intra-abdominal pressure can be voluntarily increased by vigorous contraction of the abdominal muscles against a closed glottis, creating a rigid vertical column of high pressure within the abdomen that pushes up against the diaphragm and down against the pelvic floor.[12] Acting as an inflated 'intra-abdominal balloon' this mechanism was proposed to support the spine from the front and partially reduce the demands on the lumbar extensor muscles and so lower the compression forces on the lumbar spine. However because strong abdominal activity creates a flexion torque on the spine, increased co-activity in the extensors is also necessary to counter this, creating overall increased myogenic compression and direct splinting on the lumbar spine. While a useful short term strategy to achieve postural stability and protect the spine against high loads, the vital function of respiration is sacrificed to it,[23] hence it becomes a problem if used long-term. Thompson[81] noted that global abdominal bracing may overcome pelvic floor activity causing the floor to descend. The realization that the generation of this mechanism as originally described, depended upon a strong/vigorous abdominal activation probably spawned some of the confused beliefs about the 'necessity for strong abdominals if you have back pain'.

A study by Marras and Mirka[82] found that IAP levels only significantly increased in response to significant trunk asymmetry, torque and velocity. The idea that stiffness equates to stability was further explored by Cholewicki et al.[83] who reported lumbar stability under sudden loading is augmented by voluntary increase in IAP plus increased coactivation of muscles belonging primarily to the more superficial system (SGMS). The pressure increase can only be optimal if there is sufficient coactivation of the diaphragm and pelvic floor. It is an example of a strong postural splinting role for the diaphragm and the pelvic floor. During the Valsalva, the glottis may be closed with the diaphragm in either the inspiratory (descended) position or expiratory (elevated). Hagins et al.[84] reported that during lifting, higher levels of IAP were reached by inhalation and holding the breath over natural breathing or holding in expiration.

It is important to recognize that in creating a 'rigid muscular cylinder', the spine is indeed 'stable' but the body constricted, compromising the free descent of the diaphragm and the important functions of breathing, continence and equilibrium.

The low load postural response model of IAP: a function of the SLMS

IAP is also elevated during many fairly ordinary everyday activities. Cresswell et al[85] found that in response to sudden unexpected and expected ventral and dorsal trunk perturbations, there was an automatic increase in IAP well in advance of the anticipated extensor torque production. Transversus abdominus was always the first muscle to be active in both expected and unexpected loading. They concluded that the increased IAP was part of a feed-forward postural response designed to improve trunk stability. The further work of Richardson Hodges et al[86,87] has helped provide increasing evidence about activity of certain muscles in the deep system (SLMS) and our understanding of possible mechanisms of spinal support and control in so called 'low load' states. Hodges has examined the postural support role of the diaphragm[88–91] and transversus abdominus in generating IAP.[92] Allison et al.[93] also found postural activity in the diaphragm. Similarly postural responses have been observed in the pelvic floor muscles.[94] In response to axial perturbation, co-activation between the diaphragm, transversus abdominus and the pelvic floor occur and raise IAP in the low load state as part of a feed-forward anticipatory postural control response.[92,95,96] Notably, these responses occurred both in inspiration and expiration. Hodges et al.[90] also artificially increased IAP by electrical stimulation of the diaphragm, without concurrent activity of the abdominal and back muscles, and demonstrated a trunk extensor moment the size of which was proportional to the increase in IAP, confirming the diaphragm's contribution to IAP and spinal stability. Hodges has been particularly interested in the role of transversus abdominus.[92] He describes its activity as 'reducing the circumference of the abdominal wall; flattening the abdominal wall in the lower region to increase IAP and tensioning the thoraco lumbar fascia; control of the abdominal contents and respiration'.[97] Its influence on segmental stability can only be in a general, non direction specific manner.[92] Rather than a torque producer, transversus 'is considered to have its major effects on lumbopelvic stability via increases in IAP and fascial tension and via compression of the sacroiliac joints and potentially the symphysis pubis'.[87] This author considers its role in pelvic control very significant. Hodges draws attention to the importance of coactivation of the diaphragm and pelvic floor accompanying transversus activation; otherwise there will be minimal effect upon the creation of IAP and fascial tension. This, he graphically represented by the 'abdominal canister' in Figure 6.6.

Also important is that the postural activity of transversus, diaphragm and pelvic floor muscles is also coordinated with their role in respiration. During quiet inspiration, the diaphragm and PFM concentrically contract in order to maintain the integrity of the continence mechanism against the

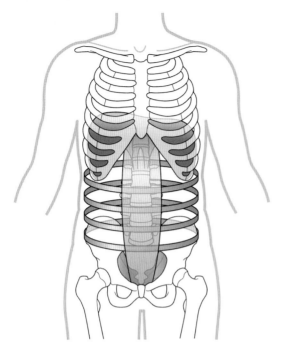

Fig 6.6 • The abdominal canister: The diaphragm, transversus abdominus muscle and pelvic floor muscles.

rise in IAP.[98] However, the inspiratory PFM activity may not be identified in all individuals, the tonic activity and passive tension in the floor being sufficient to meet the demands of IAP.[98] This PFM activity creates a slight sacro-coccygeal counter-nutation partly explaining the respiratory wave (p. 92, 108). While expiration is generally passive recoil during quiet breathing, the transversus is the first muscle recruited when expiratory flow or volume is increased.[99] When respiration is increased, IAP increases biphasically – on inspiration (as described above) and also on expiration associated with the contraction of the abdominal muscles, particularly transversus with coactivation again from the PFM to help increase IAP and elevate and lengthen the diaphragm.[98] Hence complex patterns of coordination between the diaphragm, PFM and transversus creates a modulated, oscillating concentric/eccentric interplay between them and varies according to demand. If one part of the synergy is inappropriately overactive or underactive, stability, respiration and continence will be compromised.

Hodges work demonstrates that rather than the magnitude of the response being important, it is this balanced co-activation and the early timing of IAP that is an important component in feed forward or anticipatory postural control of the spine. IAP, local muscle activity and fascial tension control vertebral movement without restricting overall movement.[98] Rather than maximal stability, dynamic control provides more optimal stability.

The breathing mechanism: the central role of the diaphragm in breathing and related postural support

Stability and control of the torso are inextricably linked with vertical posture and breathing.[1,6, 23,46,74] Breath is the most basic movement of life. Gravity is the most basic force.[100] Breath and posture influence one another. Both should be natural and effortless. This depends upon freedom and coordination of the muscles involved and no unnecessary antagonist activity. The breathing mechanism is highly sensitive to changes in the other body systems, readily reflecting the status of the psyche and the soma which includes the musculoskeletal and the internal organ/endocrine systems.

Breathing underlies the expression of us – it is the link between motion and emotion.[101] 'Breathing' is in general, poorly understood.

Normal quiet breathing at rest principally involves inspiratory activity of the diaphragm.[10] Expiration is considered to occur from the passive elastic recoil of the lungs and chest wall[97] the effects of gravity[16] and eccentric activity of the inspiratory muscles.[10,102] When the respiratory demand increases, so does the rate and depth of inspiration and expiration becomes an increasingly active component. When not exerted, the average normal breathing rate is between 10 and 14 breaths a minute.[110] Breathing rate and volume fluctuate in response to physical or emotional demands but normally return to relaxed patterns when the stimuli cease.[70] Breathing should occur through the nose which also has a facilitatory effect on the diaphragm.[102,110,111] The overall body posture and flexibility of the thoracic cage greatly affect the quality of breathing. According to Cumpelik,[103] establishing postural function is a prerequisite to addressing breathing function. If the posture is 'right' the breathing will follow.

The inspiratory muscles

The principal muscle is the diaphragm[10] aided by the external intercostals[16] and the parasternal intercostals.[104] Classified within the systemic local muscle system (SLMS) they are active at all intensities of breathing. As respiratory demand increases the *upper secondary accessory muscles of inspiration* become sequentially active – the scalenes; sternomastoid; upper trapezius, pectoralis major and minor; serratus posterior superior; superior fibres of iliocostalis; and if the upper limb is fixed or elevated, subclavius and omohyoid, the inferior fibres of serratus anterior; and the latissimus dorsi.[10,16,70] Additionally the longissimus and iliocostalis may work in synergy to extend the thoracic spine and facilitate a greater range of rib motion.[10] Note that practically all these muscles belong to the SGMS (see Ch.5). Architecturally, they are 'above' the diaphragm and assist in lifting the ribs.

The diaphragm needs stable points of attachment from which to work, and this is provided by the transversus, psoas and quadratus lumborum (as it anchors the 12th rib) and the levator ani and the coccygeus and the deep segmental extensors. It is suggested that collectively, these should be termed the *'lower primary accessory muscles of inspiration'*[6] as they form important stabilizing synergies of inferior support around the thoraco lumbar junction and lumbar spine and all share fascial connections or interdigitating fibres. Importantly they all belong to the SLMS and have an equally important postural role in supporting and adjusting the torso in response to the subtle oscillatory disturbances resulting from the breath through to the more overt dynamic adjustments. Allowing these oscillations to be reflected in the body promotes postural buoyancy and ease in movement. As these oscillations involve subtle weight shifts, the receptors in the soles of the feet are cyclically stimulated; refuelling the antigravity response which includes activation of the diaphragm[103] and so dynamic breathing and posture rhythms are set up.

The expiratory muscles

The primary muscles of active expiration are the internal intercostal muscles[16,104] and transversus thoracis.[12] As demand increases so does activity in the *lower secondary or accessory muscles of expiration*; the abdominals (transversus[10] internal and external obliques, rectus abdominis[16]); and muscles over the thoracolumbar region – the lower fibres of iliocostalis and longissimus; serratus posterior inferior and quadratus lumborum.[1] One can infer that it is the 'upper abdominals' rather than the 'lower abdominals' which are most dominantly active. The

combined muscle action around the inferior thoracic outlet strongly depresses the thoracic floor, deflates the rib cage, and narrows the diameter of the thoracic outlet. The same is involved in all expulsive acts (vomiting, coughing, sneezing etc.) as well as the Valsalva manoeuvre.[10] The central torso becomes cyclically constricted and hyperstabilized. Note that most belong to the SGMS. Spatially, they are all 'below' or lower than the diaphragm.

In summary, quiet breathing occurs because of contraction and relaxation of the diaphragm in the centre of the torso supported by appropriate SLMS activity. Of the abdominal muscles, transversus has the lowest threshold for respiratory activity.[98,99] As the respiratory demand increases so does the superficial SGMS activity above and below the diaphragm around the superior and inferior thoracic outlets in order to increase both inspiration and expiration and pump more air in and out (Fig. 6.7).

There are three primary breathing patterns[102]
- Abdominal – known also as diaphragmatic breathing. It represents the first stage of the diaphragm's activity (see p. 92). This is the most energy efficient taking up less than 5% of the body's energy to breathe. There is little or no movement of the chest at rest.
- Lateral costal breathing comes into play with increased air flow when singing or exercising etc. This represents the second stage of the diaphragm's activity. There is noticeable *lateral expansion* of the lower thorax through the 'bucket handle' action of the lower ribs.
- Apical or upper chest breathing – can take up to 30% of the body's energy as it involves a lot of secondary accessory muscle use. Here the chest expansion is more in an anteropostero direction due to the 'pump handle' action in the upper ribs.

These normal physiological responses are mixed and matched in all sorts of combinations with movement patterns appropriate to the functional task. All muscles of the body can assist in breathing when the need is great, but in the primary patterns of movement, the upper accessory muscles are the last to be called upon.

Diaphragm

The diaphragm is universally acknowledged as the prime muscle of inspiration, is responsible for about 70–80% of the work of inspiration.[12] It also provides support in postural control[89,105] (Fig. 6.8).

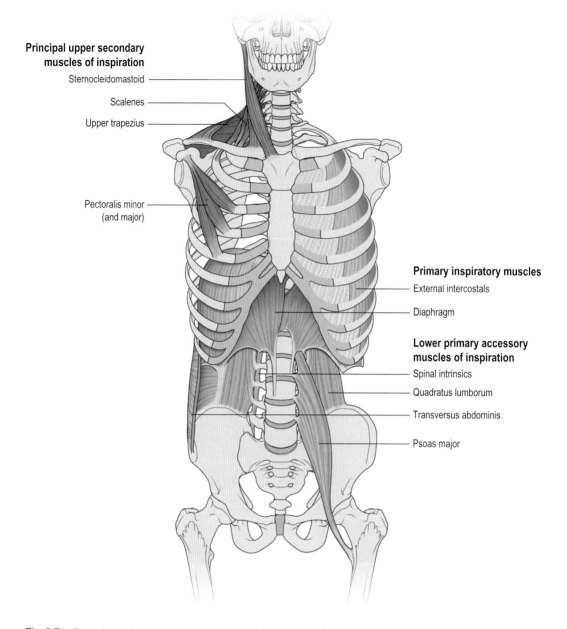

Principal upper secondary muscles of inspiration

Sternocleidomastoid

Scalenes

Upper trapezius

Pectoralis minor (and major)

Primary inspiratory muscles

External intercostals

Diaphragm

Lower primary accessory muscles of inspiration

Spinal intrinsics

Quadratus lumborum

Transversus abdominis

Psoas major

Fig 6.7 • The primary, lower primary accessory and upper secondary accessory muscles of inspiration.

Its anatomy and hence function are often difficult to grasp as it a three-dimensional musculofibrous sheet forming an irregular dome which separates the internal body space into two cavities. Its structure has been likened to a lopsided mushroom with its stem nearer to the back margin than the front[6]; the back of the irregular dome being more developed than the front.[106] The muscular fibres are on the periphery and arise from the circumference of the inferior thoracic outlet, the lumbar spine and related fascia and all converge to insert into a central sheet like tendon. The diaphragm's muscular fibres can be grouped into three parts based on their bony attachments:[10,12] sternal; costal and lumbar and have

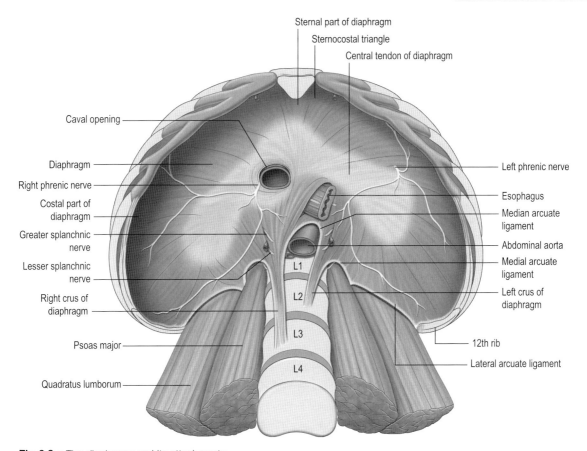

Sternal part of diaphragm
Sternocostal triangle
Central tendon of diaphragm

Caval opening

Diaphragm

Right phrenic nerve

Costal part of diaphragm

Greater splanchnic nerve

Lesser splanchnic nerve

Right crus of diaphragm

Psoas major

Quadratus lumborum

Left phrenic nerve

Esophagus

Median arcuate ligament

Abdominal aorta

Medial arcuate ligament

Left crus of diaphragm

12th rib

Lateral arcuate ligament

L1
L2
L3
L4

Fig 6.8 • The diaphragm and its attachments.

different lengths and directions and so the effects of their contractions differ.

Extending as high as the 7th rib and as low as L3, the diaphragm provides a lot of internal myofascial 'shoring up' over the thoracolumbar junction to help spread the load of the 'thoracic barrel' meeting the 'lumbar stem'. It significantly influences both static and dynamic function of the torso.

Its sole motor nerve supply is the phrenic nerve (C345), with sensory fibres coming from the lower six or seven intercostal nerves.[10] Any mechanical interference involving the nerve or its immediate relations throughout its course can influence the behavior of the diaphragm. Similarly, any acutely irritable joints between T7 and L3 can also significantly affect its function.

The intimate relationship and fascial continuity that the diaphragm enjoys with the transversus abdominus, psoas and quadratus lumborum implicate a close functional relationship between all of them in the mechanics of breathing as well as

postural control. Continuous fascial connections have also been described extending from the pelvic floor, up through the diaphragm, mediastinum up to the occiput.[70,100]

Its actions bear closer analysis. When the diaphragm contracts, it can move the tendinous central dome, the base of the rib cage, the lumbar spine or a combination of all three.[102] The costal fibres appear to play the prime role in expanding the rib cage[108] while the crural region probably provides more direct postural support through its attachment to the lumbar spine.[109] Clinically its overall action appears to lengthen the spine and 'open the centre' providing important *internal postural counter support* for the muscles of the torso. Essentially, contraction of the muscle fibres of the 'stem' and the 'rim', creates a piston like action where the musculotendinous sheet descends in the body cavity rather like the plunger in a coffee pot increasing the vertical, anteroposterior and particularly transverse diameter of the central body[16] while drawing air into the thoracic cavity. For clarity its action will be described as appearing to occur in two sequential stages. What is important to recognize is that the points of stability from which the various fibres can act change through the movement.[100]

• *First stage.* Provided that the spine and lower ribs are adequately stabilized, the crural, costal and sternal fibres contract and pull the dome towards the pelvis. This descent becomes checked by an increase in the IAP, the abdominal contents and abdominal muscle tone. This is often termed abdominal breathing and in recumbent postures when antigravity postural tone is less active, the abdomen more visibly distends. Excess or deficient abdominal activity compromises this action. When upright and moderately active the abdominals are constantly active in either concentric or eccentric mode. Thus, in stage one, the ribs and spine are stable and the abdomen moves as the diaphragm descends (Fig. 6.9).

• *Second stage.* The central tendon now rests on the abdominal contents 'held' there by continued activity in the crural fibres and counter pressure from the abdominal muscles.[23] Now it and the lumbar spine (stabilized by the lower lumbopelvic unit (LPU, see p. 110) both become the point of stable support. The ribs relinquish their support

role and instead are lifted and widened by the continuing contraction of the costal and sternal fibres. *The inferior thorax widens in the horizontal plane.* Importantly this normally includes posterior basal expansion and not just expansion forwards into the abdomen. Thus in second stage the ribs move, stabilized by the abdominal wall and a stable axial spine (Fig. 6.9). Clinically it is this second stage that patients find so difficult.

While the downward thrust of the diaphragm provides a beneficial pumping action to those organs within the peritoneum, those within the pelvic basin warrant protection. Newton[100] suggests this is achieved by biomechanics; the sum force of the diaphragm contraction pushes forward and down just below the navel, an area reinforced by the transversus abdominus. Provided that balanced neuromuscular control regulates the lumbopelvis around the 'neutral' position the pressure does not go directly into the pelvis but is shunted forward from the shape of the iliac bones. The pelvic floor muscles and obturator membrane help regulate pressure in the pelvic basin. If the lordosis is lost or the pelvis held too far back or forward, protection of the pelvic organs will be compromised.

The respiratory wave

In relaxed states, breathing ideally produces segmental movement throughout the axial spine including the pelvis. This movement can be seen when observing the prone subject. On inspiration movement commences at the sacrum, sequences through each segment and finishes at the base of the neck. However, Chaitow[70] remarks that more often than not, restricted spinal segments 'rise' simultaneously as a block, and movement of the spine occurs in two directions, caudally and cephalad from the blocked segments and often very little movement occurs above the T7/8 area.

Breathing is also reflected in movements of the pelvis (see respiratory mechanics of the pelvis). Breathing techniques can be utilized in treatment to assist in the release and reduction of activity levels of hyperactive muscles around the lower pole of the thorax and pelvic floor.

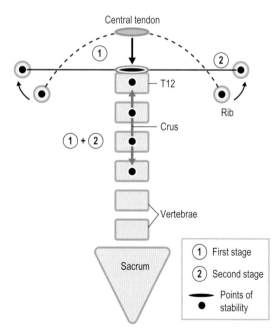

Fig 6.9 • Conceptual drawing of the apparent two stages of the diaphragm's action (CT: central tendon; C: crus; R: rib; V: vertebrae; S: sacrum).

The importance of expiration is frequently overlooked

Normally, expiration is 'passive', longer than inspiration, followed by a pause and is associated with parasympathetic activity and relaxation'[110,111] Most of us shorten this phase. At the end of expiration the diaphragm is elongated and the abdominals are in a reciprocally more shortened position. When respiratory demand increases, active expiration through abdominal activity becomes more predominant. In states of active expiration, we find the renewal of vigorous and deep inhalation. The abdominals eccentrically lengthen and the diaphragm descends. Todd [6] draws attention to the action and emergency state – jumping, fighting and so on. Here the lower primary and accessory inspiratory mechanism is also a substantial part of the power apparatus used for crouching and springing. This is reinforced by the muscles of the secondary expiratory mechanisms which increase their aid to the diaphragm and is exemplified in the judo shout, etc.

Breath holding and paradoxical breathing

When startled, frightened, or in response to 'shocks' and emotional upsets we reflexley hold our breath. We gasp, pull in the abdomen and breathe into the upper chest. There is a constriction around the centre body, the diaphragm cannot descend and the pelvic and vocal diaphragms also tighten.[112] This 'holding' can easily become a habit. Instead of the abdomen expanding with inspiration it retracts and is known as paradoxical breathing. The person becomes an upper chest breather. This is apparent when 'central cinch' behavior is operant (Ch.10).

Respiratory synkinesis

Described by Lewit,[23] respiratory synkinesis is the close association between respiration and the motor system in that certain movements are linked with inspiration or expiration. Locomotion and breathing develop together – inspiration is facilitatory, exhalation has an inhibitory effect on muscles. Breathing is automatically involved in embellishing movements of the torso. Looking up, reaching up, and trunk extension movements are associated with inspiration. Lengthening of the spine occurs in inspiration.[1] Looking down; trunk flexion movements and stooping are associated with expiration.

Lewit[23] also noted Skladal's observation that the diaphragm contracts when we stand on our toes, which led him to describe the 'diaphragm is a respiratory muscle with a postural function and the abdominal muscles are postural muscles with a respiratory function'. Janda knew of the strong functional relationship between the diaphragm and the

gastrosoleus.[113] In a MRI study, Cumpelik[103] has shown that the diaphragm reacts to changes in the posture of the head hands and feet. Activity of the diaphragm can be facilitated by activating reflex postural chain responses initiated from the hands and feet which also support and elongate the spine.

The most important thing to appreciate about the diaphragm is that it acts as a dynamic internal strut as it expands, widens and opens out the centre body from inside.

The construct of the 'body cylinder'

Todd[6] draws our attention to the principal units of body weight being the head, thorax and pelvis. She says:

The head is seen to be a trifle over a third of the breadth of the shoulders. The pelvis is approximately the width of the shoulders excluding the arms, and is as wide as the widest part of the rib cage. The three main spinal loads, heads chest and pelvis are of nearly the same diameter at their deepest points from front to back. This fact makes possible a flatter body wall both front to back than is usually imagined. If flat boards were placed at front and back so as to touch the head, chest and pelvis they could be kept approximately vertical and parallel.

At the base of each mass is a diaphragm, the vocal, abdominal and pelvic. If the 'blocks are stacked' such that the centre of mass of each unit is balanced in relation to the axis of gravity, there is minimal stress in the system. The diaphragms are in balanced relationship to one another like a series of stacked rings.

Conceptually, the torso excluding the head can be seen as a slightly irregular 'body cylinder'; the walls of which are flexible, maintained by a combination of spatially flexible bones, fascial sheets and balanced muscle activity. This principally occurs from the structural and functional integrity of the deep myofascial system (SLMS) and from the superficial SGMS as appropriate to maintaining its integral form in three dimensions[183] while at the same time allowing adaptable shaping in movement (Fig. 6.10). As it shifts, twists and distorts it remains 'open' in the centre. This requires balanced activity between the flexor and extensor muscle systems and the diaphragm. Proportional activity

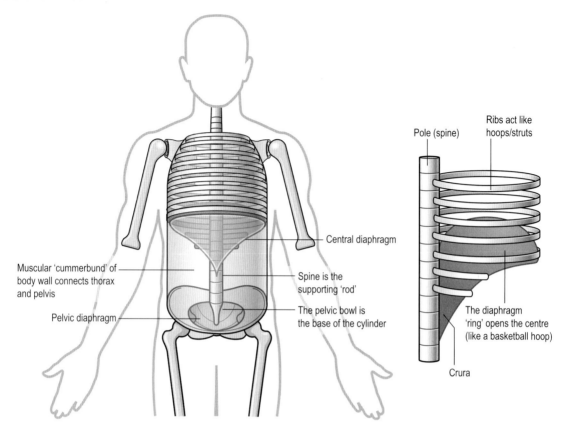

Fig 6.10 • Conceptual drawing of the 'body cylinder' – an idealized functional torso.

and correct timing of all muscles is important. The cylinder formed, has an internal cavity which houses the organ systems. These contain a lot of fluids and air. The diaphragm divides the cavity into caudal and cephalad chambers and regulates the pressures in both. These internal pressures (intra-abdominal and intra-thoracic) are important in helping create functional strength in the cylinder in much the same way that the carbonated gases inside a Coke® can stop it being crushed.[114] The maintenance of 'the line' and integrity of the body cylinder is important for correct functioning of the diaphragm in its crucial role in breathing and spinal support and control. Conversely, the diaphragm helps maintain the 'line' of the outer structure from its internal support. The body cylinder, with its base as the pelvis, the central support from the spine, cross bracing provided by the ribs; and its deep system myofascial geometry, begins to show some resemblance to a tensegrity structure. By nature, these are strong and light yet very flexible. They 'transmit loads through tension and compression only...there are no bending moments or shear'.[39] *The breath acts as the internal antagonist*, resisting the squeeze/collapse effect from activity of the 'outer musculature'. The head is an axial load centrally balanced and can be easily borne by an erect, curved and moving column'[6]... which contributes to the form of the 'body cylinder'. Control of the two proximal limb girdles contribute to the stability of the 'cylinder' centre. An important aspect is mutual function between the spinal flexors and extensors; between the abdominals and diaphragm to provide for their mutual stability; their combined activity in providing stability for psoas function;[115] and similarly balance between psoas and abdominals to provide stability for diaphragm function. When this occurs, the thoracolumbar junction including the crural arch is stabilized from deep SLMS control instead of by superficial holding patterns. This is dealt with more fully in Chapters 9 and 10.

The pelvis is the tilting platform which orients the body cylinder. Its optimal spatial arrangement facilitates the alignment of the body cylinder and optimal breathing. Effective lumbopelvic control afforded by SLMS activity in the lower pelvic unit ensures that the pelvis, the base of the cylinder can be controlled on the femoral heads and loads can be transferred through the pelvis from the legs to the trunk and vice versa. Antigravity support for the axial column comes from inside and below and not from tensioning the outer muscles, particularly those around the central torso and the upper body.

Integrated function in the SLMS helps support the diaphragm and resolve the problem of competition between its dual roles in respiration and postural control. The body wall is free to breathe in posture and movement. It is interesting to summarize the postural role of the diaphragm:

• Anterior support and stability of the lumbar spine
• Helping control the thorax on the lumbar spine
• Stabilizing the inferior thorax and the thoracolumbar junction so that the spine and ribs above are free to move
• Widening and holding open the inferior thorax – the diaphragm and abdominals provide mutual stability for each other
• Providing stability for the abdominals and psoas to act
• Contribution to the Valsalva and dealing with short term high loading.

If any of the 'blocks' are not centrally supported, an 'eccentric loading' situation is created in the spinal column, a problem dreaded by engineers for the imposed stresses this creates. Owing to the superincumbent mass of the thorax this is probable at the thoracolumbar junction and then the pelvis and thorax don't work in synchrony together. To counteract this, a combination of regional collapse and muscular holding patterns ensue with predictable consequences on postural and movement control breathing and balance (Fig. 6.11).

The three most basic functional patterns involve the pelvis orienting the body cylinder upright in hip extension; at right angles in hip flexion when sitting or in variable positions during forward bending. Standing and walking are predominantly hip extension patterns while sitting and bending/squat are predominantly hip flexion patterns (Fig. 6.12).

While all the structures contributing to the function of the body cylinder operate interdependently, the cylinder can be further conceptually viewed as consisting of upper and lower poles. The diaphragm,

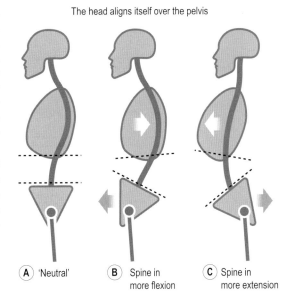

The head aligns itself over the pelvis

(A) 'Neutral'   (B) Spine in more flexion   (C) Spine in more extension

Fig 6.11 • Schematic play with altered alignment of the major body segments – the thorax and pelvis assume more oblique relationships (B) and (C).

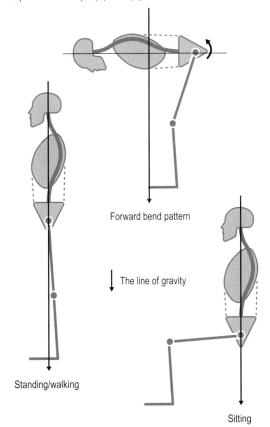

Forward bend pattern

↓ The line of gravity

Standing/walking

Sitting

Fig 6.12 • Schematic drawings of the primary posturomovement patterns which are principally sagitally oriented.

and its related function around the 'solar plexus', serves as a 'universal connecting principle' uniting upper and lower in integrated functional movement control of the whole body. Firstly the lower pole is explored.

Part B: The pelvic girdle

General features

The pelvis has the job of both balancing forces and providing movement. It is the power house of body movement, which derives from both the small movements within it and the movements of it as a whole, all of which play a decisive role for control of the legs and the spine. Continuing with the conceptual 'body cylinder', the pelvis is the base of the cylinder, a platform which orients the torso in its two principal functional alignments to gravity – vertical and through to horizontal when forward bending. It acts like a gimbal to balance the torso on the femoral heads when upright and swings and swivels on the femoral heads to initiate movements of the body cylinder into many permutations of forward, backwards and lateral bending. There is a close interrelationship between pelvic tilt, the degree of lumbar lordosis and hip position.[132] Movements of the pelvis are always closed chain, and simultaneously create corresponding forces and movements in the hips and lumbar spine which need to be managed. The architecture of the joints dictates that most movement should occur in the hip joint while the sacroiliac and lumbar spine movements are only small but need to be adequately controlled. Segmental responses can vary from minimal postural adjustments through to end range movements depending upon the particular action. The centre of gravity of the body lies within the pelvis[9,12,129] thus small alterations in its balance can have large ramifications throughout the body. Being able to control and move the pelvis around becomes a critical component of movement control of the axial spine and torso in general. Panjabi and White[116] have likened the forward bending spine to a cantilever bending load. To keep the stresses the same throughout the beam, the cross section of the beam must increase as the bending moment increases. This occurs through the lumbosacral spine. The maximum force requirement is at the fixed end of the cantilever. This can be equated to

the base of the body cylinder – the pelvis and its control both spatially and on the femoral heads become really important.

Biomechanical function

Consideration of the pelvis needs to include the hips as they are both biomechanically and functionally interlinked. The pelvis is like a rocking bridge. It marries a threefold function of bearing and transferring the weight of the upper body, moving and orienting the body on the legs and moving the legs on the body. Todd[6] suggests this is achieved through its arched structures. The pelvic bowl consisting of the sacrum and two innominates forms an arch which acts to distribute the body load. However functionally, this is in fact a double arch which behaves differently in super incumbent load transfer through the sacroiliac joints depending upon whether the person is sitting or standing.

• In standing: the forces are passed through the heavy lower parts of the ilia to the acetabulae where the head of the femur receives them and transmits them down the leg.

• In sitting: the weight, after passing into the ilia, travels through their heavy portions in line with the acetabulae, to the lowest point of the ischia, the tuberosities. Here the whole weight of the trunk is balanced.

• Considered from the ground up, the standing arch is the femoro-iliosacral; the sitting is the ischio-iliosacral.

• These two arches are the essential weight bearing portions of the pelvis and the sacrum is the keystone for both (Fig. 6.13).

Bracing the pelvic arches: re-examining the paradigm of sacroiliac stability

According to Todd,[6] for the pelvis to be balanced, the forces acting through the arches should relate in the same manner to the sacral keystone whether sitting or standing. The points of weight bearing, the ischia and acetabulae are vertically aligned. The superimposed weight of the trunk passes from the sacrum to the hip joint and tends to spread the arch. This 'is countered by the beam-action of the pubic structures upon the flaring sides of the ilia, and is

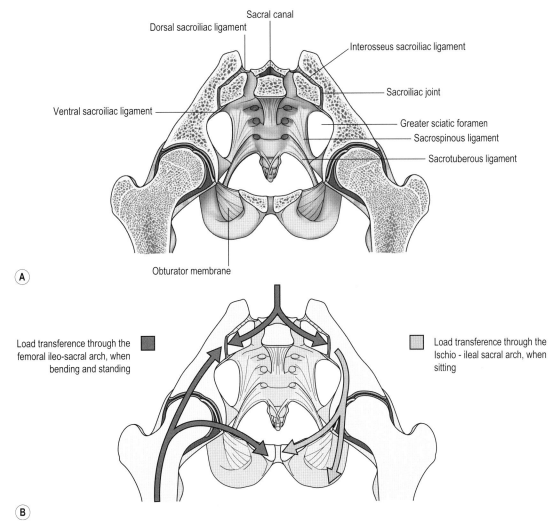

Fig 6.13 • The two pelvic arches are the essential weight bearing portions of the pelvis with the sacrum the keystone for both. Cross section through the pelvis hip in the frontal plane (A). Schematic view showing lines of force (B). Adapted from Sobotta[117], Kapandji[16] and Todd.[6]

reinforced by the tie muscles and ligaments inside the arch'.[6] Additionally, the femora act as buttresses to the ilia, which in turn buttress the key stone of the arch. The obliquity of the acetabular plane looks down, out and forward hence the thrust of the femoral head is backward in and upward.[132] The oblique lines of upward force directed up through the sacroiliac joint are tensile forces derived from the ligamentous myofascial system and meet and balance the downward compression force or weight coming through the joints of the spine and pelvis. Balanced neuromyofascial mechanisms orchestrated by appropriate activity and timing from groups of muscles and muscle systems become critically important in controlling the forces. Importantly, the bracing power of the femoral shafts is lost if the thrusts of the heads are too far forward as occurs when the hips are externally rotated. Here, the counter thrust to the body weight is no longer directed back towards the centre of the arch at the sacroiliac joint but forward and medially towards the pubic rami, increasing the tendency for the pelvic ring to spread at the sacroiliac joints[6] with associated compensatory movement at L5, generally into flexion. Todd says 'by use of tie muscles *within* (my italics) the pelvic arch, connecting lumbar vertebrae, sacrum, ilia and femora, we bind this arch together and only a slight effort is demanded to maintain the balance.[6]

Movements of the pelvis: important initiators of spinal alignment and movements

There is a void in kinematics and analytical data regarding pelvic postures and movements.[119] However, the pelvis *is* the base of support for the spine and so control of it is fundamental to all control of the lumbar spine and in many respects the spine as a whole.

Pelvic control can be distilled into:

- Intrapelvic movements occurring between the innominates and sacrum and
- Spatial movements of the pelvis as a whole.

The following impressions largely emanate from clinical practice with reference to available literature.

Intrapelvic movements

The joints within the pelvis are the sacroiliac, sacrococcygeal and the symphysis pubis. Frank movement at each joint is small. The sacroiliac joint is capable of 1–4° of angular movement and 1–3 mm of translation.[18,120] The sacroiliac junction contains the kidney shaped articulation of the joint proper, while caudally it continues as a syndesmosis[121,132] Steindler[132] describes the innominates and sacrum as fitting into the pelvic ring under considerable elastic resistance, resulting in a great amount of stored up latent energy. An intrinsic equilibrium exists between the tendency for elastic expansion of the bones which is checked by the opposing resistance of the articulation and of the syndesmosis of the ring. If this intrinsic equilibrium is destroyed by severing the pelvic ring at any point, e.g. by episiotomy or instability of the symphysis joint, its integral stability is lost. The warped surfaces of the sacroiliac joint allow the joint to exhibit a complex rotational movement not unlike the lumbar facet joints, the coupled motion of smaller magnitude, but greater force.[2] Functionally, Grieve[121] sees that the sacroiliac joint is incorporated into movement of the spine as a whole and shares in the maintenance of free motion from the occiput to the coccyx. Similarly, Gracovetsky considers we should see the spine as extending from the atlas to the acetabulum.[2] Restated, the sacrum/coccyx are important elements of the axial spine. The pelvic joints form

part of a closed system; movement at one joint affects the others and their combined movements afford strength yet pliability to the pelvis. Grieve[121] quotes a normal study on 144 male university students from 1936 which asserted that:

- In standing, with the exception of flexion and extension, all trunk motions are associated with unpaired, antagonistic movements of the innominates
- Rotation and lateral bending of the sacrum normally do not occur alone but as correlated motions that are coincidental to antagonistic movements of the innominates
- Positions of the innominates in normal standing as well as their relative mobility are affected by the dominant eye and hand.

The closed chain intrapelvic movements are fundamental to spatial control of the pelvis as a whole. They show distinct coupling patterns. To understand these, it is firstly useful to look at features of the two major composite bones involved:

The sacrum

Wedged between the two innominate bones, its principle movement is sagittal rocking as follows:

- **Nutation.** Where the coccyx at its tip moves back and up and the top of the sacrum known as the base moves forward and down. Importantly, this is associated with an increase in the lumbar lordosis and the close packed most stable position of the sacroiliac joint. Nutation, which tightens up most of the sacroiliac ligaments, occurs as a preparatory movement to prepare the pelvis for increased loading in weight bearing.[122] Lumbar multifidus and probably iliopsoas[123] directly influence this action with support from the lower pelvic unit (p. 110).

- **Counternutation.** The reverse movement where the tail bone or coccyx tucks under and the lumbar lordosis reduces. The sacroiliac joint is relatively 'gapped' and less stable. The pelvic floor muscles (PFM) and piriformis directly influence this action with synergistic activity from the hip external rotators – the obturator group and gluteus maximus. When lying supine the sacrum is passively counternutated.[18] On the pelvic aspect of the sacrospinous ligament[10] lies the coccygeus which is part of the PFM synergy which actively pulls the coccyx and sacral apex anteriorly into counternutation,[10,47]

• **Sacral torsion.** The sacrum can also rotate about an oblique or diagonal axis within the constraints of the facets of the sacroiliac joint. According to Gracovetsky,[2] these axes pass diagonally through S1 and S3 and the determination of which is in contact depends upon the lordosis. Sagittal rotation of one innominate will pull the sacrum into torsion, particularly if rotation of the other innominate is in the opposite direction. Sacral torsion is part of 'distorsion' in the pelvic ring (see p. 103). While not large movements, nutation and torsion of the sacrum are functionally important and necessary for the effective triplanar swivel action of L5/S1, (the level of the greatest rotation in the lumbar spine[5]) and further reflected in the kinematics through the rest of the lumbar spine.[120]

Innominate

The innominate consists of three fused sections, the ileum, ischium and pubis. It is irregularly shaped, constricted in the middle and expanded above and below. The acetabular cavity on the lateral surface is approximately inferior to midway between the upper and lower sections. From and through this, the pelvis swivels in multiple planes on the femoral heads (Fig. 6.14).

Several important features about the innominates are worth considering:
• The warped shape of the innominates means that rotation in one plane imparts conjunct rotations in the other planes. Conceptually the innominates have been likened to twisted discs,[17] a useful analogy in appreciating their movement capabilities (Fig. 6.15.a)
• In the sagittal plane their anterior rotation about the femoral head brings the ischium back and the front of the iliac crest forward producing anterior pelvic rotation. The reverse occurs in posterior rotation (Fig. 6.15.b).
• In the frontal plane, their contribution to forming the pelvic ring limits their range of rotation compared with sagittal plane movement however importantly the superior (ilia) and inferior (ischia) poles slightly flare in and out. Slight ischial outflare is associated with anterior sagittal rotation or tilt and ischial inflare with posterior rotation or tilt (Fig. 6.15.c).
• The inner surfaces of the innominates contribute largely to the two pelvic 'bowls' – the 'superior pelvic bowl' formed by the two iliac fossae and sacral base, and the deeper 'inferior pelvic bowl' formed by the lower part of the sacrum, coccyx

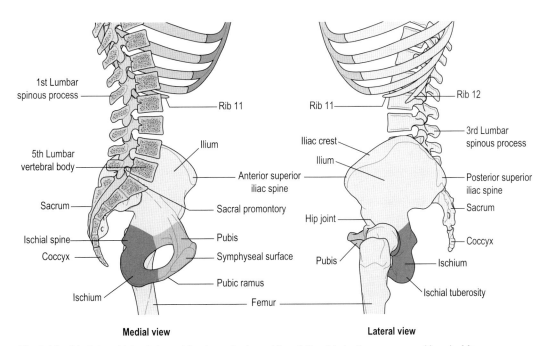

Medial view   **Lateral view**

Fig 6.14 • Medial and lateral view of the innominate and its relationship to the sacrum and head of femur.

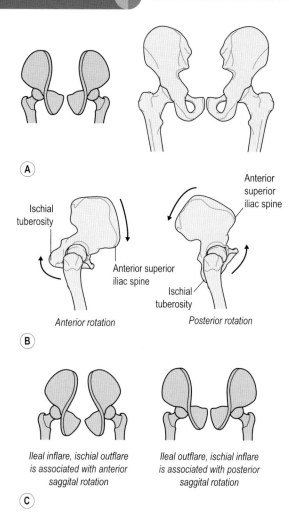

Ⓐ

Ischial
tuberosity

Anterior
superior
iliac spine

Anterior superior
iliac spine

Ischial
tuberosity

Anterior rotation

Posterior rotation

Ⓑ

*Ileal inflare, ischial outflare
is associated with anterior
saggital rotation*

*Ileal outflare, ischial inflare
is associated with posterior
saggital rotation*

Ⓒ

Fig 6.15 • Innominates as twisted discs (adapted from Franklin[17]) in neutral (A) and showing sagittal (B) and frontal plane movements (C).

pubic rami, obturator foramina, ischia and pelvic floor. Narrowing of one 'bowl' serves to widen the other and vice versa. The joints of the upper bowl are the SIJ 'proper' and symphysis pubis; the 'joint' of the lower bowl is the syndesmosis formed by the pelvic floor and the strong sacrospinous and sacrotuberous ligaments which counter excess nutation of the sacrum. The shape, length tension relationships and integrity of this syndesmosis is also affected by hip myomechanics. If the inferior syndesmosis is tight it will hold the sacrum counternutated and directly affect the stability and function in the SIJ (Fig. 6.16).

• The pubic symphysis, pubic and ischial rami and ischial tuberosities of the innominates and the

coccyx form the bony boundaries of the roughly diamond shaped inferior pelvic opening (Fig. 6.17).

• Movements of the innominates occur during both closed chain and open chain movements of the hip. Both are functionally very important yet generally poorly controlled, in particular anterior rotation in the sagittal plane.

Movements of the innominate in closed chain movements of the hip

These can be felt if you lie down on the ground on your back with knees bent and feet on the floor. Place your finger tips on the anterior iliac crests. Locate the sit bones and 'think' the movements *from* here. Imagining the innominates like wheels is helpful:[17]

• Sagittal rotation of the pelvis in supine:
  • *Anterior pelvic rotation.* When the sit bones drop back down towards the floor, the anterior iliac spines correspondingly move forward. This is anterior pelvic tilt or closed chain hip flexion.
  • *Posterior pelvic rotation.* When the sit bones lift, the anterior iliac spines correspondingly move back. This is posterior pelvic tilt or closed chain hip extension.

• Frontal plane rotation – Inflare/outflare of the innominates. Through rotation of the acetabulum around the femoral head in the frontal plane, the ischia can move closer together = 'inflare'; or further

Superior/upper bowl

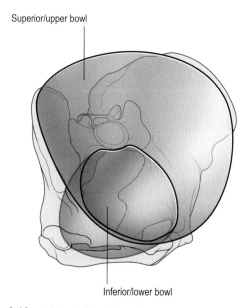

Inferior/lower bowl

Fig 6.16 • Inferior & Superior pelvic 'Bowls'.

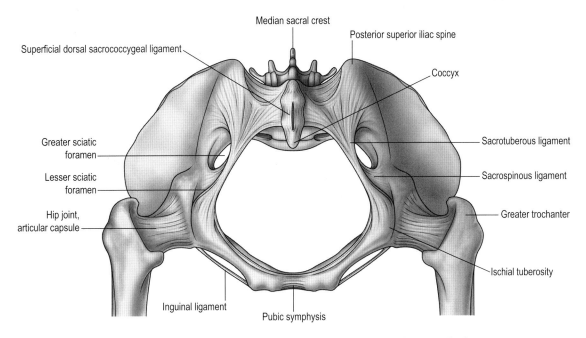

Superficial dorsal sacrococcygeal ligament

Median sacral crest

Posterior superior iliac spine

Coccyx

Greater sciatic foramen

Sacrotuberous ligament

Lesser sciatic foramen

Sacrospinous ligament

Hip joint, articular capsule

Greater trochanter

Ischial tuberosity

Inguinal ligament

Pubic symphysis

Fig 6.17 • The inferior pelvic opening viewed from behind/below with the pelvis flexed 90 ° on the femur.

apart = 'outflare'. When the ischia move 'in' the ilia correspondingly move 'out' as is shown in Fig. 6.15 and vice versa. Movement of the ischia will be used as the reference point. The innominate movements carry the sacrum with them in various ways.

The fundamental pelvic patterns

There are palpable and observable distinct patterns of kinematic coupling during sagittal closed chain pelvis on femur movements. The fundamental pelvic patterns are physiological movements which are basic to achieving modulated posturomovement control of the pelvis in space and on the legs and control of the lumbar lordosis.

First fundamental pelvic pattern (FPP1)

This involves anterior pelvic tilt and ischial outflare. When the ischia widen or move apart associated actions also occur:

• The ilia draw together in the front and anteriorly rotate in the sagittal plane. The superior pelvic bowl narrows.

• The sacrum nutates and the coccyx moves away from the symphysis pubis as it 'comes out for air'.

• The dimensions of the inferior pelvic bowl and the pelvic floor enlarge as it 'opens' (Fig. 6.20.b).

• The lumbar lordosis increases as the spine moves into extension.

• The hips move into relative flexion.

• This pattern is fundamental to any movement which requires flexing or bending *at* the hips e.g. sitting or bending forward in standing.

• This pattern is principally achieved from synergistic concentric activity of the 'lower' transversus abdominis, iliacus, and multifidus with eccentric control from the pelvic floor muscles and the obturator group. Activating the 'superior/upper pelvic bowl' serves to narrow this and open the inferior pelvic bowl'. Studies have shown that transversus activity is greater when the pelvis is neutral or in anterior pelvic tilt.[87,98] This 'squeeze' action of transversus with iliacus is important in providing pelvic stability during closed chain hip flexion loading patterns (Fig. 6.18).

• This pattern underlies control of all hip flexion movements such as sitting, sitting to stand and return, forward bending and squatting.

• Clinically, it is almost a universal finding that most people have little idea or ability to perform this action which is so fundamental to myo articular function of the lumbopelvic region. Instead they attempt the movement as Bartenieff noted 'three storeys too high'[28] from inappropriate SGMS activity around the thoracolumbar region.

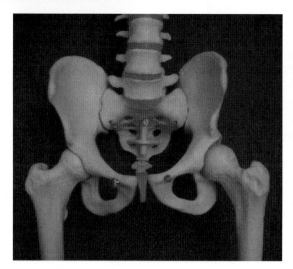

Fig 6.18 • Ischial outflare: note the 'drawing in' of the superior bowl.

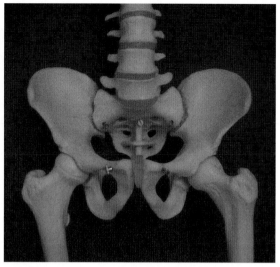

Fig 6.19 • The ischial inflare: note the flaring of the superior bowl.

Second fundamental pelvic pattern (FPP2)

FPP2 involves posterior pelvic tilt with ischial inflare. When the ischia move towards one another the following also occurs:

• The ilia not only spread apart but they also posteriorly rotate. The superior pelvic bowl 'opens' more.

• The sacrum counternutates and the coccyx moves closer to the symphysis pubis. The tail bone is 'tucked under'.

• The dimensions of the inferior bowl and pelvic floor or pelvic diaphragm become smaller – the lower pelvic bowl 'closes' (Fig. 6.20c).

• The lumbar spine moves into relative flexion.

• The hips move into relative extension.

• This pattern is fundamental to any movement requiring opening and extending *at* the hips e.g. sitting to stand; backward bending in standing.

• Ischial inflare is principally achieved from concentric action of the pelvic floor muscles, the obturator group with piriformis and even gluteus maximus with eccentric control from iliacus and transversus. Activating the lower pelvic bowl opens the upper bowl (Fig. 6.19). Bendová et al.[124] electrically stimulated the right sided pelvic floor muscles and demonstrated medial tilting (ischial inflare) and posterior rotation of the right innominate (and posterior rotation also of the left innominate). The coccyx moved ventrocaudally.

• Clinically, this pattern can usually be more easily performed by most people, as they habitually collapse in sitting and then carry the pattern forward when standing. Here they shift their pelvis forward using the hamstrings, passively 'hang' on their iliofemoral ligaments and 'hold' with the obturator group while the rest of the SLMS is relatively inactive. It is also seen in those who are 'butt grippers'.[18] Intrinsic activity is usually reduced.

• Control of this pattern underlies control of closed chain hip extension allowing us to move through postural transitions and be upright FPP1 and FPP2 *underlie all sagittal flexion and extension movements of the torso* over the legs.

Third fundamental pelvic pattern (FPP3)

FPP3 involves combined elements of FPP1 and FPP2, hence is reliant upon adequate control of these. The sagittal rotation of the innominates in opposite directions carries the sacrum into torsion. The pelvic ring or whole pelvis is in 'distorsion'.

To clarify this, sagittal rotation of one innominate creates a twist or torsion at the sacroiliac joint and the whole pelvic ring, which is greater if the other innominate is rotating in the opposite direction, e.g. if the right ileum is anteriorly rotating the top of the sacrum is carried forward with it into nutation and also twists about an oblique axis. The joints of the right lumbosacral junction move into a 'closing'

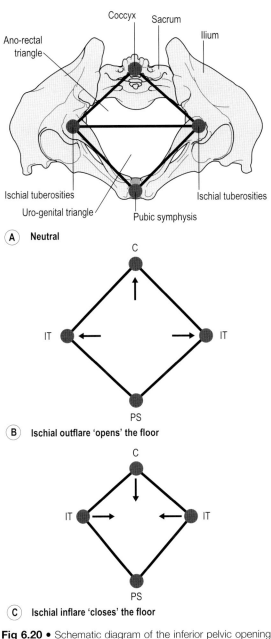

(A) Neutral

(B) Ischial outflare 'opens' the floor

(C) Ischial inflare 'closes' the floor

Fig 6.20 • Schematic diagram of the inferior pelvic opening in the neutral (A), open (B) and closed positions (C).

FPP3 *essentially underlies all weight shift and rotation through the pelvis* hence it is an important component in unilateral weight bearing, walking and balance. **'Distorsion'** The ability of the pelvic ring to sinuously distort in three planes/dimensions while maintaining its stable integrity yet facilitating hip and spinal movements is important in allowing the flexible and adaptable transmission of the movement wave and loading to proceed *through* the pelvis – both from the upper to lower body and vice versa. Contrarotation of the innominate bones carries the sacrum into torsion and occurs in most activities except pure spinal flexion and extension.[120] A force dependent oblique axis of sacral rotation is formed by the complex rotational movement between the facets of S1 and the contralateral S3.[2,147] The innominates and sacrum must be free enough to oscillate back and forth in this twisting movement so that the rotary movement wave can be transferred and dissipated through the pelvis from and to the hips. If not, the low/mid lumbar spine levels are forced to compensate.

Gracovetsky[3] has drawn attention to the importance of the lumbar lordosis (and by association, sacral nutation) in effecting axial torque through the spine in walking. Intrapelvic torsion or 'distorsion' and rotation of the whole pelvis in the transverse plane is a significant driver of axial rotation about a longitudinal axis, both important in walking, for example, and those more strenuous rotational activities such as tennis or golf. Distorsion allows

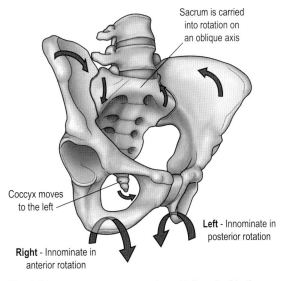

Fig 6.21 • Schematic interpretation of 'distorsion' in the pelvic ring.

pattern – extension/side bending/rotation, while those on the left are relatively 'open – flexed, side bent and rotated in the opposite direction – particularly if the left innominate is posteriorly rotating. This includes the right ischium abducting (outflare) and the left adducting (inflare) in the example above. The whole pelvic ring while stable, is distorted which we have termed 'distorsion' (Fig. 6.21).

the sacrum to 'rock n roll' and twist initiating axial rotation from the base. Problems arise when distorsion is reduced or becomes fixed in one direction. Contraction of one piriformis will bring the sacrum into torsion[134] and counternutation. Unilateral electrostimulation of the pelvic floor muscles simulating unequal activity and tension between sides has demonstrated distorsion in the pelvic ring.[124]

'Distorsion' is also involved in many lower limb movements and related change of postures, e.g. side sitting and moving to all fours and to standing. Distorsion is also required in large full range open chain movements of the hips – for example, anterior rotation of the innominate is coupled with hip extension and if the opposite is flexed, that innominate moves into posterior rotation. Inadequate control of 'distorsion' through the pelvis instead ends up shunting the movement into the lumbar spine and is a cause of much low back pain and self inflicted back problems through poor stretching and exercise programs.

Movements of the innominate in open chain movements of the hip

The rotation of the innominate in open chain hip movement is in the opposite direction to that in closed chain movements of the hip. These innominate movements serve to augment and increase the available range of the hip during 'free' hip movement. They come into play later in the range of hip movement when capsular and related hip structures become taught. Hence 'open' hip flexion is associated with posterior rotation of the innominate (while in 'closed chain hip flexion the innominate anteriorly rotates). Standing hip flexion towards 90° involves a posterior rotation of the innominate relative to the sacrum. Hungerford and Gilleard,[125,126] found that in control subjects this occurred on average around 73° of hip flexion. This is also known as the standing stork or Gillet test.[18,128]

Increasing the pelvic motion on the standing leg can be employed to functionally increase hip range of movement in the moving leg. For example, experienced dancers tend to use more anterior and posterior pelvic tilt, rather than hip flexion and extension, in order to increase the gesture leg height.[127]

However those who have posterior hip stiffness and/or habitually poor and compromised pelvic motor control will expectedly posteriorly rotate the innominate earlier in range during 'open' hip flexion. Habitual weight bearing in posterior pelvic

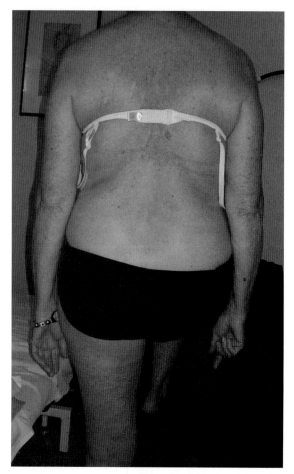

Fig 6.22 • Poor control of open chain hip flexion with posterior rotation of the whole pelvis and reduced frontal plane control.

rotation and reduced intrapelvic motion means that this posterior rotation occurs in the whole pelvis as it moves 'en bloc' (Fig. 6.22). This is common and pulls the lumbar spine into early and excess flexion and rotation to compensate with predictable effects on the tissues over time. Poorly designed exercise protocols which advocate 'knee to chest' without regard to the hip pelvis dynamic, compound the problem.

Lee[18] proposes that 'in health' open chain or free hip extension is associated by the innominate anteriorly rotating, a pattern that this author agrees with as it is readily confirmed clinically (Fig. 6.23). Again this is the reverse pattern of innominate rotation to that seen in the closed chain scenario. The presence of associated frontal plane innominate movements in open chain hip movements is unclear both clinically and in studies.[18] Generally most people, 'patients' or otherwise, display faulty open chain hip flexion and extension.

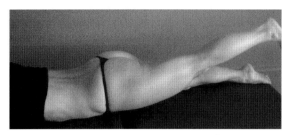

Fig 6.23 • Open chain hip extension with ipsilateral anterior pelvic rotation.

Spatial pelvic movements

These constitute movements of the pelvis as a whole while also controlling intrapelvic forces and movements, particularly during weight shift. They differ according to whether the weight bearing occurs through the femoral heads as in standing or kneeling; or through the ischia as in sitting.

Standing spatial control

Standing spatial control of the pelvis is achieved by spatial shifts and related rotations at the hip joint which serve to balance and tilt it on the femoral heads. Movements vary from slight postural adjustments in order to achieve a dynamic upright equilibrium through to large movements of the body. Due to the spherical ball and socket of the hip, three-dimensional, multiplanar movements are available; however, they will be considered within the three principal conceptual movement planes despite the fact that functional movement is rarely 'pure plane'. The magnitude of movements is far greater in the sagittal plane than in the other two planes. Their significance and the need for greater control are apparent when standing on, or mostly on one leg.

- *Sagittal plane.* The pelvis can shift forwards and backwards in space. This is coupled with a corresponding rotation on the femoral heads and consequent change in the alignment of the lumbar curve and sagittal hip position as follows:
  - Anterior shift is coupled with posterior rotation of the pelvis on the femoral heads and creates associated hip extension and relative lumbar flexion. It is dependent upon FPP2. This anterior shift pattern of movement is also used to initiate hip extension and trunk extension from forward bending[18,128] and other movements related to this pattern.

- Posterior shift is coupled with anterior rotation of the pelvis on the femoral heads, and creates associated hip flexion and lumbar extension. It is dependent upon FPP1. In movement this posterior shift pattern is used to initiate hip flexion/trunk forward bending[18,128] and other movements related to this pattern (Fig. 6.24a).[18,128]

- *Frontal plane.* The pelvis can shift to either side and is again coupled with rotation on the femoral heads and associated changes in the alignment of the hip and lumbar spine. If standing on two legs, and the pelvis shifts to the right, the pelvis assumes an oblique position, in this case higher on the right.[23,129] There is relative adduction of the right hip, abduction of the left and the lumbar spine assumes a relative right side bending alignment[129] and compensatory adaptations will occur through the spine. It is a common habit for people to shift their pelvis laterally and take the weight more on one leg and 'hang' with the weight-bearing hip in passive adduction – the SLMS is switched off! (Figs. 6.24b; 8.5.)
  - Standing on one leg is a revealing test. This is also known as the Gillet, stork or kinetic test.[18] If there is adequate control the 'neutral' pelvic position is maintained in the frontal and other two planes. In fact, there is a slight lift of the pelvis on the non weight bearing side and adjustment through the spine in the frontal plane (Fig. 6.24b). If control is inadequate, the pelvis either drops on the non-weight bearing side or the person leans the trunk over the standing leg, known as the Trendelenberg sign.[12] Both compensations create ipsilateral side flexion in the lumbar spine with potential consequences. The ability to spatially shift and control the pelvis medially under the trunk is a fundamentally important action in being able to control the lumbar spine in a reasonably neutral position during lateral weight transfer of the body over the standing leg. By our observations, this aligning of the axial spine over the weight bearing limb with a stable pelvis is principally achieved through inner support from the lower pelvic unit synergy (p. 110) providing stability for activity in the large SGMS pelvifemoral muscles – the adductors, hamstrings and glutei (see p. 119).

- *Horizontal plane.* Gracovetsky[3] draws attention to the importance of pelvic rotation in the horizontal plane in human gait. Rather than the legs

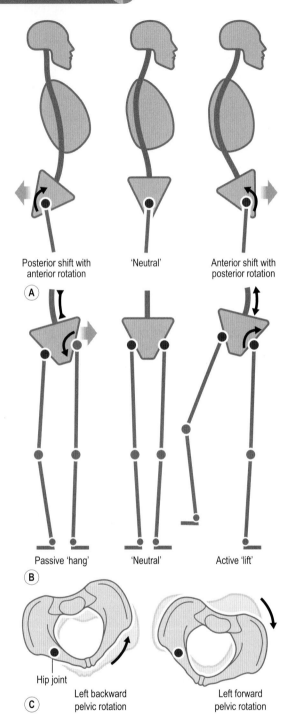

Posterior shift with anterior rotation   'Neutral'   Anterior shift with posterior rotation

(A)

Passive 'hang'   'Neutral'   Active 'lift'

(B)

Hip joint

Left backward pelvic rotation   Left forward pelvic rotation

(C)

Fig 6.24 • Triplanar spatial pelvic shifts and related rotations in the sagittal (A), frontal (B) and horizontal planes (C).

rotating the pelvis and carrying the 'passenger trunk' he considers that it is the spine that drives the pelvis to rotate. This author proposes that the *pelvis itself* is able to initiate horizontal plane rotation

which is part of 'distorsion' and closed chain hip rotation and also drives the spinal rotation. This was in fact shown by Gracovetsky: it is possible to 'walk' without legs by the ischia alternately advancing.[3] This is achieved through active control of 'distorsion' the pelvis can rotate in the transverse plane on the hips and the sacral torsion drives the spinal rotation. This movement can also be seen in sitting – weight bearing through one ischium, the other can be advanced back and forward to produce backward and forward pelvic rotation respectively. A 'stable' spine and leg allows the lower pelvic unit and abdominal and extensor system muscle synergies to create this rotation. Backward and forward pelvic rotation in the horizontal plane is the postural precursor to axial rotation needed in the body. This is an important movement as rotation in the lumbar spine itself is limited. This axial pelvic rotation is associated with movements in the hips but to a lesser degree in the lumbar spine. A reduced lordosis makes transverse plane pelvic rotation more difficult.[130] According to Gracovetsky, those muscles which operate more or less in the transverse plane – the obturator group including pyriformis and the lower fibres of gluteus maximus could conceivably axially rotate the pelvis.[131]

- Forward pelvic rotation creates ipsilateral external hip rotation relative extension and abduction and contralateral hip internal rotation.[132]
- Backward pelvic rotation creates ipsilateral internal hip rotation relative flexion and adduction and contralateral external hip rotation[132] (Fig. 6.24c).

Walking is a combination of controlling subtle multiplanar combinations of pelvic tilting and shifting. A reduction in the rotary range and control of the hips will reduce the transverse plane pelvic rotation with predictable effects through the kinetic system.

Sitting spatial control

The weight is taken through the ischia and thighs. Here the principal movement is tilting with shifting less prevalent. Sagittal tilting of the pelvis is the most dominant movement with lateral tilting and axial rotation less so though still important. Freedom to move around on the 'sit bones' is critical for spinal health. These tilts and to a lesser extent shifts, are all very important in initiating weight shift in sitting and moving from sitting to stand and are instigated through the lower pelvic unit synergy.

Sagittal plane weight shift occurs through rocking forward and back on the ischia as the acetabulae rotate on the stationary femoral heads. This creates a contra-directional lumbar rhythm[12] which is not obligatory.

• *Anterior pelvic tilt* creates hip flexion with related lumbar extension however flexion is also possible as seen at the end of range when bending forward in sitting. Transversus abdominus and the pelvic floor muscles are more active when the spine is extended.[141] Multifidus is most active when the low lumbar lordosis posture is adopted[133] (Fig. 6.25).

• *Posterior pelvic tilt* creates relative hip extension, lumbar flexion. In combination with shifting their pelvis forward in the seat, it is almost universally common habit for people to passively adopt this pattern when sitting with unfortunate long term sequelae on their tissues – a potent propagating factor in the genesis of low back pain.

• *Frontal plane or lateral tilting* of the pelvis occurs when weight is shifted laterally over one ischium, the acetabulum rolling up and over the femoral head. The base of support for the torso is one ischium and if the movement continues further as in reaching to the side, may result in the femur becoming the base of support (Fig. 6.26). Note the oblique slope of the pelvis (pants line) and that the axial spine adjusts by laterally elongating.

• *Horizontal plane movement* involves unweighting one ischium as above and moving it either forward or back in sagittal rotation creating 'distorsion' and initiating trunk rotation to orient the spine head or upper limbs (Fig. 6.27).

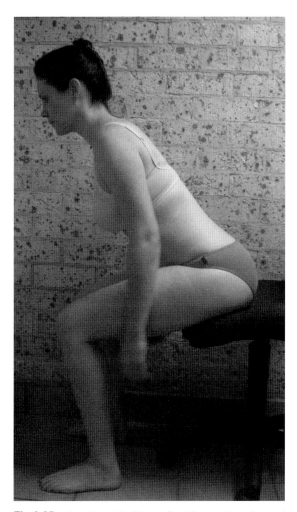

Fig 6.25 • Anterior pelvic tilt on a fixed femur allows forward weight shift of the body.

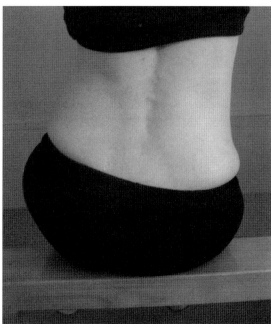

Fig 6.26 • Lateral weight shift initiated from the ischia. Note the elongation of the trunk on the weight bearing side.

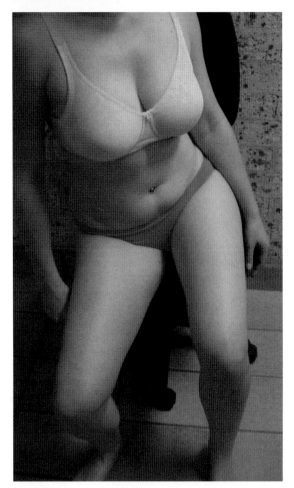

Fig 6.27 • 'Distorsion' in sitting. Note the position of the femur and the trunk rotation.

Respiratory mechanics in the pelvis

The breath creates a movement wave in the spine with a consequent oscillation of the pelvis on the femoral heads which varies according to the posture. Clinically during deep inhalation in the prone or side lying position, the sacrum and ilia posteriorly rotate[134] – the sacrum counternutates. The sacral excursion is deemed to be about 3 mm more than that of the ilia.[134] This is no doubt due to the demonstrated coactivation between the diaphragm and the PFM.[92,95] Rock maintains that during inspiration the PFM activity is an eccentric contraction.[20] In the supine 'crook' position, the sacrum is already counternutated[18] and the pelvis can be felt

or observed to anteriorly rotate on inspiration.[112] Muscular holding patterns in the pelvic floor or buttocks will damp the response. Functional movement control of the pelvis requires adaptable control independent of the breathing cycle. The respiratory mechanics of the pelvis can be utilized in manual treatment of the pelvis.

The pelvic floor or diaphragm

The boundaries of the diamond or somewhat trapezoidal shaped inferior pelvic outlet are formed by the symphysis pubis in front, the coccyx behind, on each side the inferior pubic ramus and the ramus of the ischium, the ischial tuberosity and the sacrotuberous ligament.[10] An imaginary line drawn transversely in front of the ischial tuberosities divides the region into two triangular parts. The posterior part contains the anus and is known as 'the anal triangle', while the anterior part is the 'urogenital triangle' containing the external urogenital organs (Fig. 6.20).

The pelvic diaphragm or floor is a myofascial hammock which spans the inferior opening (Fig. 6.28). It is composed of the composite levator ani and the coccygeus,[10,135] collectively known as the pelvic floor muscles (PFM).

• The levator ani forms the greater part of the floor and morphologically can be divided into:
  • Pubococcygeus (from the pubis and anterior obturator fascia to the coccyx)
  • Iliococcygeus (from the ischial spine to the coccyx).
• The coccygeus is posterosuperior to but in the same tissue plane as levator ani. It is a triangular sheet of muscle arising by its apex from the pelvic surface of the ischial spine and sacrospinous ligament and attached at its base to the margin of the coccyx and the 5th sacral segment.[10]

The coccygeus, levators ani and piriformes act in synergy to close the posterior triangle of the pelvic outlet[10] (Fig. 6.20).

The functions of the pelvic floor have been described as supportive counteracting the effects of gravity and intra-abdominal pressure; sphincteric, aiding closure of the anus vagina and urethra; and dilative during birth.[136]

The synergistic role the PFM share with the diaphragm and transversus is an important one for both the generation of IAP and also in respiration, particularly in cases of respiratory challenge.[98]

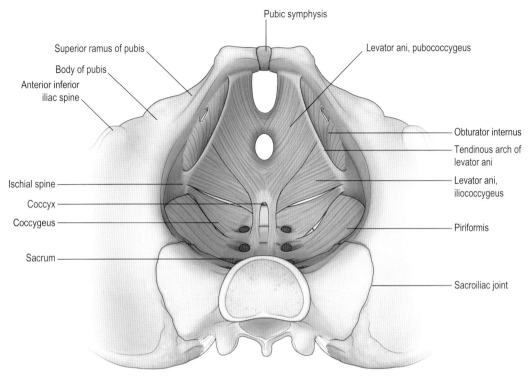

Fig 6.28 • The muscles composing the pelvic floor viewed from above.

Labels: Pubic symphysis, Superior ramus of pubis, Body of pubis, Anterior inferior iliac spine, Ischial spine, Coccyx, Coccygeus, Sacrum, Levator ani, pubococcygeus, Obturator internus, Tendinous arch of levator ani, Levator ani, iliococcygeus, Piriformis, Sacroiliac joint

Importantly, the PFM also perform an important dynamic role in helping modulate intrapelvic kinematics[124,137], to support posturomovement control of the spine and hips. They exert a powerful influence upon sacro-coccygeal mobility as well as longitudinal fascial and craniosacral mobility.[47] A predominance of type 1 fibres is indicative of their functional role in postural support. Perturbation studies of the spine show that the pelvic floor is pre-activated as part of a postural control synergy prior to upper limb movement.[94] Elevation of the pelvic floor is easier in standing than lying.[138] The spatial position and tilt of the pelvis will affect the forces imposed upon the floor and the degree of its postural reflex activity.

In continent individuals, physiological (reactive) pelvic floor activation is automatic resulting in a mid position of the floor, while voluntary activation results in elevation of the bladder neck.[20] Bø[139] points out that voluntary activation is undertaken to reach the automatic response level. She describes 'a correct pelvic floor muscle contraction' as:

• A mass contraction of the three layer muscles producing an inward movement and squeezing around the pelvic openings

• Does not involve any visible movement of the pelvis or outer body
• Can be felt by vaginal palpation and observed as movement of the perineum in a cranial direction
• Submaximal contractions can be felt in isolation.

While isolated voluntary concentric activation initially provides the 'feel' and is targeted to sphincteric closure, posturomovement activity of the floor *should* involve some *intrapelvic movement* as its contraction counternutates the sacrum[98,124,137] and closes the lower pelvic opening while opening the upper (Fig. 6.20). Importantly, the PFM must also be able to eccentrically 'let go' (see below).

Synergistic activation relationships have been shown between the PFM and the deep abdominals;[140,141] PFM and the transverse fibres of internal oblique[81]; PFM and the diaphragm.[92] Voluntary activation of the abdominal muscles activates the PFM prior to the abdominal action, indicating a pre-programmed response.[140] Clinical practice suggests lower abdominal activity may be more linked to greater activation in the anterior triangle of the floor.

Clinical practice also suggests that muscles synergistic with PFM activity – in particular the posterior floor, are the obturator group including piriformis, gluteus maximus and hamstrings. Obtaining eccentric lengthening in the posterior floor[40] and these muscles can be difficult and contributory towards pain in many. They literally have a 'tight arse'. Hartley[142] suggests balancing eccentric and concentric contractions of the PFM helps tone and strengthen its supportive function. Competent posturomovement control of the pelvis thus involves the PFM working concentrically and eccentrically in cooperative synergies with those muscles that control closing of the superior pelvic bowl – the transversus, internal oblique, multifidus, and iliacus. Rock[20] suggests that the important eccentric control of the PFM can be activated through breathing – 'physiological inspiration combined with reactive eccentric contraction of the pelvic floor muscles is only possible when concentric action of all parts of the thoracic diaphragm coincides with eccentric contraction of the abdominals'.

Imbalanced activity in the intrinsic PFM or extrinsic muscles acting upon the pelvis will affect the pelvic floor myomechanics. Spitznagle[136] suggests that the performance of the PFM is directly related to the obturator internus as the origin of pubococcygeus is from its enveloping fascia.[136] If the fascia is taught so is the pelvic floor musculature and if slack the muscles are likewise so. Accordingly changes in the position of the femur will affect the pelvic floor.[124] The typical posture of children urgently needing to urinate and attempting to inhibit this, involves a postural change that combines hip adduction and flexion. This action passively pretensions the pelvic floor by elongating the obturator internus and facilitates pelvic floor muscle activity, and when practiced has been shown to reduce cough induced incontinence by 95%.[143] If the obturators are chronically shortened as is common in back pain, pelvic floor muscle function will be compromised.

The fundamental patterns of intrapelvic control ask for eccentric/concentric/ activity of the PFM to open and close the pelvic diaphragm. They provide a functionally sound method for integrating pelvic floor muscle activity into the posturo*movement patterns* of the pelvis. Functionally meaningful movement control always involves coordinated activity of *all* muscles in the synergy to produce an appropriate pattern of response during automatic actions such as coughing or during intentional activities such as running or jumping.[144,145]

'Fundamental pelvic patterns of movement': controlled by synergies involving the 'lower pelvic unit' (LPU)

The three fundamental pelvic patterns of movement provide three-dimensional modulation of the pelvic ring which we have termed 'distorsion'. Essentially they provide for lumbopelvic control and support closed chain and open chain movements of the hip (see above). These patterns underlie all movements that the pelvis performs as it initiates and supports movement in the spine and hips while at the same time marrying control between them. They underlie all weight bearing and weight shift through the pelvis on the femur and help to control the neutral lumbar curve. So what muscles contribute to the synergies that perform those movements?

'Lower pelvic unit': support comes from within and below

These muscles all belong to the SLMS providing antigravity support and control (see Ch.5). Their coordinated synergistic activity provides a continuous myofascial sleeve of deep inner support and control from the femur through to the upper body. The muscles belonging to the LPU are shown in Table 6.1.

There is now good scientific evidence and acceptance for inclusion of all the muscles in the left hand column. Some research implicates inclusion of those in the right hand column. Clinical practice dictates that all those muscles shown merit inclusion. They all play a

Table 6.1 The principal muscles of the lower pelvic unit synergy

Transversus abdominus	Deep intersegmental muscles:
Internal oblique −1°	multifidus, interspinales
lower fibres	intertransversarii, rotatores
Diaphragm	External oblique −1° lower fibres
Pelvic diaphragm:	Iliacus
levator ani. coccygeus	Psoas major and minor
Multifidus −1° deep	Pectineus
fibres	Deep hip rotators;
Quadratus lumborum	*obturators, piriformis
−1° medial fibres	

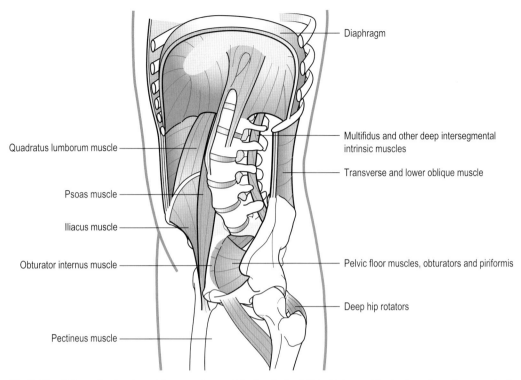

Diaphragm

Quadratus lumborum muscle

Multifidus and other deep intersegmental intrinsic muscles

Transverse and lower oblique muscle

Psoas muscle

Iliacus muscle

Obturator internus muscle

Pelvic floor muscles, obturators and piriformis

Deep hip rotators

Pectineus muscle

Fig 6.29 • Schematic drawing of the muscles contributing to the LPU which provides both an inner framework of deep anterior support to the column and 'hoop support' to the column and pelvis, functionally connecting the thorax, pelvis and hips.

role in lumbopelvic control. Referring again to the body cylinder construct, it can be seen that LPU provides both a framework of deep anterior support of 'the column' as well as providing an 'inner hoop support' which connects and integrates function between the thorax, lumbar spine, pelvis and hips. Importantly this integrated support comes from within and below (Fig. 6.29 also Fig. 6.34). What is quite extraordinary is that to date, two of the most important muscles in the synergy responsible for effective load transfer *through the pelvis*, the psoas and particularly iliacus, have been largely unrecognized and ignored by the contemporary scientific community. Poor old iliacus! It has been quietly getting on and doing such a good job – or otherwise. Maybe it's a case of out of sight out of mind. Its role deserves more attention. Likewise the obturator group serve an important function.

Activation of the lower pelvic unit involves focusing movement *from* the sit bones and tail bone – initiation from 'down in the basement of control'. Drawing the sit bones apart equates with drawing the anterior iliac spines closer together in the frontal plane. This can be *felt* to beautifully activate the

lower transversus, internal oblique and iliacus in concert with the others in the synergy. Breathing is facilitated.

Richardson et al[86,87] advocate maintaining a neutral spine and 'drawing in the lower abdomen' or abdominal hollowing to activate the deep musculofascial corset. The problem is that in the clinical setting, despite careful prompts and supervision, for many this predictably tends to activate the upper abdominals, create a flexion moment of the lumbar spine, posterior pelvic tilt and breath holding as it is an 'action that doesn't go anywhere' (Fig. 6.30). Patients generally cannot create a 'neutral spine' and 'holding patterns' are already a problem for the patient. Rather, activation of the LPU and the reintroduction of important components of *useful functional patterns of movement* help appropriate control of lumbopelvic alignment and 'stability'. At the same time activity in the diaphragm is facilitated as well as helping to achieve the 'hip hinge' control advocated by McGill[8] when forward bending.

The functional role of the LPU synergy can be summarized as contributing to:

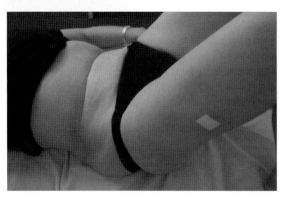

Fig 6.30 • The patient thought she was activating transversus; however, note the tendency to axial 'total flexion pattern' behavior including posterior pelvic tilt.

which acting at the sacrum, causes the innominate to posteriorly rotate through the acetabular axis. This backward tilt of the pelvis accentuates the sacral nutation. These forces are resisted by a counterbalancing tensile stress in the anterior sacroiliac, and especially the sacrospinous and sacrotuberous ligaments.[16,146] According to DonTigny,[147] a force dependent transverse axis is established through the sacrum but not necessarily through the sacroiliac joints. This axis of rotation is approximately through the S3. In fact however, this analysis relates more to the forces involved as there is little movement, any tendency being resisted by the powerful ligaments. The sacroiliac joint is 'wound up' through this self locking and so is stabilized within the pelvic rim (Fig. 6.31). If the pelvis posturally shifts forward, this mechanism is compromised.

• Providing basic antigravity support of the segments including equilibrium
• Adaptive postural presetting of the pelvis to support trunk movements
• The respiratory and postural role of the breathing mechanisms
• The generation of IAP for spinal support
• Provision of the basic movement patterns of the pelvis hip and lumbar spine
• Control of forces from legs to pelvis and torso to pelvis and load transfer *through* the pelvis
• Initiating movement *from* the pelvis on the femur
• Connecting function between the upper and lower body.

While providing fundamental support, LPU activity will obviously also involve other muscles depending upon postural, kinematic and force requirements.

Pelvic tilt – balancing the pelvis on the legs

Sacroiliac joint 'self-locking' when upright

When standing, in the 'ideal normal alignment', the weight of the trunk acts as a compression force transmitted down through the vertebral bodies. This acts upon the superior surface of the sacrum and tends to rotate it forward into nutation. At the same time the ground reaction force transmitted up through the femora to the hip joints which are more anterior, forms with the body weight, a rotary force couple

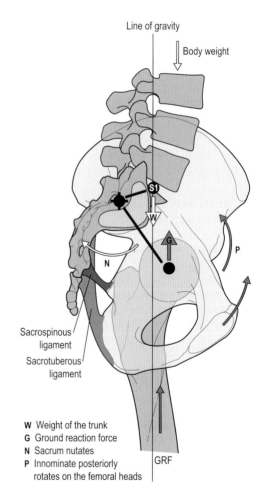

W Weight of the trunk
G Ground reaction force
N Sacrum nutates
P Innominate posteriorly rotates on the femoral heads

Fig 6.31 • Intrinsic 'self locking' and stability of the sacroiliac joint is influenced by gravitational lines of force.

Dynamic control of Sagittal pelvic tilt: the important primary role of the deep intrinsic force couple – iliopsoas and obturator group (with the hamstrings)

In the sagittal plane pelvic equilibrium is labile.[132] Gravity practically always produces moments of rotation which have to be neutralized by neuromuscular control of these forces. Nine deep muscles provide sophisticated diagonal pulls and essentially balance and adjust the pelvis with the spine on the hips and maintain hip range of motion – psoas, iliacus, and pectineus in the front, with the piriformis, obturators internus and externus, the superior and inferior gamelli and quadratus femoris forming the posterior part of the force couple.[1,6,28,148] Collectively, the posterior group are commonly termed 'the external rotators of the hip'[16] or 'the deep six' which understates their important action on the pelvis when the femur is 'fixed' (Fig. 6.32). As they are spatially positioned under the axis of the hip joint they have an important role in 'swinging'

the inferior pelvis forward at the ischia. They 'are possibly more important as postural muscles than as prime movers. . . acting as adjustable ligaments of the joint in all positions.'[10] For ease they will be collectively termed the obturator group. They all attach to the greater trochanter. Piriformis arises from the saccrum and is the most superiorly placed. The rest arise from the ischium and the membrane and rim of the obturator foramen. These six primary outward rotators form a functional muscle 'fan', each pulling at a slightly different angle to rotate the femur[28] and importantly, control the pelvis on the 'stable' femur.

Returning to the static standing construct; ideally, the line of gravity passes anterior to the sacroiliac joints but posterior to the axis of the hip joints, tending to create an extension moment at the hip, as the pelvis posteriorly tilts on the femoral heads.[9] The three strong ligaments at the front of the hip joint resist this force – passive reliance on them is a common postural habit. Dynamic control, that is, of anterior pelvic tilt at the hip is achieved by co-active control from iliacus and psoas. This has been demonstrated

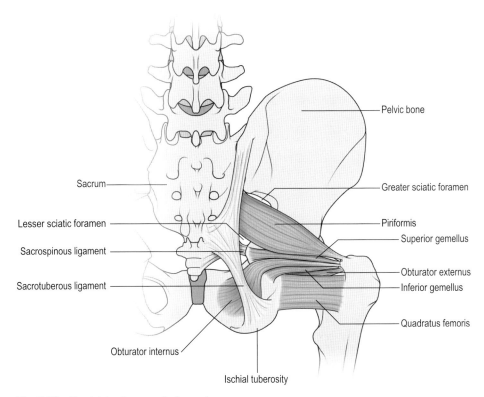

Fig 6.32 • The 'obturator group' of muscles.

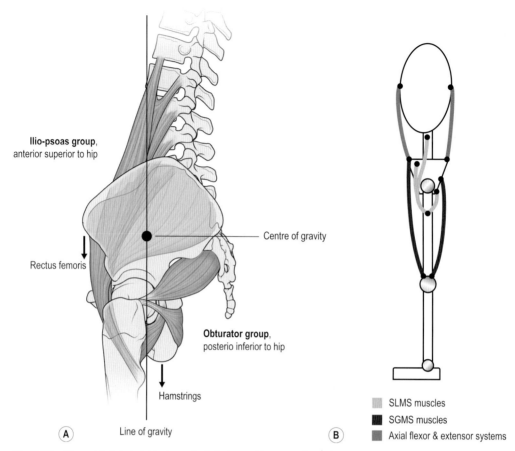

Ilio-psoas group,
anterior superior to hip

Centre of gravity

Rectus femoris

Obturator group,
posterio inferior to hip

Hamstrings

Line of gravity

(A)

(B)

SLMS muscles

SGMS muscles

Axial flexor & extensor systems

Fig 6.33 • The pelvic 'gimbals' is dynamically balanced between iliacus/psoas and obturator/hamstring groups activity (A). Schematic view (B).

by EMG in standing,[149,150] standing on one leg, and in sitting.[151] With pectineus, Todd[6] likens their activity to anterior tension members countering the posterior compression forces at the back. Their activity also thrusts the pelvis back in space.

In a dynamically balanced pelvis, activity between the obturator group and iliopsoas forms two diagonal planes of force through the pelvis which should be equal and opposite. The iliopsoas is supero-anterior, tipping the superior pelvic bowl forward. The obturators and piriformis with the hamstrings are inferoposterior tipping the inferior pelvic bowl forward. If they are overactive, the pelvis is held in posterior tilt and the lateral bracing action of the hips affording stability to the SIJ is reduced (see Aspects of normal neuromuscular behavior around the spine, above). When both groups are in a balanced relationship,

their point of intersection would fall *at* the gravity line i.e. midway between the axis of the spine and the legs (Fig. 6.33). Bartenieff[148] considers that when hamstrings action is not appropriately incorporated into pelvic-femoral rhythm by the synergistic activity of the deep external rotators the hamstrings they simply act as extensors of the knee. Some see that all the deep external rotators contribute to posterior tilt,[1,6] while others see that 'some' accompany forward tilt initiated by iliopsoas[103,148] (assumedly obturator externus). When iliopsoas is not used appropriately the rectus femoris and rectus abdominus are overused.[148]

Rolf[1] notes that psoas, iliacus, obturator internus and piriformis form a continuous steadying prevertebral web which connects the base of the thorax, lumbar spine, sacrum and pelvis to the legs. The piriformis inserting onto the greater trochanter from behind, establishes the anterioposterior position of the sacrum and so balance between sacrum and ileum and sacrum and lumbar spine and thus forms the foundation for iliacus-psoas; the iliacus-psoas attaching to the lesser trochanter in front determines balance between the hip, pelvis and lumbar spine. This prevertebral support network prevents undue anterior displacement of the spine and relieves the burden of the post vertebral extensors and helps support the thoracic structure of the body[1] (Fig. 6.34).

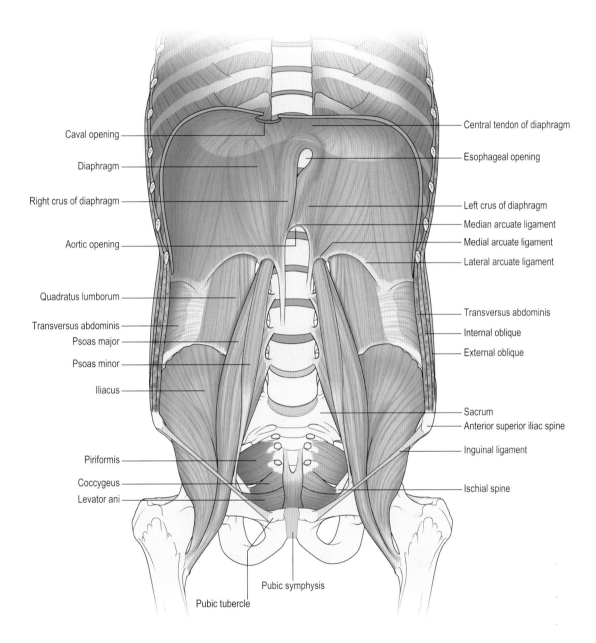

Caval opening
Diaphragm
Right crus of diaphragm
Aortic opening
Quadratus lumborum
Transversus abdominis
Psoas major
Psoas minor
Iliacus
Piriformis
Coccygeus
Levator ani

Central tendon of diaphragm
Esophageal opening
Left crus of diaphragm
Median arcuate ligament
Medial arcuate ligament
Lateral arcuate ligament
Transversus abdominis
Internal oblique
External oblique
Sacrum
Anterior superior iliac spine
Inguinal ligament
Ischial spine

Pubic symphysis
Pubic tubercle

Fig 6.34 • Much of the LPU involves a prevertebral and intrapelvic web of support.

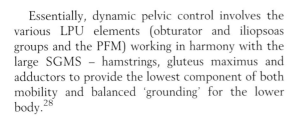

Essentially, dynamic pelvic control involves the various LPU elements (obturator and iliopsoas groups and the PFM) working in harmony with the large SGMS – hamstrings, gluteus maximus and adductors to provide the lowest component of both mobility and balanced 'grounding' for the lower body.[28]

Control of pelvic tilt is achieved from cooperative interplay between SLMS and SGMS

While convention acknowledges that pelvic rotation known as tilt affects lumbar posture, it is generally hard to find descriptions in the literature of the principal muscle force couples which are deemed responsible for controlling it. Clearly control of pelvic tilt involves complicated synergies involving both the deep and superficial systems. While certain movement educators have been aware of the important contribution of the deep intrinsic force couples in controlling sagittal pelvic tilt in both posture and movement[1,6,28,148] (see above), the medical model appears to only primarily consider the static force couples created by the large superficial muscles in the SGMS e.g. the Kendall's[129] description:

- **Posterior tilt** is achieved from the downward pull of gluteus maximus and hamstrings and the upward pull of the anterior abdominals – rectus and external oblique.
- **Anterior tilt** occurs through upward pull of the spinal extensors and the downward pull of the hip flexors – rectus femoris, tensor fascia lata, sartorius and the iliopsoas.

Often only the superior effectors are mentioned such as the abdominals create posterior tilt.[152]

A dynamic well balanced pelvis requires balanced length/tension relationships between all muscles attaching to it both inferiorly and superiorly from both the deep and superficial systems. Imbalance between the axial flexors and extensors has a significant influence on pelvic tilt control. The large common tendon of the erector spinae attaches to the sacrum and pelvis, hence their overactivity, unmatched by the abdominals can anteriorly rotate the pelvis.[12] In addition, congruent activity between iliacus/psoas and the abdominals is particularly important in providing anterior tensile support.

The deep intrinsic pelvic force couple is also very important in controlling sagittal movements further away from the gravity line in sitting and standing. DonTigny notes when bending forward the line of gravity moves forward of the acetabular axis and the sacroiliac joints are more vulnerable.[147] He recommends a strong abdominal contraction provides a self bracing of the joints affording protection during this maneuver. However, clinically activating abdominals 'alone' is more likely to create a flexion moment and 'cause a pathological release of the self bracing position'.[147] Rather, if the pelvis spatially *shifts posteriorly while anteriorly rotating*, abdominal activity in coactivation with the extensors, controls the 'body cylinder' which is carried forward in a more kinematically sound way. Inner support from the LPU allows force couple synergies to create anterior rotation of the pelvis with principal contribution from concentric activity of the iliacus and psoas[149,150] as well as lower transversus, internal oblique and multifidus, and corresponding eccentric play out from the PFM, obturator group aided and abetted by the hamstrings and gluteus maximus. The return occurs via posterior rotation of the pelvis from principal concentric gluteus maximus, hamstrings, PFM and obturator group activity and eccentric abdominal, iliacus and psoas activity. Prominent buttocks are one of the most characteristic features of the muscular system in man associated with the frequent need to bring the trunk upright.[10]

Balanced control of both the obturator and iliopsoas groups gives a free swinging pelvic base for quick postural adjustments and the ability to readily squat and return. The control of sagittal tilt is also involved in forward weight shift in sitting, moving from sitting to stand and lowering to sit and many other actions. However, clinical practice frequently reveals imbalanced and defective use and control of this force couple with altered length tension relationships in the muscles.

Influence of the thorax on sagittal pelvic tilt

Harrison et al.[153] showed that when 'normal' subjects stood with an unrestrained pelvis and performed a primary forward and backward translation of the thoracic cage, large changes in the sagittal lumbar posture and pelvic tilt were produced as well as changes in the thoracic kyphosis.

Anterior thoracic translation caused the pelvis to anteriorly tilt by 15°, while posterior translation tilted the pelvis posteriorly by nearly 16°.

Frontal plane pelvic tilt: the important contribution of obturator-iliacus concentric/eccentric activity

Iliacus lines the superior pelvic bowl while obturator internus piriformis and the PFM line the inferior pelvic bowl. The control if ischial inflare/outflare occurs from coactivity in the LPU with balanced activity between iliacus/transversus superiorly and the obturators/PFM inferiorly. This *internal control* from LPU synergies provides intrapelvic stability and a firm base of support for the pulls of the larger muscles balancing the pelvis as a whole over the standing leg (Fig. 6.35). The adductors appear synergistic with transversus and iliacus in creating ischial outflare, while the abductors are synergistic with inflare. (See further functional roles of iliacus, psoas adductors below)

The 'ischial swing'

Well developed spatial control of the pelvis as a whole is characterized by the ischia being able to freely swing in the sagittal and frontal planes. Control of this is critical to effective sagittal weight shift and frontal plane weight transfer onto one leg where the ipsilateral ischium swings medially as the leg comes under the pelvis or the pelvis moves over the leg.

The further functional roles of iliacus and psoas

The iliopsoas muscles have been long considered by certain practitioners as perhaps the most important muscles in determining upright posture.[1,6] Rolf[1] considers psoas' function is unique in unifying the torso and thigh and no other myofascial element can substitute satisfactorily.

Their actions are usually described together and conventionally as: hip flexion, bending the trunk and pelvis forward as in rising from lying to sitting;

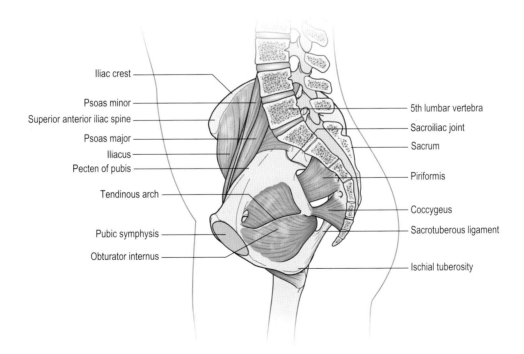

Fig 6.35 • Schematic inner view of the superior and inferior innominate bowls.

Labels (top to bottom, left): Iliac crest, Psoas minor, Superior anterior iliac spine, Psoas major, Iliacus, Pecten of pubis, Tendinous arch, Pubic symphysis, Obturator internus

Labels (right): 5th lumbar vertebra, Sacroiliac joint, Sacrum, Piriformis, Coccygeus, Sacrotuberous ligament, Ischial tuberosity and possible 'important activities' in balancing the trunk in sitting.[10] Bogduk et al.[154] proposed that the upper fascicles of psoas tend to extend the upper lumbar spine and the lower fascicles tend to flex the lower lumbar spine; otherwise it is a hip flexor. A postural stabilizing role for psoas is gaining support.[130,155,156,157] McGill describes psoas' spinal stabilizing role as resisting the forces or torques created on the spine as a result of limb movement, in particular hip flexion.[8] As far as the sacroiliac joint is concerned, Steindler[132] has been the only source found in the literature to consider that the 'mighty mass (of the sacrospinalis as well as) the iliopsoas protects the joint before it really comes to ligamentous strain'. This is particularly so with the back in motion where the iliacus and psoas help control the momentum of the back and forward pelvic swing incidental to locomotion.

Clinical practice supports agreement with all of these roles and suggests more. Iliacus' architecture allows the top of the pelvis to be pulled forward[47] hence it plays a substantial role in initiating anterior pelvic rotation during actions such as forward bending in standing. At the same time psoas is synergistically acting to control spinal intersegmental alignment – the pelvis flexes on the hip while the low back is controlled in variable extension. If the hip does not act as the fulcrum of the movement, the back is used instead with predictable consequences over time. If there is under use of iliopsoas in the flexion and support phase when walking, the obturators and piriformis compensate, become overactive, increasing hip external rotation and the stress through L4/5.[28]

Frontal plane control

In concert with psoas, iliacus conceivably also plays a crucial role in lateral weight shift and load transference through the pelvis when upright (see 'Frontal plane pelvic tilt...' above). The leg can be brought under the body or the body over the leg. It has been proposed that the SIJ is vulnerable to shear loading stress.[158] However, as has been pointed out by Gracovetsky,[2] the joint surfaces are warped and highly organized toward their functional role. He points out that the inferior part of the SIJ on the ileum is in fact a warped ledge which is part of an arch and is well suited to weight bearing. Conceivably, when the pelvis rotates in the frontal plane over the femoral head, as seen in Figure 6.36, the active line of pull of the fibres of psoas and iliacus are almost vertical between their top and bottom

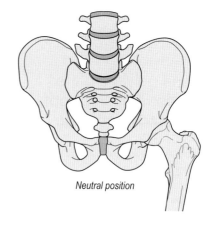

Neutral position

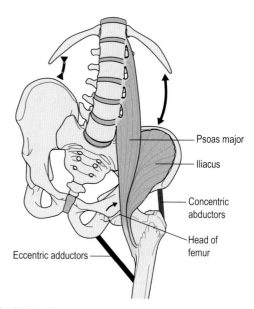

— Psoas major

— Iliacus

— Concentric abductors

— Head of femur

Eccentric adductors —

Fig 6.36 • Conceptual view of frontal plane pelvic rotation in lateral weight transfer and proposed line of pull of psoas and iliacus.

attachments and serve to provide an *internal tensile support* over the anterior SIJ, actively binding the joint surfaces together. At the same time the lumbar segments are adaptively aligned and stabilized *over the weight bearing leg*. Clinically it appears that the ipsilateral psoas is eccentrically active to 'lengthen the side' ipsilaterally while the contralateral psoas is concentrically active to help control adaptive change in the spine. In similar vein, Sims[159] cites a proposal by Bombelli that in single leg stance iliacus and the abductors balance the pelvis whilst psoas and the contralateral quadratus lumborum position the centre of gravity over the centre of rotation of the femoral head. Psoas is thus an important medial stabilizer of the hip[157] and contributing to the force couple synergy are the hip abductors helping to hold the ileum 'over' the leg while the adductors also provide important eccentric control and stability of the pelvis on the leg.

In walking, iliacus and psoas provide a complex oscillating role between stability and mobility one limb supporting, the other swinging while at the same time controlling the alignment and balance of the pelvis with the spine on the legs. An eccentric contraction occurring before a concentric contraction enables the muscle to perform more positive work with increased power.[67] This enhanced performance is attributed to the ability of the muscle to store energy during the stretch (eccentric contraction) and subsequently use some of this energy during the concentric contraction. Todd[6] suggests that because iliacus and psoas are contracting before they receive the load in either stance or swing phase, they not only assist as shock absorbers but rebounders providing an energy efficient spring in the step.

What is the role of the adductors in pelvic myomechanics?

The functional role of the adductors has in general received relatively scant attention. Kendall et al.[129] describe their actions as adduction of the hip joint; and together with pectineus, the longus and brevis flex the hip joint. The anterior fibres of the massive adductor magnus may assist in hip flexion while the posterior fibres may assist in hip extension.[10,129] They have also been assigned an essential synergistic role in the complex patterns of gait and controllers of posture.[10,160] Janda[160] showed they were active during flexion and extension of the hip and knee tested in prone, supine and sitting and particularly against resistance, demonstrating their proximal postural stabilizing role. He points out that their excitation level is relatively low; they also have with one of the shortest chronaxies of the lower limb muscles; and in cerebral palsy adductor hyper spasticity develops mainly after verticalization of the child. The magnus and longus are probably medial rotators of the thigh.[10]

Given their combined proximal attachment covers the entire lateral surface of the inferior pubic ramus from the symphysis in front to the lateral inferior ischial tuberosity below the hamstrings insertion posteriorly, they must surely play a large role in balancing the pelvis on the femur and helping stabilize the inferior bowl. Their muscle mass is enormous yet 'extensive or forcible action of the femur is not a common action'.[10] While in symmetrical easy standing their activity is minimal or absent[10] it is reasoned they come into their own when weight bearing on one leg. Hungerford et al.[161] describe their early EMG onset when standing on one leg. On a stable femur their closed chain function probably involves helping to balance the 'ischial swing' in both the sagittal and frontal planes. Also, actions where the pelvis opens away from the stable leg involve reversed origin and insertion eccentric control from the adductors and internal hip rotators.

Kendall[129] draws attention to their internal rotary action because they insert onto the femur anterior to the mechanical axis. Those which insert posterior to the mechanical axis will act as lateral rotators (Fig. 6.37).

In the frontal plane they balance activity in the glutei and tensor fascia lata and provide invaluable eccentric control as the pelvis rotates over the femoral head during lateral weight shift (see 'Further functional roles of iliacus and psoas' above). On a fixed femur in synergy with iliacus and transversus their action *abducts* the ischium and inferior pubic ramus which is counterbalanced by PFM and obturator group activity to provide stability of the inferior pelvic syndesmosis and stability of the pelvic ring.

Lee[18] notes their role in regional stabilization of the pelvis between the thorax and legs as part of the 'anterior oblique sling' of the global system.

Hip rotator balance: important for both hip and pelvic myomechanics

The deep rotators form a fan around the innominate as they encase the femoral head and variously insert onto the femur each pulling at a slightly different angle. The 'deep' internal rotators are the iliopsoas[1], gluteus medius and minimus which are anterior and superior to the hip joint – the only exception being the adductors. The deep external rotators – the obturators, the gamelli, piriformis and quadratus

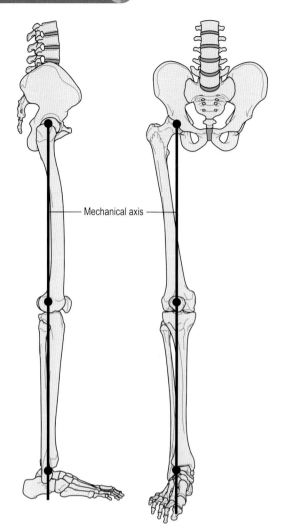

Fig 6.37 • Rotary action of the adductors acting around the mechanical axis.

chain hip movements.[28,148] More commonly the superficial gluteus maximus is used for external rotation of the leg rather than the deep rotators.[28,145] Most people don't appreciate the fact that the gluteals are rotators and are often tight.

Rolf[1] considered iliopsoas the prime internal rotator which counters principal external rotation from piriformis, and balance between them with obturator internus is important in providing the pre-vertebral support for the spine which then relieves the load on the spinal extensors.

Superficially, balance in the fascia lata is achieved from balanced activity between the anteriorly placed tensor fascia lata which is also an internal rotator and the posterior gluteus maximus which is also a lateral rotator (Fig. 6.54).

Hip rotator imbalance alters the freedom of the innominate to rotate in the sagittal and frontal planes and so disturbs pelvic myomechanics. When the internal rotators are tighter, innominate movement into posterior rotation and ischial inflare is reduced. When the external rotators are tighter, innominate movement into anterior rotation and ischial outflare is reduced. Clinically,

femoris are posterior and lie level with or below the hip joint. As their fibres are roughly horizontal they can directly modify the plane of movement of the pelvic basin and transmit tension to the pelvic bones[1]. The internal rotators are the 'upper storey' while the external rotators are the 'lower storey'[28] (Fig. 6.38). Hip external rotation is associated with elements of posterior pelvic tilt/hip extension, abduction and closing the pelvic floor while internal rotation is synergistic with hip adduction, flexion/anterior pelvic tilt and opening of the pelvic floor. These are certainly not obligatory responses. Full use of the deep hip rotators particularly the external rotators allows better range and freedom of open

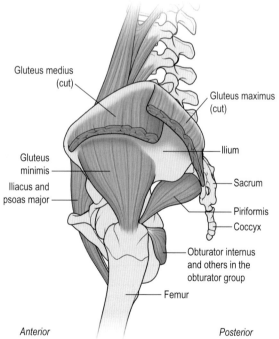

Fig 6.38 • The lateral view of the pelvis showing the 'deep rotator fan' of the hip.

it is more common for people with back pain to have more difficulty with various combinations of closed chain hip flexion, internal rotation and adduction and so related opening of the inferior pelvic bowl becomes restricted. This limits closing of the superior bowl and control of the lumbar lordosis.

Role of superficial muscle slings

Various synergistic muscle slings in the SGMS acting through fascial sheets have been proposed to provide regional stabilization of the pelvis between the thorax and legs.[18,152,162,163,164]

The posterior longitudinal sling connects the peroneii, biceps femoris, sacrotuberous ligament, the deep lamina of the thoracodorsal fascia and the erector spinae.[18]

The anterior oblique sling connects the external oblique, through the anterior abdominal fascia, to the opposite internal oblique, the transversus abdominus and the adductors.

The posterior oblique sling connects the latissimus dorsi, through the thoracolumbar fascia to the contralateral gluteus maximus. Bogduk[165] however, considers the contribution of latissimus dorsi to sacroiliac stability to be 'trivial'.

The lateral sling contains the tensor fascia lata, gluteus medius and minimus and the lateral stabilizers of the thoracopelvic region.[18]

In similar vein, Myers[166] describes functional myofascial synergies in terms of superficial front and back lines, spiral lines, lateral lines and functional lines. All of these superficial system synergies undoubtedly play a role in the panorama of movement control. However, it is suggested that without adequate preceding and more integrated tonic activity in the SLMS, their ability to provide effective control will be suboptimal.

What is core control?

No one concept has been so misunderstood, confused and abused and as that of 'core control'. The term has unfortunately become synonymous with the abdominal muscles – the need for 'strong abs' and 'holding in' and 'pulling in your stomach'. Further, the idea of 'core *strengthening*' has evolved which overemphasizes development of the superficial abdominals and

has become a major trend in rehabilitation despite meager research.[167]

Current models about back pain have proposed 'instability' of the spine as a cause. This led to thinking that in order to make the spine more stable, the abdominals needed to be strong so as to 'not let the spine move'. It appears there has been misinterpretation of some of the research. The Queensland group of Hodges and co workers have done nice research showing that in one of the abdominal muscles – transversus, activity is *reduced and delayed* in people with back pain.[86,87] In the normal state its activity is automatic and occurs *in conjunction with other muscles* such as the pelvic floor, diaphragm and multifidus as part of a postural reflex synergy *prior to* an actual movement occurring. While volitional activation of a single muscle may initially 'help get the feel' of the desired action, its synergistic activity in functionally relevant posturomovement patterns needs to be learnt. Hodges[168] makes it clear that control of the spine should be dynamic – that stability is controlled mobility. However, some of the confusion may also have arisen from the researcher's protocols which recommended the 'abdominal hollowing exercise' (AHE)[86,87,169] as a means of initially gaining simultaneous contraction of the deep muscle synergy. While a specific and controllable maneuver, it is not a particularly functional movement and certain subgroups of patients (see Ch. 9) will have great difficulty achieving the correct action. Asking for an action such as 'narrowing the waist and inwardly drawing in the abdomen',[170] tends to limit diaphragm activity, increases the tendency for central 'holding patterns' and encourages more of a 'functional disconnect' around the central torso; often doing little that it sets out to achieve. Beith[171] found that in a group of physiotherapy students, only 20% could consistently isolate the deep abdominals (IO) from external oblique in 4-point kneeling and prone raising the question as to whether elimination of EO activity during the AHE is always possible, desirable or necessary. However, interventions by 'significantly experienced' therapists who have adopted this protocol with other associated re-educative exercise[172] have shown positive outcomes.

McGill[18,59] repudiates the adoption of what he calls 'single muscle strategies' and doesn't believe that AHE ensures stability. In order that the spine can withstand steady state loading as well as sudden unexpected complex loads, McGill[173] advocates abdominal bracing involving activation of the whole lateral abdominal wall and training 'patterns of stabilization'[8] as the most effective means of achieving core control. He advises that high levels of co-contraction are not required – 5% during normal ADL and up to 10% during rigorous activity.

Abdominal bracing does provide an immediate stiffening of greater magnitude than hollowing.[174] However, creating too much stiffness is as much of a problem as too little stiffness. There is often too much bracing from hyperactivity of the abdominal or mistaken 'core' muscles[185] in certain groups of people with back pain. Clinical experience suggests that for many, both AHE and abdominal bracing represent patterns of activity that are just too close to their habitual 'central cinch' or holding patterns (see Ch.9), the action occurring 'too high' and so compromising the breathing pattern. The first sign of defective core control is defective breathing.[103] *Core control is control of the LPU at the core of the body's centre of weight.* It involves the coordinated activity of whole synergies of muscles in the control of the pelvis which *is* and supports the core and breathing. Feldenkrais[175] comments 'the dependence of proper breathing on the correct holding of the pelvis was also recognized by the Yogi long ago'. The 'core' is also the centre of weight shift. The LPU synergy, particularly iliacus and transversus stabilizes the pelvis so it can rotate on the femoral heads through all degrees of freedom in all parts of available range. Bartenieff,[148] a physiotherapist and dance movement educator talked of the importance of gaining function in this region which she termed 'the dead seven inches' so prevalent in most American's bodies.[28] Control from the *internal core* helps minimize overdependence on the external muscles. Movement at the core is basic to expressive and dynamic movement and can be seen in terms of opening and closing; expanding and condensing; concaving and convexing.[28,176] Movement at the core also begins with the breath.

When working for 'core control', which movement patterns and synergies are chosen becomes the art of the prescribing practitioner. Understanding 'what's wrong' informs the choice. Most importantly, the person needs to establish and maintain proper diaphragmatic breathing through the movement. Movements which focus on the correct activation of the LPU will generally achieve these features.

Functional role of the abdominal group of muscles

A big 'tummy' is common these days and prompts the belief that doing abdominal exercises will fix it. However, this is usually more the result of postural collapse, 'middle aged spread' and obesity. 'Curls' and 'crunches' will often aggravate rather than help the problem. The role of the abdominals is complex.

'The abdominals' consist of four muscles – the rectus abdominus suspended within the fascial sheet of the anterior abdominal wall, and the three anterolateral muscles arranged in three layers, each layer having a different fibres direction, creating a pattern of cross bracing as they form the anterolateral wall of the body, connecting the thorax to the pelvis. They are not just flexors which curl the trunk forward; they have differing yet synergistic roles. As a group they support the abdominal viscera, flex side bend and rotate the trunk, and contribute to the breathing mechanism and the stability of the spine through the generation of IAP. Importantly, they have a postural role and control the *relationship between* the thorax and pelvis and the alignment of the axial spine. They help to control forces acting upon both the spine and the pelvis. Beith and Harrison[177] report finding reflex facilitation in all four oblique muscles in response to stretch in one suggesting close synergies between the obliques in providing stability to the vertebral column. What is often not appreciated is that the architecture of the obliques and transversus is such that different regions of the one muscle show different morphology and perform different functions which become important to understand when considering axial alignment and control.

The deepest layer, **the transversus abdominis (Tr A)**, interdigitates with the diaphragm thus its function is closely intertwined with the breathing mechanism and the generation of IAP.[92] Its attachments to the lower six ribs and the pelvic rim, and fibrous attachments to large aponeurotic and fascial sheaths front and back, respectively, mean that it acts like an inner sleeve of support helping control the thorax over the pelvis. It tensions the front and back 'fascial plates,' providing postural support and stability to both the lumbar spine and ribs so the diaphragm can effectively contract. Studies have confirmed its postural role and implicate separate CNS regulation to that of

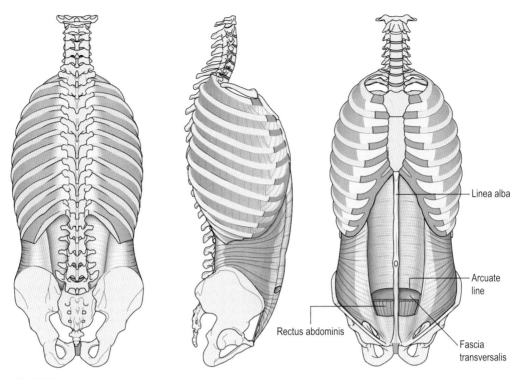

Fig 6.39 • Transversus abdominis.

Labels: Linea alba, Arcuate line, Rectus abdominis, Fascia transversalis

the rest of the group.[96,178] Urquhart[179] described three different regions (Fig. 6.39):

• The upper anterior fibres showed the least tonic activity

• The middle region was most associated with respiratory activity

• The inferior region showed more tonic postural activity. Clinically, this region plays a very important role in the synergies responsible for the control of pelvic ring myomechanics and its control on the femur.

Activation of the lower and middle regions was independent of the upper region.[180] The postural responses also varied according to body position with recruitment delayed in sitting compared to standing.[181]

The internal oblique (IO) constitutes the middle layer. Its fibre arrangement also delineates three differing regions[129] and functional roles (Fig. 6.40):

• The lower anterior fibres in conjunction with transversus support the abdominal viscera and have an important role in approximating the anterior ilia[182]

• The upper anterior fibres assist in breathing, depress the thorax, and approximate the pelvis and thorax, flexing the spine[129]

• The lateral fibres can depress and approximate the thorax and pelvis anteriorly and laterally. Clinically, these fibres are frequently tight.

The external oblique (EO) forms the superficial layer. Its fibre arrangement essentially comprises two sets of 'functional slings' with potentially different posturomovement behavioral characteristics (Fig. 6.41).

• The upper anterior fibres from ribs 5–8 pass forward and inferiorly to attach to the anterior aponeuroses and can depress the thorax and flex the thoracolumbar spine.

• The lower lateral fibres from ribs 9–12 pass down and forward. Those from the 9th rib go to the pubis and send fascial expansions towards the adductor origins; those from the 10th rib to the inguinal ligament[16] and anterior half of the ileum as do the rest of the fibres.[10] This sling can[16] flex the spine with more influence on the lumbar spine and posterior pelvic tilt.[129] If the pelvis is held stable these fibres 'help to draw the *posterior* rib cage towards the *anterior iliac crest* and in so doing tend to extend not flex the thoracic spine'.[129] These fibres thus help to maintain a good alignment of the thorax in relation to the pelvis as they counter the flexion moment of the upper anterior fibres.

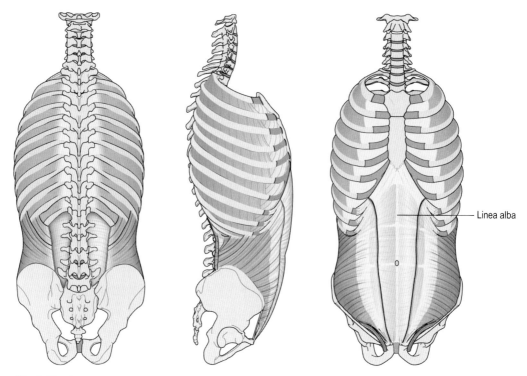

Fig 6.40 • Internal oblique.

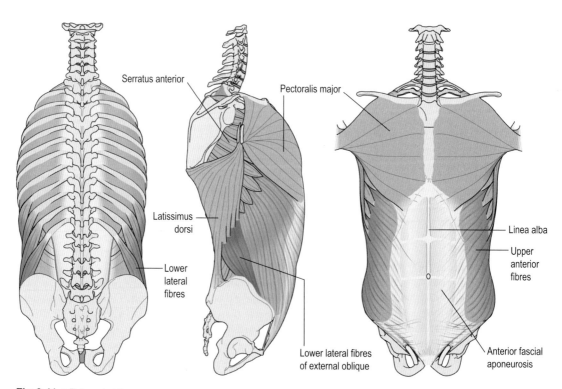

Fig 6.41 • External oblique.

Rectus abdominis activity is more straightforward in approximating the pelvis and thorax and flexing the spine. Examining abdominal wall activity during 'belly dancing', Moreside et al.[183] recently demonstrated significantly different activation levels between upper and lower rectus and that the obliques tend to work in synergy with the lower rectus more than the upper during various pelvis movements with minimal thorax motion.

Kendall[129] notes that during the trunk curl sit up, the lower lateral fibres of external oblique are elongated. Doing a lot of these, results in 'stretch weakness' of this sling and hypertrophy of the anterior sling as well as the internal oblique and rectus. This results in altered alignment in standing; either the pelvis tips anteriorly as in a kyphosis lordosis posture or anteriorly shifts with posterior deviation of the thorax in the 'sway back' posture. When the pelvis hangs or is shunted forward there is little demand for postural activity in the anterior abdominal wall. This is also related to corresponding shortness of the lateral IO in both situations.[129]

Importantly if the posterolateral sling of EO is weak, with associated deficient activity from the LPU synergy, marked difficulty in supine leg loading tests will be apparent. It is suggested that it is this mechanism which is operant during a positive active straight leg raise test (ASLR) described by Mens[184] and is not necessarily reflective of specific SIJ dysfunction. This also explains the increased SGMS fixing around the lower thorax and decreased diaphragmatic descent described by O'Sullivan et al.[185] during this test.

When both obliques are acting together in synergy, besides flexing, side bending and rotating the thorax and pelvis on one another, they help control sagittal plane alignment, bringing the thorax back when the pelvic position is controlled or 'fixed' or the pelvis forward and up when the thorax is stable. Important to control of sagittal alignment is control of lateral movements. Gracovetsky[131] considers the lateral bending motion of the torso is an archetypal and important movement pattern principally controlled by the obliques and iliocostalis. Rather than specific muscles, it has been suggested that myofascial aggregations form specific meridians[166] which create functional 'contractile fields'[186] to produce movement. Beach[186] further suggests that head, neck and torso side bending is achieved through a 'lateral contractile field' linked to sense organs in the head. Consisting of non-anatomically defined lateral tissues (including hundreds of muscles), the field extends from the eyes and ears to the pelvic floor to insert on the sides of the coccyx. This author considers that control of this lateral movement is important in 'lengthening the sides', a significant factor in controlling lateral weight shift onto one leg.

In concert with transversus and rectus, the combined upper portions of the obliques often termed 'the upper abdominals' contribute more to breathing and controlling the alignment of the thorax on the lumbar spine. Their combined lower portions – the 'lower abdominals' are more responsible for the control of intrapelvic and spatial movements of the pelvis including tilting and the alignment of the pelvis and lumbar spine.

Norris[187] draws attention to the antagonistic activity of the abdominal group where during maximal trunk extension abdominal activity can vary between 32% and 68% of the activity in longissimus.[188]

Problems for the spine ensue when abdominal activity is increased, decreased or imbalanced. Some muscles or parts become overactive and short while others become underactive and 'weak'. This affects their ability to control the relationship between pelvis and thorax amongst other things. The work of Hodges et al.[189] has shown that transversus activity is commonly decreased and delayed in people with back pain. Activity in the other three may also be decreased so that the whole abdominal wall is lax. Clinically however, while transversus is generally underactive, there may be increased activity in all or some of the others in the group – mostly the obliques.[53] Hence we have the situation of not only imbalance between the deep and superficial layers, but potentially between the obliques themselves, and/or between rectus and the obliques, reflecting changes in function.

In addition, it is common to find differences in the activity levels between the 'upper abdominals' and the 'lower abdominals'. Kendall[129] noted uppers 'strong' and lowers 'weak' was the most prevalent finding, followed by uppers and lowers both weak and this certainly accords with clinical practice findings. McGill describes the obliques as having regional neuromuscular compartments and functional separation between the upper and lower regions[8] and has recently shown the same in rectus.[183] As mentioned previously, when supine, if the uppers are stronger the person can curl the trunk but will have difficulty controlling the pelvis in leg loading actions.

Controlling the pelvis is an important component when working for abdominal control and generally poorly understood. 'Posterior pelvic tilting' is an exercise frequently practiced with little understanding of 'function' or regard to its appropriate use. It is a good example of an exercise passed on by tradition with little scientific evidence to support its effectiveness.[190] It is usually easy for most people including those with weak abdominals or a weak lateral EO to do this action! The neutral lordosis is lost in posterior tilt and the facet joints are in end range flexion. This habitual pattern generally does not need reinforcing. It is possible to posteriorly tilt the pelvis through its inferior pole at the hip via the obturators, piriformis and hamstrings without much EO activity at all. It is important that when working to improve EO activity that the pelvis is stabilized in neutral with the help of the LPU, so that the action of EO on the thorax can be appropriately worked for. Importantly, intrapelvic and spatial control of the pelvis is heavily reliant upon the 'lower abdominals' synergistically coactivating with various pelvi-femoral muscles to provide appropriate control of pelvic force couples. The control of anterior pelvic rotation is particularly important and universally deficient which explains the ubiquitous 'tummy' over the lower abdomen.

The prescription of therapeutic exercises which appropriately redress the underlying muscle imbalances in the abdominal wall is an art. Different people need different solutions. A gung ho, recipe based approach does little except to compound much prevailing dysfunction.

The bending and lifting debate – stoop or squat or something else?

The recognition that many work-related back pain incidents result from bending and lifting has engendered much research and debate on the mechanism of injury and the 'best lifting style'– stoop or squat. Stoop has been defined as 'knees straight, back bent; and squat as 'knees bent back straight'.[191] What is interesting is that neither definition mentions the *hip dynamics* yet McClure et al.[192] showed that normally return from forward bending initially occurs in the hip. McGill[8,59] notes, it is the kinematic motion patterns together with the muscle activation patterns that heavily influence the loads the spine bears. Poor patterns of movement and motor control errors can induce injury when bending to pick up a pencil.[8]

Simple mechanics informs that in 'stoop lifting' with no dynamic leg action and the spine in flexion, increased load is taken on the passive structures and if repeated enough, cumulative damage is likely.

Consequently, 'squat lifting' has generally been seen as 'the correct method' and advocated in industry training despite it being a somewhat unphysiological action. Because the emphasis has been on knee flexion rather than the hip, being less stable and more awkward for most, it has a high energetic cost, and is biomechanically hard on the knees and thus understandably compliance levels are generally low. Studies in repetitive lifting revealed subjects who began in squat reverted to stoop as they became fatigued.[193,194] Most people, including manual workers, habitually adopt stoop despite instruction to the contrary.[191] It is suggested that this is probably because it is a 'pattern of movement that they know', related in part to habitual standing and sitting postures where commonly, posterior rotation of the pelvis is consistently adopted. In 1999, Van Dieën et al.[195] extensively reviewed the biomechanical evidence and concluded that there was no justification for advocating squat technique.

Studies on self selected or freestyle lifting techniques have revealed the postures typically adopted are intermediate between stoop and squat, hence semi-squat techniques are receiving more interest. Described as 'moderate range of flexion at both knees and trunk, it allows a pattern of inter-joint coordination which appears to be functional in reducing muscular effort'.[196]

Review of the literature is fascinating in that for an action that requires initiation and control from the pelvis, this is rarely mentioned or factored into the research design, instead the focus largely being on the effect different knee positions have on the back. A recent study disallowed subjects any forward trunk inclination when squatting! Hardly a functional pattern and not surprisingly, the knee was working overtime.[197] Locking the knees in stoop limits pelvic rotation. The degree of knee flexion in squat is unphysiological as it places such high loads on them. No wonder 'the evidence' is equivocal.

Pattern of forward bending – lumbopelvic rhythm or pelvi-femoral rhythm?

While the interest has been in lifting, the *pattern of forward bending* not only underlies lifting but also many repetitive low load ADL activities such as emptying the dishwasher and gardening. Some of the confusion and clinical myths about forward bending patterns probably stems from some text book descriptions of lumbopelvic rhythm. These describe the first 60° or so of trunk flexion occurring in the lumbar spine and any further flexion occurs in the hip.[5] McGill[8] rightly refutes this as 'fiction' and instead proposes the 'hip hinge' in forward bending, citing Olympic weightlifters lock the lumbar spine close to neutral and rotate almost entirely around the hips. Hence it makes sense to adopt the term 'pelvi-femoral rhythm'.[148]

Spine in forward bending pattern resembles a cantilever

Panjabi and White[198] describe the spine in forward bending as behaving like a cantilever – where one end of a long structure is fixed and its other free end is 'loaded'. The 'fixed' end is obviously the stronger, heavier and centrally placed base of the spine within the pelvis which itself has been described as a cantilever.[6]

A simple cantilever, as Norris[187] points out, is externally supported and subject to bending load. If the spine is construed as an arch it becomes more intrinsically stable. This stability is reliant upon the musculature to modulate the lordosis and provide IAP and so keep the thrust line within the arch. When the thrust line moves outside the arch it becomes unstable. Coactivation and balanced activity between the flexors and extensors and the LPU optimizes both IAP and alignment of the 'body cylinder' functionally rendering it an effective cantilever during forward bending (Fig. 6.42).

Maneuvering the base of the cantilever is the task and this is the job of the pelvis. It should be able to swing freely between the leg axis and the spinal axis and as it does so, it carries the 'body cylinder' forward into bending and return/lifting. Effective pelvic actions allow the body cylinder to flexibly maintain its integral shape including the lumbar lordosis. The bulk of the movement occurs at the large ball and socket hip joints. Gracovetsky et al.[199] suggest that for every angle of forward flexion there is a unique degree of lordosis that will minimize and equalize the compressive stresses within the spine and at the same time will be associated with minimum muscle activity. Isometric trunk extension–flexion testing has been shown to

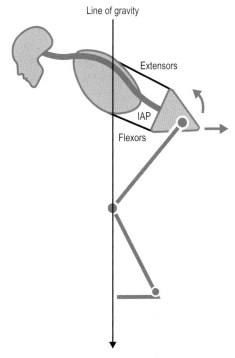

Line of gravity

Extensors

IAP

Flexors

Fig 6.42 • An effective 'body cylinder' provides both internal and three dimensional support to the spine in forward bending rendering the torso an adaptable cantilever. The centre of mass is supported over the base.

be stronger when the fulcrum for forward bending was at the hips.[200] However, achieving this pelvic control is elusive for most as it isn't an action they habitually use. It cannot happen if the knees are extended. However, flexing the knees does not necessarily solve the problem either, as a common strategy is to attempt the 'squat' with knee flexion and posterior pelvic rotation thus pulling the lumbar spine into more flexion! Habitual postural and movement patterns result in many subjects being disinclined to load the lower limb in flexion: the pelvis in hip flexion/ anterior pelvic rotation with knee flexion and dorsiflexion.

Functional forward bend pattern: semi-squat involving 'pelvic swing and shift patterns'

It is proposed that obtaining effective pelvic action in semi squat is dependent upon the initiation and support of the LPU synergy through the movement (see Dynamic control of sagittal 'Pelvic tilt' above). Reliant on active 'grounding' through the feet, the kinematics in biomechanically sound forward bending and lifting patterns involve three distinct phrases in the movement which are *led by the ischia*.

Forward bend

Forward bend is accomplished by the *ischia* assuming the following pattern:

• *Shifting posteriorly* in space and reaching backwards
• *Lifting* so the pelvis anteriorly rotates
• *Widening* into ischial outflare.

This is an extension of FPP1 and the pattern of movement involves posterior shift with anterior pelvic rotation, hip flexion and lumbosacral extension. The hip flexion provides the majority of the movement while the spine elongates through the movement and is free to perform the fine tuning and small adjustments needed for the arms to engage and carry the load (Fig. 6.43). This involves the LPU in dynamic synergism with the body cylinder which in this action also resembles a 1st class lever. The fulcrum of the movement is the hip as the acetabulum rotates around the femoral head. The spine and hips work together and Gracovetsky considers that both the erector spinae and psoas are important in control of the lordosis.[131] Incidentally, this pattern of movement is also involved in forward weight shift in sitting, moving from sitting to stand and lowering to sit and squatting as well as in many other actions.

Raising the effort arm – the ischia – is achieved from dynamic synergism between the LPU and more superficial muscles. In particular iliacus

and psoas, transversus and multifidus work concentrically and eccentric control comes from the obturator group, PFM, gluteus maximus and hamstrings acting to 'brake' the movement as the upper body is lowered. It is important to appreciate that *control of this force couple is only achieved when there is coactivation* between the anterior hip and trunk flexors and the posterior hip and trunk extensors where the pelvis can be 'driven back' from the feet and spatially controlled in order to take advantage of the extensor mechanism in the lower limb (See Ch. 4 & Fig. 6.54) Thinking about 'pushing the ischia back' in order to 'come forward' is useful in overcoming the habit of simply hanging forward (Fig. 6.44).

Lifting

The return movement continues to involve the fundamental control from the LPU, which now brings the *ischia* into the following pattern:

• *Shifting* forward in space
• *Dropping* down so that the pelvis posteriorly rotates
• *Narrowing* into ischial inflare.

This occurs in synergism with strong concentric activity of the hip/pelvic extensors[201] to 'drop' the effort arm, extend the hip and raise the body cylinder. *Co-activation from the anterior hip flexors is still important* as they eccentrically work and provide stability and control of the pelvis while the extensors 'lift' it. The magnitude of the load dictates the level of activity of the muscles in the walls of the body cylinder including the generation of appropriate levels of IAP.

The inferior pelvis is the generator and leads the movement via swings and shifts. It can only do this if the ankles and knees are simultaneously involved in the pattern. According to Pope, Borelli, the father of biomechanics understood that the levers of the musculoskeletal system magnify motion rather than force.[202] The movement role of the short stocky lever, the ischia while seemingly not large has an enormous effect on pelvic myomechanics when upright and through movement (Fig. 6.44). The hamstrings play an important role in bending and lifting, dynamically eccentrically/concentrically adjusting all through the movement to drive the ischia back/up and down/forward.

Defective control of eccentric lengthening of the obturator group and the hamstrings is the progenitor

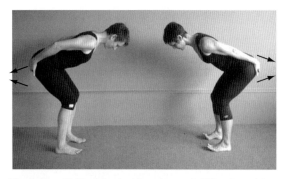

Fig 6.43 • 'Drilling' the 'pelvic swing and shift patterns' for control of the forward bend pattern; the hands help focus leading from the ischia. Note the grounding of the feet helps drive the ischia back and up where the tailbone can lengthen and the torso is well aligned.

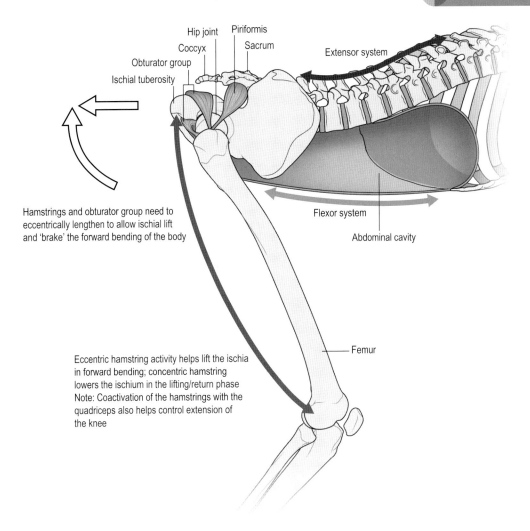

Hip joint   Piriformis
Coccyx   Sacrum
Obturator group
Ischial tuberosity

Extensor system

Hamstrings and obturator group need to
eccentrically lengthen to allow ischial lift
and 'brake' the forward bending of the body

Flexor system

Abdominal cavity

Eccentric hamstring activity helps lift the ischia
in forward bending; concentric hamstring
lowers the ischium in the lifting/return phase
Note: Coactivation of the hamstrings with the
quadriceps also helps control extension of
the knee

Femur

Fig 6.44 • Control of the 'ischial swing' is fundamental to raising and lowering the 'effort arm' in manoeuvring the 'body cylinder' in forward bending/lifting.

of many lumbopelvic pain symptoms and directly related to hamstrings 'tears'. Some studies have demonstrated flexion–relaxation in the hamstrings at the end of forward bending.[203] McGorry found that it varied[204] between individuals and in restrained or free standing postures. In the extension/lifting phase, hamstrings were recruited first indicating that pelvic motion leads the movement of trunk extension. If the legs operate as dynamic supports to assist lowering and raising the sit-bones the hamstrings should be either eccentrically or concentrically contracting throughout the movement. When the pelvis is allowed to shift backwards this facilitates this

action. It can only do this if there is co-activation from the LPU especially the lower abdominals and iliopsoas. Comparing trunk extension strength in kneeling and standing, Gallagher[205] found a reduction in kneeling which he attributed to a reduced capability to rotate the pelvis due to a disruption of the biomechanical linkage of the leg structures. While this is no doubt true, the kinematic pattern also involves a conjunct posterior spatial shift, and his testing device prevented this. Bringing the pelvis back keeps the centre of mass more within the base of support (see Ch.4, 'Basic concepts in posturomovement analysis').

Locking the knees locks the pelvis

The base of support – the feet with the ankles and knees – form an important part of the kinetic movement chain helping the pelvis to appropriately shift in space in order to present the torso to the task at hand. They must be free to dynamically adjust. Locking the knees significantly limits the important contribution of the pelvis and robs the large joints of a job they are well suited to do. One of the few lifting studies to factor the effect of pelvic tilt on lumbar posture during lifting[191] reported some increase in anterior shear and compression in lordosis and maximum segmental flexion moment in kyphosis. This led them to recommend the 'freestyle' posture – that of moderate flexion, as the safe lifting posture of choice. However, subjects were asked to keep their knees straight, significantly limiting the adaptive capability of the pelvis and the distribution of load sharing through the lower limb and increasing the load on the lumbar spine. The two joint muscles acting over the hip and knee provide effective load sharing (see Ch. 4

'Anatomical vs functional actions of muscles'). Had they allowed the dynamic action described above, it is suggested the outcome would have been more favorable (see 'The extensor mechanism' p. 142).

The importance of the feet

Being 'on your legs' and the important contribution of the feet in providing a flexible and dynamic base of support for posturomovement function is generally overlooked. Importantly, receptors in the feet are responsible for activation of significant reflex responses underlying postural stabilization and breathing.[103]

Functionally, their motion and muscular control relates to three events: shock absorption, weight bearing stability and propulsion.[206] The three foot articulations which have a major functional significance in walking are the subtalar, midtarsal and metatarsalphalangeal joints.[206] The 26 bones variously contribute to the three arches of the foot: the inner and outer longitudinal and transverse arches. These transmit weight as well as distribute it (Fig. 6.45). The medial 'unit' accepts the weight

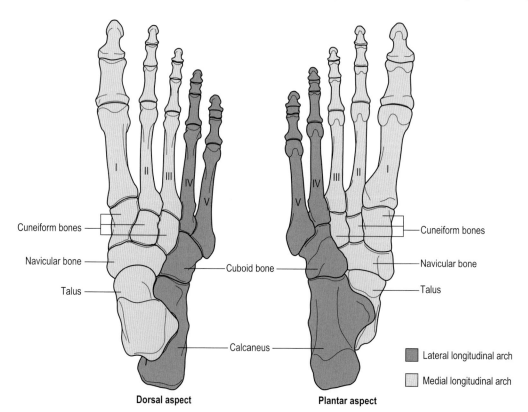

Cuneiform bones

Navicular bone

Talus

Cuboid bone

Calcaneus

Cuneiform bones

Navicular bone

Talus

Lateral longitudinal arch

Medial longitudinal arch

Dorsal aspect   **Plantar aspect**

Fig 6.45 • The structural organisation of the bones of the foot reflects its functional role.

of the leg while lateral portion function is probably more in lifting and balancing.[1] A strong myofascial matrix of tough connective tissue, tendons and small intrinsic foot muscles arranged in four layers supports the arches and gives spring and resiliency to the foot for support. In concert with the action of the calf muscles they also bring the joints of the feet into their close packed positions so that the foot is converted to a semi rigid lever for effective push off.[10] The foot oscillates between yielding to the ground and pushing away from it.

The feet are richly supplied with somatosensory inputs – proprioceptive, cutaneous and joint receptors, all contributing important information towards postural control of the body in general.[103] In neutral standing the line of gravity falls anterior to the ankle joint, hence the soleus exhibits continuous postural activity.[10] Balance requires the ability to transfer weight through the feet articulations forwards and backwards and mediolaterally hence full mobility in the hips and knees and ankles is also necessary to allow this. The arrangement of the intrinsic muscles resembles that in the hand hence the foot is capable of conforming to all manner of surfaces. Clinically, actively 'fanning the toes' and/or 'grasping' with the feet (and/or hands) directly facilitates a reflex reaction in the postural mechanism including better activation of the LPU and the diaphragm[103] (see Fig. 13.105).

However, many are functionally 'dead on their legs'. Described as 'sensory deprivation chambers'[207] the shoes we wear not only deprive us of the rich sensory bombardment that feeds and nourishes the CNS but also multiple unexpected surface changes and movements which help maintain the pliability and dexterousness of the feet. When the feet are active and well 'grounded' the SLMS is better activated and the kinetic movement chain up the legs and through the pelvis can be more effective. In this way the feet utilize the ground reaction force and assist the 'push up' against gravity. The feet affect how the pelvis can spatially shift[208] and functionally there is a strong link between heel pressure and the movement control of the ischial tuberosities and the eccentric and concentric control of the hamstrings as the pelvis is moved over the leg. Pressure through the ball of the foot also has kinetic links to activation of ilio-psoas.[28]

The control of the pelvis is also reflected in the feet such that Rolf termed them 'tattletales'. In particular, imbalance in the deep intrinsic inferior pelvic force couple with obturator group dominance creates external rotation at the hips, pronated feet, collapse of the medial longitudinal arch and possibly

hallux valgus. Many of those waddling around with foot orthotics would be better served in bare feet and addressing the disturbances obviously present in the pelvi-femoral myomechanics.

Part C: Upper pole of the body cylinder – the thorax, shoulder girdle, head and neck

The thorax provides the base of support for the head and neck and the shoulder girdle. They all operate as an interdependent system, each element reciprocally influencing all the other elements. Rolf[1] maintained that the 'pattern of the upper pole' is determined by three factors:

• The position of the thoracic spine with respect to the line of gravity
• The balance of the shoulder girdle as it distributes the physical work of the body. This girdle is more vulnerable to deformation than the pelvic girdle.
• The alignment of the cervical spine with respect to the gravity line is particularly important as it balances the head containing the prime sensing organs.

The shoulder girdle determines the position and competence of the thoracic and cervical spines and the head. The alignment of the spine dictates the placement of the girdle. Each component is explored.

Thorax

The rib cage is part of the spine's structure; a roughly ovoid shaped cage formed by the manubrium/sternum in front, 12 pairs of ribs and their adjacent vertebra. The vertebrae provide the point of stability for rib movements while at the same time embellishing rib movement – movement of one involves the other.

The thorax is capable of expansion in all dimensions, in particular the bottom half which is more flexible than the top. The upper opening or outlet is less than half the width of the capacious inferior outlet. Its structure is resilient enough to provide protection for the vital organs yet flexible enough to contribute towards movement control of the whole body. It also has the potential to be deformable.

Biomechanics

The thoracic spine is mechanically stiffer and less mobile than the other regions.[5] In general, structural and kinematic data about the thorax are limited.,[209,210] Coupling patterns between rotation and lateral bending has caused the most interest.[5] In the upper part they are strongly coupled though not as much as in the cervical spine[5] and less distinct in the middle and lower regions, although variability, and predominantly ipsilateral coupling in the middle and lower regions has been found.[211] Arm elevation produces distinct ipsilateral coupling and associated extension in the upper thoracic spine.[212]

The variability is no doubt due to the influence of different myofascial-rib states; vertebral movement is affected by the freedom or otherwise in the ribs.

Regions

Different morphological characteristics of the vertebrae and ribs have led to different regions being described in the literature. While there is no clear distinction, undoubtedly differing biomechanics serve different functions.

- Three vertebral regions have been described: T1–4; T4–8; T8–12.[5,211]
- Stokes[218] also notes three vertebral regions though different: the transitional cervicothoracic and thoracolumbar regions and an intermediate zone – T3.
- Lee[209] delineates four regions which in functional terms make sense to consider, below.

1. *Vertebromanubrial region:* consists of T1 &2; 1st and 2nd ribs and the manubrium into which they insert. The first and second ribs don't have a lot of movement and represent a firm collar or ring forming the upper thoracic outlet – 'the upper ring'. This provides a stable point of attachment for the scalenii and sternocleidomastoid to help in balancing the head and neck; a point for lifting and opening the manubrium sternum, as well as assisting in lifting the top of thorax in high demand breathing. The clavicle also attaches to the manubrium and represents the only joint directly connecting the upper limb girdle to the body. With C7 this also forms the cervicothoracic transitional zone.

2. *Vertebrosternal region:* includes T3–7; ribs 3–7 and the sternum into which they insert. The axis of the costovertebral and costotransverse in general lies closer to the frontal plane hence when the rib rotates and elevates in a 'pump handle' action, the anteroposterior dimension of the thorax is increased. This part of the cage is more flexible than that above though less than that below. With the arm by the side, the glenohumeral joint is lies approximately adjacent to the lateral 3rd 4th and 5th ribs.

3. *Vertebrochondral region:* T8–10; ribs 8–10 which share a common cartilaginous insertion which blends with that of the 7th costal cartilage. The axis of the posterior costovertebral and transverse joint largely lies more in the sagittal plane hence elevation of the rib creates a 'bucket handle' action which increases the transverse diameter of the thorax. This represents the most deformable part of the cage. Harrison et al.[153] showed that translating the thorax anteriorly/posteriorly changed the kyphosis and 60% of the movement occurred in this region.

Kapandji[16] notes that in the midzone of the thorax, the costovertebral joints lie between the sagittal and frontal planes hence elevation of the ribs increases both the anteroposterior and transverse diameters of the thorax here (Fig. 6.46)

4. *Thoracolumbar junction:* T10/11/12/L1/2; ribs 11 & 12 which are 'floating', acting like large transverse processes, they help 'feather' the transition between the thorax and the relatively mobile lumbar spine. They also provide important attachment points for numerous muscles – the diaphragm, transversus, quadratus lumborum to name a few. This region is the point of inflection between the thoracic kyphosis and the lumbar lordosis.[24] The vertebrae provide an important transition between the primary movement of rotation in the thorax and flexion/extension in the lumbar spine. The orientation of the vertebral facets through this region gradually changes from nearly coronal in the thoracic spine nearly sagittal in the lumbar spine. The first sites of ossification in the spine consistently occur in the bodies of these levels.[24] This and their resistance to

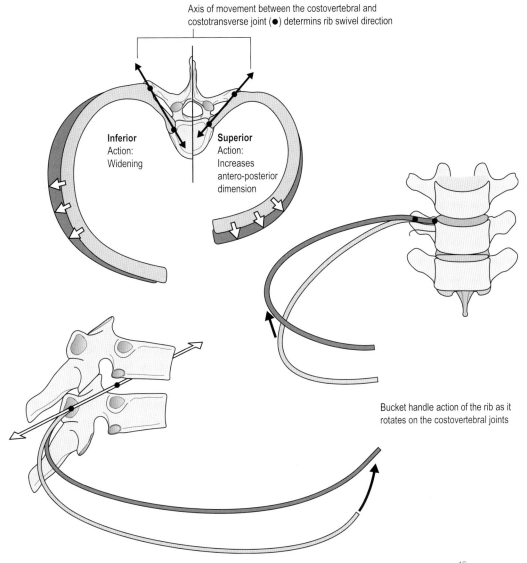

Axis of movement between the costovertebral and costotransverse joint (●) determins rib swivel direction

Inferior
Action:
Widening

Superior
Action:
Increases
antero-posterior
dimension

Bucket handle action of the rib as it rotates on the costovertebral joints

Fig 6.46 • Movements of the ribs during inspiration vary in different regions. Adapted from Kapandji[16]

rotation/torsional stresses and extension afforded by the facets[24] indicate its significance as a stable load bearing region. When laterally translating the thorax relative to a fixed pelvis, Harrison et al.[215] found lateral flexion was the largest at L1 and decreased from L1 to L5, but the segmental rotation angles for lateral flexion were largest at L3/4 (6.2°), then L4/5 (5.7°) and L2/3 (3.9°)

Scaffolding of the upper pole of the body cylinder supported by the SLMS

Acting like struts, each rib or 'hoop' is connected by the intercostals arranged in two layers, their fibres running in diagonally opposite directions. Through fascial connections they become contiguous with transversus, the diaphragm, and psoas through to the pelvis and so on, providing a continuous deep sleeve of neuromyofascial support. The line of their fibres is also continued through the obliques and further with the interdigitations of serratus and rhomboids and so on. Posteriorly the deep paraspinal intrinsic muscles control segmental movement. This myofascial cross bracing supports the structure in such a way that it can be likened to a tensegrity structure – malleable, light yet strong and dissipating forces through tension and compression.[39,213] Forces are transferred globally across the entire structure. In addition, 'a tensegrity mast like the spine, functions whether vertically or horizontal and can accept loads in any position'.[213] Studies on deep muscle control of the thoracic spine are few. Lee et al.[214] found differential activity between the deep and superficial paraspinal muscles during trunk rotation in sitting. Multifidus activity while variable, was not necessarily direction dependent, and varied in different regions of the spine probably reflecting regional biomechanical differences.

The ribs and their related fascia also provide attachment points for many of the large muscles attaching the shoulder girdle to the thorax and also the pelvic girdle to the thorax. The fibre direction in many of these is also diagonal and serves to extend and reinforce the dynamic bracing afford by the deep system muscles in a continuous myofascial 'wrapping'. The cage itself needs to be both mobile and stable as a whole as well as within it, in order that it can provide an effective and adaptable stable base of support from which these limb girdle muscles can act. Unequal length tension relationships in any one of these can 'cause distortions to occur throughout the structure in all three axes'.[213] This jeopardizes not only the alignment of the axial spine but also the intrinsic shape of the cage and its spatial relationship to the head and the pelvis.

An examination of significant aspects of the myofascial architecture of the thorax helps understand its alignment and control as part of the body cylinder.

Alignment and control of the thorax over the pelvis

Frontal plane

An important movement of the thorax is lateral translation necessary for effective weight shift and postural adjustment through the torso. Harrison et al.[215] have shown that this can be significant,

between 35 and 70 mm. This involves lengthening one side and shortening the other. 'Lengthening the sides' is an important component function in the body cylinder including weight shift, breathing and reaching.

Achieving a balanced neutral is also important where symmetry is fundamental. When disturbed, the thorax is shifted laterally and a scoliosis ensues. This may be structural – complex bio and myomechanically and more so if a double rather than a single curve. More clinically common, is the functional scoliosis or lateral list of the thorax on the pelvis. The literature is replete with motherhood statements about this condition yet nowhere could this author find a myofascial descriptor as to its genesis. Greive[216] suggests that iliopsoas may be implicated in pelvic torsion and this generally accompanies an acute list. Kendall[129] suggests 'lateral trunk muscles' are involved. Clinical practice delineates ilio-psoas, quadratus lumborum, serratus posterior inferior, the lateral abdominals and lateral latissimus dorsi can all be implicated in this changed alignment (Fig. 6.47).

Myofascial geometry helps 'shore up' the thoracolumbar junction at a potential cost

While significant control between the thorax and pelvis is afforded by the large thoracopelvic muscles – the erector spinae, anterolateral abdominals, psoas quadratus lumborum and latissimus dorsi, clinically it becomes apparent that the junction is further reinforced by a fan shaped myofascial arrangement over the junction which terminates around L2–3 (Fig. 6.48).

Anteriorly, the diaphragm attaches between T12 and L3 (on the right and L2 on the left) and extends laterally and anterosuperiorly to encircle the base of the inferior thoracic opening. It can be considered analogous to a basketball hoop on a pole. While psoas attaches to all lumbar levels and T12, Bogduk et al.[154] proposed that its lower fascicles tend to flex the lower lumbar levels and the upper fascicles extend the upper segments. Penning[156] argues that this differential action between fascicles serves to stabilize the spine. If spinal alignment is altered, their angle of pull will change and their action may become provocative.

Posteriorly, the lowest point of origin of spinalis is L3.[16] Serratus posterior inferior attaches from T11 to L2 or L3[10] and passes up to the lower four

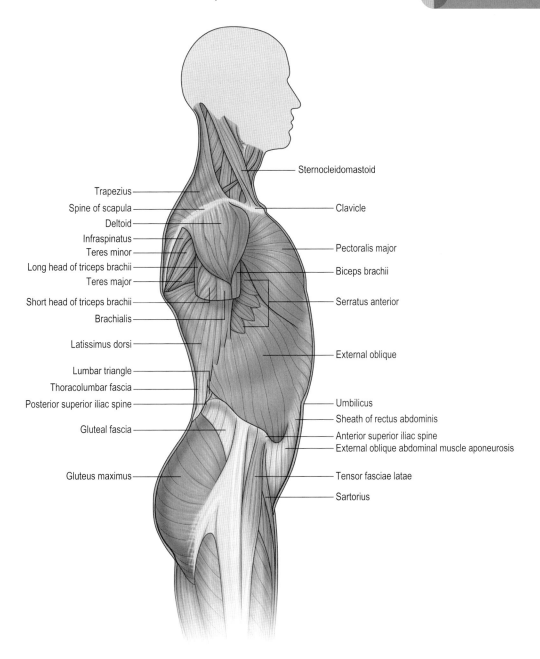

Fig 6.47 • The lateral wall of the body.

Labels:
- Sternocleidomastoid
- Trapezius
- Spine of scapula
- Deltoid
- Infraspinatus
- Teres minor
- Long head of triceps brachii
- Teres major
- Short head of triceps brachii
- Brachialis
- Latissimus dorsi
- Lumbar triangle
- Thoracolumbar fascia
- Posterior superior iliac spine
- Gluteal fascia
- Gluteus maximus
- Clavicle
- Pectoralis major
- Biceps brachii
- Serratus anterior
- External oblique
- Umbilicus
- Sheath of rectus abdominis
- Anterior superior iliac spine
- External oblique abdominal muscle aponeurosis
- Tensor fasciae latae
- Sartorius

ribs which also receive attachments from the lateral abdominals and latissimus, which itself is attached to L3. In relative terms, segments T12–L3 enjoy more myofascial stability and the lumbar segments below are potentially vulnerable in altered postur-omovement control.

Sagittal alignment of the thorax

The line of gravity passes through the upper and lower thoracic junctions and anterior to the apex of the kyphosis.[24] The attendant axial load tends to increase the thoracic curve[210] – and will certainly

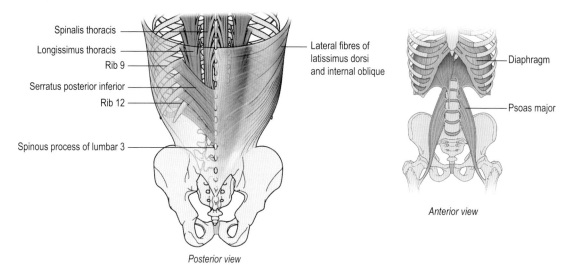

Spinalis thoracis

Longissimus thoracis

Rib 9

Serratus posterior inferior

Rib 12

Spinous process of lumbar 3

Lateral fibres of
latissimus dorsi
and internal oblique

Diaphragm

Psoas major

Anterior view

Posterior view

Fig 6.48 • Clinically an often dense myofascial fan acts to hyperstabilize the thoracolumbar region and lower pole of the thorax.

do so in the case of poor postural and movement control in the thorax. The thoracic curve varies in its magnitude[217] and is deemed to increase with age.[209,210]

The sagittal alignment of the thorax over the pelvis is dependent upon the alignment and movement capability within it which deserves attention.

Upper and lower poles of the thorax

The T6/7/8 region is interesting. The midpoint of the thoracic spine is T6/7 which is roughly the apex of the thoracic curve. Anteriorly rib 6 has a direct connection to the sternum. Rib 7 shares its insertion with ribs 8–10. The sternum or breast plate acts as an anterior strut providing more stability to the upper pole of the thorax. This creates the possibility for a functional 'hinge' between the more mobile lower pole and the more structurally reinforced upper pole of the thorax – the 'dorsal hinge'.[41] This is particularly likely to occur into flexion. The predominant pump handle A/P rib action in the upper pole and predominant bucket handle lateral rib excursion probably further reinforces this.

The more stable upper pole is more directly related to head neck and shoulder function and it is here that the major part of the axioscapulohumeral muscles attach. The lower pole being more mobile is more involved with primary breathing, controlling the alignment of the body wall,

integrating upper and lower limb function, and contributing to lower limb girdle control.

Importantly, in normal studies, rotation was found to be greatest in the mid-thoracic region around T6–7.[16,210,218] Anterior and posterior disc postural loads have been shown to be balanced at T8/9.[217]

The lower section, being relatively more mobile, is more vulnerable to potential deformation from myofascial imbalance. This will affect the myomechanics of the whole thorax and the body cylinder as a whole. Harrison et al.[153] showed that during A/P sagittal translation of the thoracic cage, 60% of this occurred between T8–12.

Myofascial control of sagittal thorax alignment

This basically depends upon balance between the flexor and extensor systems. This comprises balance of the thorax as a whole over the pelvis and between its upper and lower poles. Imbalance in the upper pole will be reflected in the lower pole and vice versa

• Balance in the upper pole is essentially represented by:

  • balance between the cervicothoracic flexors and extensors and
  • balance between the shoulder girdle flexors/ protractors anteriorly, and synergistic activity between the shoulder girdle retractors and depressors posteriorly – middle and lower

trapezius and rhomboids. Janda[53] referred to these collectively as the 'lower scapular stabilizers'.

- Balance of the lower pole is between the abdominals anterolaterally and the spinal extensors, serratus posterior inferior and latissimus dorsi posterolaterally (Fig. 6.47). Importantly, the ability to spatially move the thorax forward and back with respect to the pelvis requires adequate spatial pelvic control in order that it can provide a stable base of support for the action.

Note that while there is the tendency for a structural and functional 'hinge' in the mid thorax, nature has cleverly transitioned the attachment of the anterior shoulder muscles. The pectorals extend from the second rib to the cartilage of the 6th or 7th rib[10] and serratus anterior is generally considered to extend to rib 9,[129,219] though can be between the 8th and the 10th rib.[10] The upper attachments of the abdominals extend as high as the 5th rib. There is a direct fascial link between the sternocleidomastoid, pectoralis major and the rectus sheath of the abdominals.[10]

Posteriorly, trapezius extends from the occiput to T12 but may not extend below T8.[10] The rhomboids together attach to the spinous processes of C7 to down to T5.[10] Rolf[1] considered rhomboids central to activity of the shoulder girdle.

Changes in the shape of the thorax during inspiration

Sagittal plane

Many conventional texts such as Kapandji[16] describe the pattern of inspiration as one of raising the cage both superiorly and inferiorly and increasing the anteroposterior diameter of the upper thorax. However, well informed clinical practice[220] dictates that this pattern equates to high load auxiliary breathing using the accessory breathing muscles to lift the thorax – not a desirable state of affairs in the usual low load state. Instead, the primary action should be one of a lateral expansion of the lower ribcage with an anterior expansion of the anterior thorax and upper abdomen balancing posterolateral expansion. Importantly, all breathing aficionados[70,110] recommend *no* lifting of the cage as a whole – a pattern associated with stress, tension and hyperventilation syndrome.

Frontal plane

Normal quiet inspiration involves a lateral expansion of the lower pole of the thorax and a widening of the waist.

Shoulder girdle

The function of the shoulder girdle will in large part determine the competency and kind control in the upper thorax and its effect upon the rest of the spine. In fact, people with spinal pain always show defective control of their major ball and socket joints – the hip and the shoulder. Rather than a comprehensive treatise on the shoulder, examination of the function of the shoulder girdle as it relates to torso control will be considered.

The shoulder girdle consisting of the clavicle, scapula and head of the humerus rotating in the spherical glenoid, allows large multiplanar freedoms of movement as well as the provision for weight bearing. The girdle is suspended on top of the thorax rather like an oxen yolk, its only bony attachment via the connection of the clavicle with the sternum (Fig. 6.49). The clavicle acts like a strut or 'yard arm,' holding the girdle away from the ribs so that the arm hangs free of the body.[6] The scapulae slide and rotate on the chest wall pivoting around the lateral end of the clavicle in order to orient the arm. Movement of one is always reflected in the other.

Effective control of the claviscapular unit provides a spatially appropriate and stable platform of control to support function of the arm and hand. Like the axial column, arm use occurs as either open or closed kinetic chain movements and always involves muscle activation patterns throughout the torso as well as a degree of weight shift both within the thorax and over the base of support. Arm movements into elevation irrespective of the plane of motion produce small but arguably important segmental thoracic spinal motion.[221] This is significantly greater into side flexion and rotation with unilateral movements, whereas bilateral arm use produces a small extension displacement in the upper thoracic spine and more significant extension in the lower thoracic spine.[221] Axial muscles attaching to the scapular and humerus span every vertebral level from the occiput to the sacrum and surround the chest wall as they unite the girdle to

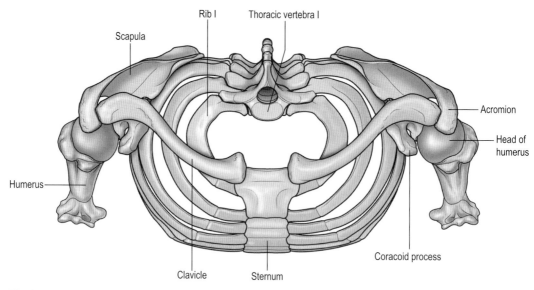

Fig 6.49 • Viewed from above, the shoulder girdle resembles a 'yoke' suspended over the thorax.

the spine and torso. Hence movement of the arms has a significant effect upon the alignment and control of the axial spine as a whole.

The position of the sternum and the rest of the thorax with respect to the line of gravity directly influence the position of the girdle. When dropped and recessed, the clavicles downwardly rotate carrying the scapula-arm so that the girdle hangs forward, down and narrows, occasioning increased holding from the suspensory muscles above. When lifted and open, the clavicles posteriorly rotate, the scapula drops back and the shoulders widen.

Similar to the pelvis, appropriate spatial positioning of the clavi-scapular position facilitates gleno-humeral movements and balanced rotator cuff action in centering the humeral head during movement. Ingenious scapular positioning can also functionally increase gleno-humeral advantage and 'reach'.

Movements of the girdle

Essentially movements of the clavi-scapular unit produce simultaneous movements in the sternoclavicular, acromioclavicular and scapulothoracic 'joint' with conjunct rotations occurring in the glenohumeral joint. All glenohumeral movements consist of rotations in the various planes which are associated with spin slide and roll in the joint. Claviscapulothoracic movements constitute movements of the whole girdle and principally consist of:

- Elevation and depression
- Retraction or adduction and protraction or abduction
- Downward or upward rotation.

Functional movement control comprises varying combinations of these movements. Like the pelvis, the scapula is the bridge marrying movement between the limb and the torso. If the arm is fixed or stable, the scapula rotates around the head of the humerus. If the scapula is fixed, the humeral head rotates in the glenoid.

However, it is critically important that the thorax and the shoulder girdle are able to move independently of one another – the ribs moving under the shoulder girdle or the girdle moving over and around the thoracic cage. The scapula can be required to perform a concurrent dual role of controlling both stability and mobility in movement. Weight shift when on all fours is an example.

Myofascial balance in the shoulder girdle ensures optimal shoulder and thorax function

Its tenuous bony attachment to the skeleton and relatively shallow glenoid fossa means that functionally, the shoulder girdle is a compromise between mobility and stability. Accordingly, it is highly dependent upon dynamic stability provided by balanced myofascial control. Balance needs to occur in all three planes of movement. For example, a winged scapula occurs with serratus anterior weakness; however, more often than not, this is indicative of disorganized spatial control of the whole girdle, part of which is due to serratus not eccentrically lengthening.

It is useful to view the girdle in the different planes in order to fully appreciate its potential dysfunction:

Sagittal plane view

The scope of upper limb activities varies from strong lifting, throwing carrying, pulling and pushing to fine movements of the hands. The manner in which the axioscapulohumeral muscles are arranged around the body wall allows lines of pull in all planes and forces can be transmitted throughout the body. Their form resembles the spokes of a wheel, which functionally converge at the shoulder, the conceptual 'hub'[6] (Fig. 6.50). Rather than pure plane movements, adjacent muscles in the 'wheel'

are able to contribute to various combinations and modulation of movement direction. If the action of any of the spokes is impaired by unequal pulls, the whole mechanism suffers. Depending upon the 'fixed point'– either the thorax/scapula or the humerus, the muscles contribute to both open and closed kinetic chain movement control similar to that seen in the pelvis. 'Open chain' movements are those where the arm moves around the stable thorax/scapula; in 'closed chain' movements, the thorax/scapula moves around the stable limb. Note movement occurs variably between the humerus, scapula and chest wall.

Balance in the muscle activation patterns and length tension relationships between antagonistic groups need to be considered as follows:

- Protraction / retraction of the girdle
  - *Anterior group* – collectively, the upper anterior chest muscles – serratus anterior and the pectorals flex and protract the girdle on the thorax. With the girdle fixed or stabilized they depress the sternum and flex the thorax. Anterior girdle fixing can also be used as a

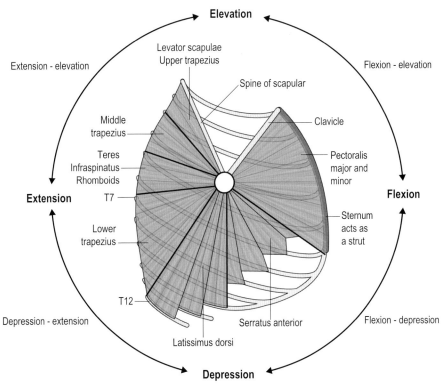

Fig 6.50 • Schematic lateral view of the thorax and the myofascial 'wheel' of the axioscapulohumeral muscles acting upon the glenohumeral 'hub' after Todd.[6]

strategy to assist in labored breathing whereby serratus and pectorals act to lift the ribs.

- **Posterior group** – rhomboids, middle and lower trapezius retract and anchor the girdle to the dorsal spine. With the girdle fixed or stabilized they assist in opening and lifting the sternum forward and extending the thoracic spine.

If the anterior group is more dominant, the girdle is forward and the upper pole of the thorax is more flexed.

- Elevation / depression of the girdle
  - **Superior group** – the upper trapezius and levator scapulae with some contribution from rhomboids[12] lift the girdle. If the girdle is fixed or stabilized they are synergistic in dropping the trunk between the girdles as in lowering oneself from sitting to the floor through the arms.
  - **Inferior group** – the serratus, pectorals, latissimus dorsi and lower trapezius depress the girdle. Subclavius also contributes. When the girdle is fixed as in weightbearing through the arms the body can be lifted through the girdles as in lifting your bottom off the seat.
  - **Activity of the anterior depressors** – the serratus, pectorals and subclavius needs to be matched by activity in the posterior depressors, the lower trapezius and latissimus, otherwise the girdle is protracted and depressed and the thorax is flexed.

Coronal plane

Given that the majority of modern man's arm use is forward, the medial scapula stabilizers – the rhomboids and middle and lower trapezius with synergistic activity in the adjacent paraspinal muscles need to provide effective eccentric and concentric control in order to balance the anterior load on the girdle (Fig. 6.51).

Balance needs to occur in the three prime movement directions:

- **Superior/inferior.** Upper trapezius, levator scapulae rhomboids activity balanced with middle and lower trapezius and latissimus.
- **Medio/lateral.** Rhomboids major and minor need to be balanced with serratus anterior and pectoralis minor and also pectoralis major acting through the humerus. Rolf[1] also draws attention to balance between rhomboids and teres. If teres is dominant scapula retraction is attempted by teres.

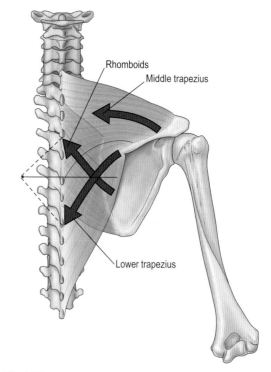

Fig 6.51 • The forces exerted by the inferomedial scapula stabilizers.

Similarly, adduction of the arm causes abduction of the scapula. Also, during glenohumeral abduction, if teres doesn't adequately lengthen and medial stabilization is inadequate the scapula is again pulled into abduction.

- **Upward and downward scapula rotation.** Upward rotation of the scapula provides the essential platform for arm elevation. It is achieved by a force couple between all three parts of trapezius and the lower fibres of serratus acting to pull the inferior angle laterally while tipping the superior angle medially and hence the glenoid up. Downward rotation is achieved through eccentric lengthening of the same synergy plus rhomboids and latissimus activity. The upper/lower and medio/lateral contributions to the force couple need to be balanced. If the upper anterior unit is dominant, the girdle becomes hitched and protracted.

Transverse plane

Forward and backward movements of one claviscapular unit produce a rotary torque in the transverse plane on the 'upper ring' – called forward and backward shoulder rotation. Essentially protraction and retraction, the upper ribs and vertebrae variably move either with[221] or independent of the girdle. When accepted by the brain, the head turns ipsilaterally, the girdle movement thus initiating and embellishing cervical movement ease and range. When resisted, for example when looking at a good sort as you reach behind, the head remains in neutral rotation. This is an important postural setting action supporting head rotation and arm actions. During walking, the transverse plane girdle rotation initiates the pendular arm swing which reduces the energy cost in walking.

- *Backward shoulder rotation (BSR).* It is important that this is primarily initiated from the medial and lower scapular stabilizers and not teres and infraspinatus. Serratus eccentrically lengthens.
- *Forward shoulder rotation (FSR).* This is primarily initiated from serratus rather than from pectorals, while rhomboids and middle and lower traps lengthen. Cervicothoracic junction and shoulder function are intimately related.

Cervical spine and head

When the axial skeleton is balanced the head is balanced and vice versa. The pelvis at the base is the key which determines the support and control of the rest of the axial spine and thorax. With well balanced support from below, the head and neck are balanced over the thorax and are free to easily lift, rotate and oscillate to orient the prime sense organs which drive motor function. The head apparently weighs some 3–4 kilos. If poorly balanced, chronic muscle activity and tension patterns are needed to 'hold' the head up. Mobility in the upper thoracic motion segments is important in facilitating movements of the cervical spine.[210]

The cervicothoracic junction represents a critical crossroads of functional cooperation between the thorax, cervical spine and shoulder. The postural fate of the neck is dependent upon the organization of the shoulder girdle[1] and in particular the related position of the 'top two rings' of the thorax; the 1st and 2nd ribs with their vertebra behind and manubrium–sternum anteriorly. Lift of the anterior strut enables a neutral cervical spine largely maintained by principal activity from the SLMS. Superficial system support is provided by the sternocleidomastoid splenius, levator scapulae, trapezius and scalenes variously attaching to the manubrium clavicle, scapula or vertebrae. They act like guy ropes and their balance is critical. However, with poor deep system control and the collapse down and forward of the thorax and shoulder girdle, they tend to become over active, hold the head forward, and shorten and extend the neck and head.

Competent inferior axial support includes competent diaphragmatic control otherwise the accessory breathing muscles are called into chronic over activity with predictable consequences on the neck.

The cervicocranial junction – the first two vertebrae are connected to each other and the skull by a complex chain of joints with three axes and three degrees of freedom.[16] The region allows the greatest triplanar mobility of any part of the spine.[12] Optimal alignment and control of the rest of the axial column allows their important contribution to nodding and rotating the head. Movements of the eyes are closely linked with facilitating head movements, generally in the same direction, though this is not obligatory and contradirectional head and eye movements are also possible. Steindler[132] draws attention to the increased functional range of rotation afforded by the eyes being able to rotate 45° on each side. When the head is carried forward, movement of the upper movement unit is hindered, and will need to occur elsewhere. The mid cervical levels risk becoming sites of relative flexibility when movement does not occur as it should in the upper and lower cervical junctions.

Part D: Functional interrelationship between the upper and lower body cylinder

It is considered that the function of the two limb girdles determines the motor competency of the whole body.[1] Inadequate proximal girdle function creates problems for the spine.[148] 'In the primary patterns of movement the thorax and pelvis work together and the breathing rhythms adjust to the coordinated whole, the shoulders and the arms follow the dictates of the head'.[6]

Rolf[1] considered that psoas provides a unique link between the legs and the upper torso. Psoas prevertebrally and rhomboids postvertebrally connect the two girdles to the spine. Functionally, however, lower trapezius is also important in the functional synergy with rhomboids and should be included particularly as both it and psoas attach to T12 (Fig. 6.52). Balance between them all ensures stability though flexibility of the girdles without disturbing the axial vertical. It also ensures correct function of the diaphragm which is fundamental to the 'open'

body cylinder. Rather than the erector spinae being the prime antagonist to the rectus abdominus, psoas and rectus abdominus need to be balanced as do psoas and rhomboids/lower trapezius. Rolf says: 'the focus of rhomboid–psoas balance is at the lumbodorsal junction which is what gives this area its unique importance in body mechanics'.[1]

The extensor mechanism of the body

Superficial to the erector spinae is an auxiliary extensor system which has interesting myofascial geometry for distributing the load between the upper and lower movement systems (Fig. 6.53).

- The three sections of the trapezius extend from the occiput to T12.
- Latissimus dorsi arises from the spines of T7–12, the spines of all the saccral and all lumbar vertebrae via the thoracolumbar fascia; as well as the posterior iliac crest; the lateral aspect of ribs 9–12; the inferior angle of the scapula. All the fibres converge into a narrow tendon to attach superiorly on the humerus. Note the trapezius and latissimus overlap between T7–12 to reinforce the mid back. Through it, the arms and the low back are functionally connected. No wonder Janda[222] considered it one of the most significant muscles in the body!
- Gracovetsky[37] considers the thoracolumbar fascia is the most important structure insuring the integrity of the spinal machinery as the viscoelastic properties of its collagen directly impacts upon the way the muscles are used and forces are channeled from the ground to the upper extremities. Its direct attachment to the spinous processes allows the powerful action of the hip extensors to be directly transmitted to the spine.[131] The ability to dynamically alter the lumbar lordosis is important in force transfer.
- Gluteus maximus extends from the iliotibial tract of the fascia lata and the femur and attaches superiorly to the iliac crest, thoracolumbar fascia, sacrum and coccyx. Its ability to bring the trunk upright has been described as the defining attribute of man.[10] Coupled motion between it and the contralateral latissimus has been shown.[223]
- Raising the body. With gluteus maximus acting over the hip, hamstrings action raises and lowers the base of the body cylinder from the ischia as though the pelvis were a draw bridge.

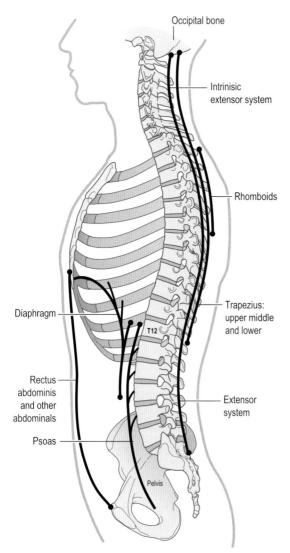

Occipital bone

Intrinisic extensor system

Rhomboids

Diaphragm

T12

Trapezius: upper middle and lower

Rectus abdominis and other abdominals

Extensor system

Psoas

Pelvis

Fig 6.52 • Schematic concept of sagittal alignment. Balanced activity between the lower scapula stabilizers, the extensors and psoas with the diaphragm and abdominals provides support and marries function between the upper and lower body.

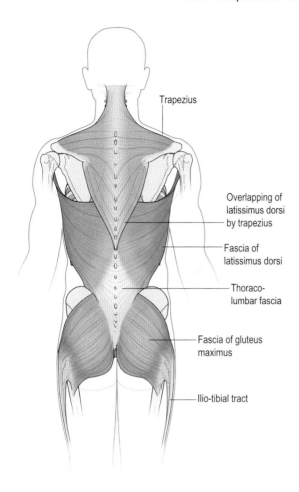

Fig 6.53 • The superficial myofascial extensor matrix.

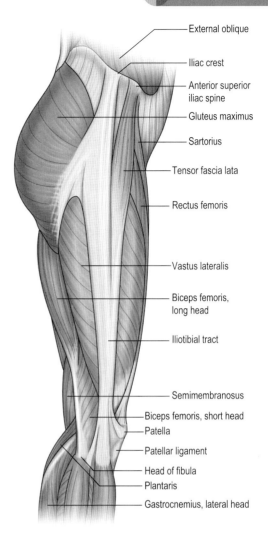

Fig 6.54 • The lower limb extensor mechanism.

• The lower limb extensor mechanism. From the ground reaction force through the feet, antigravity 'lift' is further achieved from coordinated interplay between the one and two joint leg muscles (see Ch. 4). The quadriceps mechanism and tensor fascia lata tense the fascial envelope around the thigh and help promote optimal function in the hip joint[224] including stability for gluteus maximus[7] and hamstring activity in raising and lowering the 'pelvic swing' (Fig. 6.54). Farfan[7] notes that by increasing external rotation at the hip, the hip extensors gain mechanical advantage. The extensive fascia lata with the reinforced iliotibial tract is distally attached to the lateral tibial condyle, fibula head and femoral condyles and extends proximally to attach to the back of the sacrum and coccyx, iliac crest, inguinal ligament and superior and inferior pubic rami,

ischial tuberosity and the lower border of the sacrotuberous ligament.[10]

The main functional roles of the upper and lower body

Helped by Bartenieff's observations[148] one can delineate the essentially different roles between the upper and lower units of the body.

• The lower unit as the controller of the centre of weight essentially 'grounds' the 'base of support' for antigravity control and postural changes for locomotor activity.

- 'The upper unit essentially serves exploring, manipulating gesturing activities. It initiates and extends reach space, communicates through spatial gesture, body touch grasp, enveloping dispersing and intertwining'.

It is common to see a certain 'role reversal' in many of our patients which is associated with a 'central disconnect' between the upper and lower poles of the body cylinder.

Walking

Locomotion is basic to survival. A fundamental physiological movement, walking involves integrated function of the legs, both proximal limb girdles and the axial spine while allowing independent motion of the head in order to focus the senses. Many in the world still walk many miles a day to gather food and work. 'Exercise' is a matter of course.

The greatest amount of motion occurs at the pelvis.[225] Pelvic motion is initiated by the base of the trunk mass (sacroiliac joint) being eccentric to the centre of the supporting hip joints. Pelvic movement is restrained by the hip muscles while the axial muscles control trunk alignment over the pelvis.[225] During each stride, the pelvis rotates asynchronously in three directions: sagittal 4°, coronal 7° and in the transverse plane 10°.[225] This involves 'distorsion'. With increasing stride, 'the horizontal components become greatly increased. The backward leg develops a forward, and the forward leg a backward, rotating thrust creating a force couple which rotates the pelvis in the transverse plane. These forces are essential to producing the propulsion and restraint of human gait'.[132] Transverse plane rotation thus occurs at the hip joint, sacroiliac joint and the lumbosacral joint. Lumbar motion occurs in all segments, is triaxial and although small, the complex multiplanar motion allows the lower extremities to remain in a largely planar pattern.[13]

Gracovetsky[130] has proposed the spine as an engine which drives the primary movement of the pelvis.[131] Walking is possible without legs – the legs only amplify movements of the pelvis. However, in energy efficient walking the extensor power from the legs is transmitted by the hip extensors through the pelvis to the spine taking advantage of a lordotic spine that compresses and twists driving rotation of the pelvis and counter rotation in the shoulder. This counter rotation between the limb girdles enables the connecting link – the spine and its viscoelastic tissues, to store and release kinetic energy – the body becoming an oscillator resonating in the gravitational field. The viscoelasticity of the spinal tissues and the inertia of the limbs are important features of the system. In his model, psoas is the controller of the spine enhanced by the combined action of the erectors, latissimus and trapezius.[130] 'In this model, the arms and legs need to be evenly developed, smoothly interrelated'.[226] Overdevelopment and imbalance of superficial SGMS muscles in the proximal girdles and body wall including the abdominals, will limit freedom of movement in axial rotation in the limb girdles and the spine reducing the rhythmical movement and energy transfer. As Newton suggests, the result will be 'visible homologous (sagittal) or homolateral (lateral flexion) patterns of spinal motion[226] during walking'.

Studies on walking have confirmed that the pelvic and shoulder girdles rotate in the transverse plane. This is initially synchronous in the same direction and evolves toward counterrotation with increasing walking velocity.[227] Bruijn et al.[228] found this is due to the pelvis beginning to move in-phase with the femur while the thorax continued to counter rotate with respect to the femur. Moreover, pelvic and thoracic contributions to total body angular momentum were low, the contributions of the legs and arms being much larger. Crosbie et al.[229] found small but definite segmental axial rotation and lateral flexion movements occur through the lower thorax during walking. Lumbopelvic movements were greatest in the sagittal and frontal planes which led them to suggest that spinal segments move more in response to the lower limbs, due in large part to iliopsoas activity. They also showed that the amplitude of spinal motion increased with increased walking speed particularly in the sagittal plane. Significant reduction in spinal range of motion occurred with advancing age.[230] However, they did find that thoracic spine axial rotation was less in males. Walking on an incline exerts major influences on the thoracic spine by increasing the amplitudes of the axial rotations.[231]

Ideally walking is effortless and flowing because of a coordinated sequence of interconnected functions between the proximal limb girdles and spine.

References

[1] Rolf IP. Rolfing: the integration of human structures. New York: Harper and Row; 1977.

[2] Gracovetsky S. Stability or controlled instability? In: Vleeming A, Mooney V, Stoeckart R, editors. Movement, stability & lumbopelvic pain: integration of research and therapy. 2nd ed Churchill Livingstone; 2007.

[3] Gracovetsky S. Linking the spinal engine with the legs: a theory of human gait. In: Vleeming, et al., editors. Movement, stability and low back pain: the essential role of the pelvis. New York: Churchill Livingstone; 1997. p. 243–51.

[4] Janda V. Introduction to functional pathology of the motor system. In: Proc. V11 Commonwealth and International Conference on Sport Physical Education, Recreation and Dance vol. 3; 1982.

[5] White AA, Panjabi MM. Clinical biomechanics of the spine. Philadelphia: J. B. Lippincott Company; 1990.

[6] Todd ME. The thinking body. Hightstown: Dance Horizons-Princeton Book Company; 1937.

[7] Farfan H. The biomechanical advantage of lordosis and hip extension for upright activity. Spine 1978;3(4):336–42.

[8] McGill SM. Ultimate back fitness and performance. Waterloo: Wabuno Pub.; 2004.

[9] Norkin CC, Levangie PK. Joint structure and function: A comprehensive analysis. 2nd ed Philadelphia: F.A. Davis Company; 1992.

[10] Williams PL, Warwick R. Gray's Anatomy. 36th ed Edinburgh: Churchill Livingstone; 1980.

[11] Indahl A, et al. Interaction between the porcine lumbar intervertebral disc, zygapophysial joints, and paraspinal muscles. Spine 1997;22(24):2834–40.

[12] Neumann DA. Kinesiology of the musculoskeletal system: Foundations for physical rehabilitation. Mosby; 2002.

[13] Rozumalski A, et al. The in vivo three dimensional motion of the human lumbar spine during gait. Gait Posture 2008;28(3):378–84.

[14] Pearcy MJ. Twisting mobility of the human back in flexed postures. Spine 1993;18 (1):114–9.

[15] Burnett A, et al. Lower lumbar spine axial rotation is reduced in end range sagittal postures when compared to a neutral spine position. Man Ther 2008;13 (4):300–6.

[16] Kapandji IA. The physiology of the joints. Vol.3: the trunk and the vertebral column. 2nd ed, Edinburgh: Churchill Livingstone; 1974.

[17] Franklin E. Pelvic power: mind/body exercises for strength, flexibility, posture and balance. New Jersey: Princeton Book Company; 2002.

[18] Lee D. The pelvic girdle: An approach to the examination and treatment of the lumbo-pelvic-hip region. 3rd ed Edinburgh: Churchill Livingstone; 2004.

[19] Twomey L. The effects of age on the ranges of motions of the lumbar region. Aust J Physiother 1979;25(6):257–63.

[20] Rock C-M. Reflex incontinence caused by underlying functional disorders. In: Carrière B, Markel Feldt C, editors. The pelvic floor. Stuttgart: Thieme; 2006.

[21] Levine D, Whittle MW. The effects of pelvic movement on lumbar lordosis in the standing position. J Orthopaedic & Sports Physiotherapy 1996;24(3): 130–135.

[22] Black KM, McClure P, Polansky M. The influence of different sitting positions on cervical and lumbar posture. Spine 1996;21(1):65–70.

[23] Lewit K. Manipulative therapy in rehabilitation of the motor system. London: Butterworths; 1985.

[24] Singer KP, Malmivarra A. Pathoanatomical characteristics of the thoracolumbar junctional region. In: Giles LGF, Singer KP,

editors. Clinical anatomy and management of thoracic spine pain. Oxford: Butterworth Heinemann; 2000.

[25] Boyle JJW, Milne N, Singer KP. Influence of age on cervicothoracic spinal curvature: an ex vivo radiographic study. Clin Biomech 2002;17(5): 361–367.

[26] McCouch GP, Deering ID, Ling TH. Location of receptors for tonic neck reflexes. J Neurophysiol 1951;14:191–5.

[27] Bergmark A. Stability of the lumbar spine: a study in mechanical engineering. Acta Orthop. Scand. Suppl. 1989;230 (60):1–54.

[28] Hackney P. Making connections: Total body integration through Bartenieff Fundamentals. New York: Routledge; 2002.

[29] Twomey L, Taylor J. Flexion creep deformation and hysteresis in the lumbar vertebral column. Spine 1982;7(2):116–22.

[30] Bogduk N, Twomey LT. Clinical anatomy of the lumbar spine. Melbourne: Churchill Livingstone; 1987.

[31] Granhead H, Jonson R, Hansson T. The loads on the lumbar spine during extreme weight lifting. Spine 1987;12 (2):146–9.

[32] Adams MA, Dolan P, Hutton WC. The lumbar spine in backward bending. Spine 1988;13(9): 1019–26.

[33] Claus A, et al. Sitting versus standing: Does intradiscal pressure cause disc degeneration or low back pain?. J Electromyogr Kinesiol 2008;18(4):550–7.

[34] Solomonow M. Ligaments: a source of work related musculoskeletal disorders. J Electromyogr Kinesiol 2004;14:49–60.

[35] Solomonow M. Ligaments: a source of musculoskeletal disorders. J of Bodywork and Movement Therapies (IN PRESS).

[36] Solomonow M, et al. The ligamento-muscular stabilising system of the spine. Spine 1998;23(23):2552–62.

[37] Gracovetsky S. Is the lumbodorsal fascia necessary? J Bodywork and Movement Therapies 2008;12(3):194–7.

[38] Findley T, Schleip R, editors. Fascia Research: basic science and implications for conventional and complementary health care. Elsevier; 2007 Introduction.

[39] Levin SM. A suspensory system for the sacrum in pelvic mechanics: biotensegrity. In: Vleeming A, Mooney V, Stoeckart R, editors. Movement, stability and lumbopelvic pain: integration of research and therapy. New York: Churchill Livingstone; 2007.

[40] Bond M. The new rules of posture: How to sit stand and move in the modern world. Rochester: Healing Arts Press; 2007.

[41] Schultz RL, Feitis R. The endless web: Fascial anatomy and physical reality. Berkeley: North Atlantic Books; 1996.

[42] Robertson S. Integrating the fascial system into contemporary concepts on movement dysfunction. The J of Manual and Manipulative Therapy 2001;9(1):40–7.

[43] Guggenheimer KT, Barker PJ, Briggs CA. Effects of tensioning the lumbar fascia on segmental sagittal motion and instability factor during flexion and extension. In: Fascia Research: basic science and implications for conventional and complementary health care. Elsevier; 2007.

[44] Langevin HM, Sherman KJ. Pathophysiological model for chronic low back pain integrating connective tissue and nervous system mechanisms. Med Hypotheses 2007;68:74–80.

[45] Schleip R, Klingler W, Lehmann-Horn F. Fascia is able to contract in a smooth muscle like manner and thereby influence musculoskeletal mechanics. In: Fascia Research: basic science and implications for conventional and complementary health care. Elsevier; 2007.

[46] Smith J. The oscillatory properties of the structural body. IASI Year Book; 2006.

[47] Upledger JE, Vredevoogd. Craniosacral therapy. Seattle: Eastland Press; 1983.

[48] Gracovetsky S. Is the lumbodorsal fascia necessary? In: Fascia Research: basic science and implications for conventional and complementary health care. Elsevier; 2007.

[49] Gandevia SC, McCloskey DI, Burke D. Kinaesthetic signals and muscle contraction Trends. Neurosci 1992;15:62–5.

[50] Dolan KJ, Green A. Lumbar spine reposition sense: the effect of a 'slouched' posture. Man Ther 2006;11:202–7.

[51] Swinkels A, Dolan P. Spinal position sense is independent of the magnitude of movement. Spine 2000;25(1):98.

[52] Brumagne S, et al. Effect of paraspinal muscle vibration on position sense of the lumbosacral spine. Spine 1999;24(13):1328–33.

[53] Janda V. Muscles as a pathogenic factor in back pain. In: Proc. IFOMPT. New Zealand; 1980.

[54] Cholewicki J, Panjabi MM, Khachatryan A. Stabilising function of trunk flexor extensor muscles around a neutral spine posture. Spine 1997;22(19):2207–12.

[55] Potvin JR, O'Brien PR. Trunk muscle co-contraction increases during fatiguing isometric lateral bend exertions: possible implications for spine stability. Spine 1998;23(7):774–80.

[56] Radebold A, et al. Muscle response pattern to sudden trunk loading in healthy individuals and in patients with low back pain. Spine 2000;25(8):947–54.

[57] Quint U, et al. Importance of the intersegmental trunk muscles for the stability of the lumbar spine: a biomechanical study. Spine 1998;23(18):1937–45.

[58] Reeves NP, et al. The effects of trunk stiffness on postural control during unstable seated balance. Exp Brain Res 2006;174:694–700.

[59] McGill S. Low back disorders: evidenced based prevention and rehabilitation. Champaign: Human Kinetics Publ.; 2002.

[60] Adams M, et al. The biomechanics of back pain. 2nd ed. Edinburgh: Churchill Livingstone; 2006.

[61] Kippers V, Parker AW. Posture related to myoelectric silence of erectors spinae during trunkflexion. Spine 1984;9(7):740–5.

[62] Toussaint HB, Winter A, de Haas Y, et al. Flexion relaxation during lifting: implications for torque production by muscle activity and tissue strain at the lumbo-sacral joint. J Biomech 1995;28:199–210.

[63] Bogduk N, Macintosh J, Pearcy MJ. A universal model of the lumbar back muscles in the upright position. Spine 1992;17(8):897–913.

[64] Andersson, et al. EMG activities of the quadratus lumborum and erector spinae muscles during flexion-relaxation and other motor tasks. Clin Biomech 1996;11:392–400.

[65] Gupta A. Analyses of myo-electrical silence of erectors spinae. J Biomech 2001;34(4):491–6.

[66] O'sullivan P, et al. Evaluation of the flexion relaxation phenomenon of the trunk muscles in sitting. Spine 2006;31(17):2009–16.

[67] Enoka RM. Neuromechanics of human movement. 3rd ed Human Kinetics; 2002.

[68] Trew M, Everett T. Human movement: an introductory text. 5th ed Edinburgh: Elsevier; 2005.

[69] Bradley D. Hyperventilation Syndrome: breathing pattern disorders. 3rd ed New Zealand: Tandem Press; 1998.

[70] Chaitow L, Bradley D, Gilbert C. Multidisciplinary approaches to breathing pattern disorders. Edinburgh: Churchill Livingstone; 2002.

[71] Chaitow L. Breathing and altered motor control. In: 5th Interdisciplinary Congress on Low Back and Pelvic Pain: Effective diagnosis and treatment of lumbopelvic pain. Melbourne; 2004.

[72] Hanna T. Somatics: reawakening the mind's control of movement, flexibility and health. Cambridge MA: Da Capo Press; 1988.

[73] Laban R, Lawrence FC. Effort: Economy of human movement. 2nd ed London: Macdonald and Evans Ltd; 1974.

[74] Feldenkrais M. The Elusive Obvious. California: Meta Publications; 1981.

[75] Shumway Cook A, Woollacott MH. Motor control: Theory and practical applications. 2nd ed. Philadelphia: Lippincott Williams and Wilkins; 2001.

[76] Gruneberg C, et al. The influence of artificially increased hip and trunk stiffness on balance control in man. Exp Brain Res 2004;157:472–85.

[77] Mok NW, Brauer SG, Hodges PW. Hip strategy for balance control in quiet standing is reduced in people with low back pain. Spine 2004;29(6): E107–12.

[78] Panjabi MM. The stabilising system of the spine. Part 1. Function, dysfunction, adaptation and enhancement. J Spinal Disord 1992;5:383–9.

[79] Panjabi MM. The stabilising system of the spine. Part 11. Neutral zone and stability hypothesis. J Spinal Disord 1992;5:390–7.

[80] Bartelink DL. The role of abdominal pressure in relieving the pressure on the lumbar intervertebral discs. J Bone Joint Surg 1957;39B:718–25.

[81] Thompson J, et al. Motor control strategies for activation of the pelvic floor. In: Proc. 5th Interdisciplinary World Congress on Low Back and Pelvic Pain. Melbourne; 2004.

[82] Marras WS, Mirka GA. Intra-abdominal pressure during trunk extension motions. Clin Biomech 1996;11(5):267–74.

[83] Cholewicki, et al. Lumbar spine stability can be augmented with an abdominal belt and/or increased intra-abdominal pressure. Eur Spine J 1999;8:388–95.

[84] Hagins M, et al. The effects of breath control on intra-abdominal pressure during lifting tasks. Spine 2004;29(4):464–9.

[85] Cresswell AG, Oddsson L, Thorstensson A. The influence of sudden perturbations on trunk muscle activity and intra-abdominal pressure while standing. Exp Brain Res 1994;98:336–41.

[86] Richardson C, et al. Therapeutic exercise for spinal segmental stabilisation in low back pain: scientific basis and clinical approach. Edinburgh: Churchill Livingstone; 1999.

[87] Richardson C, Hodges P, Hides J. Therapeutic exercise for lumbopelvic stabilisation: A motor control approach foe the treatment and prevention of low back pain. 2nd ed Edinburgh: Churchill Livingstone; 2004.

[88] Hodges PW, Gandevia S. Changes in intra-abdominal pressure during postural and respiratory activation of the human diaphragm. J Appl Physiol 2000;89:967–76.

[89] Hodges PW, Gandevia SC. Activation of the human diaphragm during a repetitive postural task. J Physiol 2000;522:165–75.

[90] Hodges PW, et al. In vivo measurement of the effect of intra-abdominal pressure on the human spine. J Biomech 2001;34 (3):347–53.

[91] Hodges PW, Heijnen, Gandevia SC. Postural activity of the diaphragm is reduced in humans when respiratory demand increases. J Physiol 2001;537(3):999–1008.

[92] Hodges PW. Is there a role for transversus abdominis in lumbo-pelvic stability? Man Ther 1999;4(2):74–86.

[93] Allison G, et al. The role of the diaphragm during abdominal hollowing exercises. Aust J Physiother 1998;44(2): 95–102.

[94] Hodges PW, Sapsford RR, Pengel HM. Feedforward activity of the pelvic floor muscles precedes rapid upper limb movements. In: Proc. VIIth. International Physiotherapy Congress. Sydney, Australia; 2002.

[95] Hodges PW, Richardson CA. Contraction of the abdominal muscles associated with movement of the lower limb. Phys Ther 1997;77:132–44.

[96] Hodges PW, Richardson CA. Feedforward contraction of transversus abdominis is not influenced by the direction of arm movement. Exp Brain Res 1997;114(2):362–70.

[97] Hodges P. Abdominal mechanism and support of the lumbar spine and pelvis. In: Richardson C, Hodges P, Hides J, editors. Therapeutic exercise for lumbopelvic stabilisation: A motor control approach foe the treatment and prevention of low back pain. 2nd ed Edinburgh: Churchill Livingstone; 2004.

[98] Hodges PW. Low Back Pain and the Pelvic Floor. In: Carrière B, Markel Feldt C, editors. The pelvic floor. Stuttgart: Thieme; 2006.

[99] De Troyer A, et al. Transversus muscle function in humans. J Appl Physiol 1990;68:1010–6.

[100] Newton A. Breathing in the gravity field. Part 1. Rolf Lines 1997; Fall.

[101] Wildman F. The brain as the core of strength and stability. Sydney: Feldenkrais workshop; 2003.

[102] Bartley J. Breathing matters: a New Zealand guide. New Zealand: Random House; 2006.

[103] Cumpelik J. Breathing mechanics in postural stabilisation. Sydney: Course notes; 2008.

[104] De Troyer A, Kirkwood PA, Wilson TA. Respiratory action of the intercostal muscles. Physiol Rev 2005;85:717–56.

[105] Hodges, et al. Contraction of the human diaphragm during rapid postural adjustments. J Physiol 1997;505:539–48.

[106] Netter FH. Atlas of Human Anatomy. 4th ed Philadelphia, Pennsylvania: Saunders Elsevier; 2006.

[107] Calais-Germain B. Anatomy of breathing. Seattle: Eastland Press Inc; 2006.

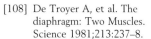
[108] De Troyer A, et al. The diaphragm: Two Muscles. Science 1981;213:237–8.

[109] Shirley D, et al. Spinal stiffness changes throughout the respiratory cycle. J Appl Physiol 2003;95:1467–75.

[110] Clifton smith T. Breathe to succeed. New Zealand: Penguin; 1999.

[111] Ameisen P. Every breath you take; Facts about the Buteyko Method. Sydney: Lansdowne; 1997.

[112] Farhi D. The breathing book: good health and vitality through essential breath work. New York: Henry Holt and Company; 1996.

[113] Janda V. Sydney: Course notes; 1995.

[114] Massery M. Breathing: is it really necessary? – Integrating cardiopulmonary and postural control strategies (paediatric and adult populations) In: Sydney: Course notes; 2008.

[115] Kolar P. Facilitation of agonist-antagonist co-activation by reflex stimulation methods. In: Liebenson C, editor. Rehabilitation of the spine: a practitioner's manual. 2nd ed Philadelphia: Lippincott Williams and Wilkins; 2007.

[116] Panjabi MM, White AA. Biomechanics in the musculoskeletal system. New York: Churchill Livingstone; 2001.

[117] Putz R, Pabst R, editors. Sobotta: Atlas of Human Anatomy. Volume 2: Thorax, Abdomen, Pelvis, Lower Limb. 12th English ed. Baltimore, Philadelphia: Williams & Wilkins; 1997.

[118] Putz R, Pabst R. (Eds). Sobotta Atlas of Human Anatomy Vol. 2. 12th English-Edition. Williams & Wilkins; Baltimore, 1997.

[119] Harrison DE, et al. Upright static pelvic posture as rotations and translations in 3-dimensional from three 2-dimensional digital images: Validation and computer analysis. J Manipulative Physiol Ther 2008;31(2):137–45.

[120] Smidt GL. Interinnominate range of motion. In: Movement, stability and low back pain: the essential role of the pelvis. New York: Churchill Livingstone; 1997.

[121] Grieve GP. The sacro-iliac joint. Physiotherapy 1976;62(12):384–400.

[122] Vleeming A, Stoeckart R. The role of the pelvic girdle in coupling the spine and the legs: a clinical anatomical perspective on pelvic stability. In: Vleeming A, Mooney V, Stoeckart R, editors. Movement stability and lumbopelvic pain: integration of research and therapy. Edinburgh: Churchill Livingstone; 2007.

[123] Snijders CJ, et al. Biomechanics of the interface between spine and pelvis in different postures. In: Vleeming, et al. editors. Movement, stability and Low Back Pain: The essential role of the pelvis. New York: Churchill Livingstone; 1997.

[124] Bendová, et al. MRI based registration of pelvic alignment affected by altered pelvic floor muscle characteristics. Clin Biomech 2007;22(9):980–7.

[125] Hungerford B, Gilleard W. Sacroiliac joint angular rotation during the stork test and hip drop test in normal subjects: pilot study results. In: Proc. 3rd Interdisciplinary Congress on Low Back and Pelvic Pain. Vienna; 1998. p. 332–4.

[126] Hungerford B, Gilleard W. The pattern of intrapelvic motion and lumbopelvic muscle recruitment alters in the prescence of pelvic girdle pain. In: Vleeming A, Mooney V, Stoeckart R, editors. Movement, Stability & Lumbopelvic pain: Integration of research and therapy. Edinburgh: Churchill Livingstone; 2007.

[127] Wilson M, Ryu J-H, Kwon Y-H. Contribution of the pelvis to gesture leg range of motion in a complex ballet movement. J Dance Medicine & Science 2007;11(4):118–23.

[128] Lee D. The pelvic girdle: an approach to the examination and treatment of the lumbo-pelvic-hip region. 2nd ed. Edinburgh: Churchill Livingstone; 1999.

[129] Kendall FP, McCreary EK, Provance PG. Muscles: testing and function. 4th ed Baltimore: Williams and Wilkins; 1993.

[130] Gracovetsky S. An hypothesis for the role of the spine in human locomotion: a challenge to current thinking. J Biomed Eng 1985;7:205–16.

[131] Gracovetsky S. The Spinal Engine. Austria: Springer-Verlag/Wien; 1988.

[132] Steindler A. Kinesiology of the Human Body under Normal and Pathological conditions. Springfield Illinois: Charles C Thomas; 1955.

[133] Claus A, et al. Activity of the paraspinal muscles is differentially affected by changes in spinal curves in sitting in people with and without low back pain. In: Proc. 6th Interdisciplinary World Congress on Low Back and Pelvic Pain. Barcelona; 2007.

[134] Mitchell FL, Moran PS, Pruzzo NA. An evaluation and treatment manual of osteopathic muscle energy procedures. 1st ed. Valley Park Mo: Mitchell, Moran and Pruzzo Assoc. Publishers; 1979.

[135] Fritsch O. Anatomy and Physiology of the Pelvic Floor. In: Carrière B, Markel Feldt C, editors. The pelvic floor. Stuttgart: Thieme; 2006.

[136] Spitznagle TM. Musculoskeletal chronic pelvic pain. In: Carrière B, Markel Feldt C, editors. The pelvic floor. Stuttgart: Thieme; 2006.

[137] Pool-Goudzwaard A, et al. Contribution of pelvic floor muscles to stiffness of the pelvic ring. Clin Biomech 2004;19(6):564–71.

[138] Kelly M, et al. Healthy adults can more easily elevate the pelvic floor in standing than in crook lying: an experimental study. Aust J Physiother 2007;53(3):187–91.

[139] Bø K. Evidence-based Physical Therapy for stress and urge incontinence. In: Carrière B, Markel Feldt C (Eds). The Pelvic floor. Stuttgart: Thieme; 2006.

[140] Sapsford RR, Hodges PW. Contraction of the pelvic floor muscles during abdominal manoeuvres. Arch Phys Med Rehabil 2001;82:1081–8.

[141] Sapsford RR, et al. Co-activation of the abdominal and pelvic floor muscles during voluntary exercises. Neurol Urodyn 2001;20:31–42.

[142] Hartley L. Wisdom of the Body Moving: An introduction to Body-Mind Centering. Berkeley: North Atlantic Books; 1995.

[143] Norton PA, Baker JE. Postural changes can reduce leakage in women with stress urinary incontinence. Obstet Gynecol 1994;84:770–4.

[144] Umphred D. The nervous system and motor learning. In: Carrière B, Markel Feldt C, editors. The pelvic floor. Stuttgart: Thieme; 2006.

[145] Sapsford R. Rehabilitation of the pelvic floor muscles utilising trunk stabilisation. Man Ther 2004;9(1):3–12.

[146] DonTigny RL. Mechanics and treatment of the sacroiliac joint. In: Vleeming A, et al., editors. Movement, stability and low back pain: the essential role of the pelvis. New York: Churchill Livingstone; 1997.

[147] DonTigny RL. A detailed and critical biomechanical analysis of the sacroiliac joints and relevant kinesiology: the implications for lumbopelvic function and dysfunction. In: Vleeming A, Mooney V, Stoeckart R, editors. Movement, Stability & Lumbopelvic Pain: Integration of research and Therapy. Edinburgh: Churchill Livingstone; 2007.

[148] Bartenieff I, Lewis D. Body movement: coping with the environment. Australia: Gordon and Breach Science Publishers; 2002.

[149] Basmajian JV. Muscles Alive. 4th ed. Baltimore: Williams and Wilkins; 1978.

[150] Nachemson A. Electromyographic studies on the vertebral portion of psoas muscle. Acta Orthop Scand 1966;37:177–90.

[151] Andersson E, et al. The role of psoas and iliacus muscles for stability and movement of the lumbar spine, pelvis and hip. Scand J Med Sci Sports 1995;5:10–6.

[152] Porterfield JA, DeRosa C. Mechanical low back pain: perspectives in functional anatomy. 2nd ed. Philadelphia: Saunders; 1998.

[153] Harrison DE, et al. How do anterior/posterior translations of the thoracic cage affect the sagittal lumbar spine, pelvic tilt, and thoracic kyphosis? Eur Spine J 2002;11:287–93.

[154] Bogduk N, Pearcy M, Hadfield G. Anatomy and biomechanics of psoas major. Clin Biomech 1992;7:109–19.

[155] Santaguida PL, McGill SM. The psoas major muscle: a three dimensional geometric study. J Biomech 1995;28(3):339–45.

[156] Penning L. Psoas muscle and lumbar spine stability: a concept uniting existing controversies. Critical review and hypothesis. Eur Spine J 2000;9:577–85.

[157] Gibbons SGT. The model of psoas Major stability Function. In: Proc. 1st International Conference on Movement Dysfunction. Edinburgh; 2001.

[158] Vleeming A, et al. Relationship between form and function in the SI joint part 11. Spine 1990;15:133–6.

[159] Sims K. The development of hip osteoarthritis: implications for conservative management. Man Ther 1999;4(3):127–35.

[160] Janda V. The role of the thigh adductors in movement patterns of the hip and knee joint. Courrier 1965;(Sept):563–5.

[161] Hungerford B, et al. Altered lumbo-pelvic muscle recruitment occurs in the prescence of sacroiliac joint pain. In: Proc. 5th Interdisciplinary World Congress on Low Back and Pelvic Pain. Melbourne; 2004.

[162] Vleeming A, et al. The posterior layer of the thoracolumbar fascia: its function in load transfer from spine to legs. Spine 1995;20:753.

[163] Snijders CJ, Vleeming A, Stoeckart R. Transfer of lumbosacral load to iliac bones and legs. 1. Biomechanics of self bracing of the sacroiliac joints and its significance for treatment and exercise. Clin Biomech 1993;8:285.

[164] Pool-Goudzwaard AL, et al. Inefficient lumbopelvic stability: a clinical, anatomical and biomechanical approach to 'a-specific' low back pain. Man Ther 1998;3(1):12–20.

[165] Bogduk N. The morphology and biomechanics of latissimus dorsi. Clin Biomech 1998;13(6):377–85.

[166] Myers TW. Anatomy trains: myofascial meridians for manual and movement therapists. Edinburgh: Churchill Livingstone; 2001.

[167] Akuthota V, Nadler SF. Core strengthening. Arch Phys Med Rehabil 2003;85(1):86–92.

[168] Hodges PW, Cholewicki J. Functional control of the spine. In: Vleeming A, Mooney V, Stoeckart R editors. Movement, stability & lumbopelvic pain: integration of research and therapy. 2nd ed. Churchill Livingstone; 2007.

[169] Richardson CA, Jull GA. Muscle control – pain control. What exercises would you prescribe. Man Ther 1995;1(1):2–10.

[170] Hodges PW, Jull GA. Spinal segmental stabilisation training. In: Liebenson C, editor. Rehabilitation of the spine: a practitioner's manual. 2nd ed. Philadelphia: Lippincott Williams and Wilkins; 2007.

[171] Beith ID, Synnott RE, Newman SA. Abdominal muscle activity during the abdominal hollowing manoeuvre in the four point kneeling and prone position. Man Ther 2001;6(2):82–7.

[172] O'sullivan PB, Twomey LT, Allison GT. Evaluation of specific stabilising exercise in the treatment of chronic low back pain with radiologic diagnosis of spondylolysis or spondylolisthesis. Spine 1997;22(24):2959–67.

[173] McGill SM. Lumbar spine stability: Mechanism of injury and restabilisation. In: Liebenson C, editor. Rehabilitation of the spine: a practitioner's manual. 2nd ed. Philadelphia: Lippincott Williams and Wilkins; 2007.

[174] Stanton T, Kawchuk G. The effect of abdominal stabilisation contractions on postero-anterior spinal stiffness. Spine 2008;33 (6):694–701.

[175] Feldenkrais M. Body and Mature Behaviour; A study of anxiety, sex, gravitation and learning. New York: International Universities Press Inc; 1949.

[176] Bainbridge-Cohen B. Sensing, Feeling and Action; The experiential anatomy of body-mind centreing. Northampton MA: Contact Editions; 1993.

[177] Beith ID, Harrison PJ. Reflex control of human trunk muscles. In: Proc. 1st International Conference on Movement Dysfunction. Edinburgh; 2001.

[178] Hodges PW, Richardson CA. Transversus abdominus and the superficial abdominals are controlled independently in a postural task. Neurosci Lett 1999;265:91–4.

[179] Urquhart DM, et al. Regional morphology of transversus abdominis and internal oblique. In: Proc. Musculoskeletal Physiotherapy Australia Twelfth Biennial conference. Adelaide; 2001.

[180] Urquhart D. Regional variation in the morphology and recruitment of transversus abdominus: implications for control and movement of the lumbar spine. In: Proc. 5th Interdisciplinary World Congress on Low Back and Pelvic Pain. Melbourne; 2004.

[181] Urquhart DM, Hodges PW, Story IH. Postural activity of the abdominal muscles varies between regions of these muscles and between body positions. Gait Posture 2005;22 (4):295–301.

[182] Snijders CJ, et al. Biomechanical modelling of sacroiliac stability in different postures. Spine:

State of the art reviews 1995;9:419–32.

[183] Moreside JM, Vera-Garcia FJ, McGill SM. Neuromuscular independence of abdominal wall muscles as demonstrated by middle-eastern style dancers. J Electromyogr Kinesiol 2008;18 (4):527–37.

[184] Mens J, et al. The active straight leg raise test and mobility of the pelvic joints. Eur Spine J 1999;8:468–73.

[185] O'Sullivan PB, et al. Altered motor control strategies in subjects with sacroiliac joint pain during the active straight leg raise test. Spine 2002;27(1): E1–8.

[186] Beach P. The contractile field: a new model of human movement. J Bodywork and Movement Therapies 2007;11 (4):308–17.

[187] Norris CM. Spinal stabilisation: stabilisation mechanisms of the lumbar spine. Physiotherapy 1995;81(2):72–9.

[188] Zetterberg C, Andersson GB, Schultz. The activity of individual trunk muscles during heavy physical loading. Spine 1987;12(10):1035–40.

[189] Hodges PW, Richardson CA. Inefficient muscular stabilisation of the lumbar spine associated with low back pain: a motor control evaluation of transversus abdominus. Spine 1996; 21:2640–50.

[190] Vézina MJ, Hubley-Kozey CL, Egan DA. A review of the muscle activation patterns associated with the pelvic tilt exercise used in the treatment of low back pain. The J of Manual and Manipulative Therapy 1998;6(4):191–201.

[191] Arjmand N, Shirazi-Adl A. Biomechanics of changes in lumbar posture in static lifting. Spine 2005;30 (23):2637–48.

[192] McClure PW, et al. Kinematic analysis of lumbar and hip motion while rising from a forward flexed position in patients with and without a history of low back pain. Spine 1997;22(5):552–8.

[193] Sparto PJ, et al. The effect of fatigue on multijoint kinematics and load sharing during a repetitive lifting task. Spine 1997;22(22):2647–54.

[194] Van Dieën JH. Effects of repetitive lifting on the kinematics, inadequate anticipatory control or adaptive changes? J Motor Behaviour 1998;30(1):20–32.

[195] Van Dieën J, Hoozemans MJM, Toussaint HM. Stoop or squat: a review of biomechanical studies on lifting technique. Clin Biomech 1999;14 (10):685–96.

[196] Burgess-Limerick R. Squat, stoop or something in between? Int J of Industrial Ergonomics 2003;31(3):143–8.

[197] Dionisio VC, et al. Kinematic, kinetic and EMG patterns during downward squatting. J Electromyogr Kinesiol 2008;18 (1):134–43.

[198] Panjabi MM, White AA. Biomechanics in the musculoskeletal system. New York: Churchill Livingstone; 2001.

[199] Gracovetsky S, et al. The importance of pelvic tilt in reducing compressive stress in the spine during flexion and extension exercises. Spine 1989;14(4):412–6.

[200] Rantanen P, Nykvist F. Optimal sagittal motion axis for trunk extension and flexion tests in chronic low back trouble. Clin Biomech 2000;15(9):665–71.

[201] Gracovetsky S, et al. Analysis of spinal muscular activity during flexion/extension and free lifts. Spine 1990;15 (12):1333–9.

[202] Pope M. Giovanni Alfonso Borelli- The father of biomechanics. Spine 2005;30 (20):2350–5.

[203] Sihvonen T. Flexion relation of the hamstring muscles during lumbar-pelvic rhythm. Arch Phys Med Rehab 1997;78 (5):487–90.

[204] McGorry R, et al. Timing of activation of the erector spinae and hamstrings during a trunk flexion and extension task. Spine 2001;26(4):418–25.

[205] Gallagher S. Trunk extension strength and muscle activity in standing and kneeling postures. Spine 1997;22 (16):1864–72.

[206] Perry J. Gait analysis: normal and pathological function. New Jersey: Slack Incorp; 1992.

[207] Beach P. The contractile field: a new model of human movement – Part 2. J of Bodywork and Movement Therapies 2008;12(1):76–85.

[208] Pinto RZA, et al. Bilateral and unilateral increases in calcaneal eversion affect pelvic alignment in standing position. Man Ther 2008;13(6):513–9.

[209] Lee D. Manual therapy for the thorax: a biomechanical approach. DOPC Delta; 1994.

[210] Edmondston SJ, Singer KP. Thoracic spine: anatomical and biomechanical considerations for manual therapy. Man Ther 1997;2(3):132–43.

[211] Willems JM, Jull GA, Ng JK-F. An in vivo study of the primary coupled rotations of the thoracic spine. Clin Biomech 1996;11 (6):311–6.

[212] Theodoridis D, Ruston S. The effect of shoulder movements on thoracic spine 3D motion. Clin Biomech 2002;17 (5):418–21.

[213] Flemons T. A biotensegrity explanation for structural dysfunction in the human torso. http://www.intensiondesigns. com.

[214] Lee LJ, Coppieters M, Hodges PW. Differential activation of the thoracic multifidus and longissimus thoracis during trunk rotation. Spine 2005;30(8):870–6.

[215] Harrison D, et al. Lumbar coupling during lateral translations of the thoracic cage relative to a fixed pelvis. Clin Biomech 1999;14(10):704–9.

[216] Grieve GP. Common Vertebral Joint Problems. Edinburgh: Churchill Livingstone; 1981.

[217] Keller TS, et al. Influence of spine morphology on intervertebral disc loads and stresses in asymptomatic adults: implications for the ideal spine. Spine J 2005;5(3):297–309.

[218] Stokes IAF. Biomechanics of the thoracic spine and rib cage. In: Giles LGF, Singer KP, editor. Clinical anatomy and management of thoracic spine pain. Oxford: Butterworth Heinemann; 2000.

[219] Travell JG, Simons DG. Myofascial pain and dysfunction: The trigger point manual. Baltimore: Williams and Wilkins; 1983.

[220] Kolar P. In: Dynamic neuromuscular stabilisation: according to Kolar. Presented by Safarova M. Conducted by C E A Ltd. Sydney: Course notes; 2008.

[221] Crosbie J, et al. Scapulohumeral rhythm and associated spinal motion. Clin Biomech 2008;23 (2):184–92.

[222] Janda V. Sydney: Course notes; 1995.

[223] Mooney V, et al. Coupled motion of the contralateral latissimus dorsi and gluteus maximus: its role in sacroiliac stabilisation. In: Vleeming A, et al., editors. Movement, stability and low back pain: the essential role of the pelvis. New York: Churchill Livingstone; 1997.

[224] Fairclough J, et al. Is iliotibial band syndrome really a friction syndrome? J Sci Med Sport 2007;10(2):74–6.

[225] Perry J. Gait analysis: Normal and Pathological Function. New Jersey: SLACK Incorporated; 1992.

[226] Newton A. Gracovetsky on walking. Structural Integration 3003, February:4–8.

[227] Lamoth CJC, et al. Spine 2002;27(4):E92–9.

[228] Bruijn SM, et al. Coordination of leg swing, thorax rotations, and pelvis rotations during gait: the organization of total body angular momentum. Gait Posture 2008;27(3):455–62.

[229] Crosbie J, Vachalathiti R, Smith R. Patterns of spinal motion during walking. Gait Posture 1997;5:6–12.

[230] Crosbie J, Vachalathiti R, Smith R. Patterns of spinal motion during walking. Gait Posture 1997;5:13–20.

[231] Vogt L, Banzer W. Measurement of lumbar spine kinematics in incline treadmill walking. Gait Posture 1999;9(1):18–23.

7

Changed control of posture and movement: the dysfunctional state

Cholewicki and van Dieën[1] comment that while there is an emerging consensus in the literature that muscle activation patterns are different in people with back pain, the interpretations of these findings are divergent. By and large the scientific community has little considered whether altered motor control might be significant in causing back pain.

Some 30 years ago Janda,[2,3] Lewit[4] and others in the Prague school of manual medicine introduced the concept of 'functional pathology of the motor system' to explain the development and perpetuation of pain in the musculoskeletal system. Some more recent studies have implicated pre existing functional changes in the development of later pain[5–8] or in the recurrence of low back pain.[9]

Functional pathology of the motor system[2]

Excluding insidious pathology, Janda[2] considered that most musculoskeletal pain syndromes are the result of impaired motor system function. This functional pathology of the motor system and its interactions with the whole organism, mainly of a reflex nature,[3] is regularly involved in many organic diseases and underpins most spinal pain and related disorders.

In essence, the motor system comprises three functionally interdependent systems. Dysfunction in any one system will influence function in the other systems, perpetuating further impairment.

A pattern generating mechanism can be set in train. The systems are:

- *The corticosubcortical motor regulatory centers of the CNS*. Phylogenetically the youngest and most fragile part of the motor system. Impaired function at this level results in defective and uneconomical movement patterns,[10] poor adjustment of fine movements, and the progressive switch from complicated movement patterns to the more primitive ones regulated at the subcortical level.[2]
- *The muscle system.* This represents perhaps the most exposed part of the motor system, having to 'extensively respond to changes due to civilization or more exactly to the technicalization of our living conditions'.[11] As the main movement effectors, they must respond quickly to all stimuli coming from the neural system, reacting to changes in the periphery especially from the articular system.[2] Clinically, evident changes in the muscle system are generally apparent for some time before the onset of pain. The presence of pain further compounds the muscle dysfunction creating further change throughout the whole motor system.
- *The articular system.* The welfare of the joints is dependent upon balanced neuromuscular control. 'Joint dysfunctions are only one expression of impairment of motor system as a whole i.e. of both neuromuscular and osteoarticular systems'.[3] Further, any changes in the joints will be reflected in changes in both the neural and muscle systems.

Motor control impairments precede the onset of pain

The quality of muscle function depends directly on the central nervous system activity.[12] While functional impairment of the motor system is the most frequent cause of pain in the motor system it is not identical with pain and may remain clinically silent. Depending upon the primary locus, the impairment is generally clinically discernable either in palpable changes at the spinal joint and observable changes in movement patterns, the early onset of fatigue and faster switch into more primitive movement patterns in fatigue of the motor system.[2] Gregory et al.[7] demonstrated altered motor control characteristics that can distinguish the likelihood of an individual developing back during common tasks such as standing.

Significantly, Janda says, 'the high incidence of functional impairment makes it extremely difficult to estimate the borders between the norm and evident pathology'.[2]

According to Janda,[2] the development of impairment follows two basic rules as follows:

1. *The rule of vertical generalization.* A local impairment, for instance in a joint, provokes reaction and adaptation processes in all other parts of the motor system i.e. in the muscular or neural system. Similarly, any alteration in motor regulation as in stress, depression and neurotic reactions involves simultaneously and preferably the muscles and then the joints. In this respect, the limbic system has particular relevance in motor control.

2. *The rule of horizontal generalization.* Impaired function in one joint or muscle provokes a reaction and adaptation in related other joints or muscles and spreads so that finally the whole system, articular or muscular will be involved. This is particularly evident in the axial spine and proximal limb girdles. Restriction of a spinal segment or a number creates relative flexibility at adjacent segments. A stiff hip joint creates a compensatory relative flexibility[13] in the low back. Clinically it is common to see the coexistence of back pain with a plethora of other overt or covert symptoms such shoulder and neck symptoms, hip and knee pain etc.

A local pain symptom is generally the expression of a regional and general neuromyoarticular problem.

Importantly, recognizing the significance of these 'rules' allows the clinician to *predict* the development of functional impairments and introduce prophylactic and rational therapeutic interventions.

The muscle system mirrors the state of sensory motor integration

Movement patterns are one of the basic elements of movement. The patterning process is the most important way that movement develops. According to Janda,[14] these involve a chain of conditioned and unconditioned reflexes which are constant over a short period of time but change, sometimes considerably, over life. Changes occur in response to changing conditions of the 'inner milieu' as well as the outer environment. 'The degree of activity and time synchronization of various muscle groups within the movement are thus characteristic of such patterns'.[14]

Hodges[15] remarks that with regard to lumbopelvic pain, 'two relatively consistent research findings have been observed: increased activity in the superficial muscles and decreased activity of the abdominal canister'.

Clinical observation of patients with spinal pain syndromes, supported in part by frank and extrapolative research findings, demonstrates changes in the typical activation patterns and altered functional roles of muscles in each of the two proposed principal *muscle systems*. This results in imbalanced activity between the two systems which is reflected in altered motor control responses to perturbation and for organizing body alignment, postural control and movement.

In time this leads to structural changes and changes in other co-dependent systems.

Altered qualities of function in each muscle system

Conceptually and generally speaking, we tend to see a change in the timing and level of activity – too little activity and more phasic activity in the deep system and too much, more tonic activity of certain muscles in the superficial system. However, muscles in the deep system can be overactive and those in the superficial system underactive.

Systemic local muscle system (SLMS; see Ch.5)

Altered responses which variably occur in muscles classified within this system as muscles of the SLMS demonstrate:

• *Delayed feedforward postural responses* have been demonstrated in transversus abdominus,[16,17] internal oblique and transversus,[18] internal oblique, multifidus and gluteus maximus.[19] Transversus activity changes from direction independent to direction specific activity in the control of reactive forces of the trunk.[16] Mok et al.[20] found decreased preparatory movement of the lumbopelvis and increased corrective movements in response to perturbation from rapid arm movement.

• *Inadequate*. Relative *underactivity, inhibition, weakness* has been shown in the abdominals;[18] transversus abdominus;[21] multifidus;[22,23] the diaphragm.[24] Functionally they act like 'shy muscles'. Also, arthrogenic inhibition, e.g. of multifidus due to pain or directly impaired proprioception of an injured joint is clinically common. Isolated segmental wasting of multifidus ipsilateral to symptoms has been shown.[25] Simulated microgravity/spinal un-loading/bed rest studies have also shown selective atrophy of multifidus.[26]

• *Diminished patterns of coactivation in the SLMS* affect spinal support and control mechanisms. O'Sullivan et al.[24] found poor coactivation of the diaphragm and pelvic floor in subjects with sacroiliac pain. During the active straight leg raise test diaphragm splinting, respiratory disruption and pelvic floor descent occurred.

• Muscle system *activity is poorly sustained*. Low load sustained postures become difficult as the more usual SLMS tonic yet variable activity becomes more phasic. Subjects with back pain have also demonstrated more phasic activity in transversus while walking[27] and a shift from locomotor to primarily respiratory activity.[28]

Systemic global muscle system (SGMS)

In conjunction with the changed activity in the SLMS, altered timing and degree of activation occurs inversely in muscles within this system as follows:

• *Early onset* of activity precedes SLMS muscles.[19] This means that these muscles are activated from a non stable, poorly controlled foundation tending to create yanking stresses within the axial skeleton.

• Muscles within this system become variably *overactive and dominant in movement patterns*[7,29] irrespective of pain.[30] In the presence of underlying irritable segmental joint restrictions and/or frank pain they are predictably overactive. Normal studies have indicated that these muscles become more active in situations involving reduced gravitational loading and related decreased sensory input.[31,32]

• These muscles are *easily strengthened, hypertrophy and become tight and short*[33] – the functional 'bullies', they are generally over active and those that everyone is obsessively stretching!

• SGMS muscles become *more tonically active* rather than phasic, a changed role from phasic activity to more tonic activity as the system becomes co-opted into a more postural role.[34] When abnormally activated for antigravity control[35], the patient 'holds himself up' against gravity rather like scaffolding holding up a building. He then often can't voluntarily let them go, particularly around the body's centre of gravity, and evidenced in a lack of the flexion–relaxation response seen in many people with back pain.[36,37] Muscles such as external oblique and thoracic erector spinae form part of this system.[38]

In general terms, Janda[39] considered that at least five types of increased muscle tone can result from either:

• Dysfunction of the limbic system
• Impaired function at the segmental (interneuronal) level
• Impaired coordination of muscle contraction (trigger points)
• As a response to pain irritation
• Overuse of the muscles – this is as a rule combined with changed elasticity of the muscle and usually described as muscle tightness.

Muscle imbalance

Janda proposed that clinically developed imbalance between different muscle groups was probably the result of both reflex and mechanical mechanisms.[3] He was initially more interested in the effect of the tight overactive muscles (SGMS) and their inhibitory action upon their antagonists e.g. overactive erector spinae may inhibit abdominal activity.[3] Stretching and other inhibitory techniques applied to the tight muscles often spontaneously improved the weakened antagonist. With respect to the imbalanced muscle system response, he questioned whether there was any difference of innervation between the two systems and noted that the tight muscles were often those involved in flexor reflexes and those with a tendency to be underactive or weaken were those mainly participating in extensor reflexes.[3] *Importantly, pain, injury, fatigue or stress and the working out of new movement patterns tends to reduce activity in the SLMS and increase activity in the SGMS.*

Clinically, in the dysfunctional state, a reciprocal relationship evolves whereby reduced deep system activity necessitates the adoption of more superficial system strategies, which in turn inhibits or disallows effective deep system activation. The dysfunction becomes reinforced, perpetuated and entrenched.

The poorly coordinated activity between the two muscle systems creates muscle imbalance throughout the body. This can occur in a number of ways:

• Between the two systems which begin to work counter to one another instead of in a mutually supportive relationship
• Within each system, particularly the SGMS e.g. between the rectus femoris and hamstrings
• Between the axial flexor and extensor systems.

When overactive, the global muscles of the trunk can act to shorten, compress and constrict parts of the torso acting rather like very tight outer clothing, while the behavior of the SLMS resembles loose old underwear!

Imbalanced activity between the two muscle systems: direct ramifications for underlying control of NPRM

Research interest is increasingly concerned with the quality of postural and movement control in the presence of back pain. However, to date, Dankaerts et al.[40] are one of the few who have suggested that inherent postural control faults may predispose one to the development of pain syndromes.[40]

The main features of dysfunction in the postural reflex mechanism can be summarized as:

• *Reduced endurance in antigravity posture and movement* because of poorly organized and sustained synergies of low grade tonic activity from muscles within the SLMS. While some studies have shown that people with chronic back pain develop a higher ratio of fast to slow twitch fibres and extensor muscle activity becomes more phasic,[41] it is suggested that clinically this inability to *organize* appropriate patterns of underlying response also contributes to reduced staying power in movement.

• *Reduced, imbalanced and delayed patterns of SLMS coactivation* affects joint protection and control of spinal support mechanisms such as low load IAP; jeopardizes effective weight shift and appropriate adaptive postural presetting of the limb girdles necessary to facilitate the ensuing pattern of movement. Ineffective deep system coactivation diminishes effective SGMS activity.

• Effective postural control and precisely coordinated and discrete movements are highly dependent upon adequate proprioception. *Diminished proprioception* in subjects with back pain has been reported.[42,43] Taimela et al.[44] found reduced ability to sense rotational position change in the lumbar spine when sitting, particularly when fatigued. O'Sullivan et al.[45] found significant deficits when patients attempted to reposition the lumbar spine into a neutral lordosis when sitting. Postural and gait stability is reduced in astronauts following in-flight adaptation of CNS processing of altered sensory inputs from the vestibular, proprioceptive and visual systems.[46] Bed rest studies involving reduced antigravity sensory input demonstrate reduced activity in certain SLMS muscles particularly the one joint extensors[26,47] and increased activity in certain SGMS muscles.[31,32]

• *Poorer balance* has been found with greater postural sway,[48] the predominant use of the hip strategy over the ankle strategy.[49] Mok et al.[50] found inability to initiate and reduced control of the hip strategy for balance. Conversely, increased trunk muscle stiffening has been shown to degrade postural control[51] as it limits adaptive segmental adjustments. This has been shown in sitting[52] and particularly so in the sagittal plane.[72]

• *Disturbed motion patterns* become more stereotyped and show predictable change in kinematics e.g. back pain subjects used increased lumbar flexion when forward bending.[9,53,54,67]

• *Variably increased patterns of SGMS co-contraction act to splint some regions of the spine*. Reduced postural support from the deep system and increased SGMS activity leads to the adoption of coarse central holding or 'cinch' patterns in posture and movement. These have also been described by O'Sullivan as fixing and splinting strategies.[24,29] Radebold et al.[55] found increased co-contraction of the superficial trunk muscles in response to multidirectional sudden load release while subjects were generating isometric forces of 20%–30% maximal exertions. SGMS activity typically increases with load, exertion and speed. Incidentally subjects were semi seated and the pelvis was restrained allowing no postural adjustment of the pelvis in controlling the perturbation to the torso – hardly a functional pattern and co-contraction can be expected. Gregory[7] found greater responses of the superficial trunk extensors and flexors in response to unexpected perturbations in subjects who developed back discomfort when standing for 2 hours. After 8 weeks of bed rest simulating a microgravity environment, Belavey et al.[32] found increased activity but decreased co-activation of the superficial lumbopelvic muscles in stabilizing the pelvis during a repetitive leg movement. Clinically, patterns of both increased and decreased SGMS co-activation are found and better understood when patients are sub grouped into the two principal clinical pictures. This helps explain the variance in the various research studies (see Ch. 9).

• *Altered performance of other functionally related systems* such as continence, breathing and cardiovascular deconditioning. Studies by Smith[56] have shown that people with respiratory disease and incontinence have increased activity of the superficial trunk muscles, restricted rib expansion and diaphragm descent.

Further findings in back pain research influencing motor control

Muscle fatigue

The subject of fatigue has attracted a lot of research interest. Enoka[57] describes fatigue as 'the activity related impairment of physiological processes that reduce muscle force… after the onset of sustained physical activity'. Fatigue involves a variety of elements throughout the motor system and Neumann[58] suggests it is useful to consider fatigue as primarily occurring centrally or peripherally. Central fatigue can involve the limbic system, activation of the primary motor cortex, or descending CNS control over neurons and motoneurons in the spinal cord. Peripheral fatigue relates to neurophysiologic factors related to action potential propagation in motor nerves and transmission of activation to muscle fibres.[58] Normally the nervous system compensates for muscle fatigue by either increasing the rate of activation or recruiting assistive motor units thereby maintaining a stable force level.[58] Slow twitch motor units can sustain an isometric force longer than fast twitch. Slow twitch muscle can sustain a greater force during isovelocity shortening contractions, while fast twitch muscle is able to sustain greater power production.

Janda[59] maintained 40 years ago that fatigue increased the differential timing and activity level in the two muscle systems adversely affecting coordination and the quality of the motor patterns (see Ch.5).

More recent research on fatigue has shown various effects on neuromuscular performance; in brief: altered latency of the stretch reflex;[60] the loss of force generation of the back muscles[61,62] and the subsequent effect on the bending moments acting on the lumbar spine.[63] Fatigue occasions a preferential loss of fast twitch fibres in the shift to lower frequencies and so increases the muscle reaction time and reduces the magnitude of the EMG, potentially affecting the response to sudden loads.[64] Other studies have looked at the effects of isodynamic fatiguing on movement patterns and trunk motor output but restrained the subjects into equipment such as triaxial dynamometers.[65] Research design such as this does not allow for the natural kinematic patterns which should accompany trunk forward bending. Van Dieën et al.[66] and Sparto et al.[67] examined the kinematic patterns of motion during repetitive lifting, importantly allowing free body movement which equate more to activities of daily living. Both groups found that with increasing fatigue, hip and knee motion decreased, the legs becoming more extended while the lumbar spine became increasingly flexed. Postural stability is also reduced under fatigue conditions[68] particularly when more proximal muscles are fatigued.[69,70] Lumbar fatigue impairs lumbar spatial position sense and so the ability to anticipate and respond to altered postural events.[44] Some studies have indicated that fatigue experienced with eccentric muscle contractions is less than during concentric contractions particularly if performed slowly.[57] This is interesting as clinical impressions seem to indicate a disinclination for people with spinal pain and related disorders to perform slow eccentric movements when weight bearing through the limbs, while fast concentric actions appear much easier.

Delayed reaction times

Hodges[16–18] found direction independent delayed responses in deep system muscles, and direction specific delay in superficial trunk muscles.[17] Most other studies have only examined responses in the superficial trunk muscles. Radebold[55] showed longer reaction times in response to sudden load release both in switching muscles on and off. Descarreaux et al.[71] found low back pain subjects could generate flexion and extension forces equal to controls however some of their sample took longer time to reach peak force. Longer latencies were also correlated with reduced balance.[72] In a prospective study, Cholewicki et al.[5] found delayed muscle reflex responses appear to be a pre-existing risk factor that significantly increases the risk of sustaining a low back injury.

Luoto et al.[73,74] found deficits in information processing and delayed psychomotor speed in chronic low back pain patients and among women. This was also related to impaired postural control.

Effect of pain on altered motor control

Altered motor control leads to spinal joints and related soft tissues including the nerves to become pain producing over time. Once pain is present – whatever the source, further changes in motor control can be expected. Janda[75] maintained that 'trunk muscle activity can be inhibited to prevent motion into a painful posture or direction and to avoid stresses on motion segment pathology. Conversely, the trunk muscles may go into spasm to fulfil a similar protective role'. Pain has been shown to increase the amplitude of the stretch reflex[76] and muscle activity[77] which in turn will increase pain and has led to the 'pain-spasm-pain model[78] proposed for perpetuating spinal disorders. However,

experimental pain has also been shown to delay postural adjustments with decreased activation of deep system muscles such as transversus abdominus.[79,80] Lund et al.[81] proposed a 'pain adaptation' model which proposed that pain reduces the activation of muscles when active as agonists and increases their activation when antagonistically active. Van Dieën et al.[82] point out that the theory is somewhat aspecific and interpret antagonists as those eccentrically lengthening muscles and agonists as those that are shortening. This serves to reduce the velocity and range of motion and prevent mechanical provocation of sensitive tissues. In a review of the literature on the effect of pain on the activation of the lumbar extensor muscles, van Dieën et al.[82] conclude that neither model is unequivocally supported by the literature. High pain-related fear of movement has been shown to alter movement strategies in limiting lumbar motion while reaching.[83] Hodges et al.[79] showed that experimental pain delayed feedforward postural responses and that these changes persist after the resolution of the pain leading them to conclude that the changes in motor control were more complex than simple inhibition and include changes in motor planning. Leinonen et al.[84] also demonstrated impaired anticipatory feedforward control in subjects with sciatica. Significant in this study was the fact that the impairment was only apparent when subjects stood unsupported as against supported standing.

It is proposed that in general terms pain will tend to inhibit SLMS function and increase SGMS function. Hodges and Moseley[85] report consistent differential effects of pain on the deep and superficial lumbopelvic muscles. Mosely et al.[86] showed that the anticipation of experimental back pain delayed activity in the deep trunk muscles and augmented at least one of the superficial muscles.

Clinically an acute, irritable and 'hot' spinal joint will certainly fire up the local intersegmental as well as the long multisegmental muscles. This is what often makes effective assessment and treatment of spinal joints especially difficult as the joint becomes hard to access, particularly in some regions. In more subacute or chronic states, pain may be more related to chronic neural irritation from either a blocked or relatively over mobile joint and local and long muscle spasm may not be so apparent. In all stages, marked local reactive changes are apparent in the surrounding soft tissues and over the joint itself. The irritability, complexity and stage of disorder thus affect the responses found.

Back pain patients appear to demonstrate features of less well integrated sensorimotor and perceptuomotor behavior

The quality of mature motor behavior is variable. In some, full integration and transformation of the primitive reflexes and early responses fails to occur, despite normal development in other areas, resulting in less effective proprioceptive and motor integration.

Janda[3] performed a detailed analysis of 100 patients who were 'therapeutic failures' and found subtle sensorimotor dysfunction attributable to 'minimal brain dysfunction'. Three striking findings emerged:

1. In the ***neurological examination***, subtle 'soft' neurological symptoms were evident which while often combined, could be divided into three groups:

- Microspasticity: with increased muscle tonus, tendon reflexes, a decreased threshold for provoking spastic phenomena and slight developmental asymmetries such as slight hemipareisis
- Hypotonia: usually asymmetrical with irregular tendon reflexes mostly decreased, evident instability in static functions, lack of coordination and evidence of involuntary movements similar to that in slight choreoathetoid syndrome
- Proprioceptive deficits: with failure in tests requiring greater demand upon afferent pathways such as standing on one leg, especially if the eyes were closed; and alterations in discriminative sensitivity

2. Evaluation of ***the ability to work out new movement patterns***.[14] Clinically, assisted by multichannel EMG, he found they had difficulty with:

- Alterations in the ability to work out finely adjusted coordination so that they activated more muscles than expected
- Inability to activate one side of the body only with a tendency to mirror movements

3. ***Psychological evaluation***. Besides examining the usual personality characteristics he evaluated perceptuomotor coordination, visual and space orientation and motor memory and learning. He found:

- Poor fine motor coordination with frequent tremor, uncertain timing, and overshooting with reduced visual-perception ability
- While no intellectual deficits were found, subjects displayed poor sustained attention and concentration and had difficulty changing from one working method to another and abstracting from simple sensory ideas.

In addition to the motor and perceptuomotor dysfunctions, two other characteristics stood out:

- Wide variations in the general activation level. A higher activation level with medium or poor control was evident in some e.g. superfluous movements. Another group was evidently slower with delayed reactions, long reaction times and slow in pace and language.
- Low tolerance to stress was a striking finding in more than half the subjects, living in high tension, worrying over trifles and coping with daily problems with undue strain. "Some might be said to even produce these stresses by their own 'over-reactivity', 'over-excitability'".[3]

Janda summarized these patients as 'unable to adjust or adapt themselves adequately to altered physiological conditions'.[3]

Altered muscle tonus and flexor/extensor proclivity

In local terms, Janda[11] maintained that one of the factors influencing the irritability of muscles in the vicinity of a joint is change in the intraarticular pressures. Traction or separation facilitates the flexor muscle groups whereas compression in the longitudinal axis of the joint facilitates the extensors.

In more global terms, we have noticed in our spinal pain population, a tendency for two main forms of basic muscle tonus – those who have 'lower tone' and are 'looser' who tend more to antigravity collapse, and those whose tone is more hyperactive with general tightness, tension and stiffness. Those with low tone were often 'hyper mobile' as children. These differences in tone could be an expression of subtle primary CNS dysfunction alluded to above[3,33] – the clumsy kid. Janda has also drawn attention to the similar patterns of excess 'postural muscle' (SGMS) activity seen in postural problems and those with spastic syndromes.[14,33,87] Further, in agreement with Janda[33,59] secondary, subtle CNS dysfunction appears to also result from altered demand and inadequate sensory input and proprioceptive control related to modern living, resulting in imbalanced action between the SLMS and the SGMS.

Whatever the cause, adequate muscle coactivation is more difficult in those with a tendency to low tone, while inhibition of overactive muscles is more difficult in the higher tone group. All will have difficulty with activation of the deep system and inhibition of the superficial system albeit to varying degrees.

Clinically it is also apparent that some show a tendency for flexor muscle system dominance while others are more robust in their extensor systems impeding balanced co-activation.

Schleip[88] ruminated upon the evolution of an individual's structure or posturomovement patterns from a neurobiological perspective and noted two primary reaction patterns involving two opposing sets of muscles – the genetic flexors and the genetic extensors. These differ neurologically, functionally and morphologically and are innervated from separate areas of the spinal cord, as seen in Table 7.1.

In the process of development, balance between the flexors and extensors needs to be achieved for optimal posturomovement control (see Ch. 3). If this does not occur, one of the genetic extensor/flexor patterns will tend to dominate and can act as a basis for chronic muscle shortening and so influence adult human structure. The integrity of the body cylinder is altered (see Ch. 6).

Table 7.1 Classification of genetic extensors and flexors according to Schleip[88]

Genetic extensor muscles	Genetic flexor muscles
• Mainly tonic muscles with a lot of slow twitch Type 1 fibres. Red meat color	• Mainly phasic with a lot of fast twitch type 11 fibres. White meat color
• Innervated from the ventral part of the anterior horn of the spinal cord – either the dorsal primary ramus or by a dorsal ramus of the plexi	• Innervated from the dorsal part of the anterior horn of spinal cord
• Located on the dorsal trunk and arms and on the ventral leg and plantar side of the foot	• Located on the ventral side of the trunk and arms, on the dorsal leg and dorsal side of the foot

Clinically, flexor dominance appears more apparent in those with low tone while extensor dominance is associated more with higher tone. This helps explain the increased extensor EMG findings in some and not all low back pain patients.[36,37]

Hanna[89] felt that a person's structure was influenced by neuromuscular adaptations in response to chronic stress which resulted in primary flexor or extensor activity (see Ch. 6). Sustained negative stress (distress) provoked a flexor withdrawal response which activated muscles on the front of the body. Sustained positive stress (eustress) activates the extensors for 'get up and go' and is related to assertion. Both responses are basic adaptive reflexes necessary to survival. They involve the entire body musculature and the whole nervous system in a specific orientation of either negative withdrawal or positive action and mobility.

The presence of the two primary flexor and extensor patterns are not exclusive of one another and can overlap in the one individual. This is a common finding in people with back pain (see Ch. 9).

Is altered motor behavior observed in people with back pain functional or dysfunctional – adaptive or maladaptive?

In a very comprehensive presentation, Van Dieën[90] argues a theory of 'contingent adaptations' to help explain the changed motor behavior seen in patients with back pain. Many aspects of his theory are compelling and concur with clinical experience of people with back pain. In particular this author agrees with his contention that patients adhere to preferred motor strategies, are less responsive to changing task constraints and that these altered strategies involve costs relative to other constraints that negatively affect outcome (Fig. 7.1). Also the relationship between the disorder and adaptive motor behavior is non deterministic. However, he also states:

1. 'A (pain) disorder triggers adapted motor strategies that help cope with the *new situation* (my italics)'.[90]

2. 'The adaptive changes in motor behavior are generally aimed at increasing 'more robust (i.e. resistant to internal and external perturbation) control over motion of afflicted joints or body parts is a common goal of adaptive strategies in musculoskeletal disorders'.[90]

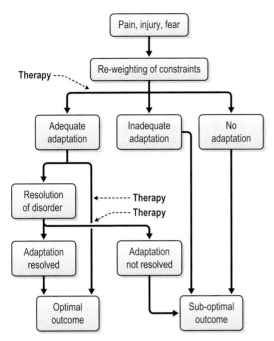

Fig 7.1 • Van Dieën's depiction[90] of the potential role of motor behavior adaptations in outcome of musculoskeletal disorders.

In other words in response to pain, he says: 'the alterations in trunk muscle recruitment in patients are **functional** as they reduce the probability of noxious tissue stresses by limiting range of motion and stabilizing the spine'.[82]

However, this author would like to enter the debate and build upon van Dieën's model in suggesting that the altered motor behavior seen in people with back pain is principally **dysfunctional** (albeit with functional aspects) as it *both causes and serves to further perpetuate* the patient's problem. To expound this further in response to points 1 and 2 above:

1. Low back pain is in general, a developmental disorder. The pain is not necessarily 'new' but develops over time as a result of habitual altered postural control and more primitive and stereotyped movement patterns which jeopardize spinal support and control mechanisms and alter the spinal joint kinematics over time. This represents a *dysfunctional maladaptive* response to the patient's internal and external environment over time. Clinically there are always the early warning signs which herald developing pain. These are usually unaccounted for and their significance ignored until finally '*the straw that breaks the camels/patient's back*' comes into play (Fig. 7.2).

2. The patient now has 'acute' or 'sub-acute' back pain which in van Dieën's terms requires a *further* re-weighting of constraints. Depending upon the stage of disorder, learning effect, and the neuromyoarticular status of the person, responses accounted for in the 'pain-spasm-pain' and 'pain adaptation'[82] models variably become apparent. The patient brings into play the best '*functional adaptive* changes' in motor behavior that he can muster, many of which are in fact provocative. The problem is that he is trying to 'functionally adapt' on a platform of already substandard quality motor control and he has limited choices based on the experience of prior motor learning history. He still needs to get up against gravity and move as best he can as he shops, walks and dresses etc. He will habitually do so in the 'way that he knows' and is familiar with – even though it may be detrimental to his musculoskeletal well being. He now demonstrates a combination of 'functional adaptive' and 'dysfunctional maladaptive' motor behavior. The sensorimotor dysfunction becomes perpetuated. Van Dieën's model appears to assume that prior to the onset of pain, motor control was 'normal'. While the motor system *is* highly redundant, it would appear that many who develop back pain utilize fewer motor pattern options. Their motor behavior is more 'primitive'. The 'more robust strategies' have usually been already been brought in to play *before* pain is apparent, serve to 'bring it to the surface', and then perpetuate it. Clinically one finds different responses in different regions of the spine – some are hyperstabilized while others are hypostabilized. What seems to be generally unaccounted for is the influence of the 'facilitated segment' as described by Korr[91] in facilitating (or inhibiting) local and regional muscle responses further affecting motor control. Altered afference to the CNS even further changes motor behavior. The neuromyoarticular dysfunction becomes compounded and the patient now wears the label of 'chronic non specific back pain'.

Movement behavior quality: characteristic of more primitive and coarse motor control

The quality of movement patterns is dependent upon the cerebral cortex. Fine motor coordination is needed to prevent damage of a joint and especially

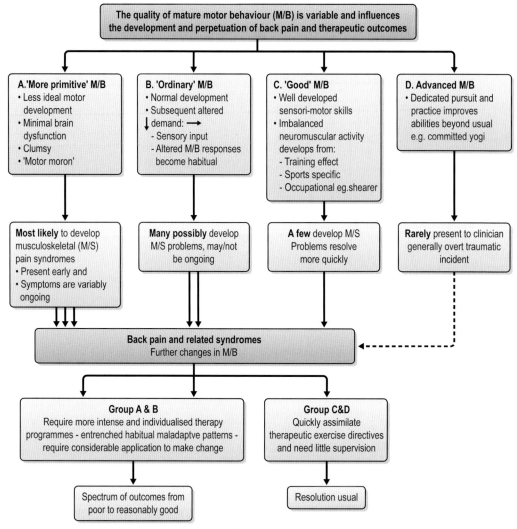

Fig 7.2 • Building upon van Dieën's model[90]: suggested prior influences on the development and subsequent perpetuation of back pain syndromes.

so during a fast movement.[3] At the end of a fast movement, the active inhibition of the antagonist switches into rapid facilitation and contraction in order to slow down the movement and prevent injury. If this reciprocal interplay is altered, the joint is endangered. This reciprocal reflex mechanism occurs at the spinal segmental level.[3]

Clinical observation of *how* people with spinal pain syndromes move can reveal certain quite *subtle yet typically common* altered qualities in the organization of their movement behavior. In some respects their responses resemble those attributable to a more primitive state of development or less well integrated development. This is not to say that

they did not develop normally, but for some reason or other their current motor behavior shows the hallmarks of less well integrated control.

These features have mostly emanated from clinical observation; however researchers such as van Dieën[90] are recognizing the importance of quality of response in motor control.

Altered features of movement

The motor system is deemed to be highly redundant in that there are an infinite number of different muscle activity patterns that can be drawn upon to satisfy mechanical requirements.[90,92] However, the movements of many with back pain can display variable subtle combinations of the following less ideal qualities:

• Certain responses are stereotypical and more obligatory e.g. central cinch patterns.

• Less flexibility and adaptability in responses to internal and external perturbation. Responses fall into more predictable patterns.

• Reduction in movement pattern abilities. A more limited movement repertoire[93] with less variety in those used. Responses are less differentiated.

• Adherence to the motor strategies they know[90] which may in fact be provocative

• In limiting the repertoire of movement options, they further reduce sensorimotor learning experience and stimulation.

Altered qualities of movement

Examining movement quality more closely reveals an array of possible strategies:

• Adopt a more fixed and less flexible use of the vertical

• Altered alignment of head and pelvis as they balance on the occipital and femoral condyles alters alignment of whole spine in relation to the vertical

• Poor integration of flexor/extensor balance with a tendency of one to dominate over the other

• Tendency to more mass movements in 'more total flexor/extensor pattern response'

• Movements tend to be more jerky, are grosser, coarser and clumsier; less differentiated, less refined

• Use of unnecessary movements and effort – being upright and moving is often hard work

• Importantly, see reduced use of lateral and rotary movements which affects weight shift and balance

• The increased use of central fixing, holding or cinch strategies with a functional 'disconnect' between the upper and lower body and poor sequencing of movements from the limbs to torso and torso to limbs[94]

• Tendency to 'propping' when weight bearing through limbs

• More symmetrical limb use and tendency to remain within the body's centre of mass; reciprocal limb movements are often not automatically well organized

• Reduced distal initiation – head, tail bone, hands and feet

• Limited use of reaching actions away from the body and exploration of movements into the surrounding space

• Predominance of upper body over lower body muscle activity

• Movements are heavy, laboured 'bound' rather than light, easy and free flowing

• Reduced stability/mobility element interaction means weight shift suffers in all positions

• Reduced internal body awareness and ability to discretely modulate movement

• Increased use of protective and defensive responses either learned through habit, pain[95] or emotionally driven

• Some difficulty with actions requiring antigravity eccentric muscle control in the trunk and limbs.

Altered patterns of motor control become habitual and learned

As posture and movement control is largely an automatic function, the repeated adoption of the abnormal strategies means they become *habitual, learned* and begin to *feel normal*. 'Habituation is the simplest form of learning – a slow, relentless adaptive act, which ingrains itself into the functional patterns of the central nervous system'.[89] Their repeated use means that over time, subjects simply forget to draw upon and maintain the array of other available motor pattern options. Many of these become relegated to the functional archive department and rust away from disuse while they continue to use those few they 'know'.

References

[1] Cholewicki J, van Dieën JH. Muscle function and dysfunction in the spine. Editorial J Electromyogr Kinesiology 2003;13:303–4.

[2] Janda V. Introduction to functional pathology of the motor system. In: Proc. Vol. 3. V11 Commonwealth and International Conference on Sport, Physical Education, Recreation and Dance; 1982.

[3] Janda V. Muscles, central nervous motor regulation and back problems. In: Korr IM, editor.

Neurobiologic Mechanisms in Manipulative Therapy. New York: Plenum Press; 1978. p. 27–41.

[4] Lewit K. Manipulative Therapy in Rehabilitation of the Motor System. Butterworths; 1985.

[5] Cholewicki, et al. Delayed trunk muscle reflex responses increase the risk of low back injuries. Spine 2005;30(23):2614–20.

[6] Sihvonen T, et al. Functional changes in back muscle activity correlate with pain intensity and prediction of low back pain during pregnanc. Arch Phys Med Rehabil 1998;79(10):1210–2.

[7] Gregory DE, Brown SHM, Callaghan JP. Trunk muscle responses to suddenly applied loads: Do individuals who develop discomfort during prolonged standing respond differently? J Electromyogr Kinesiol 2008; 18(3):495–502.

[8] Moseley GL. Impaired trunk muscle function in subacute neck pain: etiologic in the subsequent development of low back pain? Man Ther 2004;9:157–63.

[9] McClure PW, et al. Kinematic analysis of lumbar ad hip motion while rising from a forward, flexed position in patients with and without a history of low back pain. Spine 1997;22(5):552–8.

[10] Janda V. Muscles as a pathogenic factor in back pain. In: Proc. I.F.O.M.P.T. New Zealand; 1980.

[11] Janda V. Muscle and joint correlations. In: Proc. 1Vth Congress F.I.M.M. Prague; 1975. p. 154–8.

[12] Janda V. Muscle weakness and inhibition (pseudoparesis) in back pain syndromes. In: Greive G, editor. Modern manual Therapy of the vertebral column. Edinburgh: Churchill; 1986.

[13] Sahrmann SA. Diagnosis and treatment of movement impairment syndromes. St Louis: Mosby; 2002.

[14] Janda V, Stara V. Comparison of movement patterns in healthy and spastic children. In: Proc. 2nd International Symposium on Cerebral Palsy. Prague; 1987. p. 119–22.

[15] Hodges PW. Low back pain and the pelvic floor. In: Carrière B,

Markel Feldt C, editors. The Pelvic Floor. Stuttgart: Thieme; 2006.

[16] Hodges PW, Richardson CA. Inefficient muscular stabilisation of the lumbar spine associated with low back pain: a motor control evaluation of transversus abdominus. Spine 1996; 21(22):2640–50.

[17] Hodges PW, Richardson CA. Delayed postural contraction of transversus abdominus in low back pain associated with movement of the lower limb. J Spinal Disord 1998;11(1): 46–56.

[18] Hodges PW, Richardson CA. Altered trunk muscle recruitment in people with low back pain with upper limb movements at different speeds. Arch Phys Med Rehabil 1999;80(9):1005–12.

[19] Hungerford B, Gilleard W, Hodges P. Evidence of altered lumbopelvic muscle recruitment in the presence of sacroiliac pain. Spine 2003;28(14):1593–600.

[20] Mok N, Hodges P, Brauer S. Different range and temporal pattern of lumbopelvic motion accompanies rapid upper arm flexion in people with low back pain. In: Proc. 5th Interdisciplinary World Congress on Low Back and Pelvic Pain. Melbourne; 2004.

[21] Ferreira PH, Ferreira ML, Hodges PW. Changes in the recruitment of the abdominal muscles in people with low back pain: ultrasound measurement of muscle activity. Spine 2004; 29(22):2560–6.

[22] Hides JA, Richardson CA, Jull GA. Multifidus muscle recovery is not automatic following resolution of acute first episode low back pain. Spine 1996;21:2763–9.

[23] Danneels LA, et al. Differences in Electromyographic activity in the multifidus muscle and the iliocostalis lumborum between healthy subjects and patients with sub-acute and chronic low back pain. Eur Spine J 2002;11:13–9.

[24] O'Sullivan PB, et al. Altered motor control strategies in subjects with sacroiliac joint pain during active straight leg raise test. Spine 2002;27(1):E1–8.

[25] Hides JA, et al. Evidence of lumbar multifidus muscle wasting ipsilateral to symptoms in patients with acute/Subacute low back pain. Spine 1994; 19(2):165–72.

[26] Hides JA, et al. Magnetic resonance imaging assessment of trunk muscles during prolonged bed rest. Spine 2007; 32(15):1687–92.

[27] Saunders S. Lumbo-pelvic control during human bipedal locomotion. Doctoral thesis abstract. In: MPA Intouch magazine. 2 Publication of Musculoskeletal Physiotherapy. Australia; 2008.

[28] Saunders SW, et al. Reduced tonic activity of transversus abdominus muscle during locomotion in people with low back pain. In: Proc. 5th Interdisciplinary World Congress on Low Back and Pelvic Pain. Melbourne; 2004.

[29] Silfies SP, et al. Trunk muscle recruitment patterns in specific low back pain populations. Clin Biomech 2005;20(5):465–73.

[30] Arena J, et al. Electromyographic recordings of low back pain subjects and non pain controls in six different positions: effect of pain levels. Pain 1991; 45(1):23–8.

[31] Belavey D, et al. Long term over activity in the oblique muscles after 8 weeks of bed rest – implications for inactivity, lumbar spine stability and sedentary lifestyle. In: Proc. 14th Biennial Conference MPA. Brisbane; 2005.

[32] Belavey DL, et al. Superficial lumbopelvic muscle overactivity and decreased cocontraction after eight weeks of bed rest. Spine 2007;32(1):E23–29.

[33] Janda V. Muscles and motor control in low back pain – assessment and management. In: Twomey L, editor. Physical Therapy of the low back. 1st ed. New York: Churchill Livingstone; 1987.

[34] Gleeson MG. The alexander technique. In: Proc. 1st International Conference on Movement Dysfunction. Edinburgh; 2001.

[35] Dankaerts W, et al. Differences in sitting postures are associated with non specific low back pain disorders when patients are sub classified. Spine 2006; 31(6):674–98.

[36] Ahern DK, et al. Comparison of lumbar Paravertebral EMG patterns in chronic low back pain patients and non patient controls. Pain 1988;34(2):153–60.

[37] Watson PJ, et al. Surface electromyography in the identification of chronic low back pain patients: the development of the flexion relaxation ratio. Clin Biomech 1997; 12(3):165–71.

[38] O'Sullivan P. Motor control and the lumbo-pelvic region. Proc. 5th Interdisciplinary World Congress on Low Back and Pelvic Pain. Melbourne; 2004.

[39] Janda V. Differential diagnosis of muscle tone in respect to inhibitory techniques. In: Paterson JK, Burn I, editors. Back pain, an international review. London: Kluwer Academic Press; 1990. p. 196–9.

[40] Dankaerts W, O'Sullivan P, Burnett A, Straker L. Differences in sitting postures are associated with non-specific chronic low back pain disorders when patients are subclassified. Spine 2006; 31(6):698–704.

[41] Mannion AF, et al. Fibre type characteristics of the lumbar paraspinal muscles in normal healthy subjects and in patients with low back pain. J Orthop Res 1997;15:881–7.

[42] Gill KP, Callaghan MJ. The measurement of lumbar proprioception in individuals with and without low back pain. Spine 1998;23(3):371–7.

[43] Brumagne S, et al. The role of paraspinal muscle spindles in lumbosacral position sense in individuals with and without low back pain. Spine 2000; 25(8):989–94.

[44] Taimela S, Kankaanpää M, Luoto S. The effect of lumbar fatigue on the ability to sense a change in lumbar position: a controlled study. Spine 1999;24(13):1322–7.

[45] O'Sullivan PB, et al. Lumbar repositioning deficit in a specific low back pain population. Spine 2003;28(10):1074–9.

[46] Speers RA, Paloski WH, Kuo AD. Multivariate changes in coordination of postural control following spaceflight. J Biomech 1998;31:883–9.

[47] Belavy DL. (F)lying to Mars: how spaceflight research helps healthcare. In: MPA Intouch magazine. Issue 2. Australia: National APA; 2008.

[48] Mientjes MIV, Frank JS. Balance in chronic low back pain patients compared to healthy people under various conditions in upright sitting. Clin Biomech 1999;14(10):710–6.

[49] Byl NN, Sinnott P. Variations in balance and body sway in middle aged adults: subjects with healthy backs compared with subjects with low back dysfunction. Spine 1991;16(3):325–30.

[50] Mok NW, Brauer SG, Hodges PW. Hip strategy for balance control in quiet standing is reduced in people with low back pain. Spine 2004;29(6): E107–12.

[51] Reeves NP, et al. The effects of trunk stiffness on postural control during unstable seated balance. Exp Brain Res 2006;174: 694–700.

[52] Hamaoui A, et al. Does postural chain stiffness reduce postural steadiness in a sitting posture? Gait Posture 2007;25(2): 199–204.

[53] Esola M, et al. Analysis of lumbar spine and hip motion during forward bending in subjects with and without a history of low back pain. Spine 1996;21(1):71–8.

[54] Porter J, Wilkinson A. Lumbar-hip flexion motion: a comparative study between asymptomatic and chronic low back pain in 18 to 36 year old men. Spine 1997;22(13): 1508–13.

[55] Radebold A, et al. Muscle response pattern to sudden trunk loading in healthy individuals and in patients with chronic low back pain. Spine 2000;25(8):947–54.

[56] Smith M. Competing demands on the trunk muscles: effects consequences and mechanisms. Thesis abstract. In: MPA Intouch Magazine.Issue 2. Australia: A.P.A; 2008.

[57] Enoka RM. Neuromechanics of human movement. 3rd ed. United States: Human Kinetics; 2002.

[58] Neumann DA. Kinesiology of the musculoskeletal system: Foundations for physical rehabilitation. St Louis: Mosby; 2002.

[59] Janda V. Postural and phasic muscles in the pathogenesis of low back pain. In: Proc: X1th Congress I.S.R.D. Dublin; 1968. p. 553–4.

[60] Jackson ND, Gutierrez GM, Kaminski T. The effect of fatigue and habituation on the stretch reflex of the ankle musculature. J Electromyogr Kinesiology (IN PRESS).

[61] Mannion AF, et al. The influence of muscle fibre size and type distribution on electromyography measures of back muscle fatigability. Spine 2395: 1998;576–84.

[62] Ng JK, et al. Fatigue related changes in torque output and Electromyographic parameters of trunk muscles during isometric axial rotation exertion: an investigation in patients with back pain and healthy subjects. Spine 2002;27(6): 637–646.

[63] Dolan P, Adams MA. Repetitive lifting tasks fatigue the back muscles and increase the bending moment acting on the lumbar spine. J Biomech 1998;31(8): 713–21.

[64] Wilder DG, et al. Muscular response to sudden load: a tool to evaluate fatigue and rehabilitation. Spine 1996;21(22):2628–39.

[65] Parnianpour M, et al. The triaxial coupling of torque generation of trunk muscles during isometric exertions and the effect of fatiguing isoinertial movements on motor output and movement patterns.

[66] Van Dieën JH, et al. Effects of repetitive lifting on kinematics: Inadequate anticipatory control or adaptive changes? J Motor Behav 1998;30(1):20–32.

[67] Sparto PJ, et al. The affect of Fatigue on Multijoint Kinematics

and Load Sharing During a Repetitive Lifting Test. Spine 1997;22(22):2647–54.

[68] Sparto P, et al. The effect of fatigue on multijoint kinematics, coordination and postural stability during a repetitive lifting task. J Orthopaedic & Sports Physical Therapy 1997;25(1):3–12.

[69] Gribble PA, Hertel J. Effect of hip and ankle muscle fatigue on unipedal postural control. J Electromyogr Kinesiol 2004; 14(6):641–6.

[70] Salavati M, et al. Changes in postural stability with fatigue of lower extremity frontal and sagittal plane movers. Gait Posture 2007;26(2):214–8.

[71] Descarreaux M, Blouin JS., Teasdale N. Force production parameters in patients with low back pain and healthy control participants. Spine 2004; 29(3):311–7.

[72] Radebold A, et al. Impaired postural control of the lumbar spine is associated with delayed muscle response times in patients with chronic idiopathic low back pain. Spine 2001;26(7):724–30.

[73] Luoto S, et al. Psychomotor speed and postural control in chronic low back pain patients: a controlled follow-up study.

[74] Luoto S, et al. Mechanisms explaining the association between low back trouble and deficits in information processing: a controlled study with follow up. Spine 1999;24(3):255–61.

[75] Jull G, Janda V. Muscles and motor control in low back pain: assessment and management. In: Twomey LT, editor. Physical Therapy of the low back. New York: Churchill Livingstone; 1987.

[76] Matre DA, et al. Experimental muscle pain increases the human stretch reflex. Pain 1998;75(2–3): 331–9.

[77] Arendt-Nielson L, et al. The influence of low back pain on muscle activity and coordination during gait: a clinical and experimental study. Pain 1996; 64(2):231–40.

[78] Roland MO. A critical review of the evidence for a pain-spasm-pain cycle in spinal disorders. Clin Biomech 1986;1(2):102–9.

[79] Hodges PW, et al. Experimental muscle pain changes feedforward postural responses of the trunk muscles. Exp Brain Res 2003;151:262–71.

[80] Moseley GL, Hodges PW. Are the changes in postural control associated with low back pain caused by pain interference? Clin J Pain 2005;21(4):323–9.

[81] Lund JP, et al. The pain adaptation model: a discussion of the relationship between chronic musculoskeletal pain and motor activity. Can J Physiol Pharmacol 1991;69:683–94.

[82] Van Dieën JH, Selen LPJ, Cholewicki J. Trunk muscle activation in low-back pain patients, an analysis of the literature. J Electromyogr Kinesiol 2003;13:333–51.

[83] Thomas J, France C. Pain-related fear is associated with avoidance of spinal motion during recovery from low back pain. Spine 2007;32(16):E460–66.

[84] Leinonen V, et al. Disc herniation-related back pain impairs feedforward control of paraspinal muscles. Spine 2001;26(16):E367–72.

[85] Hodges PW, Moseley LG. Pain and motor control of the lumbopelvic region: affect and possible mechanisms. J Electromyogr Kinesiol 2003; 13(4):361–70.

[86] Moseley LG, Nicholas MK, Hodges PW. Does anticipation of back pain predispose to back trouble? Brain 2004; 127(10):2339–47.

[87] Janda V. Comparison of spastic syndromes of cerebral origin with the distribution of muscular tightness in postural defects. Int. Symposium on Rehabilitation in Neurology Rehabilitacia Suppl. 1977;14–5.

[88] Schleip R. Primary reflexes and structural typology. Sourced at http://www.somatics.de/ flexextens/primrefl.html

[89] Hanna T. Somatics: reawakening the mind's control of movement, flexibility and health. Cambridge MA: Da Capo Press: Perseus Books; 1988.

[90] Van Dieën JH. Low back pain and motor behavior: contingent adaptations, a common goal. In: Proc. 6th Interdisciplinary World Congress on Low Back and Pelvic Pain. Barcelona; 2007. p. 3–14.

[91] Korr IM. The facilitated segment. In: Korr IM, editor. Neurobiologic Mechanisms in Manipulative Therapy. New York: Plenum Press; 1978. p. 27–41.

[92] Bergmark A. Stability of the lumbar spine: a study in mechanical engineering. Acta Orthop Scand 1989;230(60 Suppl.):2–54.

[93] Edwards I, Jones M, Hillier. The interpretation of experience and its relationship to body movement: A clinical reasoning perspective. Man Ther 2006;11:2–10.

[94] Hackney P. Making Connections: Total body Integration through Bartenieff Fundamentals. New York: Routledge; 2002.

[95] Moseley LG, Hodges PW. Reduced variability of postural strategy prevents normalization of motor changes induced by back pain: a risk factor for chronic trouble? Behav Neurosci 2006;120(2):474–6.

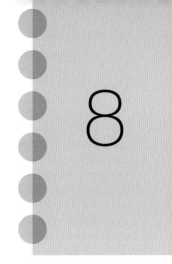

Chapter **Eight**

Common features of posturomovement dysfunction

The imbalanced activity between the deep and superficial muscle systems and between the flexor and extensor systems is expressed in a number of clinically observable altered features of postural and movement control, which appear to be more or less common in those with spinal pain and related disorders.

It is important to appreciate that these features are interrelated and variable in their presence, effect and mutual reinforcement of one another.

Defective antigravity support and control

A general or regional lack of axial extension control

The manner in which the spine is postured when upright highly influences patterns of trunk muscle activity.[1] Conversely, patterns of muscle activity determine how the spine is postured. By and large people with spinal pain syndromes can move but they can't 'posture' very well: if they manage to align the spine in neutral they have difficulty maintaining it in movement.

Poor control of a 'dynamic antigravity neutral' means the patient finds sitting or standing difficult to do in an easy non effortful way. He will tend to adopt either of two extremes – passive collapse or overactive 'holding'. Both affect function around the body's centre:

• *Passive strategy:* he hangs/sags/collapses relying more upon passive ligamentous support and where possible seeks external support such as leaning

against the kitchen bench when standing, or the back of the seat when sitting. Relaxing becomes more a state of collapsing. The spine tends towards a functional 'buckling' or 'folding'. 'Hanging the head' is common.

• *Overactive strategy:* he 'holds himself up' principally utilizing superficial SGMS muscles particularly those around the body's centre, such as the thoracolumbar erector spinae. Usually this quickly becomes tiring and so he collapses again. However, some have developed such entrenched 'holding' or 'fixing' strategies that they then 'cannot let go'. 'Holding strategies' create constant regional muscle tension in the torso and hyperstabilization of the underlying joints.

Poor pelvic base of support

The requirement for any column 'to be up' is an appropriate and well grounded foundation and the spinal column is no exception. Effective support comes from below and yet most have a 'dead tailbone' and poor control of the base of the spine. As the sacrum is part of the pelvis it is this that provides the important active base of support for the entire axial spinal column. Inadequate deep system activity, particularly of the Lower Pelvic Unit, reduces the ability of the pelvis to spatially adapt and provide an appropriate and effective base of support to initiate, lift and direct control of the spine from its base – the sacrum and coccyx.

The alignment and control of the spine in sitting, standing and bending forward is compromised, jeopardizing its safety. See defective pelvic control (p.170)

Common altered strategies for sitting and standing

The habitual adoption of poor sitting positions is probably the single most significant instigator and perpetuator of the postural and related movement dysfunction associated with the development of spinal pain and related disorders. In a modern industrial society long periods of sitting and relatively reduced general activity levels begin with schooling. The advent of computers and increasing sedentary work and leisure practices mean we do even more of it. The central nervous system (CNS) is relatively starved of decent proprioceptive inputs and automatic responses begin to suffer (see Ch.11). Altered alignment changes the motor memory, affects muscle activation demand, the line of pull of muscles, creates the need for 'holding patterns' and leads to changes in the myofascial matrix.

Passive strategy

Sitting. The common strategy involves rolling back onto the posterior ischia and staying there. Repeated enough, the person begins to lose options for varied position change in sitting. Poor initiation and control of the base of support through the ischial tuberosities compromises the ability of the axial spine to adjust and move. This is particularly so when the commonly habitual strategy of crossing the legs is adopted. Even worse is 'putting the feet up' on stools or similar, often advised when the 'circulation is bad' which only serves to worsen it! The alignment and control of the whole spinal column is affected (Fig. 8.1).

Collapsed sitting switches off demand in the systemic local muscle system (SLMS), rendering the joints and soft tissues vulnerable. In 'normal' pain free subjects, slump sitting has been shown to decrease activity in the internal oblique and multifidus[1–3] transversus and internal oblique,[4] particularly if the legs are crossed[5] or higher than the pelvis. Some normative studies have reported increased lumbar extensor muscle activity[6,7] in slump sitting, yet the subjects shown in the study by Callaghan and Dunk[7] are not in the position that most potentially or actually symptomatic subjects commonly adopt.

The posterior pelvic tilt creates hyper flexion of the spine[8] – particularly over the lower levels, including the lumbosacral junction with well documented detrimental consequences. Cadaveric studies of lumbosacral motion segments have demonstrated the

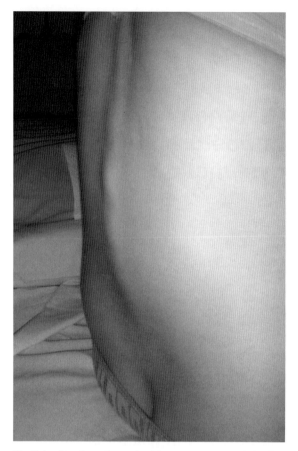

Fig 8.1 • Passive collapse in sitting creates eccentric loading in the spine of a 15 year old (also in Fig 8.10).

dramatic impact of increased segmental flexion on fatigue failure.[9] Solomonow et al.[10] showed induced flexion creep in feline viscoelastic tissues desensitized the mechanoreceptors and dramatically diminished muscular activity in multifidus. Later studies[11] showed prolonged flexion results in tension-relaxation and laxity of viscoelastic structures, loss of reflexive muscular activity within 3 minutes and EMG spasms in multifidus and other posterior muscles. The spasms and muscular hyperexcitability in response to 20 minutes static loading even when very light loads were applied were still evident after 7 hours of rest[12] and lasted for more than 24 hours.[13] In addition, the micro-damage from sustained loading of the viscoelastic tissues results in time dependent development of inflammation[14] setting the stage for chronic neural irritation and a plethora of referred symptoms of which pain is just one.

Usually, any attempts to 'sit up straight' are not initiated from the pelvic base of support but by intermittent systemic global muscle system (SGMS) activity of the muscle groups over the thoracolumbar junction.[15] O'Sullivan[2] draws attention to the critical role of pelvic position in determining spinal muscle activation patterns. 'Holding oneself up' is tiring and poorly sustained and so shortly the patient collapses again. In 'normal' subjects, significantly less superficial lumbar multifidus and internal oblique activity has been demonstrated in this postural strategy.[16]

The work of Solomonow and colleagues clearly demonstrates that a cumulative neuromuscular disorder develops because of repetition of static lumbar flexion, the severity of which is magnified by the number of repetitions. Full recovery of creep may not occur.[17] O'Sullivan et al.[18] showed a relationship between flexed sitting postures, reduced back muscle endurance, physical inactivity and flexion provoked low back pain. In sitting, twisting mobility significantly increases when the spine is flexed further increasing vulnerability of the posterior annulus to injury.[19]

Importantly, collapse of the lumbopelvic spine will affect the alignment of the rest of the spine including the head and neck, a fact which is often overlooked in some studies on cervicothoracic posture.[20] It also contributes to the development of the shoulder crossed syndrome[21] (see Ch.10).

In *standing*, the same postural pattern of posterior pelvic rotation is invariably carried through from sitting – the tendency being, to shift the pelvis forward with posterior rotation, hang off the iliofemoral ligaments in hip external rotation, with hyperextended knees and a collapsed spine. The sacrum is counternutated and L5 in relative flexion – an unfavorable loading state of the lumbosacral and SIJ region. This 'locking' of the lower limb kinetic chain limits the pelvis' ability to be an adaptable and appropriate base of support for movement control of the spine. Further, when the pelvis is shunted forward, there is reduced lumbopelvic SLMS demand. Snijders et al.[22] showed posterior pelvic rotation decreased activity in internal oblique. There is little buoyancy or 'lift' in the axial column or through the pelvis-leg base of support– the whole SLMS is relatively 'switched off.

Overactive strategy

Sitting. The person 'holds himself up' (Fig. 8.2) – from extensor system dominance and often also as a result of a mistaken belief that it is 'good posture'

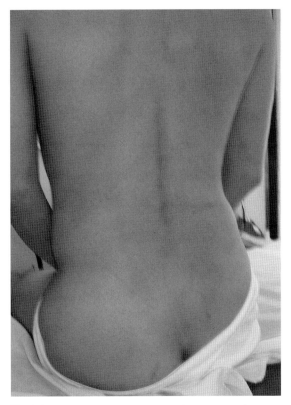

Fig 8.2 • An ineffectual pelvic base of support requires 'holding oneself up'. Note the poor lateral abdominal tone.

to do so. This is generally achieved by more consistent over activity of SGMS muscles – particularly the extensor groups over the thoracolumbar junction.[3,15] However, control of the pelvis as an effective and adaptable base of support for the axial skeleton is still deficient. Dankaerts et al,[23] using an electromagnetic measuring device, examined sitting postures in those low back pain subjects who actively extend in sitting and reported an increased lumbar lordosis. While the low lordosis was reported as greater than the controls, it is suggested that clinically, even this group usually demonstrate reduced intersegmental joint play into extension over the lower levels when assessed by skilled palpation. Appearances can be deceptive. In a radiographic study, Roussouly et al.[24] showed that while lordosis was increased, segmental extension between L5 and S1 was reduced. In the main, reduced extension over the lower levels (relative to the upper levels) and associated deficient intersegmental neuromuscular control is clinically apparent.

The superficial muscle overactivity reduces the ability to posturally adjust and shift weight over the support base. Intentionally stiffening the trunk by co-activating the superficial muscles has been shown to degrade postural control in unstable sitting.[25]

Standing. The standing overactive patterns are again a reflection of the sitting posture patterns – primarily relying upon dominant activity of thoraco-lumbar extensor groups and related considerable underactivity of the anterior abdominal wall. The thorax is shunted forward in relation to the pelvis. In an important and really nice 'normal' study, Harrison et al.[26] demonstrated that anterior translation of the thorax resulted in posterior displacement and anterior tilt of the pelvis with extension of the upper lumbars and flexion of the lower lumbars. Reduced SLMS activity in the lower pelvic unit means that the dynamic base of support through the pelvis-leg kinetic chain is still inadequate.

The superficial muscle hyperactivity splints the spine and further disallows it to adequately prepare for, dissipate and dampen the forces created by head movement breathing and particularly in response to limb movements. Reduced segmental adjustments mean balance suffers. Mok et al.[27] showed decreased preparatory and resultant increased correctional lumbopelvic movements in response to rapid arm movements. Smith et al.[28] experimentally induced low back pain and found reduced motion of the trunk associated with breathing.

Thus in upright activities, some regions of the spine are subjected to collapse, compression and a functional 'buckling'– they become relatively uncontrolled or 'unstable' while other regions become stiff or 'over stable' and fixed. This interrupts or damps the transference of the movement wave up through the spine.

The tendency to uneven patterns of control is also apparent in the asymptomatic population as Gregory and Callaghan[29] found when 'university population' subjects stood for 2 hours as they performed four light manual tasks. 13 of the 16 subjects developed some level of low back pain during that time. One of only three variables to significantly change was an increase in lumbar spine flexion. When central support is reduced because of inadequate deep local muscle system activity, the person is forced to rely more on abnormal SGMS activity in low load activities. Gregory et al.[30] had a group of college students stand for 2 hours and found that those who developed substantial back discomfort showed greater superficial extensor trunk muscle activity at the beginning and end of the standing period with further increased responses to sudden trunk perturbations. After discomfort developed, the superficial abdominal activity also increased.

Defective pelvic control

In the clinical setting, it is an almost universal finding that those people with spinal pain and related disorders demonstrate to a greater or lesser extent, inadequate neuromotor control of the pelvis in many, if not all, of the different aspects of its functional movement repertoire. This affects pelvic joint kinematics and transmission of forces and loads through the pelvis. Joint findings generally reflect the movement difficulties. Mechanical dysfunction of the pelvic joints is generally in the form of a 'functional biomechanical block' where 'distorsion' is reduced or fixed. This may not necessarily be directly pain producing but is accompanied by associated signs when palpating the ligaments and myofascia and for joint 'play'. This 'functional block' may be symmetrical or asymmetrical and affects segments higher up and down the kinetic chain. Pelvic asymmetry has been shown to create functional kinematic compensations not only in the lumbar spine but also in the thoracic region.[31] Pelvic dysfunction acts as a potent and important contributor to the development and perpetuation of many lumbopelvic and related pain disorders including hip and knee pain as well as underpinning a lot of mid and upper torso dysfunction syndromes.

Pelvic control *is* core control. It is the lack of *this* core control which needs to be better appreciated and more appropriately addressed in many treatment interventions.

Understanding the various aspects of altered pelvic control which will be present in varying degrees is assisted by examining each separately. They are as follows:

Defective intrapelvic control (refer to Ch. 6 Part B)

Inadequate control of Lower Pelvic Unit (LPU) muscle synergies result in difficulty performing the Fundamental Patterns of Pelvic Control. Attempts to do so invariably utilize strategies involving a lot of SGMS activity – either from large pelvi-femoral muscles and/or those higher up the torso normally responsible for controlling the relationship between the thorax and pelvis. Manual movement testing predictably reveals patterns of joint hypomobility which are also reflective of the motor control difficulties.

Fundamental Pelvic Pattern 1 (FPP1)

FPP1 is consistently the pattern that most if not all have little idea of the action and the most difficulty performing. Low lumbar segmental movement into extension is generally reduced with underactivity in multifidus, lower transversus, internal oblique, iliacus and probably psoas. The prime movers responsible for FPP2 are generally hyperactive and do not adequately eccentrically lengthen further hindering the proper performance of this pattern. Instead the action is more likely attempted by activating the thoracolumbar erector spinae, serratus posterior inferior higher up around the mid torso – a bilateral 'posterior cinch' which serves to 'fix' the thoracolumbar segments, thrust the lower anterior pole of the thorax forward and limit diaphragm activity and basal chest expansion. This may be overt or subtle yet readily discernable by palpation (Fig. 8.3). Because of difficulty with or habitual non use of this pattern, the pelvis is generally more posteriorly rotated, the sacrum counter-nutated and posterior hip opening is reduced as is low lumbar extension and control.

Fundamental Pelvic Pattern 2 (FPP2)

Generally this movement seems easier though appearances can be deceptive. Commonly, poor eccentric co-activation from those muscle groups with a prime role in FPP1 means there is imbalance

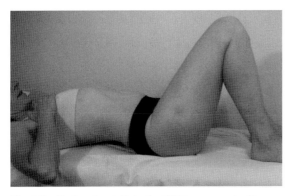

Fig 8.3 • Rather than initiate the FPP1 movement with a subtle anterior pelvic rotation, there is just discernable central posterior cinch pattern activity.

in the force couple producing the movement. Principal activity involving the pelvic floor and obturator group including piriformis, is augmented by the tendency to create the habitual 'dysfunctional posterior pelvic tilt' by pushing through the feet, clenching the buttocks or 'butt gripping'[32] with associated overactivity from hamstrings. The underactivity of the lower abdominals is associated with over activity of the upper abdominals in some subgroups (Fig. 6.30).

Difficulty performing these two fundamental patterns means that spatial modulation of the two pelvic bowls is deficient. This affects the myomechanics of the pelvic floor and the ability of the pelvic ring to adapt its internal shape as well as the whole unit in space in order to provide a stable base of support for torso and lower limb movements.

Fundamental Pelvic Pattern 3 (FPP3)

Deficient control of FPP1 and FPP2 accordingly affects the ability to perform FPP3 and achieve and modulate pelvic ring 'distortion' necessary for contra-lateral innominate rotation in the sagittal plane and pelvic rotation in the transverse plane, both involved in walking and most movements. This further affects the ability to control movements of the pelvis such that it is a spatially adaptable yet stable platform to support movements in the hips and torso.

Defective spatial control of the pelvis

Normally, the lumbopelvic stabilizing muscles including the pelvic floor are active when maintaining optimally aligned erect postures.[1,3,33] Hodges[34] states 'there is considerable debate as to whether pelvic and lumbar positions are different in low back and pelvic pain although changes have been identified in specific subgroups'. Clinical observation reveals definite patterns of altered spatial position and control and this is described.

Reduced intrapelvic control compromises the ability to spatially align and adjust the pelvis when weight bearing. Rather than control the pelvis around a 'dynamic neutral', the tendency is to assume postures in more passive, end range positions. The motor control difficulties are apparent in all three planes of spatial pelvic control, but are particularly obvious in the sagittal plane.

Sagittal plane

Here the observed preference is to posture and initiate subsequent movement from either an anteriorly or posteriorly shifted spatial relationship to the vertical neutral. The habitual preference for either forms the basis for a clinical classification system based on altered function (see Ch. 9). While whole synergies of muscles control the spatial position of the pelvis, psoas appears to play a large role. When underactive the pelvis shifts forward and when overactive it shifts back. The postural shift is always accompanied by a coexistent sagittal rotation as shown in Figure 8.4:

• Anterior shift and related posterior pelvic rotation with a corresponding diminished ability to posteriorly shift and counter rotate the pelvis into anterior pelvic rotation

• Posterior shift and related anterior pelvic rotation – with corresponding difficulty in anteriorly shifting and counter rotating the pelvis into posterior sagittal rotation.

While the anterior and posterior pelvic shifts and associated sagittal rotations are clinically apparent, there is little acknowledgement found in the literature except in a personal article by Schleip on the structural typology of Hans Flury.[35] In a very recent paper, Brumagne et al.[36] discuss the inconsistent results in the small amount of studies which report altered body inclination in relation to postural control. Two studies found a more anterior centre of mass[36,37] with related increased back muscle activation, while two others reported a more posteriorly located centre of mass.[38,39] Clinical classification into the two primary pictures of dysfunction may help explain these diverse findings (Ch. 9).

Coronal plane

The postural habit of passively 'hanging' the body predominantly on one leg is common and partly contributes towards the high incidence of hip 'bursitis' (Fig. 8.5). Reduced LPU activity subsequently

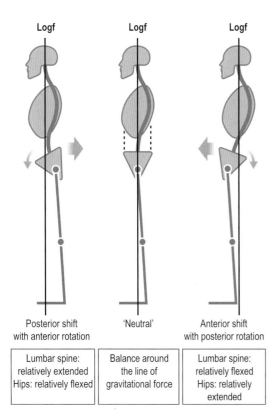

Fig 8.4 • Conceptual schematic sagittal view showing pelvic shifts and associated rotations (exaggerated for clarity).

Posterior shift with anterior rotation	'Neutral'	Anterior shift with posterior rotation
Lumbar spine: relatively extended Hips: relatively flexed	Balance around the line of gravitational force	Lumbar spine: relatively flexed Hips: relatively extended

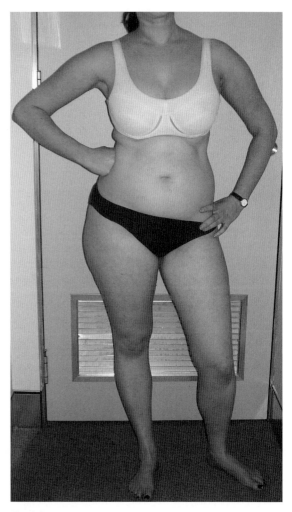

Fig 8.5 • Passive lateral 'hang' in standing – the deep system is 'off'.

affects the ability to laterally shift weight *through the hip* joints; either the pelvis over the weight bearing leg, or the leg medially under the pelvis. Instead control is attempted higher up via a bilateral 'cinch' which then affects the spines ability to posturally adapt in the coronal plane and maintain three dimensional control of its alignment.

Horizontal plane

Diminished control of backward and forward pelvic rotation affects adaptive postural pre- positioning of the pelvis to support lower limb movements as well as rotation in the horizontal plane and related spinal rotation. Gracovetsky draws attention to the importance of pelvic rotation in walking.[40] Tightness and/or imbalance in the hip rotators, particularly tighter external rotators, limit transverse plane pelvic rotation. A combination of reduced intrapelvic rotation or 'distorsion' and reduced rotation of the pelvis as a whole on the hips means that the mid lumbar spine becomes the site of relative rotary flexibility. Because of the poor spatial control, the pelvis is easily shunted around and movements of the hips invariably end up being movements of the low back.

Poor pelvic control affects the ability of the sacrum to direct alignment and control of the rest of the spine

Regional or general reduction of the lumbar lordosis is universally common clinically,[41] and as noted by Adams et al.[42] particularly in the lower lumbar spine. Poor control of anterior pelvic rotation and the habitual adoption of posterior pelvic rotation or tilt means the sacrum is carried into flexion and the lumbosacral region moves more into relative flexion in posture and movement. Generally, closed chain hip flexion and open chain hip extension are more difficult. Both rely on control of sagittal anterior pelvic rotation which is coupled with lordosis in the lumbar spine. The importance of being able to control posture and movement around the neutral lordosis for a healthily functioning spine is acknowledged by clinicians and has been stressed by noted researchers such as McGill[43] and Adams.[42] Loss of control of the neutral lumbosacral position jeopardizes local segmental control,[44] and also transmission of the movement wave and control up and down the whole axial spine, including coupled rotation and side bending amongst other things.

Altered control of sagittal pelvic tilt generally reflects imbalanced activity between the iliopsoas and obturator/hamstrings groups

Sagittal tilting movements of the pelvis on the femur are the largest and most employed in functional movement. It is necessary that each muscle in the LPU synergy works enough but not too much so each can effectively contribute to the synergy and co coordinated movement patterns ensue (see Ch. 6).

The ability to readily tilt or swing the pelvis forward and back on the femoral heads is influenced by the habitual posturomovement patterns used which in turn affects balance in the length/tension relationships between the obturator/hamstrings and iliopsoas groups. Unfortunately imbalance in the 'ischial swing' is clinically common. The obturator/hamstrings group is generally tight and the iliopsoas group can show underactivity, overactivity or imbalance between iliacus and psoas activity.

The imbalance is reflected in the pattern of the standing posture and contributes to clinical functional classification which is covered in the next chapter.

The relationship between back pain syndromes and hypo or hyper tonus of iliacus and psoas is understood by clinicians yet there is a dearth in the literature. Mostly considered as open chain hip flexors,[45] a postural stabilizing role is increasingly accorded to psoas[46–49] particularly if hip flexion is part of the movement.[50] Except for inclusion with psoas as the 'iliopsoas', iliacus barely rates a mention. However the two muscles differ anatomically, neurally and functionally.[50] Andersson et al.[47] demonstrated individual and task specific activation patterns between iliacus and psoas which varied according to the particular demands for stability and movement at the lumbar spine, pelvis and hip. The scant attention paid to iliacus in the literature is indicative of paucity in the understanding of functional movement control around the lumbopelvic region. Both these muscles provide important internal bracing of forces and movements within the pelvis[51] including stability of the sacroiliac joint as well as controlling the pelvis on the femur and the alignment and stability of the spine over the legs. Unilateral spasm of iliacus and psoas can contribute to a fixed intrapelvic 'distorsion'.[52,53]

The influence of the deep external hip rotators on modulating pelvic tilt control is practically nowhere to be found in the literature. Their influence is also important in transverse plane rotation of the pelvis on the fixed femur.

The myomechanics of the pelvic floor muscles (PFM) are dependent upon the reciprocal relationship between the ilio/psoas and the obturator groups as they balance and modulate the dimensions of the superior and inferior pelvic bowls. Because of the close functional synergism between the PFM and the obturator group, dominance of the latter renders the PFM likely to overactivity and shortness also. When the more superiorly spatially placed iliacus/transversus synergy is sufficiently active to balance the obturator group, the PFM are functionally required and better able to both concentrically and eccentrically contract and lengthen.

Imbalance in the 'swing' is also reflected in the position of the hips. When the obturator group dominates, the hips are more externally rotated and internal rotation is reduced. When the iliacus/psoas are tighter (less common), the hips move more freely into internal rotation and less into external rotation. Both groups can be tight where the neutral rotation position is more balanced but range into rotation, flexion and extension is more limited (see Ch.10 'Mixed syndrome').

When adaptive pelvic tilt support for functional spinal movement is insufficient, compensatory regional hyperactivity around the centre of the body is seen, serving to further limit spinal control mechanisms as the region becomes hyperstabilized. Increased activity in the superficial abdominals is increasingly reported[30,54–57] as well as extensor hyperactivity[30,58,59] (see Ch. 10, 'Central cinch patterns').

Difficulty controlling closed chain movements of the hip joint and subsequent effect on lumbar spine (see Ch. 6, Part B)

It is interesting to ponder the manner in which we personally and conceptually view dysfunction. The noted researcher McGill states 'I am continually surprised at the number of people with back troubles who also have hip troubles'.[50] They are always interrelated; and emanate from defective pelvic control. The huge numbers of people with back pain and those increasingly undergoing hip replacement surgery attest to the extent of the communal dysfunction.

Sagittal plane

Related to control of sagittal pelvic tilt movements, patients generally demonstrate poor alignment and control of the segments when executing the two most functionally significant patterns used in performing usual everyday activities:

Forward bend pattern

Ideally this is achieved from a 'pelvic swing and shift pattern' based upon FPP1 (see p.127). However, habitual buttock clenching and not 'letting go' of the posterior pelvic floor[60] and pelvi-femoral muscles contribute to difficulty initiating and controlling this action *from* the pelvis. Instead the pelvis commonly rolls into posterior rotation where the sacroiliac joint and the mid/low lumbar spine levels are the victim as they are pulled into hyper flexion to compensate (Fig. 8.6). This is common and has also been described as a 'click-clack' movement.[5,61]

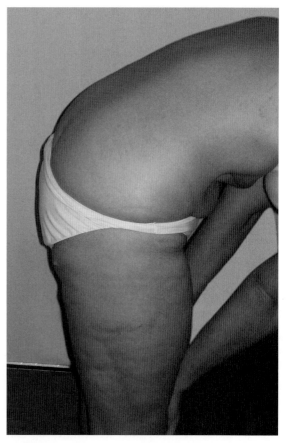

Fig 8.6 • Habitual poor forward bend pattern – note the use of the arms.

The sacroiliac joint is especially prone to shear forces if loaded in the counter-nutated position.[71]

Roussel et al.[62] described a study which found that reduced control of this pattern in dancers as a basis for performing open and closed chain hip flexion was predictive of risk for developing future musculoskeletal injuries. A large epidemiology study by Vingård et al.[63] found the strongest risk factor for LBP of biomechanical origin in men was working in a forward bent position. It makes no sense to attempt to 'stabilize' the lumbar spine – or the sacroiliac joint for that matter, if they are being constantly forced to abnormally compensate for movements which should be initiated from the pelvis during our many and varied activities of daily living. The disinclination to shift the pelvis posteriorly and weight bear through a flexed hip is also apparent in kneeling, all fours and variations of these positions. In fact loading weight through a flexed hip in any position such as supine is usually challenging e.g. 'bridging' is generally only achieved by posterior pelvic rotation. Achieving functional lengthening in the hamstrings and obturator group can only occur when the pelvis can be controlled in anterior rotation.[64]

Lifting or return from forward bend pattern

Ideally this is based upon control of FPP2 which brings the pelvis forward and extends the hips while balanced activity of the flexors and extensors controls the 'body cylinder' alignment. When control is defective, the patient tends to principally rely upon the hamstrings and passive tension in the posterior myofascial structures with the spine in flexion and posterior pelvic rotation or conversely, he excessively relies upon the back extensors (see Ch.9).

Transverse plane

In the transverse plane it is common to see:
Decreased ipsilateral backward pelvic rotation, hip internal rotation and lumbosacral 'closing'. This is usually more compromised than:

• Decreased ipsilateral forward pelvic rotation and associated hip external rotation and lumbosacral 'opening'.

Cibulka et al.[65] found subjects with sacroiliac joint pain has significantly more hip external rotation with a limitation of internal rotation on the side of the posterior innominate.

Coronal plane

In the coronal plane, reduced control of the LPU and lateral and medial weight shift *at* the hip engenders the need for holding patterns higher up in the torso or for excess activity in the large pelvi-femoral muscles. Underactivity in iliacus-psoas reduces control of lateral weight shift while overactivity disrupts the neutral pelvic position and feeds into central 'cinch posterior cinch' behavior (Ch.10; Fig. 8.7). Reduced intrapelvic

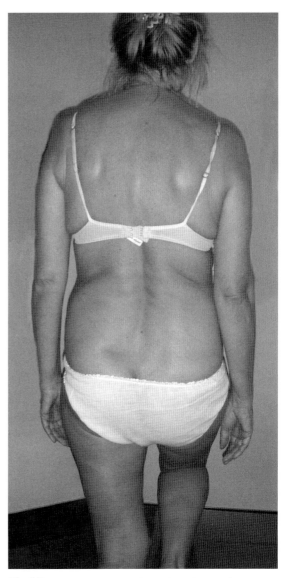

Fig 8.7 • Defective control of lateral weight transfer in standing becomes 'hanging' and 'holding'.

control provides a less stable base to support well controlled activity of the large SGMS pelvifemoral muscles – in particular the adductors and hamstrings both of which are notorious for 'sprains'. Mens[66,67] draws attention to the fact that 'adduction-related groin pain' in the athlete may not be caused by adductor tendonitis but by instability of the pelvic ring. In a study of 44 athletes with groin pain clinically elicited by resisting the adductors in crook lying, he then applied a pelvic belt placed inferior to the iliac spines and just above the greater trochanter. Subsequent retesting generally but variably improved adductor force and lessened pain during the maneuver. It is suggested that the pelvic belt is performing the action that would otherwise be provided by the synergy of the LPU in performing the first fundamental pelvic pattern. In particular the lower abdominals and iliacus provide intrinsic medial stability of the upper pelvic bowl and ipso facto mediolateral stability of the inferior bowl to support actions of the large pelvifemoral muscles. He notes the strong association between groin pain and abdominal wall weakness. He also describes[67] two other studies where cases of osteitis pubis, instability of the symphysis and adduction related groin pain were treated either by surgical fusion of the symphysis or intraarticular injections into the symphysis with improvement in the adductor related groin pain. Increased adductor tension/activity possibly not only causes tendonitis but overstress of the ligaments of the joints of the pelvic ring.

Three-dimensional control of closed chain movements of the hip is not only critical in being able to functionally move *at* the hips but is also particularly important when 'stretching the hips'. The 'catch 22' is that the hips are tight *because* of poor control of the fundamental patterns, yet often, subsequent hip stretching is performed as 'stupid stretches' (Fig. 8.8) with no attention paid to initiation and control *from* the pelvis. The lumbar spine is generally pulled into end range flexion or extension and rotation and becomes the site of relative flexibility[68] and even more vulnerable, setting up a vicious cycle where the dysfunction is perpetuated. This is particularly so in the case of tightness of the hamstrings and piriformis (see the 'hamstrings/hip conundrum' (Ch.12).

Reduced pelvic control at the hip particularly during dynamic single leg exertions has also been associated with patellofemoral pain syndromes.[69]

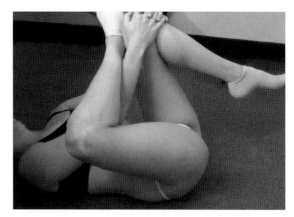

Fig 8.8 • This common stretch perpetuates her problem. Note the axis of movement in the stretch is the lumbo pelvic junction rather than the hip. See Fig 8.26 and text.

Impaired movements of the femur on a stable pelvis

Movements at the hip are generally better understood and considered in terms of 'open chain' movements – the pelvis providing a stable platform for the moving femur. This is also an important component of pelvic function and most contemporary rehabilitation strategies do focus on this aspect. However attention to the ability to control sagittal pelvic rotation and the neutral lumbar lordosis, as well as isolating the movement to the hip is frequently overlooked in practice. Reduced lumbo-pelvic or intra/extra pelvic control means that the pelvis is an ineffectual platform to support open chain hip movements. This is particularly important with large long lever actions of the leg such as the ASLR test and particularly so if they are ballistic as in kicking a football. The lumbar spine again becomes overstressed setting up a vicious cycle where the dysfunction is perpetuated. Tightness of the pelvifemoral muscles further compounds the problem. This helps explain the prevalence of various 'diagnoses' of hamstring problems in the sporting arena – pulls, tightness, tears, tendinopathies etc. is (see 'The hamstrings conundrum' Ch.12).

The close functional relationship between hip–pelvis myomechanics

The more common patterns of habitual posturo-movement tend to underutilize available hip range of movement and control and certain patterns of movement become more prevalent. Reduced activity and imbalance *within* the LPU and an over reliance on the outer SGMS muscles affects intrapelvic stability and control e.g. dominance of rectus femoris over psoas for hip flexion; of TFL over gluteals for abduction. The tendency is to 'hang' relying on the 'outer' muscles rather than find 'inner' support. The neuromuscular predominance of closed chain hip extension, abduction external rotation patterns *with reduced antagonist activity*, causes the inferior pelvic bowl to become hyperstabilized and more 'closed' and the sacrum counternutated. Altered loading stresses and reduced 'distorsion' in the pelvic ring ensue. Articular and neuromuscular freedom of patterns of hip movement into various combinations of flexion, internal rotation and adduction and related opening of the inferior bowl begin to show restriction. This limits closing of the superior bowl and control of the lumbar lordosis. Clinically, this is more common (Fig. 8.9).

If there is then a requirement for sudden or explosive muscular activity involving patterns of hip flexion, internal rotation and particularly adduction such as in kicking, the decreased eccentric lengthening in the extensor/external rotators/abductors can potentially lead to 'tears' as they are forced to lengthen. On the other hand, any of the flexor/internal rotator/adductors may also potentially 'tear' as they are forced to contract against antagonists which do not 'let go'. Particularly in the sportsman, actions that suddenly require large opening hip/leg movements or those requiring a sudden change of direction on a fixed leg, risk yanking the proximal muscle attachments and the pelvic bones themselves at the inferior pubic ramus and ischial tuberosities. This jeopardizes the stability of the pelvic floor and the syndesmosis of the SIJ. Clinically, the association between adductor hyperactivity 'osteitis pubis' and other related 'unstable' conditions of the symphysis become probable. In likewise manner the incidence of 'groin pain' syndromes can be partially explained. The influence of altered segmental function and related 'facilitation' in these muscles should also not be overlooked.

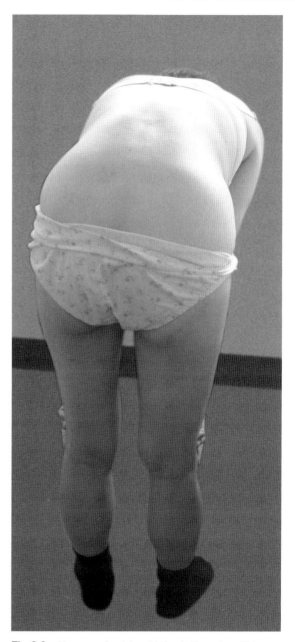

Fig 8.9 • Neuromyofascial restriction in the external hip rotators and hamstrings act to inferiorly 'tether' the pelvis during forward bending. The axis of movement becomes the low lumbar spine.

Sacroiliac Instability?

Vleeming et al.[70,71] considered that the articular surfaces of the sacroiliac joint (SIJ) were relatively flat and as large forces needed to be transferred across the joints, they were potentially unstable. They introduced the notion of a self locking or self bracing mechanism which acted to stabilize the joint. This model comprised a combination of 'form closure'– the specific anatomic features of the joint, and 'force closure' – compression generated by lateral muscle forces and ligaments with friction, in order to withstand potential shear at the joint from gravitational forces and during load transfer. Nutation of the saccrum is crucial in this self locking mechanism and tensions most SIJ ligaments.[70] The four muscles they listed as specifically important in providing joint compression were erector spinae, gluteus maximus, latissimus dorsi and biceps femoris. Through their attachments including those to the thoracolumbar fascia, they were considered to form part of three muscle slings: the longitudinal, posterior oblique and anterior oblique slings (see p.121) which acted to compress the joint[70] and provide support. Van Wingerden et al.[72] managed to show that sacroiliac joint stiffness did increase when individual muscles were activated, especially the erector spinae. Failure in the system is said to occur when erector spinae and gluteus maximus become weak with an increase in hamstrings tension which serves to hold the sacroiliac joint in counternutation, and so more vulnerable to shear forces in loading.[70] Note that practically all these muscles belong within the SGMS and are not intimately related to pelvic ring myomechanics, hence are unlikely to provide a truly effective postural pre-stabilizing role to support integrated load transfer through the pelvis. As those authors suggest, the superficial slings *will* play an important role in gross motor activities such as walking and running, but it is suggested only if they are able to act on a stable base of support provided by deep system preactivation. With the benefit of more recent evidence by Australian researchers[73–77] into function of various muscles within the deep system, the authors later suggested including the contribution of 'core muscles' to the self bracing mechanism.[71]

The instability model was further developed when in 1999 Mens et al.[78] published a paper which showed that impairment of the active straight leg raise test (ASLR) correlated strongly with instability of the pelvic ring in patients with peripartum pelvic girdle pain (PPPGP). The increased mobility was demonstrated on X-ray and occurred at the *symphysis pubis* and was most evident when passively hanging the symptomatic leg while standing on a raised box. The ASLR was improved by the application of a pelvic belt either just below the anterior superior iliac spines or at the level of the symphysis pubis. This external compression provides pelvic ring stability either above or below the hip joint. The researchers surmised that the caudal shift of the pubic

bone seen on X-ray was possibly caused by an anterior rotation of the innominate about a horizontal axis near the sacroiliac joint. However, normally, weight bearing is considered to produce a posterior rotation of the weight-bearing innominate while the superincumbent body weight causes the sacrum to nutate.[79,80] It can be reasoned that hanging the contralateral leg will produce further physiological 'distorsion' in the pelvic ring. If the pelvic ring is unstable at the symphysis, this will 'appear to be' excessive anterior rotation of the free innominate. While this study does show instability at the symphysis it does not necessarily show it at the SIJ. However, largely through it, a positive ASLR has somehow become construed as indicative of 'SIJ instability'.

Furthermore, clinically there is also a danger that pelvic girdle pain and the associated finding of a positive ASLR test have become readily interpreted as confirming 'sacroiliac instability'. This author agrees with O'Sullivan[56] who suggests many clinicians hold confused beliefs that the pelvis is unstable or displaced, which are then transferred to their patients with unfortunate consequences. While Mens et al.[78] found a strong correlation between positive ASLR and actual demonstrated pubic joint laxity in PPPGP, the test can also be positive in cases of pelvic joint stiffness. Clinically in a general population, the joint is more often symptomatic because of stiffness which may or not be directly pain producing. Pain provocation tests are not necessarily clinically reliable and it is generally necessary to apply composite tests to arrive at a diagnosis.[81] Examining the quality and 'feel' of the tissues and specific movement testing of the spinal, hip and pelvic joints including control of key functional movement patterns without necessarily reproducing 'the pain,' generally delineates the source and reasons for the pain and informs appropriate treatment direction. O'Sullivan et al.[77] identified altered motor control in subjects who had pain over the sacroiliac joint, positive pain provocation tests and a positive ASLR. During the active ASLR test, not only did the pelvic floor descend but this was associated with bracing and decreased descent of the diaphragm and alterations in respiration which improved with external pressure over the ilia. Rather than necessarily indicating 'sacroiliac instability', this study nicely showed that it is the operant suboptimal motor control strategies of the whole torso that are 'unstable' in many with pelvic girdle pain syndromes.

The Netherlands model of 'sacroiliac instability' has been popular and adopted by clinicians [32,82,83] and researchers.[84-86] An improved understanding of function in the deep system has led to the inclusion of those muscles responsible for generating IAP, also considered to have a role in maintaining pelvic stability and respiration (transversus, internal oblique diaphragm and pelvic floor).[77] However, highly significant is that apart from the pelvic floor and piriformis muscles, the influence of the very functionally important 'other internal pelvic muscles' – the iliacus and obturator group have to date not yet been well considered. Andersson et al.[47] showed that during ASLR, moderate to high activity was present for both psoas and iliacus. Clearly they contribute to providing *internal support* for load transfer through the pelvis. Eminent clinicians[87,88] describe spasm of iliacus as a potent factor in maintaining sacroiliac dysfunction. In the Mens study the raised leg was 'relaxed in lateral rotation'.[78] Clinically, preactivation of the FPP1 with the hip in neutral rotation can impressively change the ASLR test result. Interestingly, in an earlier paper documenting the results of a survey of 518 women with PPPGP, Mens et al.[89] noted the high frequency of delivery positions with a bent spine. They concluded a flexed position during delivery may enhance the risk for PPPGP. Post partum tasks involve constant flexion patterns, undoubtedly further feeding the dysfunction.

Gracovetsky[90] refutes the Netherlands 'instability model' suggesting that there is an evolutionary advantage to instability – function drives the anatomy and not the other way around; 'the viscoelastic nature of biomechanical material precludes straightforward application of these engineering concepts'. Even a steady erect stance is maintained by cycling through a sequence of different but closely related postures so that no one structure is continuously loaded. He proposes a 'SG ridge' on the sacrum locks into a corresponding shape in the innominates allowing coupled motion similar to that seen in the lumbar facets, but of smaller magnitude though greater force. The SG ridge acts as a fulcrum transferring the vertical loads, leaving the SIJ relatively free to rotate around the hinge in two planes, thus allowing axial rotation of the pelvis and nutation. The joint surfaces are warped and so do not slip past each other; the ligaments are strong and the geometry of the joint is such that there is no need for additional force closure to keep it together. The spine needs to be impulse loaded[40] with oscillating load sharing roles between the passive and active tissues.

This proposed model is appealing both clinically and in terms of function allowing the pelvic ring to slightly twist or distort ('distorsion') in the basic functional movement – walking, as well as numerous other activities involving the lower limbs. Dysfunctional spatial and particularly intrapelvic control as described will disrupt the kinematic chain controlling and transferring forces and movements between the hips and spine through the pelvis.

Neuromyo-articular dysfunction of the spinopelvic–hip complex underlies most pelvic girdle pain and related disorders

Pain in the pelvic girdle can either arise from the local joints or myofascia including the hip, or be referred from the spine or manifest from a combination of the above. Groin pain in the sporting population can be associated with pathology in the hip, pubic symphysis[91] and associated dysfunction in the lumbar spine and SIJ. While traumatic injuries including childbirth can precipitate the development of symptoms, more often than not their onset is insidious, seemingly occurring for no apparent reason. The pelvic organs receive sympathetic supply from the thoracolumbar outflow while the parasympathetic is via the sacral outflow. It should also be borne in mind that psoas is innervated by L123[94] and iliacus by L23[94], and the adductors by L234.[94] Spasm in iliacus can result from L23 and/or SIJ dysfunction. Palpation of joints over the thoracolumbar spine can reproduce scrotal, haunch, hip and pelvic pain. The functional relationship between the thoracic and pelvic diaphragms means that clinically, thoracolumbar dysfunction is usually part of the dysfunction picture in many pelvic girdle pain disorders. Clinical assessment readily delineates underlying patterns of neuromyo-articular dysfunction precipitating and perpetuating symptoms. In an excellent review synthesizing current evidence with clinical observation, O'Sullivan and Beales[56,92] make the case for clinically classifying and diagnosing pelvic girdle pain disorders based upon the dysfunctional mechanisms underlying the disorder. Currently, theories about the sacroiliac joint are popular yet confused and poorly validated, and these authors attempt to clarify the known facts. Importantly they suggest that 'directional strain' may be more significant than positional changes. In agreement with these authors, clinical findings generally delineate patterns of both neuromuscular hyperactivity and hypoactivity with a tendency for two main clinical subgroups. Those they classify as having 'reduced force closure' fairly much equates to the anterior pelvic crossed syndrome group (APXS; see Ch. 9) while those with 'excessive force closure' bear similarity to the mixed syndrome (MS; see Ch.10). Assessing and redressing joint function and activation and control of the fundamental pelvic movements and functional patterns generally ensures symptom amelioration.

Postural asymmetry of the pelvis

Clinically this is quite common[87,88] even in children, where Lewit found approximately 40% prevalence in children from nursery school age onwards. The asymmetry may be directly or indirectly responsible for the patient's symptoms. Lewit[87] considers that pelvic distortion is always secondary to some other lesion which must be found and treated, atlanto-occipital joint dysfunction being common, particularly in children. As Lewit[87] describes it: viewed from behind, the pelvis deviates slightly to one side (usually the right) and is slightly rotated (usually to the left). There is a fixed 'distorsion' where one innominate is anteriorly rotated against the other (usually the right) where the PSIS is higher and the ipsilateral ASIS is lower. Related to this is the 'overtake' phenomenon where in forward bending in sitting or standing, the lower PSIS (usually the left) overtakes the other becoming more cranial for about 20s after which the two spines return to a symmetrical position. There is usually muscle imbalance in the pelvic region and spasm of iliacus is frequent on the side of the lower PSIS, gluteal muscle bulk and activity is usually asymmetrical as is PFM activity. Clinically, the side of the lower PSIS is usually the painful side.[88] When torsion is present the leg lengths appear unequal.[88]

Pelvic floor dysfunction

Effective function of the pelvic myofascial floor requires the ability to coordinate the static, 'opening' and 'closing' actions appropriate to the combined situational demands of breathing, continence and posturomovement control. Much of the interest

generated in pelvic floor function stems from the problem of stress urinary incontinence (SUI). A recent longitudinal study by Smith et al.[93] provides evidence of a relationship between back pain, incontinence and respiratory problems, suggesting a common underlying mechanism.

Pelvic floor and continence

Good coordination is required between the pelvic diaphragm (levator ani and coccygeus[94]) and the urogenital diaphragm as the floor may need to open spatially in movement such as the dancer's high kick, while the sphincters remain closed. Pelvic posturomotor control dysfunction is likely to have consequences for the continence mechanism.[34] When the pelvic floor muscles (PFM) lose their automatic coordinated function, it is the timing of muscle recruitment, as well as the endurance and strength which is deficient[95] and activation may be asymmetrical.[99]

The incidence of stress incontinence is, or apparently was, low in Chinese women and cadaver studies have shown better developed levator ani muscle mass when compared to occidentals. This was attributed to hard work, minimal obesity and squatting.[95] Altered spatial control of the pelvis and its inclination affect the gravitational forces acting on the floor[33,96] and the line of pull of the muscles. When habitually forward and posteriorly tilted, postural demand is reduced. Increased sustained vertical loading on the PFM and increase stretch weakness is likely.[97]

A close functional interrelationship exists between the PFM and the abdominals and co-activation has been shown.[98] Given the underactivity of the entire abdominal wall in some groups reasoning suggests probable associated underactivity of the PFM.

An association between uterovaginal collapse and decreased lumbar lordosis has been described.[99] Similarly, postural collapse has been shown to relate to decreased PFM activity.[100] Lordosis facilitates activation.[57,95,100] Incompetent PFM response to sudden increases in IAP have been observed to be greater in spinal flexion in both sitting and standing.[95] Poor tonic PFM activity is likely if tonic holding ability in transversus is reduced.[33] Carrière[101] notes weakness of the PFM can occur from damage to the pudendal nerve from heavy falls onto the bottom, and if the parasympathetic nerves are also injured, various pain syndromes can also occur. SUI has a general connotation of a 'weak pelvic floor' and the need to strengthen it. While low muscle tone, reduced or delayed activity may relate to prolapse[102] and defective sphincter control,[32] subjects with SUI can also have EMG-demonstrated increased activity of all the PFM.[57,95] This is related to problems in the coordination and timing of activity between the abdominals and PFM[57,103] The abdominal activity can be either decreased or increased. When decreased, the increased PFM activity is probably more likely in those who attempt to control the pelvis by the posterior inferior pelvic force couple (see Altered control of sagittal pelvic tilt p.173) with or without buttock clenching and related underactivity of the lower or entire abdominal wall. The obturator group is hyperactive and shortened and the pelvic diaphragm is in the 'closed', shortened position and hyperactivity more likely. The coccyx becomes hyperstabilized creating an inferior 'tether' of the syndesmosis part of the SIJ which restricts nutation of the sacrum and the lumbar spine moving into lordosis. When abdominal activity is increased, particularly the external oblique,[95,103,104] the associated PFM hyperactivity may be in response to the increased intra-abdominal pressure so created. Retraining diaphragmatic breathing is indicated as a first step.[33] The current fad of inappropriate overtraining the abdominals as 'core muscles' is compounding a lot of spinopelvic girdle dysfunction syndromes and probably contributing to SUI incidence. Furthermore, there is a subgroup of patients with SUI who have diligently performed 'PFM exercises' only to experience increasing leakage. Freeing the sacrum-coccyx and mastering the 1st fundamental pelvic pattern which opens the floor, coupled with complementary postural advice can lead to dramatic improvement in one treatment.

Importantly, Rock[105] draws attention to 'reflex incontinence' whereby changes in PFM tone occur from reflex changes which occur in response to disorders of neuromyo-articular function elsewhere in the body e.g. functional disorders of the diaphragm can result in a reduction in both the elasticity and strength of the PFM due to diminished eccentric and concentric contractility respectively.

Pelvic floor and breathing

The close functional synergy between the diaphragm and PFM is disturbed when diaphragmatic breathing is compromised and can be further reflected in altered tone in the pelvic floor.[105,106] Chaitow[102] draws attention to the effects of PFM trigger points which in the main serve to increase PFM tone. Rock[105] describes a study where external palpation of the PFM in continent male and female physiotherapists found all cases were hypertonic with painful trigger points and clear cut differences in

tone between the two sides. Local PFM pain from trigger points cleared after 2–5 inspirations which focused upon 'pushing the palpating finger away'. Improving diaphragm activity can thus change the tonus of the PFM. Clinical correlations between pelvic myo-articular dysfunction, PFM dysfunction and thoracolumbar dysfunction are common and treating either can affect the other.[106] The complex innervation to the pelvic organs and pelvic floor includes somatic nerve fibres from S234, sympathetic nerves which originate T10 – L2, and parasympathetic supply originating in spinal segments S2-S4.[107] Trigger points, altered muscle tone, SUI and various pain syndromes are often associated with disturbed related spinal segmental function and associated irritation of the spinal nerve roots supplying that particular pelvic muscle or tissue. The clinical findings of symptomatic segmental dysfunction can extend higher than the thoracolumbar junction and certainly appears to implicate autonomic contributions to PFM dysfunction and symptoms.

Pelvic floor and posturomotor control

Because the PFM forms part of the ligamentous/myofascial syndesmosis[119] contributing to the mechanics of the sacroiliac joint, their altered length/tension relationships and coordination will affect intra-pelvic alignment and control and moderation of the dimensions the inferior pelvic bowl. Electrical stimulation of one side of the PFM demonstrated altered pelvic alignment with significant displacement of the coccyx, femur and innominate on the stimulated side.[108] During the ASLR test, PFM hypoactivity has been demonstrated[77] while others have reported increased activity.[103] Unfortunately many sufferers have been taught to activate the PFM by 'pull up and in' in isolation without incorporation into appropriate synergistic and functional patterns of posturomovement control. This risks further imprinting the tendency for axial 'holding patterns', further disturbing motor control in the torso.

Movement control becomes coarser resembling more primitive and total flexion/ extension movement patterns

In Chapter 7 we noted features of more primitive movement behavior, which can be variably apparent in subjects with spinal pain disorders and this is further explored. Instead of an infinite variety of adaptable postural sets, and movements, the patient often demonstrates a reduced repertoire, tending to adopt more primitive and stereotyped postur-omovement strategies reminiscent of aspects of earlier developmental stages and possibly reflecting less than ideal integration; the early postural reflexes. The person tends to posture and move from say a pattern of more dominant flexion and will have some difficulty achieving pattern break up into combinations of flexion and extension such as hip flexion with spinal extension. This is associated with imbalanced muscle co-activation in the proximal limb girdles with poor regional or general axial control and patchy SGMS dominance. For example:

Flexor pattern influence

A common tendency is for both proximal limb girdles and the spine to contribute towards more 'total pattern synergies' probably as a result of habitual postures and use and perhaps also reflecting developmental aspects e.g:

* *Habitual sitting postures* often reflect a generalized flexion pattern which is maintained by a combination of gross flexor activity and collapse of the whole spine instead of hip flexion with spinal extension in the normal curves (Fig. 8.10). Sustained forward arm use compounds the picture

e.g. computer use; knitting. More total axial flexion then becomes the postural set for initiating movement such as initial forward weight shift in sitting in order to stand up.

* *Standing forward flexion* frequently becomes a pattern of 'more total flexion' of the trunk and shoulder girdle with poor pattern break up of hip flexion, lumbosacral neutral / and axial extension with upper limb girdle posterior engagement and control. The person adopts an 'axial folding pattern' initiated from the centre rather than the hip. (Fig. 8.11)

* *Limb movements* also show a total pattern tendency e.g. hip flexion is generally associated with excess lumbar flexion with loss of control of

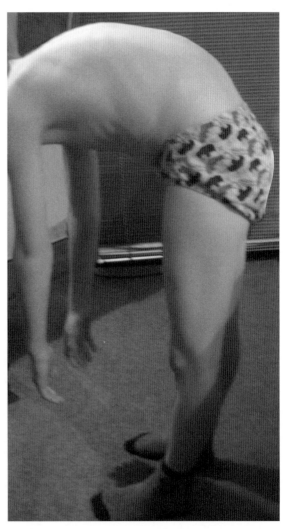

Fig 8.11 • Axial folding pattern in forward bending. The patient is 9 years old.

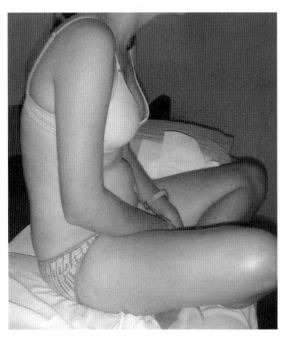

Fig 8.10 • Habitual 'more total flexor' collapse in sitting.

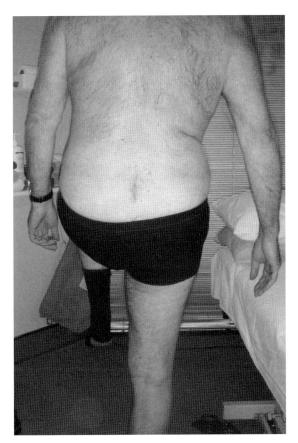

Fig 8.12 • Hip flexion also becomes lumbar flexion (side bending).

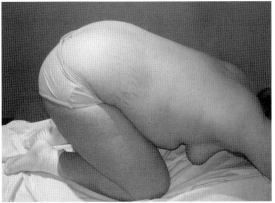

Fig 8.13 • Tendency to collapse into more total flexion in 'Allah' on all fours with marked posterior pelvic rotation and lumbosacral flexion (also see Fig.13.71).

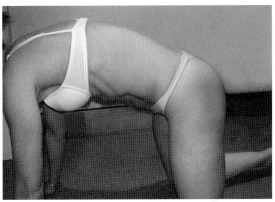

Fig 8.14 • Observable more total flexion pattern in all fours with dominance of 'pectoral cinch and propping'.

the neutral lordosis. Arm flexion is associated with excess shoulder girdle flexion. Limb stretches become axial flexion (Fig. 8.12)

• **When on all fours** there is often a tendency towards posturing in a more total flexion pattern, either tonus shift or overt posture. This may be intrinsic (Fig. 8.13) or increased through training effect (Fig. 8.14). The pelvis is posteriorly rotated on the femora and lumbar spine in relative flexion. Asking for weight bearing through the hands will generally be actioned by 'propping' through the arms with the elbows usually locked in extension. This is more a reflection of pectoral and anterior chest muscle 'flexor lock in' which does not allow for balanced co-activation of the shoulder girdle needed for good stable weight bearing control. The patient finds it difficult to break up this pattern and achieve proximal girdle control and proper axial alignment with elongation between the head and the tail bone. Similar difficulty maybe encountered in the kneeling alignment and control test (Ch.13).

• **Supine activities.** Care needs to be exercised when working for activation of transversus as advocated by Richardson et al.[109] not to reinforce the tendency for more total flexion responses with increased proximal girdle flexion seen in unnecessary pectoral overactivity and posterior pelvic tilt.

• Many so called 'hip stretching' activities become total flexion patterns of both proximal limb girdles and the spine (Fig. 8.8) and/or often involves general collapse into flexion (Fig. 8.15).

Extensor pattern influence

While torso flexion patterns can be more 'total', extension is patchier but can be 'mega' when and where it occurs:

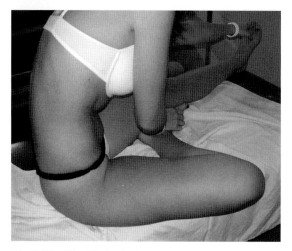

Fig 8.15 • 'Total flexion' collapse during stretching. The stretch is in the back rather than the legs.

In standing, the patient tends to adopt a more total extension pattern in the lower limb locking the knees into extension with a disinclination for flexible control between the ankles, knees pelvis–hip[36] (Fig. 8.16). This is particularly so if the pelvis is carried forward and/or he 'butt grips' (see Ch.10). Janda[110] likened the subtle changes which are seen, to the more obligatory synergies seen in lesions of the upper motor neuron – for example, movements of the upper limb tend to favor over activation of the flexors and internal rotators and those of the lower limb the extensors and external rotators and this is clinically apparent. Locking the legs limits postural shifts of the pelvis (see Ch. 6, Part B).

In the torso, more patchy yet coarse extensor activity is seen in consistent patterns of cervical hyperextension and especially thoracolumbar extensor 'fixing' which respectively shunt the chin and the lower rib cage forward.

When on all fours, because of poor pelvic control, attempts to anteriorly rotate the pelvis on the femora are generally attempted by a dominant thoracolumbar strategy (Fig. 8.17). Attempts at hip extension again result in a thoracolumbar fixing or a central posterior cinch (CPC) (see Ch. 10) with movement poorly isolated to the hip joint and associated poor patterns of axial alignment and control.

In prone the hyperactivity in the cervicothoracic and particularly the thoracolumbar extensors is readily apparent e.g. lifting the head results in CPC behavior with little activity in the upper thorax to support the movement (Fig. 8.18). Therapist

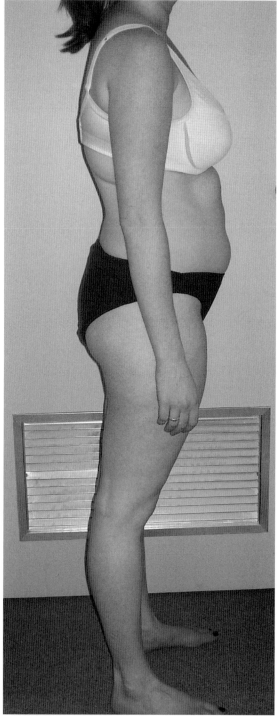

Fig 8.16 • Locking the legs and 'hanging'.

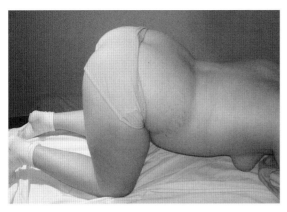

Fig 8.17 • The same patient as in Fig.8.13 attempting to anteriorly rotate the pelvis does so from a dominant central posterior cinch strategy. The patient is aged 17. The same difficulty is seen in Fig. 9.17.

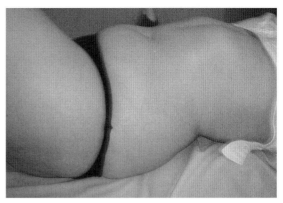

Fig 8.19 • Central posterior cinch activity when entrenched can still prevail when the patient is in the supine 'relaxed' position.

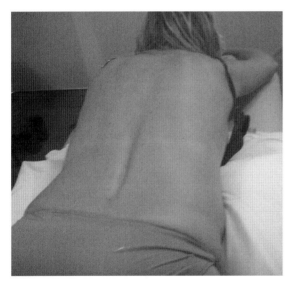

Fig 8.18 • Central posterior cinch behavior as a result of lifting the head in prone. Note the 'dead space' in activity over the mid thorax.

Patterns of upper limb weight bearing can suggest lingering influences from the tonic neck reflexes (see Figs 3.6 & 3.7). Upper limb weight bearing often involves 'propping' associated with either hyperextension of the head or hanging the head possibly further indicating incomplete integration of the tonic labyrinthine reflex (see Ch. 3) and adequate development of the Landau reaction. Habitual head forward posturing may also contribute (Fig. 8.20).

More primitive control is also seen in the tendency for bilateral activation in the limbs. Elements of reduced crossed pattern ability where dissociation between them is required, shows up as difficulty in seemingly simple tasks such as flexing one hip while extending the other with a neutral lumbo-pelvic posture or alternate plantar and dorsiflexion.

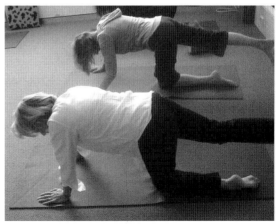

Fig 8.20 • The tendency for retracting the neck or hanging the head on all fours. Notice the different tonus in the arms in relation to head position.

skill is required in directing motor relearning in order to counter and not further reinforce these patterns.

In supine, hyperactivity in the cervicothoracic and thoraco lumbar extensors can be so fixed as to be operative in supine e.g. ASLR test may involve an increase in CPC behavior and cervical hyperextension. This can even be present at rest (Fig. 8.19) and could partly represent influences from incomplete integration of the tonic labyrinthine reflex (see Ch. 3).

The person becomes more of what we have termed a 'Primary A-P mover'– a rather crude flexor/extender in posture and movement. He finds it difficult to modulate co-activation of the deep flexors and extensors to achieve balanced alignment, elongation and discrete movement control of his torso in a multitude of different actions. These reflex responses resulting in variations in muscle tonus and more obvious flexor/extensor proclivity are subtle yet quite apparent in more loaded situations and those requiring greater antigravity response, the use of effort and upper limb use (See Ch. 7).

Importantly, the proclivity for the more bilateral flexor/extensor response limits use of the lateral and rotary components of movement needed for weight shift and balance and which provide for three-dimensional control.

Further changed muscle activation patterns within the dominant flexor/extensor patterns reduce selective movement control in the torso and affect alignment

Underactivity in the deep systemic system and altered control of the postural reflex mechanism is associated with uneven patterns of torso muscle activation between the two systems and within the superficial system which can be further mapped. Janda[110,111] was the first to clinically observe a tendency to alternate layers or strata of muscle hyper and hypo-activity in the extensor and flexor systems of the body. He termed this the layer or stratification syndrome (Ch.10). Best seen in the extensor muscle system it is evidenced by changes in the muscle bulk and contours and changed sequence and particularly degree of muscle activation. The following classification of the torso flexor and extensor systems in Tables 8.1 and 8.2 is extrapolated from Janda's classification[110–112] with some additions, based upon the clinical patterns consistently recognized.

The imbalanced development between the flexors and extensors leads to imbalanced co-activation in the proximal limb girdles and axial spine. This uneven patterning of torso muscle activity has significant consequences for spinal health and well-being. When any of these superficial muscle groups e.g. the thoracolumbar extensors, work harder,

Table 8.1 Altered muscle activation patterns in the torso extensor system

Hyperactive extensors	Underactive extensors
• Cervicothoracic extensors to T2 • Upper trapezius, levator scapulae • Thoracolumbar extensors T8–L2 or so +++ • ?obturator group including piriformis • Hamstrings	• Mid/upper dorsal erector spinae T2–7 • Shoulder girdle medial and lower scapular stabilizers • Middle trapezius • Lower trapezius • Rhomboids • Lumbosacral extensors: multifidus significantly underactive in **all** • Glutei

Table 8.2 Altered muscle activation patterns in the torso flexor system

Hyperactive flexors	Underactive flexors
• Sternocleidomastoid • Scaleni • Shoulder girdle flexors: pectorals; serratus anterior?; lateral latissimus dorsi • Upper abdominals in some subgroups (see APXS, Ch.9) • Hip flexors: psoas; rectus femoris in some subgroups (see PPXS, Ch.9)	• Craniocervical/deep neck flexors • Whole abdominal wall in some groups (see PPXS) • Lower abdominal wall in **all** groups is significantly underactive • Iliacus underactive in most and psoas in some groups

faster, longer and more often, then a number of the underlying joints are not free to move properly but are functionally 'straightjacketed'– they become *hyperstabilized*. Segmental movement becomes limited in one or more planes. Over time this will result in these joints becoming stiff from lack of variety in their movement repertoire. We start to see regions or 'blocks' of stiff segments forming. Movement tends to be shunted into more mobile regions e.g. the lumbar spine. At the same time we see a consistent pattern of underactivity over the lumbosacral junction – of both the deep and superficial systems (Figs 8.21 & 8.22). The lumbar spine becomes even more vulnerable. The SLMS is generally underactive throughout the axial spine and loss of SLMS co-activation with uneven superficial muscle activity pulls the spine 'off centre' creating eccentric loading states and altered stresses through the spine. The person then finds it *difficult to get intersegmental movement in the stiff regions*, e.g. the thoracic spine while at the *same time* he finds it *hard to control movement in the relatively mobile regions*, e.g. lumbar and cervical spines. This is a really important concept to grasp and will be discussed further on in relation to O'Sullivan's work (see p.188).

Imbalanced activity between the two systemic muscle systems occurs in differing proportions

It was noted in Ch.7 that there are two basic scenarios in the picture of systemic muscle system imbalance. Both display a reduction in SLMS activity and an increase in SGMS activity although in differing proportions as follows:

- *Flexor inclined*: here the reduced SLMS system activity is probably more pronounced. These demonstrate more flexion pattern proclivity and their increased extensor SGMS activity is more intermittent.
- *Extensor inclined*: here the increased SGMS extensor activity is more pronounced and constant with still evident decreased SLMS contribution to movement.

Both pictures play into the layered patterns of altered torso muscle response and in particular around the central torso we see a significant increase in muscle activity – a dominance of thoracolumbar extensor activity albeit more intermittent in the flexor inclined group. We see a predominance of upper abdominal activity in the flexor inclined groups. When these extensors and flexors are regionally activated it appears that it is more in the manner of a *'bilateral total response'* pattern – likened to a 'cinch' which serves to anchor or somewhat immobilize the thoracolumbar region towards extension or flexion keeping it in a more sagittal orientation. We have termed the regional extensor hyperactivity around the thoracolumbar junction a 'Central Posterior Cinch' (CPC); the regional flexor hyperactivity over the lower thorax a 'Central Anterior Cinch' (CAC) and when both are hyperactive, a 'Central Conical Cinch' (CCC) (see Ch.10).

During everyday functional activities, the adoption of these Central Cinch Patterns (CCPs) will

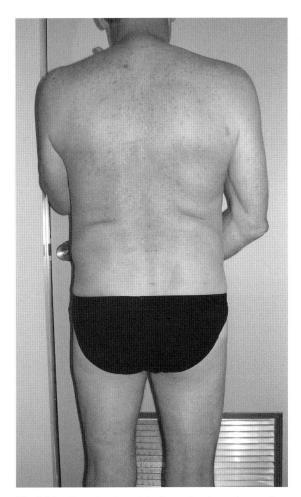

Fig 8.21 • Posterior view of the Layer Syndrome in standing.

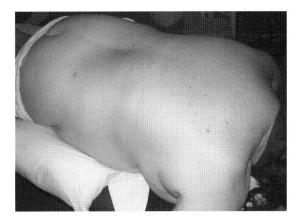

Fig 8.22 • Layer Syndrome in the prone patient. Even at rest, note dominant neuromuscular activity over the thoracolumbar region with 'emptiness' over the posterior proximal limb girdles.

tend to shunt the movement that should occur in this region more into the lumbar region. At the same time, we also see a significant reduction in lower abdominal and lumbosacral extensor activity across all groups. Control of the pelvis is diminished and the lumbar spine is under controlled or 'under protected' and becomes more vulnerable still (see 'Belted torso syndrome', Ch.10).

It becomes apparent then, that in the spinal column as a general principle, a pattern emerges where there are regions of muscular over control, or hyperstability whereby the underlying joints become stiffer; and adjacent regions which are under controlled or hypostable (or relatively 'unstable' to use the contemporary parlance). Here, the joints and soft tissues become more vulnerable to the effects of attrition because of the relatively excess and changed movement. A plethora of various clinical 'diagnoses' begin to develop.

Are movement impairments and control impairments co-related?

While there is increasing evidence that subjects with chronic low back pain have associated motor control impairments, these are generally seen as a response to pain. O'Sullivan[113–115] proposes that painful movement will be reflected in altered motor control as either adaptive (protective) or maladaptive (provocative) responses producing excessive or reduced spinal stability respectively. Adaptive behavior serves to splint the injured tissue and is synonymous with the pain-spasm-pain model. Van Dieën et al[116] would argue that this adaptive motor behavior is functional in order to reduce the probability of noxious tissue stress by limiting range of motion and providing stabilization of the spine. According to O'Sullivan,[114,115] the maladaptive movement patterns present as either:

'*Movement impairment*': movements which are painful are avoided and are associated with an exaggerated reflex withdrawal motor response, high levels of cocontraction and guarding resulting in high levels of compressive joint loading, muscle fatigue hypervigilance and fear of movement. This appears to fit the acute stage of disorder and severe pain states. He argues that the compensations for the pain become the mechanism that drives the disorder.

'*Control impairments*': more common clinically, postures and movements which are pain

provocative are not avoided, thus subjects maximally stress their pain sensitive tissues and are unaware of their role in perpetuation of the problem. Pain onset is gradual and associated with specific functional segmental control deficits and more chronic pain states. The non compensations for the pain become the mechanism that drives the disorder.

O'Sullivan's classification rests on a movement response to pain. However, it is suggested that most spinal pain patients *develop their pain because of the pre-existing underlying posturomotor problems* the nature of which is partly the subject of this book. Spinal pain syndromes are usually a developmental disorder, and over time as *a result of altered muscle activation patterns* and enough attrition to the joints and soft tissues, pain develops. If it is severe enough and acute enough splinting behavior is always present. Inflamed and angry spinal joints effectively facilitate or inhibit the muscle system. Clinically the local SLMS muscles are more prone to inhibition e.g. multifidus,[117] although not always. Depending upon the stage of disorder and joint irritability, the local muscles can be in spasm. Those of the SGMS are more prone to facilitation and hyperactivity in pain states e.g. lack of flexion relation phenomenon in the erector spinae. The presenting stage of disorder again becomes a significant element. If the joint problem is not addressed, the muscle activation patterns risk becoming entrenched and fear of movement, psychological sensitization etc all begin to kick in. Once pain is present it can certainly drive the motor control in the manner O'Sullivan suggests. However, this is a superimposition on underlying defective control. Clinically, most patients demonstrate a variable mixture of both movement and control impairments; they exist together, each influencing the other and creating the tendency to regions of hyperstability and hypostability in the spine. A pattern generating mechanism is set in train and will continue in the absence of effective therapeutic interventions which address the underlying pain producing mechanisms.

Deficient initiation and sequencing of axial rotation

It is well acknowledged that most functional activities require transverse plane motion.[118] Rotation is an important component of all movement, and particularly in functional control of the torso. Normally, it is variously initiated through the eyes and head and the proximal limb girdles, the movement sequencing though the spine – yet in movement dysfunction it is lacking.

In 1955 Steindler[119] wrote 'we know from clinical experience that it is particularly the length rotary movements of the trunk which, when blocked in their purpose of carrying through visible motion by an intrinsic rigidity of the body or by external resistance, are most apt to lead to structural damage'.

Clinically, the reduced axial rotation is not constant throughout the spine, but observed as too little in some regions and too much in others – both a reflection of inadequate neuromuscular control. While the morphology of the cervical and thoracic regions indicates that rotation should be greatest here, thoracic rotation is universally somewhat woeful, cervical is reduced and the lumbar region is forced into a major role for which it is not suited. A number of factors play out to adversely affect rotary control in the torso as follows:

• Sahrmann drew attention to the notion of 'compensatory relative flexibility'[120] and Janda[121] to the Rule of Horizontal Generalization (Ch.7). Both concepts involve the notion that in a segmented structure such as the human musculoskeletal system, if some structure or regions are stiff, then adjacent or further removed structures or regions will be required to compensate with a relative increase in movement. This concept is evidenced in altered control of rotation in the torso.

• The combination of passive sagittal collapse and coarse more general flexor/extensor synergies in posturomovement and has the effect of shortening and mal aligning the axial spine, limiting spinal control to a more sagittal orientation e.g. CPC behavior holds that region of the spine in more extension limiting flexion, lateral flexion and rotation through the thoracolumbar region of the spine. When rotation is required in the system it will generally occur below this hyperstabilized region – the mid-low lumbar levels.

The component parts are examined more closely below.

Head

The head initiates rotation from the top of the spine. Disturbed axial alignment impedes the rotary freedom of the head. Contemporary occupational demands require long hours of head down and forward postures with related eye hand activities. Neurologically we begin to habituate to these postures and 'forget' to utilize all the other available movement options of which rotation is an important one. In particular, eye movements as initiators of head movements are neglected. Conversely the hunter gatherer is constantly varying his head postures to orient his prime organs of sense towards survival.

Shoulder girdle

Most contemporary occupations involve bilateral arm use low down in front of the body with a relative paucity of outer spatial reaching actions. This leads to common patterns of neuromuscular dysfunction seen in the shoulder girdle with over activity and related shortening of the large anterior SGMS chest muscles with associated underactivity in the shoulder girdle extensors creating a consequent bias for protraction and depression of the shoulder girdle in posture and movement. Over time the girdle may lose freedom into elevation, and rotating forwards and particularly backwards on the thorax.

Limited backward and forward shoulder girdle rotation control will affect a number of torso functions:

• These movements are coupled with intersegmental thoracic rotation and their limitation also limits movement in the thorax and vice versa. This compromises the function of the upper limb and underpins the genesis of many developmental shoulder problems which are often given the dubious diagnosis of 'rotator cuff' tear, etc.

• Restricted rotation in the shoulder-thorax unit requires compensatory movement in the cervical spine above and the lumbar spine below e.g. actions requiring body patterns of rotation such as hitting a forehand or back hand tennis shot or a golf swing then become a potential or actual problem for the low back and neck.

• Reduced shoulder girdle rotation and arm swing interferes with the natural counter rotation between the proximal girdles when walking. Normally, the viscoelastic properties of the tissues and the counter rotary oscillation between the girdles affords an energy storing and releasing mechanism and ensures no one structure is continuously loaded such that walking can be done for a long time.[90] The energy load of walking increases while endurance decreases.

- McGill[122] notes the important role of arm swing in assisting counter rotation between the girdles, which effectively decreases the actual loading stress in the lumbar spine by up to 10%.

- Latissimus dorsi is an important member of the synergy forming part of the posterior oblique muscle sling[30,70,82] deemed an important factor in helping stabilize the lumbar spine and pelvis during load transfer between the upper and lower body. When its line of pull is altered and/or its shoulder firing patterns change, the effectiveness of this posterior system begins to decrease.

Neuromuscular imbalance in the shoulder girdle has far reaching effects through the torso as it impedes the transference of movement between the upper limb and the spine and interferes with movement within the whole spine.

Pelvic-hip girdle

The initiation of axial rotation from the base of the spine occurs through pelvic 'distorsion' rotating the sacrum, the movement then sequencing up the spine. Distorsion is part of axial rotation of the pelvis, a key functional component of many movement patterns. Gracovetsky[40] notes: 'In its elementary form, human gait can be reduced to rotating the pelvis in the horizontal plane'. In dysfunction there is always some reduction in the ability to accomplish forward and particularly backward pelvic rotation in the transverse plane. Reduction in the multiplanar range and control of hip movements, particularly the deep hip rotators is an important factor in limiting transverse plane pelvic rotation. Experimentally fixating the pelvis in the horizontal plane has been shown to result in altered gait and excessive trunk rotation.[123] Lumbar spine morphology renders it less suited to this role. If the sacrum is blocked, so will the lumbosacral junction levels, owing to their corresponding functional relationship. The movement will then tend to occur more around the mid lumbar levels – the lumbar spine again becomes the site of 'relative flexibility'. This is particularly likely in sports which require repeated rotary actions.[124] Grieve[88] notes 'that it is not rare for a sacroiliac problem to be accompanied by abnormalities at L3'. Clinically, many of those presenting with knee pain yet minimal local signs, are found to have a functional lumbosacral junction/pelvic block and associated chronic low grade L3/4 nerve irritation producing somatic pain referral syndromes to the knee. This is a common cause of much non traumatic knee pain and often not recognized as back and or pelvic pain is not necessarily a feature. Conversely, the altered pelvic myomechanics also helps explain why some people notice increased back pain when they walk.

Axial spine

The flexibility of the spine is crucial to all torso movement.[125] Regions of segmental hyper and hypostability interfere with the even sequencing of rotation through the spine.

Cervical spine

The common clinical presentation of the head forward posture creates relative hype flexion of the joints over the cervicothoracic junction and relative extension in the joints in the cervicocranial complex. Invariably this is associated with a pattern of restricted rotation at the C1/2 joint (where 50% of cervical rotation is deemed to occur)[126] and restricted movement in the joints over the cervicothoracic junction. The mid cervical spine then becomes the site of relative flexibility, with relatively excess segmental movement. Restriction in the shoulder girdle and upper thoracic spine as noted above compounds the picture of dysfunction.

Thoracic spine

Despite anatomy favoring side bending and particularly rotation here, clinically, the thoracic spine is predictably stiff in these movements with extension. Posterior or anterior translation can also be reduced.[127] The axial movement wave is damped or blocked through the thorax further shunting the movement into the lumbar and cervical regions (Fig. 8.23).

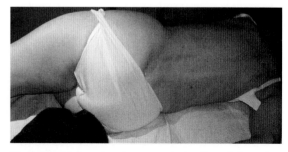

Fig 8.23 • Reduced and uneven rotation through the spine with evident 'wind' over the low lumbar levels.

Lumbar spine

The collective influences of restricted function within the thorax–shoulder girdle, the hip–pelvic girdle and over the thoracolumbar junction, and corresponding inadequate SLMS activity shunts the movement into the lumbar spine, particularly over the mid/low lumbar levels. Caution needs to be exercised in the manner of guiding improved torso rotation as the patient will tend to reflexley initiate the action through 'central cinch' strategies 'wringing the waist', limiting the diaphragm and requiring the lumbar spine to further accommodate the movement.

Farfan[128] postulated that loss of the lumbar lordosis and excess torsion or rotation of the lumbar spine were a provocative cause of disc pathology. He was correct – the low back being forced to unfairly bear the brunt for example in lifting and twisting actions because other functional links in the kinetic chain do not adequately contribute to the pattern of movement. However, he also pointed out[129] that upright and lifting activities were subserved by a strong hip extensor mechanism which helped protect the integrity of the lordosis. However, somehow the message was lost and the trend in therapeutic advice to patients became to limit or *avoid* flexion and rotation activities of the trunk. This is unrealistic as so many ordinary activities of daily living involve aspects of trunk flexion and rotation. When thoracic and pelvic posturomovement dysfunctions are addressed, the lumbar spine can align and function more normally, only having to take its fair share of the movement load (see Ch. 6).

In more general terms, loss of rotary ability makes is difficult to roll over in lying and transition through postural sets e.g. getting up and down from the floor. It also compromises the ability for postural adjustments needed in balance control. Being able to control rotation through all links in the functional kinetic chain is necessary for walking. Studies have shown that people with back pain walk at a slower pace with shorter steps,[130,131] with a reduced ability to adapt trunk pelvis coordinationto changes in velocity.[132] The altered motor control showed a more rigid, less flexible pelvis-thorax coordination[133,134] which was also less variable and showed irregular movements of the thorax[131] and increased fluctuations in dynamic thoracic and pelvic oscillations.[135]

Reduced use of lateral movements

Lateral spinal movements are an important feature in the development of our patterns of spinal control (Ch. 3). They help achieve balance between the flexors and extensors, control of all the sagittal curves while lengthening the side of the body cylinder for frontal plane weight shift. Gracovetsky[136] suggests the phylogenetic importance of lateral bending and its role in coupled motion of the spine helping drive axial rotation of the spine and pelvis.

The tendency for more predominant posturomovements in the sagittal plane including 'fixing strategies' from the CCPs means that in general, spinal pain subjects show disinclination and poor ability for lateral weight shift/transfer and 'body half' activities where the weight bearing occurs through one side of the body and the other side is free to move e.g. in all fours or standing on one leg. Weight bearing through one side involves adaptive ipsilateral *eccentric* activity in the 'lateral contractile field'[137] of the body cylinder to allow 'lengthening the side', in particular from erector spinae, psoas, quadratus lumborum, lateral latissimus and the anterolateral abdominals. CCP behavior limits this. The difficulty is in both initiating and controlling the shift through the pelvic base and allowing adaptive lateral shift through the torso including the thorax (Fig. 8.24). In addition, imbalance between the flexors and extensors jeopardizes able control of the sagittal alignment between thorax and pelvis with anterior 'rib shunt' of the lower pole of the thorax common.

Reduced weight shifts over the base of support and through the spine affect equilibrium control

The SLMS (Ch.5) in its role of moderating the normal postural reflex mechanism is the primary agent of weight shift and equilibrium control in the body. Its relative underactivity, the consequent over use of more superficial SGMS activity towards the coarse flexor and extensor synergies and the consequent reduced ability for lateral and rotary control,

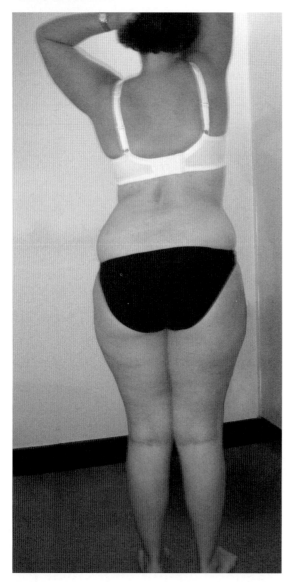

Fig 8.24 • The patient has been asked to grow the right elbow to the ceiling to facilitate ipsilateral weight shift. Note poor spatial shift through the pelvis and reliance upon central posterior cinch behavior which stops ipsilateral lengthening in the torso. Note how she also compensates in the neck.

serve to limit effective weight shifts over the person's base of support and through their proximal limb girdles and spine – *whatever position they are in*. Most spinal pain patients are loathe to shift the body over and around the particular base of support. The base of support is in general poorly 'grounded' with resultant collapse or 'propping'. Control of weight shift **is** control. Weight shifts underpin all movements of the body and particularly those of

the limbs (Ch.3). The person's balance suffers. 'Falls in the elderly' become more likely in the future.

Research has variously shown defective equilibrium control in chronic low back pain subjects. In standing, significantly increased anteroposterior postural sway [138,139] is apparent and more so when combined with task complexity and removal of visual cues.[39] The internal perturbation of respiration exerts a greater disturbing effect on standing equilibrium in back pain subjects[140] with a tendency to less hip motion to counteract the postural disturbances.[141] During bilateral and single leg stance balance control tasks, Mok et al.[142] found decreased ability to initiate and control the anteroposterior hip strategy responses with increased visual dependence. Luoto et al.[143] found a relationship between impaired psychomotor speed and impaired postural control among females. In another study Luoto et al.[144] found a strong relationship between severe low back pain and poor ability to balance on one leg.

When standing, it is common for spinal pain subjects to adopt a wide base of support and 'lock in' with the obturator group/buttock clench. Rather than stand over the legs they stand between them which is much more stable, limiting perturbations to the system which otherwise help to refuel the sensorimotor apparatus (Fig. 8.25). Lack of opportunity and 'practice' in equilibrium responses reduces system smartness. If weight shifts and equilibrium are not well integrated – particularly the ability to *initiate the shift from and through the base of support*, the person will compensate by combinations of propping through his limbs, and utilizing collapsing and/or 'holding' strategies in his body. Clinically, the ability to control weight shift even in prone and supine is frequently so impressively reduced that some patients find it hard to turn over! Needless to say, subsequent positions such as all fours, kneeling etc. also show poor control.

The pelvis is the base of support for the 'body cylinder'. When upright, the prime centre of weight shift is through the pelvis – of itself in sitting or through the legs when standing.

• *In sitting.* It's all about what the sit bones do or don't do – the person's ability to direct and control how the ischial tuberosities present and change the base of support and so direct movement of the torso. Reduced intra and extra pelvic control makes this more difficult. Doing it improves control. Balanced activity in iliacus-psoas is critical to sagittal and lateral weight shift control. When underactive

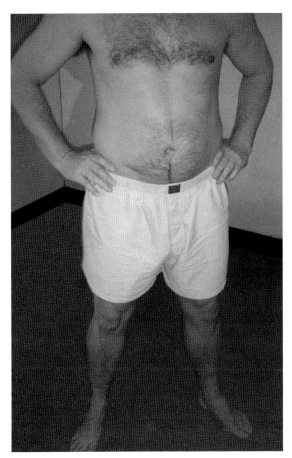

Fig 8.25 • Despite the fact this person 'works out' he finds it hard to adopt dynamic antigravity postures choosing to hang between abducted legs.

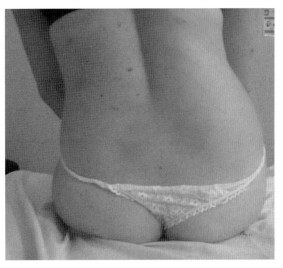

Fig 8.26 • This patient does 'physical culture' yet cannot weight shift through the pelvis, instead she is trying to do it from higher up. This then also limits appropriate lateral elongation in the torso. The reason is apparent in Figs 8.8, 9.18 & 11.4.

the pelvis falls back and the spine collapses. When overactive the pelvis tilts forward and the spine is 'held' as reduced eccentric lengthening does not let the spine posturally adjust. Attempted weight shifts predictably occur higher up via CCP behavior around the mid torso (Fig. 8.26). The spine is not free to adjust and breathing is compromised. Axial collapse is not conducive to active weight shifts either. An inactive base of support for sagittal weight shift helps explain incidents such as 'I did my back in when all I was doing was putting on my shoes!'

• *In standing.* Apart from the wide base of support through the feet, the person locks their knees into extension and habitually positions the pelvis forward or back from the midline. This defacilitates active pelvic control and the readiness for balance reactions and weight shifts. It is

becoming so prevalent for people to habitually stand this way – just stand on a station platform or any public place and note this – particularly in the young! The deep system becomes rustier from lack of demand and disuse. When perturbations do occur, rather than resolving the postural challenge through a flexible torso on a dynamic base of support, he tends to react by stepping to widen his base of support, stiffening his trunk and grabbing with his arms. Importantly disallowing freedom of the 'ischial swing' means that capability in the large sagittal pelvic weight shifts needed in bending and lifting becomes reduced.

Lateral weight transfer also suffers. Reduced sagittal control of the 'ischial swing' correspondingly limits control of lateral weight shift through the pelvis. Again iliacus-psoas activity tends to be either inadequate or increased with predictable effects in the spine and pelvis. Unilateral limb activities involve lateral weight shift whatever the posture. The patient is disinclined to shift his weight onto one leg and if he does, it is usually a passive strategy of lateral pelvic shift and passive 'hanging' with the hip in relative adduction. The de-tuned pelvis–hip myomechanics mean actively shifting his weight onto one leg *through the pelvis* with 'postural lift' and flexible control through the kinetic chain is not good. He has to hold himself up from higher up (Figs 8.27 & 8.28). There may be asymmetry in

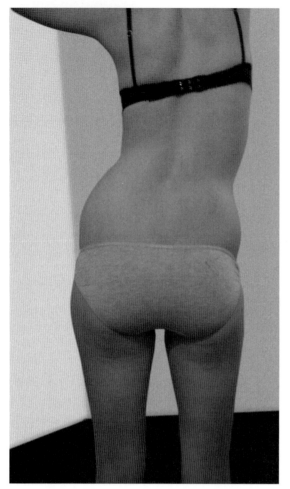

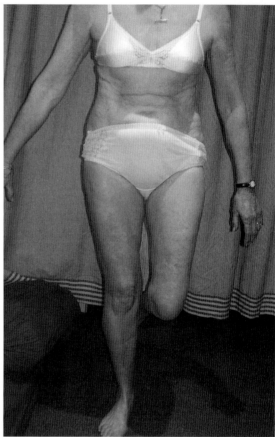

Fig 8.28 • Defective control of pelvic rotation in the sagittal and frontal planes again reduces weight shift through the pelvis and the need for 'holding strategies' higher up.

Fig 8.27 • Disability in frontal plane pelvic rotation limits lateral weight transfer through the pelvis and creates the need for compensations higher up. The patient is 21 years old and complaining of right sacroiliac joint pain.

Poor proprioceptive, spatial, kinesthetic awareness

the action. Not surprisingly balance on one leg is difficult and involves sag and grip in the kinetic system. He may move into a slight crouch in an attempt to lower his centre of gravity and also try and grab and 'fix' with his arms to compensate through his upper body for that stability and control which his lower body is not providing. Clinical tests such as the Trendelenberg and Gillet may/not test positive.[32] Even if the pelvis remains level reduced spatial shift and central cinch behavior shows the poor quality of LPU support.

To recap, poor control of multiplanar weight shift *from the base of support* and the adoption of central cinch patterns stops movement sequencing through the torso, thus affecting equilibrium.

Effective SLMS activity is dependent upon good afference. Reduced perceptual awareness is variably apparent in subjects with spinal pain. In general their 'senses' appear to be less well attuned to both their intrinsic and extrinsic state. This may be due to subtle CNS dysfunction (Ch.7) or subsequently 'acquired'. This compromises effective motor planning and control, the appreciation of various spatial relationships of the limbs to the torso as well as spatial positioning of the pelvis and torso. When the postural system is 'on', the small oscillating adjustments serve to continually recharge the system. The adoption of sustained collapsed or 'held' postures subverts the system. Sitting slouched for 5 minutes has been shown to alter lumbar spine

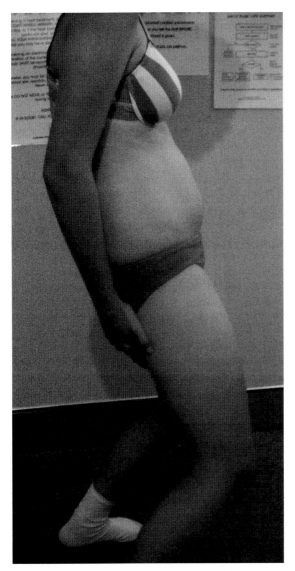

Fig 8.29 • The same patient in Fig. 8.1 & Fig. 8.10 has been asked to move her pelvis back in space in order to bend forward and instead she initially does what she 'knows' which is to bring it forward and into posterior tilt.

reposition sense in pain free subjects,[145] thus the habitual adoption of collapsed postures in LBP subjects can be expected to significantly limit their ability in appreciating and finding a neutral alignment of the pelvis spine and head. Hyperkyphosis in young subjects has been associated with disturbed integration of proprioception and in sensory interaction which may result in postural instability especially in a mediolateral direction.[146] The abnormal state is perceived as normal which often makes 'exercise

therapy' difficult as the patient 'thought they were doing it right' when their performance frequently indicates otherwise. Diminished use of space can mean they 'have no idea' how to do an unfamiliar movement (Fig. 8.29).

Low back pain research has demonstrated proprioceptive deficits in the form of significantly degraded lumbosacral position sense in sitting.[147,148,149] Similar difficulties with spinal repositioning have been shown in standing and four point kneeling.[150] Lumbar fatigue further impairs ability.[148] Evidence suggests that reduced sensory feedback particularly diminishes eccentric muscle control[151] and is also reflected in difficulties with sustaining antigravity postures, motor impersistence, the ability to selectively move parts of the body, force modulation and fine tuning of movements. Movement control becomes more primitive (Ch.7). At times they appear the 'motor moron'. 'Sensation seekers' in exercise classes may be trying to redress their deficits.

The importance of head control in postural control is frequently overlooked. Sensorimotor disturbances in neck disorders can affect postural stability, head and eye movement control.[152] Previous trauma can wield insidious effects shown by subjects who had suffered QTF grade II whiplash injuries and demonstrated postural control deficits despite not complaining of symptoms, indicating that when postural control disturbances become clinically symptomatic, several subsystems involved with balance control fail.[153]

Movement quality reflects excess effort and stress/tension patterns (see Ch. 6, Part A)

While there is generally 'emptiness' in the SLMS, muscular patterns of stress, tension and 'holding' are usually apparent. These are SGMS dominant and are more active around the centre of the body, the neck jaw and shoulder area. Patients can exhibit signs of hyper-arousal, are often tense, reflexley overactive and find it difficult to 'let go' and relax.[154] Asking for an action invariably results in 'overkill' – they have lost the sense of discrete movement. When stress is a chronic event, the patient tends to posture and move with a strong underlying influence from these patterns. He tends to move in a more gross explosive way, using too much unnecessary effort and breath holding.

He wants to move quickly as he finds sustained low load from activity of the systemic deep muscles difficult to achieve. Grading and modulating the motor response is difficult as he is relying more on the superficial system whose actions are more characterized by quick, large and strong actions. Underactivity in the SLMS is probably in part due to reduced afferent input.[155–157] He does not have much experience of soft sequential pleasurable and easy movement but instead his posturomovement control ricochets between collapse and trying too hard with evident superficial muscle activity.

Dysfunctional breathing patterns (DBP) emerge
(see Ch. 6, Part A)

In essence, breathing is altered both in *where* the patient breathes and also *how* he breathes in terms of the pattern of breathing, his ability to coordinate breathing with moving and an altered rate and volume.

In a study of 38000 women, Smith et al.[158] found that disorders of continence and respiration had a stronger association with frequent back pain than obesity and physical activity. Clinically, patients with spinal pain disorders always have some form of DBP – a fact that most are surprised to hear and resistant to embrace. Breathing and movement are inextricably intertwined hence disturbed movement control will also be reflected in dysfunctional breathing. Inadequate SLMS control of axial alignment and the 'internal cylinder' means a poor 'spatial ring' to support effective function of the diaphragm. This is compounded by the adoption of consistently poor sitting postures with passive collapse of the thorax towards the pelvis. Otherwise, active holding via the CCPs serve to restrict the torso and render diaphragmatic descent and consequent basal expansion more difficult. Stiffness within the thorax itself also further hampers diaphragm activity with related reduced intercostal action. These factors all contribute to the person beginning to display various altered breathing characteristics as follows:

- Inefficient activity of the diaphragm with consequent *reduced opening and widening* of the lower pole of the thorax on inspiration[159,160] and an inability to breathe into the posterior wall of the

thorax[87], hence posterior basal expansion is poor as is the postural support from the diaphragm towards patterns of axial stabilization and control (Fig. 8.30). The thoracic spine shows little or no

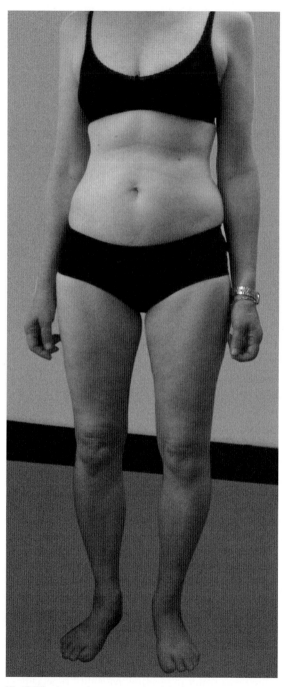

Fig 8.30 • Internal support and activity from the diaphragm is wanting.

respiratory wave.[87] In fact the breathing wave is reduced throughout the spine and pelvis.

• *Lifting of the whole thorax* on inspiration is considered by Lewit[87,160] to be a most serious finding. Imbalance between the primary and secondary accessory breathing muscles where the secondary predominate results in upper chest breathing and can result in the thorax being chronically held in the inspiratory position.[159] In those with insufficient or no activity in the abdominal muscles, the spinal column loses the support from the diaphragm.[87]

The poor breathing stereotype is thus too much lifting and too little widening of the lower pole of the thorax.

• *Habitual upper chest breathing* can be observed at rest, while the subject gasps as they talk or when asking them to inhale. The contours of the sternocleidomastoidei, upper trapezius and scalenii are variably prominent with noticeably increased activity, the upper clavicular grooves are deep and during inspiration the clavicles are lifted too[87] (Fig. 8.31). In marked cases of secondary accessory muscle dominance, the scapulae can be seen to protract from pectoral activity. While this method of breathing is a useful short term solution in states of high demand and arousal such as in 'running away from the tiger', if habitually adopted in low demand situations it comes with a high energy cost and stresses the cervical and shoulder structures. Upper chest breathing occurs both when there is insufficient abdominal activity to anchor the inferior thorax to provide stability for the diaphragm and in cases of overactivity of the abdominals which disallows proper diaphragm descent. It is common in those who have learned to hold in their abdomen through vanity or fashion[161] – as Farhi[162] suggests: 'feeling bad in order to look good'; those who are habitually stressed and anxious,[163] or who have over trained their abdominals in the misguided pursuit of 'core control'.

• Upledger[53] notes an abnormal state of hypertonus or contracture of the respiratory diaphragm may occur unilaterally or bilaterally as a result of problems with the lower four thoracic nerves and/or the phrenic nerve which collectively innervate the diaphragm. Dysfunction of the diaphragm may also occur secondary to somatic dysfunction which involves the lower six ribs, the sternum, xiphoid, the upper three lumbar vertebrae, psoas, quadratus lumborum and/or

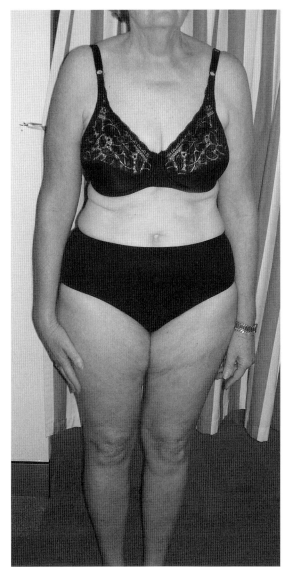

Fig 8.31 • Reduced activity in the diaphragm is associated with increased use of the accessory breathing muscles and neck tension and pain syndromes.

the fasciae related to any of the above structures. Frequently after the primary problem is cleared the diaphragm autonomously maintains and continues the asymmetrical tension patterns and abnormal hypertonus created within it interfering not only the breathing patterns but also with craniosacral system function and freedom of fascial mobility

• Respiration can be so badly coordinated that trying to 'deep breathe' can instead result in paradoxical breathing where the patient will draw in the abdomen on inspiration and push it out while breathing out.[87,160]

• During movement, an altered breathing rate is frequently adopted at different times in the following manner:

    • The patient will often initiate a movement with a *'central cinch' or breath hold* and related central fixing by the global muscles around the body's centre in association with unnecessary effort which further favors mid-upper torso global muscle activation. The abdominals are accessory muscles of expiration in high respiratory demand situations yet are often over employed in low demand situations. We have noted that attempts to control the pelvis are frequently attempted by abnormal global system activity around the body's centre. This superficial muscle overactivation creates a central 'squeeze' effect which hampers diaphragm descent and its valuable contribution in control of torso stability. Breath holding thus becomes a compensatory postural control strategy in the case of deficient SLMS control which includes the diaphragm. O'Sullivan et al.[77] nicely showed decreased diaphragmatic excursion, altered breathing patterns and pelvic floor descent during the ASLR test in subjects with sacroiliac pain. Thompson et al.[164] describe the negative effects of global abdominal bracing combined with an increase in chest wall activity and breath holding, on effective pelvic floor function.

    • Variable increase in breathing rate and volume inappropriate to the level of activity. This is associated with a shorter expiratory phase and little if no post expiratory pause. This can be observed when subjects are working out new motor patterns and particularly so when redressing movement restrictions in stiff regions or 'stretching' tight muscles. They often find it difficult to disassociate the action from the breathing – to organize the dual roles of breathing and movement in a harmonious way. It is widely held that muscular activity is facilitated during inspiration and inhibited during expiration.[87] 'Stretching' is often accompanied by short inspiratory gasps, breath holding and a general increase in muscle tension where the patient invariably works against himself –'central intelligence' and control is more often than not, fundamentally disturbed.

• The habitual upper chest breathing pattern is generally associated with *hyperventilation syndrome* (HVS) or over breathing. Chronic HVS is an insidious condition which may not be readily apparent, is more prevalent in females and deemed responsible for a plethora of medical symptoms[165] and has been estimated to affect 10% of the American population.[166] The altered breathing patterns are caused by physical, environmental, behavioral or psychological stimuli which override the automatic activity of the respiratory centers resulting in over breathing at rest[161] or where the breathing depth and rate are in excess of the metabolic needs.[165] This leads to a reduction in the arterial partial pressure of carbon dioxide known as hypocapnia. Bradley[165] states that hypocapnia reduces blood flow to the brain in the order of 2% decrease in flow per 1 mm Hg reduction in arterial CO^2, causing a multitude of symptoms including poor concentration and memory lapses, headaches, sympathetic dominance, tingling, paresthesia, weakness dizziness, tremor and confusion. Further, according to Chaitow,[167] the evidence points to breathing pattern disorders (BPD) causing a variety of negative psychological, biochemical, neurological and biomechanical influences and interferences capable of modifying neuromuscular control mechanisms and low back function in general. Chaitow[166] also includes HVS as causing an automatic increase in levels of anxiety and apprehension, affecting balance, heightened pain perception, speeding up of spinal reflexes, increased excitability of the corticospinal system, hyperirritability of motor and sensory axons, changes in serum calcium and magnesium levels and encouragement of the development of myofascial trigger points. Addressing our patient's breathing problems will clearly help right many of their ills! McLaughlin and Goldsmith[168] reported a case series of 24 patients with low back/pelvic pain who all showed lower than normal end tidal carbon dioxide levels via capnography. Breathing retraining improved CO_2 levels to normal in all but one patient, as well as improvements in pain, functional activity and breathing with decreased anxiety. Clinically, the state of chronic hypocapnia appears to create hypertonus in the diaphragm and secondary expiratory muscles – the abdominals – which can make it very difficult for the subject to reduce the inspiratory rate and volume during breathing retraining. This can be seen on the capnograph as spikes in diaphragm activity when attempting to lengthen the exhalation and expiratory pause.

Demonstrating the close link between SLMS activity, diaphragmatic breathing and postural stability, Cumpelik[169] describes a pilot study where those who were upper chest breathers took longer to restabilize their posture in response to external perturbation than those who were abdominal breathers.

'Breathing is the link between motion and emotion'.[170] It is important to recognize the potent influence of emotional stress and anxiety on the development and maintenance of DBP. However DBP further serve to increase arousal states and a vicious cycle risks being activated. If you don't breathe well, you can't move well. If you don't move well, you can't breathe well. Lewit[87] considers DBP the most disastrous of all faulty patterns and if allowed to remain, may jeopardize any treatment of the locomotor system.

Thoracic dysfunction

The thoracic spine represents somewhat of an enigma in that it comprises the largest region of the axial spine yet accounts for the smallest proportion of published studies on the spine as a whole.[171] This is probably due to the focus on pain rather than dysfunction as the principal driver of much of the research to date.

In general, thoracic musculoskeletal pain complaints are not disabling, do not significantly occasion absence from work and so are not seen as such a cost burden. Local thoracic joint dysfunction is not necessarily highly pain producing, but often seen as a relatively unimportant associated complaint ('just' tightness or stiffness) to another more flagrant presenting pain symptom. This ignores the enormous biomechanical influence of the thorax on the functional movement control of the rest of the axial spine. Clinically, posturomovement dysfunction of the thorax is always implicated in some degree to presenting spinal pain syndromes and related disorders including many of those in the upper and lower limb. Thoracic function plays a large role in healthy function of the autonomic nervous system as the sympathetic outflow extends from T1 to L2.[172] Both somatic and autonomic dysfunction are implicated in many and varied bodily symptoms possibly accounting for a significant proportion of the complaints presenting to the general medical practitioner. Generally, as a basic underlying functional problem, its role needs to be understood and addressed for effective therapeutic outcomes.

Common clinically observed features of thoracic dysfunction help provide a functional working model

Lee[173] describes rotational instability of the mid thoracic spine after trauma, however in clinical practice this is a relatively uncommon event. Generally the thorax as a whole is found to be functionally stiff and in time, becomes structurally stiff. The coexistence thoracic stiffness and chronic low back pain is clinically known.[174] An under active deep system, antigravity collapse and imbalanced overactivity of the large SGMS muscles attaching to the thorax, serve to functionally convert it to a 'distorted semi-rigid barrel'. This means that postural shifts, selective movement and segmental control *within the thorax* are reduced. These must be compensated for elsewhere in the spine and usually occur in the cervical and lumbar spine[127,171,175] which helps explain the high clinical incidence of both lumbar and cervical pain and related syndromes in the one patient. Achieving a proper neutral lumbar and cervical lordosis is difficult.

Characteristic changes are apparent and fall into certain patterns further affecting thoracic and related bio and myomechanics. They are best understood examining the thorax as a whole unit as well as regionally.

The thorax as a whole. The shape and function of the thorax is partly dependent upon the inherent myomechanics operating through it. The large axioscapular and thoracopelvic muscles have extensive rib attachments and if their function changes have the propensity to significantly alter thorax function. In particular the abdominal muscle group has a significant effect on the lower pole of the thorax as they extend as high as the 5th rib, while the anterior shoulder girdle muscles significantly affect the upper pole of the thorax as they extend down to the 7th rib with serratus going as low as the 9th (see Ch.6, Part C).

The more common features can be generally attributed to imbalanced activity between the flexor and extensor systems:

• The thorax tends to be spatially postured either forward or back relative to the pelvis and the line of gravity:

  • when more anterior, increased activity of posterior erector spinae is evident

  • when more posterior relative to the forward (sway) of the pelvis, upper abdominal activity rather than lower is more prevalent.

• An increase in the thoracic kyphosis both functional and structural (Fig. 8.32) is clinically very common and strongly influences the alignment of the rest of the spine, patterns of load bearing and segmental movement[171] and trunk muscle forces.[176] Hyperkyphosis has been associated with lowered static and dynamic postural stability.[146]

• Clinically, the patient commonly demonstrates a '*dome*'. This describes an increased local kyphosis with stiff reactive segments around T6/7/8 (Fig. 8.33). While this region represents the apex of the thoracic curve[177,178] it also the functional junction between the upper and lower poles of the thorax – the 'dorsal hinge' between regions 2 and 3 (Ch. 6, Part C). Loading studies in those with an increased kyphosis showed the peak mean flexion moment occurred at T8.[176] A significant decrease in the range of thoracic rotation has been shown in flexion compared with neutral and extended postures in pain free subjects.[179] Mid thoracic hypomobility disorders are the most common thoracic presentation, the primary movement restriction is rotation and to a lesser extent

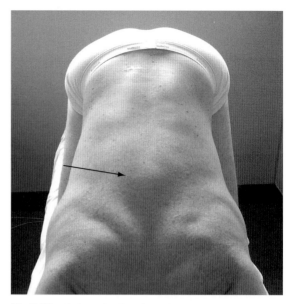

Fig 8.33 • A thoracic 'dome' is evident when doing the "Allah" stretch.

extension.[171,180] Al-Eisa et al.[181] describe an 'incidental finding' of significantly reduced range of thoracic lateral flexion and axial rotation in LBP subjects! Energy efficient walking requires a derotation between the pelvis and shoulder girdle. Normally, most segmental rotation occurs at T6/7[182]. Gracovetsky[40] and Kapandji[183] cite a normal study performed by Gregerson and Lucas in 1967 which impressively shows that this derotation occurs maximally at T7 (Fig. 8.34). The presence of a 'dome' limits this movement occurring which must then be compensated for somewhere else – usually the lumbar or cervical spine, which in function are then required to become the site of relative flexibility.[68] Addressing the dome in management is necessary in lessening CCP behavior.

A 'dome' appears to result from and be maintained by a combination of factors:

• passive axial collapse and 'hinging' between the upper and lower poles

• imbalanced activation of the myofascial fan which anchors the shoulder girdle to the thorax (Ch.6, Part C) – increased activity and shortness in the anterior chest muscles and

• related poor medial scapular and adjacent deep intersegmental muscle activity

• changed muscle activation strategies acting around the lower pole of the thorax

• altered breathing patterns (see Fig. 8.36).

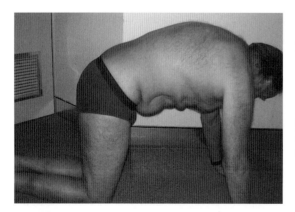

Fig 8.32 • A thoracic kyphosis effects the alignment of the rest of the spine.

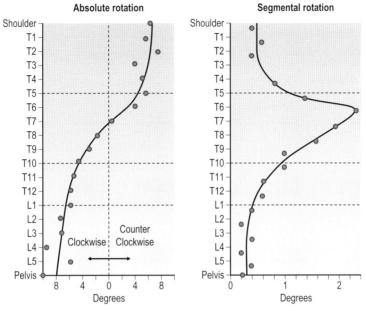

Fig 8.34 • Gregerson and Lucas [40,183] showed that maximal segmental rotation occurred around T7 when walking.

Alterations in the spatial and movement properties of each region

While regional distinctions are somewhat arbitrary, functional differences can be observed to commonly occur:

1. *The vertebromanubrial region* or 'upper ring' drops anteriorly and assumes more vertical orientation with less flexibility within it. This affects regional segmental function and posturomovement control of the head and neck and shoulder girdle.

2. *The vertebrosternal region* becomes stiffer. This appears to be a consequence of:

- sustained static postures involving axial collapse associated with
- repetitive bilateral arm use in the forward and down position primarily involves the anterior chest muscles being over activated in their shortened position. The axial attachments of these muscles are significant: pectoralis minor attaches to the 3rd – 5th rib (and frequently between ribs 2 and 4[94]); pectoralis major from the medial clavicle, sternum and ribs 2 – 6 or 7;[94] serratus anterior has

extensive costal attachments from all ribs in this region and those of the upper ring with some slips also extending down as far as rib 8 or even 10.[94] Shortening of these large shoulder girdle protractors and depressors results in the shoulder girdle hanging more down and forward with 'stretch weakness'[68] and a reduction in the activity of the lower scapular stabilizers and associated spinal intrinsics. Balance in the axioscapular force couples is disturbed. This results in related increased activity in the levator scapulae upper trapezii. Szeto et al.[184] found increased upper trapezius activity preceded the onset of neck and shoulder discomfort in keyboard operators and was also associated with increased head neck and shoulder flexion angles.[185] In a healthy population Crosbie et al.[186] found decreased upward rotation of the scapula in all planes on the dominant side. Scapulothoracic neuromyofascial imbalance also limits spinal segmental movements, costovertebral movements, and movements of the ribs independent of the scapula and spatial positioning of the shoulder girdle over the chest wall. The kyphosis increases and the sternum drops and is recessed. Movements of the upper limb into elevation, extension and retraction become reduced. Thoracic and shoulder girdle 'opening' and movement options are hampered and become the genesis of many shoulder pain syndromes including many of the increasingly prevalent so called 'rotator cuff' problems.

Together, the two regions above constitute the *upper pole of the thorax* and when stiff create local pain syndromes as well as exerting significant biomechanical influences on adjacent functionally interdependent structures. The segmental dysfunction can lead to clinical patterns such as T4 syndrome[187] contribute to headaches and symptoms emanating from autonomic irritation simulating visceral disease such as palpitations.[188] Reduced adaptive postural adjustments of the vertebrae and ribs within the upper pole directly affect load bearing and movements of the cervical spine[175] and orienting and control of the head on the neck. Cervical pain syndromes are a predictable consequence. When shoulder stiffness and pain develop this serves to further limit movements within the upper pole.

3. The *vertebrochondral region* begins to show variable deformation of its internal cavity and external shape due to the combined effects of either passive or overactive antigravity postural strategies and related changed activation patterns of the thoraco-pelvic muscles. Essentially two main patterns appear to result:

• *Passive antigravity collapse* particularly in sitting, results in an increased kyphosis around the midpoint of the curve from the 'dome' and down through this region to the thoracolumbar junction. This is associated with the anterior ribs from about the 7th, being shunted forward at around the level of the xiphoid where the strut effect of the sternum terminates. There is a recess below the breasts. Observing the lateral wall of the thorax, a 'windswept appearance' of ribs 7–10 can result where their anterior part almost resemble the 'shunters' on the front of a train (Fig. 8.35). The infra-sternal angle is often narrower and there is also a reduction in the anterior-posterior volume of the cage. Rotary and lateral movements become even more difficult. Postural collapse and overactivity or adaptive shortening of the upper abdominal muscles means that diaphragmatic descent is hampered and its postural and respiratory support is reduced. The circumference of the

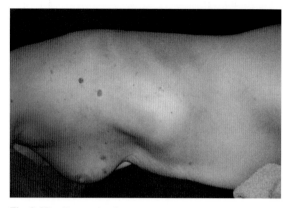

Fig 8.35 • Postural collapse and a 'dome' can lead to deformation of the thorax and anterior 'shunters' (the photo is post treatment hence the skin reaction).

lower ring of the thorax is diminished (Fig. 8.36B).

• *Overactive antigravity strategies* generally involve hyperactivity in the erector spinae and serratus posterior inferior with either related underactivity in the whole abdominal wall or overactivity.

• Abdominal underactivity particularly of upper external oblique, results in the anterior ribs in this region flaring out with a wide infra-sternal angle and more open inferior thoracic outlet or 'ring' which is more oblique and hyperstabilized posteriorly and hypostabilized anteriorly. (Figs 8.36C & 8.37)

• Abdominal overactivity combined with overactivity in the extensors acts to 'squeeze' or constrict this region including narrowing the infra-sternal angle and especially the lower thoracic aperture. The lower pole of the thorax is hyperstabilized and becomes more conical in shape. The 'body cylinder' resembles an hourglass. Diaphragmatic descent is really hampered (Figs 8.36B & 8.38)

4. *The thoracolumbar junction.* Clinically, the importance of segmental dysfunction in this region as a contributor to lumbar pain and a variety of diffuse pain syndromes [180,189,190,194] cannot be overestimated. Its functional disturbances and altered joint kinematics exert a biomechanical influence over joints in the lumbar spine while pain from here is also usually referred distally and can extend to the low back, buttocks, hip groin, and lateral thigh.[189] Segmental dysfunction in this region is particularly implicated in the really nasty and severe acute back pain presentations including

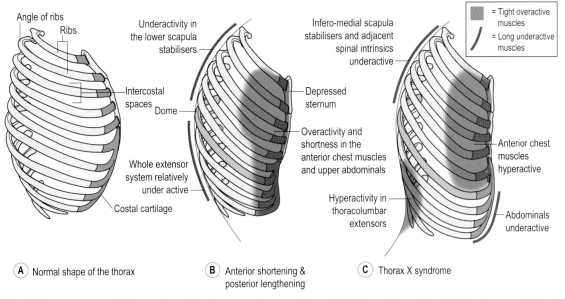

Fig 8.36 • The upper and lower poles of the thorax can become differently 'deformed' through postural collapse and altered myofascial length / tension relationships. Both scenarios explain the development of a 'dome'.

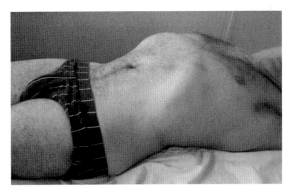

Fig 8.37 • Open lower anterior pole of the thorax.

those with a trunk list. The region is vulnerable to both compressive and torsional forces and in particular T12 as it checks and marries rotation in the thorax above with a relative lack of it below in the lumbar spine. Singer[180] and Stokes[182] describe a study by Malmivarra et al. which found particular patterns of degenerative pathologies through the region no doubt in response to the loading stresses incurred at each level: at T10/11 there was primarily anterior degeneration characterized by disc degeneration, vertebral body osteophytosis and Schmorl's nodes; the T11/12 segment showed both anterior and posterior degeneration involving the facet and costovertebral joints; while the T12/L1 level was characterized by

primarily posterior facet joint degeneration (Fig. 8.39).

Collapsed sitting postures place a lot of imbalanced compression loading on these levels. Clinically, regional erector spinae hyperactivity is usual. This probably results for two reasons. Local or regional joint dysfunction will result in 'firing up' the adjacent muscles and those which receive innervation from these segments. Secondly, the habitual strategies adopted in posturomovement control act to further hyperstabilize the region. Depending upon the proclivity for flexor or extensor system dominance, the region is functionally 'held' or hyperstabilized in more flexion or extension or 'straight-jacketed' between both. The joints become more symptomatic and a vicious self generating cycle is set in train.

Regions 3 and 4 together constitute the ***lower pole of the thorax***. While selective movement control is deficient within this region it is also subject to external deformation as it compensates for inadequate movement in the upper pole. This is appreciated when trying to move or stretch the shoulders towards their end range which invariably results in a reflex SGMS dominant 'cinch' of muscles acting around the lower pole posteriorly, anteriorly or both. This central 'cinch' also occurs in response to inadequate lumbopelvic control further splinting the thorax and serving to increase the load on lumbar segments.

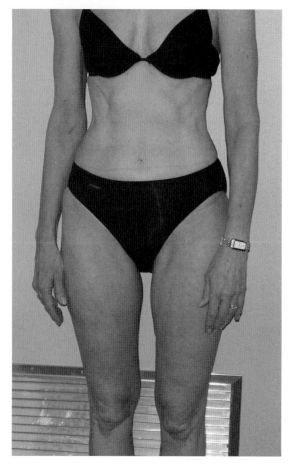

Fig 8.38 • Closed lower anterior pole of the thorax.

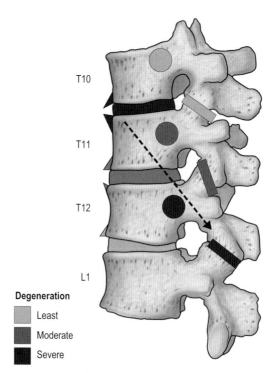

Fig 8.39 • Pattern of segmental degeneration over thoracolumbar levels. A schematic depiction of the transition (arrow) in degeneration from anterior elements at T10, to a posterior element pattern of degeneration at T12–L1. Vertebral body osteophytes and disk degeneration were more prevalent in the T10–T11 and T11–T12 levels, in contrast with costovertebral joint reactive changes which was least at T12–L1, where the zygapophysical joints acted to constrain torsion.

Disturbance in the form and function of the lower pole from an over reliance on various SGMS dominant cinching, gripping holding and fixing strategies in the mid torso compromises important functions:

• the central postural support and respiratory role of the breathing mechanism

• alignment of the body wall and 'core' central stability mechanisms including IAP

• connecting and sequencing movements between the upper and lower pole of the body cylinder including that between the limbs

• equilibrium responses and weight shift through the torso. Importantly the bilateral 'cinch' responses limit lateral bending and lateral weight shift and segmental adjustments through the region

• lower limb function is compromised because of poor adaptive support for control of the lumbopelvic complex – lumbar, hip and lower limb pain syndromes are a predictable consequence.

Largely, the movement restrictions within the thorax tend to render it a functional 'carapace' and to compensate, the patient is further obliged to employ variable increased global muscle activity around the thoracolumbar junction as he attempts to control movements of the upper torso and limb girdle; the 'thoracic barrel' on the lumbar spine; while at the same time trying to control the pelvis in space. This helps explain why treating and improving function in the thorax deloads the lumbar spine and usually contributes towards pain relief.

Biomechanical and articular changes become predictable over time

Dysfunctional posturomovement control creates predictable changes in skeletal alignment and function over time. Sagittal plane postural collapse is probably the most pernicious influence:

Change in the normal physiological spinal curves

Altered pelvic position; reduced lumbar lordosis; increased thoracic kyphosis; altered alignment of the head and neck and shoulder girdle eventually become apparent. Depending upon the stage of disorder, functional problems become structural and begin to mutually reinforce one another. Altered loading stress on the joints and soft tissues predictably lead to neural irritation and pain syndromes.

General/regional loss of extension through spine

Most of our activities are axial flexor pattern dominant and extension loss is significant in spinal pain disorders. This is particularly prevalent in the thoracic spine and while the cervical and lumbar spines are required to compensate, they too generally show reduced passive and active intersegmental movement into extension. Protocols advocated by McKenzie[191,192] partly address this aspect. Consistently adopted flexed postures can so stretch the superficial tissues that when assuming an extended position there is puckering of the tissues (Fig. 8.40). One can easily guess the joint problems!

The development of functional 'hinges' and 'blocks'

Regions of segmental stiffness can act like 'blocks', while the abnormally, relatively flexible/hyper

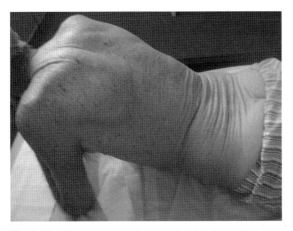

Fig 8.40 • Simple observation reveals a lot about this person's potential or actual joint problems.

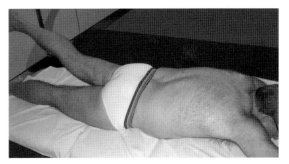

Fig 8.41 • Functionally, when the thoracic spine becomes a 'block' the lumbar spine becomes more of a 'hinge' in function.

mobile segment(s) act like 'hinges' in posture and movement (Fig. 8.41). They feed off one another. Inadequate deep system and regional control means the patient finds it difficult to get movement into the stiff regions and he can't adequately control the relatively mobile segments or regions. This creates further compensations up and down the spine. Clinically, symptomatic joints occur in both the stiff regions and the relatively over mobile regions.

This phenomenon plays out in many clinical presentations e.g. 'spinal stenosis' where segments become symptomatic because of the abnormal loading stress placed upon them over time. Frequently patients are ill advised to avoid extension and undertake passive flexion maneuvers which only serve to further bother levels which are already struggling and iatrogenic perpetuation of the problem. Gaining function, in particular extension, rotation and side bending *through the kinetic chain* - through the thorax, and hip/pelvis/lumbosacral junction and the symptomatic levels usually ameliorates symptoms despite significant radiological changes. (Fig. 8.42)

Clinically observed and found regions of stiffness

Stiffness is a general feature, however some regions are consistently found to be more hypomobile and so in function, shunt the movement responsibility to adjacent structures creating regions of compensatory relative flexibility.[68] Sahrmann also coined the term 'directional susceptibility to movement' if this compensatory movement or applied stress is in a consistent specific direction.[68] Both are exemplified in the tendency for the lumbar spine to flex early in

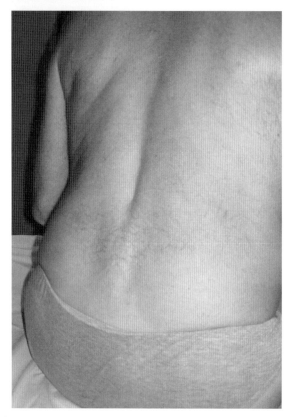

Fig 8.42 • This physician was diagnosed with spinal stenosis and told to avoid extension! He had been doing 'flexion exercises'. He could not walk the length of a ward to do his rounds. Restoring intersegmental movement into 'closing patterns' and addressing 'function around the junctions', particularly the lumbosacral, allowed him to walk 8km without pain 10 days after presentation.

movement relative to the hip and thoracic spine. Sahrmann believed that the site of compensatory movement was the site of pain. However, this author would argue than in respect to the spine while this may be so, it is certainly not necessarily so. For instance pain felt over the mid lumbar spine may emanate from T12/L1 or higher. We are never absolved from the responsibility to fully assess all structures.

Thoracic spine and rib cage

To generalize, the common findings include a variable segmental and regional reduction of mobility into extension, rotation and side bending, the presence of a 'dome' and related myofascial tightness.

The junctional regions

Ideally the line of gravity passes through each of these regions, but when spinal alignment and control changes, these transitional regions are more vulnerable and prone to develop hypomobility. Experienced practitioners note problems in these regions.[87,190] In general, there is an altered flexion/extension relationship and a significant loss of rotation and side bending through the junctions. By and large, all clinical presentations can be found have some 'defective function in the junction(s)' which produces compensations in adjacent functional segments or regions e.g. cervical and lumbar spines, shoulders etc. Sahrmann[193] reminds us to consider 'what are the sources, and what are the causes of the pain'– the 'criminals' and the 'victims'.

- *Craniocervical junction* – C0/1/2/3 – is complex biomechanically and has an important functional role in mediating postural tone throughout the body. The most common articular restrictions are reduced *flexion*/extension (0/1); rotation (1/2); side bending (2/3).
- *Cervicothoracic junction* – C7/T1/2 and ribs 1 and 2 – most commonly lose extension (widow's hump); rotation and side bending in these levels.
- *The dome* – T/6/7/8. While not strictly a junction as described, it is clinically significant with a common loss of extension, rotation and side bending.
- *Thoracolumbar junction* – T10/11/12 /L1/2 – usually hyper stabilized which can be in flexion, neutral or extension; variable loss of flexion, extension, and notable loss of rotation, lateral shift / side bending. In particular, T12 is a segment of frequent dysfunction.[189,194] Dysfunction in various of these levels can refer to the abdomen hip and pubis[195] as well as the groin, scrotum and into the leg.
- *Lumbosacral junction* – L5 and sacrum are closely linked to sacroiliac function. Clinically most lumbopelvic pain disorders are associated with some loss of extension and 'swivel' between L5/S1 with related loss of freedom in sacral nutation and torsion.

Note three of the five junctional regions relate to the thorax.

A cervical or lumbar problem will usually show local and regional neuromuscular dysfunction with attendant symptomatic joint restrictions at the superior and inferior junction, although usually one will be dominant.

Intrapelvic joints: principally sacroiliac joint

While cases of sacroiliac instability occur, these are usually related to trauma or post partum. The biomechanical effects of a stiff sacroiliac are clinically compelling. In most 'developmental' back pain syndromes, it is common to find a somewhat counternutated sacrum with reduced mobility which may/not be stuck in torsion and related contrarotation of the innominates.

The large ball and socket joints are often the criminals

The importance of the shoulder and hip joints in providing the biggest source of rotation in the body and allowing multiplanar movements in all three dimensions is generally not appreciated. However, they are always stiff in varying degrees in those with spinal pain and related disorders and require compensations which significantly impact upon posturomovement control of the torso. A pattern generating cycle appears to prevail: changed shoulder/hip function requires compensations in the spine. Over time, segmental irritation begins to occur and further affects change in the facilitation /inhibition of muscles controlling these large joints. This may not include somatic pain referral. The stiffer the hip/shoulder, the more the axial stress and so on. Habitual provocative movement strategies become further modified and so the dysfunction becomes more entrenched. The increasing amount of hip and shoulder surgery attests to the extent of the dysfunction in contemporary sedentary society.

Shoulder stiffness not only changes cervical and thoracic and kinematics but ipso facto through its affect upon the thorax also significantly impinges on proper function in the low back. Many cannot even elevate their arms above their head and attempts to do so invariably result in compensatory cervical movements and thoracolumbar cinching strategies which affect the lumbar spine (Fig. 4.5). Clinically one also finds an impressive incidence of coexisting shoulder and low back pain syndromes. When large shoulder girdle muscles such as latissimus and serratus are tight, adaptive lengthening of the lateral body wall is compromised affecting standing on one leg and reach patterns.

Rolf[196] stated 'it is impossible to overemphasize the importance of a free hip joint'. The clinical incidence of concurrent hip and spine symptoms is common and has been described as Hip-Spine Syndrome.[197] However, restriction in the hip is usually sub-clinical and painless yet exerts significant biomechanical effects upon the sacroiliac and lumbar joints because of their close functional interdependence. Commonly the hips show restriction into flexion, internal rotation and extension. The functional interrelationship between low back pain and hip dysfunction has increasing recognition.[198,199] Recurrent lateral hip pain and conditions such as trochanteric bursitis have been correlated with lumbar degenerative disease.[200] Early intraarticular hip disease may present with similar symptoms to that of posterior pelvic pain attributable to SIJ dysfunction[201] or referred from the lumbar spine. McGill[202] states 'sufficient hip and knee flexibility is imperative in sparing the spine excessive motion during tasks of daily living'. Forward bending studies have found altered patterns of flexion motion with reduced hip motion and increased lumbar motion.[203–206] Positive correlations were found between loss of hip internal rotation lumbar extension and back pain in a cohort of professional golfers.[207] Associations between reduced hip internal rotation and low back pain have been found[65,208] as have decreased passive hip extension mobility.[209,210] Subjects with unilateral sacroiliac dysfunction had significantly more external than internal rotation of the hip on the side of the posterior innominate.[65] Artificially increasing hip stiffness in normal subjects caused profound changes in the profile of trunk movements and balance control.[211]

The lower kinetic chain

The legs need both flexibility and strength in order to provide an adaptable yet stable base from which pelvic control can be executed. While there is often joint restriction in the hip and ankle, the stiffness in the lower kinetic chain is more 'neural pattern rustiness'. Generally the feet resemble dead little paddles with poor intrinsic myomechanics, stiffness of the ankle joints and imbalance in the mediolateral stirrup between peroneus longus and tibialis posterior. The common habit of standing with the legs abducted, externally rotated with hyperextended knees and hips mean the feet tend to pronate with collapse of the medial arch. There is poor grounding through the feet to provide and active base of support. This is particularly evident through the heel where reduced push from here affects the ability to direct and control movement from the ischia.

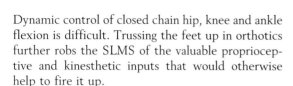

Dynamic control of closed chain hip, knee and ankle flexion is difficult. Trussing the feet up in orthotics further robs the SLMS of the valuable proprioceptive and kinesthetic inputs that would otherwise help to fire it up.

The brain

While this may appear a fatuous inclusion it *is* actually the heart of the problem and the most complex and difficult to change. Feldenkrais[212] said 'the stiffness is only in the head' – our brains are stiff to change. Posturomovement control is largely reflex and automatic with the option for voluntary control. Habitual patterns of response become ingrained and require focus, perceptual awareness application and determination to change them. Whether psychological, emotional or physical, 'old habits die hard'. Knowing what the bad habit is and its deleterious effect to ones being is the first task. However, making change is more difficult but necessary if sustained improvement is to occur: 'You can't fix the problem with the same bad habits that created it'.

Role reversal in aspects of upper and lower body function

Bartenieff[125] describes 'distinctively diverse roles' between the upper and lower body which when integrated into one unit, provide for effective movement function.

The prime role of the lower unit is weight support, groundedness through the feet and the crucial role of weight shift which centers the body at any moment and provides an anchor for the upper unit. The pelvis houses the centre of gravity in the body and is fundamentally the base of weight support.[51]

The upper unit contains our principal organs of perception and its principal role is manipulative and communicative. Nowadays, man has become absorbed with the upper unit in intellectual pursuits and in the development of skill of hand and speech;[51] the brain and the hands have become the most predominant 'workers'.[213] Work generally happens in sitting and function changes.

In people with back pain and poor movement habits, the lower unit is underactive. They show a distinct disinclination and disability in effectively controlling their pelvis for physiological support and weight shift. This includes loading the lower limb in patterns of flexion. Conversely the upper unit is overactive and the arms are used more for antigravity support, and grab to regain balance. The 'centre' has become maladaptive and the sense of power has been transferred from the base to the top of his structure. As Todd[51] says: 'to a great extent he has also lost both the fine sensory capacity of the animal and its control of power centered in the lower spinal and pelvic muscles ... the crouch muscles which should still be employed for spring or take off and for shock absorption'. This is readily apparent – even in a yoga class! It inevitably leads to an over reliance on 'pushing down' with the arms when 'coming up' from sitting or from the floor. We need to truly find and stand on our own two feet!

References

[1] O'Sullivan PB, et al. The effect of different standing and sitting postures on trunk muscle activity in a pain free population. Spine 2002;27(11):1238–44.

[2] O'Sullivan PB, et al. Evaluation of flexion relaxation phenomenon of the trunk muscles in sitting. Spine 2006;31(17):2009–16.

[3] O'Sullivan PB, et al. Effect of different upright sitting postures on spinal-pelvic curvature and trunk muscle activation in a pain free population. Spine 2006;31 (19):E707–12.

[4] Ainscough–Potts AM, Morrissey MC, Critchley D. The response of transverse abdominis and internal oblique muscles to different postures. Man Ther 2006;11:54–60.

[5] Snijders CJ, et al. Biomechanics of the interface between spine and pelvis in different postures. In: Vleeming A, et al., editors. Movement, stability and low back pain: the essential role of the pelvis. New York: Churchill Livingstone; 1997. p. 103–13.

[6] Dolan P, Adams MA, Mutton WC. Commonly adopted postures and their effect on the lumbar spine. Spine 1988;13(2):197–201.

[7] Callaghan JP, Dunk NM. Examination of flexion relaxation phenomenon in erector spinae during short duration slump sitting. Clin Biomech 2002;17 (5):353–60.

[8] O'Sullivan P, et al. Trunk kinematics and EMG during static and dynamic sitting. In: Proc. 5th Interdisciplinary World Congress on Low Back and Pelvic Pain. Melbourne; 2004.

[9] Gallagher S, et al. Torso flexion loads and the fatigue failure of human lumbosacral motion segments. Spine 2005;30 (20):2265–73.

[10] Solomonow M, et al. Volvo award winner in biomechanical studies: Biomechanics of increased exposure to lumbar injury caused by cyclic loading: Part 1. Loss of reflexive muscular stabilisation. Spine 1999;24(23):2426.

[11] Williams M, et al. Multifidus spasms elicited by prolonged lumbar flexion. Spine 2000;25 (22):2916–24.

[12] Jackson M, et al. Multifidus EMG and tension-relaxation recovery after prolonged static lumbar flexion. Spine 2001;26 (7):715–23.

[13] Solomonow M, et al. Biomechanics and Electromyography of a common idiopathic low back disorder. Spine 2003;28(12):1235–48.

[14] Solomonow M, et al. Muscular dysfunction elicited by creep of lumbar viscoelastic tissue. J Electromyogr Kinesiol 2003;13 (4):381–96.

[15] Dankaerts W, et al. Altered patterns of superficial trunk muscle activation during sitting in nonspecific chronic low back pain patients. Spine 2006;31 (17):2017–23.

[16] O'Sullivan P, et al. Effect of different upright sitting postures on trunk muscles activity in a pain free population. In: Proc. 6th Interdisciplinary World Congress on Low Back and Pelvic Pain. Barcelona; 2007.

[17] Sbriccoli P, et al. Static load repetition is a risk factor in the development of lumbar cumulative musculoskeletal disorder. Spine 2004;29 (23):2643–53.

[18] O'Sullivan PB, et al. The relationship between posture and back muscle endurance in industrial workers with flexion-related back pain. Man Ther 2006;11:264–71.

[19] Pearcy MJ. Twisting mobility of the human back in flexed postures. Spine 1993;18 (1):114–9.

[20] Edmondston SJ, et al. Postural neck pain: an investigation of habitual sitting posture, perception of 'good' posture and cervicothoracic kinaesthesia. Man Ther 2007;12(4):363–71.

[21] Janda V. Sydney: Course notes; 1995.

[22] Snijders CJ, et al. EMG recordings of abdominal and back muscles in various standing postures: validation of a biomechanical model on sacroiliac stability. J Electromyogr Kinesiol 1998;8(4):205–14.

[23] Dankaerts W, et al. Differences in sitting postures are associated with nonspecific chronic low back pain disorders when patients are subclassified. Spine 2006;31 (6):698–704.

[24] Roussouly, et al. Sagittal alignment of the spine and pelvis in the prescence of L5-S1 isthmic lysis and low grade spondylolisthesis. Spine 2006;31 (21):2484–90.

[25] Reeves NP, et al. The effects of trunk stiffness on postural control during unstable seated balance. Exp Brain Res 2006;174:694–700.

[26] Harrison DE, et al. How do anterior/posterior translations of the thoracic cage affect the sagittal lumbar spine, pelvic tilt, and thoracic kyphosis? Eur Spine J 2002;11:287–93.

[27] Mok N, Hodges PW, Brauer S. Different range and temporal pattern of lumbopelvic motion accompanies rapid upper limb flexion in people with low back pain. In: Proc. 5th Interdisciplinary World Congress on Low Back and Pelvic Pain. Melbourne; 2004.

[28] Smith MD, Coppieters MW, Hodges PW. Effect of experimentally induced low back pain on postural sway with breathing. In: Proc. 5th Interdisciplinary World Congress on Low Back and Pelvic Pain. Melbourne; 2004.

[29] Gregory DE, Callaghan JP. Prolonged standing as a precursor for the development of low back discomfort: An investigation of possible mechanisms. Gait Posture 2008;28(1):86–92.

[30] Gregory DE, Brown SHM. Callaghan. Trunk muscle responses to suddenly applied loads: Do individuals who develop discomfort during prolonged standing respond differently. J Electromyogr Kinesiol 2008;18 (3):495–502.

[31] Al-Eisa E, et al. Effects of pelvic asymmetry and low back pain on trunk kinematics during sitting: a comparison with standing. Spine 2006;31(5):E135–43.

[32] Lee D. The Pelvic Girdle. 3rd ed. Edinburgh: Churchill Livingstone; 2004.

[33] Sapsford R. Rehabilitation of pelvic floor muscles utilising trunk stabilisation. Man Ther 2004;9:3–12.

[34] Hodges PW. Low back Pain and the Pelvic Floor. In: Carrière B, Markel Feldt C, editors. The Pelvic Floor. Stuttgart: Thieme; 2006.

[35] Schleip R. The structural typology of Hans Flury. Sourced: http://www.somatics.de/Flury. html

[36] Brumagne S, et al. Altered postural control in anticipation of postural instability in persons with recurrent low back pain. Gait Posture 2008;28(4):657–62.

[37] Brumagne S, Cordo P, Verschueren S. Proprioceptive weighting changes in persons with low back pain and elderly persons. Neurosci Lett 2004;366:63–6.

[38] Nies N, Sinnott PL. Variations in balance and body sway in middle-aged adults: subjects with healthy backs compared with low back dysfunction. Spine 1991;16:325–30.

[39] Mientjes MIV, Frank JS. Balance in chronic low back pain patients compared to healthy people under various conditions of upright standing. Clin Biomech 1999;14(10):710–6.

[40] Gracovetsky SA. Linking the spinal engine with the legs: a theory of human gait. In: Vleeming A, et al., editors. Movement, stability and low back pain. New York: Churchill Livingstone; 1997.

[41] McKenzie RA. The lumbar spine: mechanical diagnosis and therapy. New Zealand: Waikanae Spinal Publications; 1981.

[42] Adams M, et al. The biomechanics of back pain. 2nd ed. Edinburgh: Churchill Livingstone; 2006.

[43] McGill SM. The functional anatomy of stability – What are the critical components? In: Proc. 5th Interdisciplinary Congress on Low Back and Pelvic Pain. Melbourne; 2004.

[44] Cholewicki J, Panjabi MM, Khachatryan A. Stabilising function of trunk flexor-extensor muscles around a neutral spine posture. Spine 1997;22 (19):2207–12.

[45] Bogduk N, Pearcy M, Hadfield G. Anatomy and biomechanics of psoas major. Clin Biomech 1992;7:109–19.

[46] Nachemson A. The possible importance of the psoas muscle for stabilisation of the lumbar spine. Acta Orthop Scand 1968;39:47–57.

[47] Andersson E, et al. The role of psoas and iliacus muscles for stability and movement of the lumbar spine pelvis and hip. Scand J Med Sci Sports 1995;5:10–6.

[48] Hadjipavlou AG, Farfan HF, Simmons JW. The functioning spine. In: Farfan HF, Simmons JW, Hadjipavlou AG, editors. The sciatic syndrome Slack. Thorofare.

[49] Penning L. Psoas muscle and lumbar spine stability: a concept uniting existing controversies. Critical review and hypothesis. Eur Spine J 2000;9:577–85.

[50] McGill SM. Low back disorders: Evidence based prevention and rehabilitation. USA: Human Kinetics; 2002.

[51] Todd ME. The thinking body. NJ: Princeton Book Company; 1937.

[52] Grieve GP. Common Vertebral Joint Problems. Edinburgh: Churchill Livingstone; 1981.

[53] Upledger JE, Vredevoogd JD. Craniosacral Therapy. Seattle: Eastland Press; 1983.

[54] Hanna T. Somatics: reawakening the mind's control of movement, flexibility and health. Cambridge MA: Da Capo Press; 1988.

[55] Stuge B, et al. Abdominal and pelvic floor muscle function in women with and without long lasting pelvic girdle pain. Man Ther 2006;11:287–96.

[56] O'Sullivan PB, Beales DJ. Diagnosis and classification of pelvic girdle pain disorders – Part 1. A mechanism based approach within a biopsychosocial framework. Man Ther 2007;12:86–97.

[57] Hodges P. In: MPA Workshop: Australian Physiotherapy Association National Conference Week. Cairns; November 2007; November 2007.

[58] O'Sullivan PB. Lumbar segmental 'instability': clinical presentation and specific stabilising exercise management. Man Ther 2000;5 (1):2–12.

[59] Dankaerts W, et al. Altered patterns of superficial trunk muscle activation during sitting in non specific low back pain patients. Spine 2006;31 (17):2017–23.

[60] Bond M. The New Rules of Posture: how to sit, stand and move in the modern world. Rochester: Healing Arts Press; 2007.

[61] Snijders CJ, et al. Effects of slouching and muscle contraction on the strain of the iliolumbar ligament. Man Ther 2008;13 (4):325–33.

[62] Roussel N, et al. Altered motor control patterns of the lumbopelvic region are able to predict musculoskeletal symptoms and injuries in dancers. In: Proc. 6th Interdisciplinary World Congress on Low Back and Pelvic Pain. Barcelona; 2007.

[63] Vingård E, et al. To what extent do current and past physical and psychosocial occupational factors explain care-seeking for low back pain in a working population?: results from the Musculoskeletal Intervention Centre-Norrtälje Study. Spine 2000;25 (4):493–500.

[64] Sullivan MK, Dejulia JJ, Worrell TW. Effect of pelvic position and stretching method on hamstring muscle flexibility. Medicine & Science in Sports and Exercise 1992;24 (12):1383–9.

[65] Cibulka MT, et al. Unilateral hip rotation range of motion asymmetry in patients with sacroiliac joint regional pain. Spine 1998;23(9):1009–15.

[66] Mens J, et al. A new view on adduction-related groin pain. Clin J Sport Med 2006;16:15–9.

[67] Mens JMA. Groin pain in the athlete: a new perspective. In: Proc. 6th Interdisciplinary World Congress on Low Back and Pelvic Pain. Barcelona; 2007.

[68] Sahrmann SA. Diagnosis and treatment of movement impairment syndromes. Mosby; 2002.

[69] Willson JD, Binder-Macleod S, Davis IS. Lower extremity jumping mechanics of female athletes with and without patellofemoral pain before and after exertion. Am J Sports Med 2008; April 30.

[70] Vleeming A, et al. The role of the sacroiliac joints in coupling between spine, pelvis legs and arms. In: Vleeming A, et al., editors. Movement, stability & low back pain: The essential role of the pelvis. New York: Churchill Livingstone; 1997.

[71] Vleeming A, Stoeckart R. The role of the pelvic girdle in coupling the spine and the legs: a clinical anatomical perspective on pelvic stability. In: Vleeming A, Mooney V, Stoeckart, editors. Movement Stability & Lumbopelvic Pain: Integration of research and therapy. Edinburgh: Churchill Livingstone; 2007.

[72] Van Wingerden JP, et al. Stabilisation of the sacroiliac joint in vivo: verification of muscular contribution to force closure of the pelvis. Eur Spine J 2004;13:199–205.

[73] Hodges PW. Feedforward contraction of transversus abdominis is not influenced by the direction of arm movement. Exp Brain Res 1997;114:362–70.

[74] Hodges PW, Richardson CA. Contraction of the abdominal muscles associated with movement of the lower limb. Phys Ther 1997;77:132–44.

[75] Hodges PW, Kaigle A, Holm S, et al. Intervertebral stiffness of the spine is increased by evoked contraction of transverse abdominis and the diaphragm;

in vivo porcine studies. Spine 1998;23:2594–601.

[76] Richardson CA, et al. The relationship between the transversus abdominus muscle, sacroiliac joint mechanics and LBP. Spine 2002;27(4):399–405.

[77] O'Sullivan PB, et al. Altered motor control strategies in subjects with sacroiliac pain during active straight leg raise test. Spine 2002;27(1):E1–8.

[78] Mens JM, et al. The active straight leg raise test and mobility of the pelvic joints. Eur Spine J 1999;8:468–73.

[79] Snijders C, Vleeming A, Stoeckart R. Transfer of lumbosacral load to iliac bones and legs. Pt. 1: Biomechanics of self bracing and its significance for treatment and exercise. Clin Biomech 1993;8:285–94.

[80] Don Tigny RL. A detailed and critical biomechanical analysis of the sacroiliac joints and relevant kinesiology: the implications for lumbopelvic function and dysfunction. In: Vleeming A, Mooney V, Stoeckart R, editors. Movement, Stability and lumbopelvic pain: Integration of research and therapy. Edinburgh: Churchill Livingstone Elsevier; 2007.

[81] Laslett M, et al. Diagnosis of sacroiliac joint pain: validity of individual provocation tests and composites of tests. Man Ther 2005;10(3):207–18.

[82] Pool-Goudzwaard AL, et al. Insufficient lumbopelvic stability: a clinical, anatomical and biomechanical approach to 'a-specific' low back pain. Man Ther 1998;3(1):12–20.

[83] Lee D. The Pelvic Girdle: an approach to the examination and treatment of the lumbo-pelvic-hip region. 2nd ed. Edinburgh: Churchill Livingstone; 1999.

[84] Hungerford B, Gilleard W, Hodges PW. Evidence of altered lumbopelvic muscle recruitment in the prescence of sacroiliac joint pain. Spine 2003;28 (14):1593–600.

[85] Stuge B, et al. Abdominal and pelvic floor muscle function in women with and without long

lasting pelvic girdle pain. Man Ther 2006;11:287–96.

[86] de Groot M, et al. The active straight leg raising test (ASLR) in pregnant women: differences in muscle activity and force between patients and healthy subjects. Man Ther 2008;13:68–74.

[87] Lewit K. Rehabilitation of the Motor System. London: Butterworths; 1987.

[88] Grieve GP. The sacroiliac joint. Physiotherapy 1976;62 (12):384–401.

[89] Mens JM, et al. Understanding peripartum pelvic pain: implications of a patient survey. Spine 1996;21(11):1363–9.

[90] Gracovetsky S. Stability or controlled instability. In: Vleeming A, Mooney V, Stoeckart, editors. Movement Stability & Lumbopelvic Pain: Integration of research and therapy. Edinburgh: Churchill Livingstone; 2007.

[91] Bradshaw CJ, Bundy M, Falvey E. The diagnosis of longstanding groin pain – a prospective clinical cohort study. Br J Sports Med 2008; Apr 1.

[92] O'Sullivan PB, Beales DJ. Diagnosis and classification of pelvic girdle pain disorders, Part 2: Illustration of the utility of a classification system via case studies. Man Ther 2007;12(2): e1–12.

[93] Smith MD, Russell A, Hodges PW. Incontinence, breathing disorders and back pain: an inseparable triad? In: Proc. 6th Interdisciplinary World Congress on Low Back and Pelvic Pain. Barcelona; 2007. p. 69.

[94] Williams PL, Warwick R. Grays Anatomy. 36th ed. Edinburgh: Churchill Livingstone; 1980.

[95] Sapsford R. The pelvic floor: a clinical model for function and rehabilitation. Physiotherapy 2001;87(12):620–30.

[96] Spitznagle TM. Musculoskeletal chronic pelvic pain. In: Carrière B, Markel Feldt C, editors. The Pelvic Floor. Stuttgart: Thieme; 2006.

[97] Grewer H, McLean L. The integrated continence system: a manual therapy approach to the treatment of stress urinary

incontinence. Man Ther 2008;13 (5):375–86.

[98] Sapsford RR, Hodges PW. Contraction of the pelvic floor muscles during abdominal maneuvers. Arch Phys Med Rehab 2001;82(8):1081–8.

[99] Lee D, Lee L-J. Stress urinary incontinence – a consequence of failed load transfer through the pelvis. In: Proc. 5th Interdisciplinary World Congress on Low Back and Pelvic Pain. Melbourne; 2004.

[100] Sapsford RR, Richardson CA, Stanton WR. Sitting posture affects pelvic floor muscle activity in parous women: an observational study. Aust J Physiother 2006;52:219–22.

[101] Carrière B. Interdependence of Posture and the pelvic floor. In: Carrière B, Markel Feldt C, editors. The Pelvic Floor. Stuttgart: Thieme; 2006.

[102] Chaitow L. Chronic pelvic pain: pelvic floor problems, sacroiliac dysfunction and the trigger point connection. J Bodywork & Movement Therapies 2007;11 (4):327–39.

[103] Hodges PW. Women's Health Workshop Australian Physiotherapy Association National Conference Week. Cairns; November 2007.

[104] Thompson J, O'Sullivan P, et al. Motor control strategies for activation of the pelvic floor. In: 5th Interdisciplinary World Congress on Low Back and Pelvic Pain. Melbourne; 2004.

[105] Rock C_M. Reflex incontinence cause by underlying functional disorders. In: Carrière B, Markel Feldt C, editors. The Pelvic Floor. Stuttgart: Thieme; 2006.

[106] Lewit K. Palpation of the pelvic floor. In: Liebenson C, editor. Companion DVD for Rehabilitation of the spine: A practitioner's manual. Philadelphia: Lippincott Williams and Wilkins; 2007.

[107] Fritsch H. Anatomy and physiology of the pelvic floor. In: Carrière B, Markel Feldt C, editors. The Pelvic Floor. Stuttgart: Thieme; 2006.

[108] Bendová P, et al. MRI-based registration of pelvic alignment

affected by altered pelvic floor muscle characteristics. Clin Biomech 2007;22(9):980–7.

[109] Richardson C, Hodges P, Hides J. Therapeutic exercise for lumbopelvic stabilisation: A motor control approach for the treatment and prevention of low back pain. 2nd ed. Edinburgh: Churchill Livingstone; 2004.

[110] Janda V. Muscles and motor control in low back pain: assessment and management. In: Twomey LT, editor. Physical Therapy of the Low Back. New York: Churchill Livingstone; 1987. p. 253–78.

[111] Janda V, Frank C, Liebenson C. Evaluation of Muscular Imbalance. In: Liebenson C, editor. Rehabilitation of the Spine: A Practitioner's Manual. 2nd ed. Philadelphia: Lippincott Williams and Wilkins; 2007.

[112] Janda V. Muscles as a pathogenic factor in back pain. In: Proc. I.F.O.M.T New Zealand; 1980.

[113] O'Sullivan P. Motor control and pain disorders of the lumbo-pelvic region. In: Proc. 5th Interdisciplinary World Congress on Low Back and Pelvic Pain. Melbourne; 2004.

[114] O'Sullivan P. Diagnosis and classification of chronic low back pain disorders: Maladaptive movement and motor control impairments as underlying mechanism. Man Ther 2005;10:242–55.

[115] O'Sullivan P. Classification of lumbopelvic pain disorders Why is it essential for management. Man Ther 2006;11:169–70.

[116] Dieën Van, Selen LPJ, Cholewicki J. Trunk muscle activation in low-back pain patients, an analysis of the literature. J Electromyogr Kinesiol 2003;13:333–51.

[117] Hides JA, Richardson CA, Jull GA. Multifidus muscle recovery is not automatic following resolution of acute first episode low back pain. Spine 1996;21:2763–9.

[118] Liebenson C. Core training: the importance of the diaphragm.

Dynamic Chiropractic 2007;13 (25):30–3.

[119] Steindler A. Kinesiology of the Human Body under Normal and Pathological Conditions. Springfield Illinois: Charles C Thomas; 1955.

[120] Sahrmann SA. Diagnosis and treatment of Movement Impairment Syndromes. St. Louis: Mosby; 2002.

[121] Janda V. Introduction to functional pathology of the motor system. In: Proc. Vol. 3. V11 Commonwealth and International Conference on Sport, Physical Education, Recreation and Dance; 1982.

[122] McGill S. Ultimate Back Fitness and Performance. Ontario: Wabuno Publishers; 2004.

[123] Veneman JF, et al. Fixating the pelvis in the horizontal plane affects gait characteristics. Gait Posture 2008;28 (1):157–63.

[124] Van Dillen LR, et al. Trunk rotation-related impairments in people with low back pain who participate in rotational sports activities. In: Proc. 5th Interdisciplinary World Congress on Low Back and Pelvic Pain. Melbourne; 2004.

[125] Bartenieff I, Lewis D. Body Movement: Coping with the environment. Australia: Gordon and Breach Science Publishers; 2002.

[126] White AA, Panjabi MM. Clinical biomechanics of the spine. Philadelphia: J. B. Lippincott Company; 1990.

[127] Lee LJ. Is it time for a closer look at the thorax? In Touch 2008;1:13–6 Musculoskeletal Physiotherapy Australia.

[128] Farfan H. Normal Function and Biomechanics of the lumbar spine. Source unknown p. 127–34. Copy available on request.

[129] Farfan HF. The biomechanical advantage of lordosis and hip extension for upright activity. Spine 1978;3(4):336–42.

[130] Keefe FJ, Hill RW. An objective approach to quantifying pain behavior and gait patterns in low back pain patients. Pain 1985;21 (2):153–61.

[131] Lamoth CJ, et al. Effects of chronic low back pain on trunk co-ordination and back muscle activity during walking: changes in motor control. Eur Spine J 2006;15(1):23–40.

[132] Lamoth CJ, et al. How do persons with chronic low back pain speed up and slow down? Trunk pelvis co-ordination and lumbar erector spinae activity during gait. Gait Posture 2006;23(2):230–9.

[133] Lamoth CJ, et al. Pelvis-thorax co-ordination in the transverse plane during walking in persons with non-specific low back pain. Spine 2002;27(4):E92–9.

[134] Selles RW, et al. Disorders in trunk rotation during walking in patients with low back pain: a dynamical systems approach. Clin Biomech 2001;16 (3):175–81.

[135] Vogt L, et al. Influences of non specific low back pain on three dimensional lumbar spine kinematics in locomotion. Spine 2001;26(17):1910–9.

[136] Gracovetsky S. The Spinal Engine. Austria: Springer-Verlag/ Wien; 1988.

[137] Beach P. The contractile field: A new model of human movement. J Bodywork and Movement Therapies 2007;11 (4):308–17.

[138] Byl NN, Sinnott P. Variations in balance and body sway in middle aged adults: subjects with healthy backs compared with low back dysfunction. Spine 1991;16(3):325–30.

[139] Della Volpe R, et al. Changes in coordination of postural control during dynamic stance in chronic low back pain patients. Gait Posture 2006;24 (3):349–55.

[140] Hamaoui MC. Poupard l, Bouisset S. Does respiration perturb body balance more in chronic low back pain subjects. Clin Biomech 2002;17 (7):548–50.

[141] Grimstone SK, Hodges PW. Impaired postural compensation for respiration in people with recurrent low back pain. Exp Brain Res 2003;151:218–24.

[142] Mok NW, Brauer SG, Hodges PW. Hip strategy for balance control in quiet standing is reduced in people with low back pain. Spine 2004;29(6): E107–12.

[143] Luoto S, Taimela S, et al. Psychomotor speed and postural control in chronic low back pain patients: A controlled follow-up study. Spine 1996;21 (22):2621–7.

[144] Luoto S, Heikki A, et al. One-footed and externally disturbed two-footed postural control in patients with chronic low back pain and healthy control subjects: a controlled study with follow-up. Spine 1998;23 (19):2081–9.

[145] Dolan K, Green A. Lumbar reposition sense: the effect of slouched posture. Man Ther 2006;11:202–7.

[146] Khalkhali Z, et al. Quantification of the effects of postural hyper-kyphosis on postural stability and spinal proprioception. In: Proc. 6th Interdisciplinary World Congress on Low Back and Pelvic Pain. Barcelona; 2007.

[147] Brumagne S, et al. The role of the paraspinal muscle spindles in lumbosacral position sense in individuals with and without low back pain. Spine 2000;25 (8):989–94.

[148] Taimela S, Kankaanpää M, Luoto S. The effect of lumbar fatigue on the ability to sense a changer in lumbar position. Spine 1999;24(13):1322.

[149] O'Sullivan PB, et al. Lumbar repositioning deficit in a specific low back pain population. Spine 2003;28(10):1074–9.

[150] Gill KP, Callaghan MJ. The measurement of lumbar proprioception in individuals with and without low back pain. Spine 1998;23(3):371–7.

[151] Enoka RM. Neuromechanics of Human Movement. 3rd ed. USA: Human Kinetics; 2002.

[152] Treleaven J. Sensorimotor disturbances in neck disorders affecting postural stability, head and eye movement control. Man Ther 2008;13(1):2–11.

[153] Dehner C, et al. Postural control deficit in acute QTF grade II whiplash injuries. Gait Posture 2008;28(1):113–9.

[154] Hannon JC. Wartenberg Part 3: Relaxation training, centration and skeletal opposition: a conceptual model. J Bodywork and Movement Therapies 2006;10:179–96.

[155] Belavey D, et al. Long term over activity in the oblique muscles after 8 weeks of bed rest – implications for inactivity, lumbar spine stability and sedentary lifestyle. In: Proc. 14th Biennial Conference Brisbane: MPA; 2005.

[156] Belavey DL, et al. Superficial lumbopelvic muscle overactivity and decreased cocontraction after eight weeks of bed rest. Spine 2007;32(1):E23–9.

[157] Comerford M, Mottram S. Movement and stability dysfunction – contemporary developments. Man Ther 2001;6(1):15–26.

[158] Smith MD, Russell A, Hodges PW. Disorders of breathing and continence have a stronger association with back pain than obesity and physical activity. Aust J Physiother 2006;52(1):11–6.

[159] Kolar P. Dynamic neuromuscular stabilisation: According to Kolar – an introduction. Course presented by Safarova M. Sydney; 2008.

[160] Lewit K. Managing common syndromes and finding the key link. In: Liebenson C, editor. Rehabilitation of the Spine: A Practitioner's Manual. 2nd ed. Philadelphia: Lippincott Williams and Wilkins; 2007.

[161] Clifton-Smith T. Breathe to Succeed. New Zealand: Penguin; 1999.

[162] Farhi D. The Breathing Book. New York: Henry Holt and Company; 1996.

[163] Hanna T. Somatics. Cambridge MA: Da Capo; 1988.

[164] Thompson J, O'Sullivan PB, et al. Motor control strategies for activation of the pelvic floor. In: Proc. 5th Interdisciplinary World Congress on Low Back

and Pelvic Pain. Melbourne; 2004.

[165] Bradley D. Patterns of breathing dysfunction in hyperventilation syndrome and breathing pattern disorders. In: Chaitow L, Bradley D, Gilbert C, editors. Multidisciplinary approaches to breathing pattern disorders. Edinburgh: Churchill Livingstone; 2002.

[166] Chaitow L. Breathing Pattern Disorders (BPD), motor control, and low back pain. In: Proc. 5th Interdisciplinary World Congress on Low Back and Pelvic Pain. Melbourne; 2004.

[167] Chaitow L. Breathing pattern disorders, motor control and low back pain. J Osteopathic Medicine 2004;7(1):33–40.

[168] McLaughlin L, Goldsmith CH. Altered respiration in a case series of low back/pelvic pain patients. In: Proc. 6th Interdisciplinary World Congress on Low Back and Pelvic Pain. Barcelona; 2007.

[169] Cumpelik J, Véle F. Yoga-based training for spinal stability. In: Liebenson C, editor. Rehabilitation of the Spine: A Practitioner's Manual. 2nd ed. Philadelphia: Lippincott Williams and Wilkins; 2007.

[170] Wildman F. The brain as the core of strength and stability. Sydney: Feldenkrais workshop; 2003.

[171] Singer KP, Edmondston SJ. Introduction: the enigma of the thoracic spine. In: Giles LGF, Singer KP, editors. The clinical anatomy and management of back pain series; Volume 2: Clinical anatomy and management of thoracic spine pain. Oxford: Butterworth Heinemann; 2000.

[172] Bogduk N, Twomey LT. Clinical anatomy of the lumbar spine. Melbourne: Churchill Livingstone; 1987.

[173] Lee DG. Rotational instability of the midthoracic spine: assessment and management. In: Beeton KS, editor. Manual Therapy Masterclasses: The vertebral column. Edinburgh: Churchill Livingstone; 2003.

[174] McConnell J. Recalcitrant chronic low back and leg pain – a new theory and different approach to management. In: Beeton KS, editor. Manual Therapy Masterclasses: The vertebral column. Edinburgh: Churchill Livingstone; 2003.

[175] Edmondston SJ, Singer KP. Thoracic spine: anatomical and biomechanical considerations for manual therapy. Man Ther 1997;2(3):132–43.

[176] Briggs AM, van Dieën JH, et al. Thoracic kyphosis affects spinal loads and trunk muscle force. Phys Ther 2007;87(5):595–607.

[177] Singer KP, Goh S. Anatomy of the thoracic spine. In: Giles LGF, Singer KP, editors. The clinical anatomy and management of back pain series; Volume 2: Clinical anatomy and management of thoracic spine pain. Oxford: Butterworth Heinemann; 2000.

[178] Boyle JW, Milne N, Singer KP. Influence of age on cervicothoracic spinal curvature: An ex vivo radiographic study. Clin Biomech 2002;17 (5):361–7.

[179] Edmondston S, et al. The influence of posture on range of axial rotation and coupled lateral flexion of the thoracic spine. J Manipulative Physiol Ther 2007;30(3):193–9.

[180] Singer K. Pathology of the thoracic spine. In: Giles LGF, Singer KP, editors. The clinical anatomy and management of back pain series; Volume 2: Clinical anatomy and management of thoracic spine pain. Oxford: Butterworth Heinemann; 2000.

[181] Al-Eisa E, et al. Effects of pelvic skeletal asymmetry on trunk movement: three dimensional analysis in healthy individuals versus patients with mechanical low back pain. Spine 2006; 31(3):E71–9.

[182] Stokes IAF. Biomechanics of the thoracic spine and rib cage. In: Giles LGF, Singer KP, editors. The clinical anatomy and management of back pain series; Volume 2: Clinical anatomy and management of thoracic spine pain. Oxford: Butterworth Heinemann; 2000.

[183] Kapandji IA. The physiology of the joints. Vol. 3 The trunk and vertebral column. New York: Churchill Livingstone; 1974.

[184] Szeto GPY, Straker LM, O'Sullivan PBA. Comparison of symptomatic and asymptomatic office workers performing monotonous keyboard work – 1. Neck and shoulder muscle recruitment patterns. Man Ther 2005;10(4):270–80.

[185] Szeto GPY, Straker LM, O'Sullivan PB. A comparison of symptomatic and asymptomatic office workers performing monotonous key board work – 2. Neck and shoulder kinematics.

[186] Crosbie J, et al. Scapulohumeral rhythm and associated spinal motion. Clin Biomech 2008;23 (2):184–92.

[187] Conroy JL, Schneiders AG. The t4 syndrome. Man Ther 2005;10 (4):292–6.

[188] Grieve GP. The autonomic nervous system in vertebral pain syndromes. In: Grieve GP, editor. Modern Manual Therapy of the Vertebral Column. Edinburgh: Churchill Livingstone; 1986.

[189] Maigne J-Y. Cervicothoracic and thoracolumbar spinal pain syndromes. In: Giles LGF, Singer KP, editors. The clinical anatomy and management of back pain series; Volume 2: Clinical anatomy and management of thoracic spine pain. Oxford: Butterworth Heinemann; 2000.

[190] Bourdillon JF, Day EA. Spinal Manipulation. 4th ed. Oxford: Heinemann Medical Books; 1987.

[191] McKenzie RA. The lumbar spine: Mechanical diagnosis and therapy. New Zealand: Spinal Publications; 1989.

[192] McKenzie RA. The cervical and thoracic spine: Mechanical diagnosis and therapy. New Zealand: Spinal Publications; 1998.

[193] Sahrmann S. Effects on muscle of repeated movements and sustained postures. In: Proc. 1st International Conference on Movement Dysfunction. Edinburgh; 2001.

[194] Greenman PE. Principles of manual medicine. 2nd ed. Baltimore: Williams and Wilkins; 1996.

[195] Jiménez L, et al. High origin of lumbopelvic pain. In: Proc. 6th Interdisciplinary World Congress on Low Back and Pelvic Pain. Barcelona; 2007.

[196] Rolf IP. Rolfing: The integration of human structures. New York: Harper and Row; 1977.

[197] Offierski CM, McNab IMB. Hip-spine syndrome. Spine 1983;8(3):316–21.

[198] Liebenson C. Hip dysfunction and back pain. J of Bodywork and Movement Therapies 2007;11(2):111–5.

[199] Sims K. The hip is back. Musculoskeletal Physiotherapy Australia Intouch magazine 2007;4:8–9.

[200] Wong L, et al. Is recurrent trochanteric bursitis due to lumbar degenerative disease?. In: Proc. 6th Interdisciplinary World Congress on Low Back and Pelvic Pain. Barcelona; 2007.

[201] Prather H, et al. The association of posterior pelvic pain with early intra-articular hip disease. In: Proc. 6th Interdisciplinary World Congress on Low Back and Pelvic Pain. Barcelona; 2007.

[202] McGill SM. Low back exercises: evidence for improving exercise regimens. Phys Ther 1998;78 (7):754–65.

[203] Esola M, et al. Analysis of lumbar spine and hip motion during forward bending in subjects with and without a history of low back pain. Spine 1996;21(1):71–8.

[204] Porter JL, Wilkinson A. Lumbar-hip flexion-motion: a comparative study between asymptomatic and chronic low back pain in 18-to-36 year old men. Spine 1997;22 (13):1508–13.

[205] Sparto PJ, et al. The effect of fatigue on multijoint kinematics and load sharing during a repetitive lifting task. Spine 1997;22 (22):2647–54.

[206] McLure PW, et al. Kinematic
analysis of lumbar and hip
motion while rising from a
forward flexed position in
patients with and without a
history of low back pain. Spine
1997;22(5):552–8.

[207] Vad V, et al. Low back pain in
professional golfers. The role of
associated hip and low back
range of motion deficits. Am J
Sports Med 2004;32(2):494–7.

[208] Ellison JB, Rose SJ,
Sahrmann SA. Patterns of
rotation range of motion: a
comparison between healthy
subjects and patients with low

back pain. Phys Ther
1990;70:537–41.

[209] Kujala UM, et al. Baseline
anthropometry, flexibility and
strength characteristics and
future low back pain in
adolescent athletes and non
athletes. A prospective, one year
follow up study. Scand J Med
Sci Sports 1994;4:200–5.

[210] Van Dillen LR, et al. The effect
of hip and knee position on hip
extension range of motion
measures in individuals with and
without low back pain. J Orthop
Sports Phys Ther 2000;
30(6):307–16.

[211] Grüneberg C, et al. The
influence of artificially
increased hip and trunk stiffness
on balance control in man. Exp
Brain Res 2004;157:472–85.

[212] Feldenkrais M. Awareness
through movement. In: San
Francisco Evening Class
Workshop, vol. 1. Berkeley:
Feldenkrais resources; 1976.
p. 7.

[213] Hackney P. Making
Connections: Total body
integration through Bartenieff
Fundamentals. New York:
Routledge; 1998.

Chapter **Nine**

9

The two primary patterns of torso dysfunction

Altered function in the posturomovement system is observable in the manner in which we relate to gravity. The pelvis, in housing the centre of gravity of the body plays a central role in posturomovement control and its position when standing is the key to good or faulty postural alignment.[1] Small shifts can exert significant changes throughout the body.

While each person with back pain has an individual presentation; in general, the altered neuromuscular responses fall into certain predictable, common patterns of response which can be distilled into the two primary pictures of torso dysfunction. These are characterized by a changed sagittal plane spatial position of the pelvis in standing and corresponding alterations in the postural alignment of the body in relation to the line of gravity (see Ch. 8). They afford a simple clinical classification system and underlie a working model or paradigm to help understand the *development and perpetuation* of posturomovement disorders responsible for many musculoskeletal pain syndromes. Before examining these two proposed primary patterns more closely, it is useful to consider clinical classification systems suggested by other authors.

The case for a clinical classification based upon underlying motor control impairments

The premise that impairments in the way people posture and move are the underlying factor driving the patient's presenting musculoskeletal pain and dysfunction is central to the approach of this model and is one shared by Sahrmann,[2,3] O'Sullivan,[4,5] and Dankaerts et al.[6] Based upon this premise, those authors have argued for a clinical classification system to assist in the diagnosis and management of chronic non specific low back pain disorders (CNSLBPD). They advocate classification into clinical subgroups which are determined by 'the alignment, stress, or movement direction that most consistently reproduces pain.[3] When the mechanism or cause of a disorder is known treatment of the cause is usually considered more effective.[6]

Sahrmann[3] arrived at five diagnostic categories for CNSLBP based upon the direction of movement causing the pain, which in order of her observed frequency are:

- rotation–extension
- extension
- rotation
- rotation–flexion
- flexion syndromes.

Sahrmann says: 'The diagnosis is designed to direct the intervention. The primary strategy for an intervention program is eliminating the alignment stress or movement in the symptom producing direction. The program does not emphasize movement in the opposite direction, except where the alignment impairment is excessive'.[3]

Similarly, O'Sullivan[7,8] and Dankaerts et al.,[6] no doubt influenced by Sahrmann, suggest a mechanism based classification in the diagnosis and treatment of CNSLBPD. They also proposed five distinct yet different clinical patterns based upon a *specific direction of motor control impairment which*

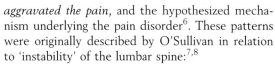

aggravated the pain, and the hypothesized mechanism underlying the pain disorder[6]. These patterns were originally described by O'Sullivan in relation to 'instability' of the lumbar spine:[7,8]

- flexion pattern – this appears to be most common pattern[8]
- lateral shift pattern
- active extension pattern
- passive extension pattern
- multidirectional pattern.

O'Sullivan[4,5] further elaborated his classification based upon the mechanism underlying the disorder, proposing that three broad subgroups of NSCLBP disorders exist. The directional patterns appear to be a subgroup of Group 3.

1. In this group, the underlying pathological processes drive the pain and the patient's motor responses are secondary and adaptive to this, e.g. inflammatory pain disorders, severe structural disorders, neuropathic or centrally mediated pain.

2. In this, a dominance of psychological and/or social factors represents the primary mechanism underlying the disorder. Altered central processing, and amplification of pain result in disordered movement and motor dysfunction. The patient's coping and motor control strategies are maladaptive in nature.

3. In this large group, maladaptive movement patterns result in chronic abnormal tissue loading and ongoing pain. They present in *either* of two ways:

- *Movement impairments* characterized by *avoidant pain behavior* associated with a loss of normal physiological lumbopelvic mobility in the direction of pain. They present with abnormally high levels of muscle guarding and cocontraction of the lumbopelvic muscles and fear of movement. The neuromuscular splinting and pain avoidance behavior is considered to be the mechanism which drives the pain.
- *Control impairments* demonstrate no impairment to mobility of the symptomatic spinal segment in the direction of pain provocation. This is associated with inability to effectively control the neutral zone.
  The *pain provocation behavior* is considered to represent the mechanism driving ongoing symptoms.

This author concurs with O'Sullivan's three broad subgroups and that maladaptive movement patterns are responsible for chronic abnormal tissue loading and ongoing pain. However, this author considers that movement and control impairments are not necessarily exclusive, but generally co-exist in some measure, albeit with one dominating, depending upon the subgroup classification to be presented in this chapter (see also Ch. 8). The patterns of altered neuromuscular response (movement impairments) may well be the heightened responses of chronically dysfunctional movement pattern behavior and indicative of the severity of pain, tissue irritability as well as the stage of the disorder. It is suggested that clinically, symptom reproduction with movement is not necessarily always achieved nor a reliable guide to the *underlying reason why* that person's movement problems have developed and are further feeding his pain picture. Nor is it necessarily always desirable to reproduce the pain as the testing in doing so can be potentially very provocative.

This proposed model, while resonant with O'Sullivan's work, offers a somewhat different view around the notion that maladaptive movement patterns result in chronic abnormal tissue loading and ongoing pain. Rather than rely upon symptom provocation, it offers a simple clinical classification system which initially relies upon observation of the quality of movement. Concerned with basic function, it delineates the more common postural and related movement impairments which appear to constitute the *underlying mechanism responsible for* the development and perpetuation of most axial and related pain syndromes including those of the lumbopelvic region. It would appear that there is an inherent tendency for these maladaptive motor responses to develop in us all under certain conditions. Various elements can be fairly consistently observed in the young and old, from the elite sportsman, yoga practitioner to the office worker and the 'couch potato'. The maladaptive responses are just more numerous, developed and obvious in people with frank musculoskeletal pain disorders.

Appreciating the features of the model as outlined not only provides a clinical classification but also guides the assessment process and provides a functional diagnosis based on the pattern of neuromyoarticular dysfunction responsible for the pain disorder. It also provides predictive and preventative insights – the presenting symptom picture usually being an acute or subacute episode on a variable picture of underlying neuromusculoskeletal dysfunction at various stages of disorder.

The two primary pictures of torso dysfunction

Observing the habitual standing posture provides a convenient 'road map' of the way in which the patient has adaptively organized herself against gravity.

In the sagittal view optimal posturomotor control has the pelvis balanced within the line of gravity, but when disturbed, the pelvis is postured either more anteriorly or posteriorly from the line of gravity (Fig. 9.1 & also Fig. 8.4).

This constitutes the basis of the two primary pictures of dysfunction – the pelvic crossed syndromes. When pelvic alignment changes so do the spinal curves in a predictable fashion. The thoracolumbar junction is considered the inflexion point between the thoracic kyphosis and the lumbar lordosis and through which the line of gravity passes.[9] Its position has a marked effect on the distribution of the intersegmental rotations of the lumbar vertebrae and upon the magnitude of the sagittal moments carried by the passive spine.[10] When more anterior, a constant extension torque ensues; when more posterior, a flexion torque results.[11]

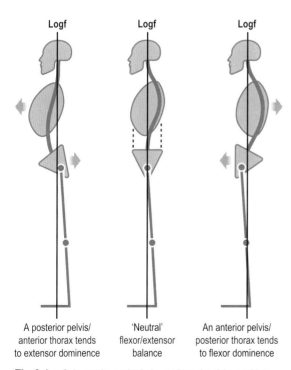

Logf	Logf	Logf

A posterior pelvis/anterior thorax tends to extensor dominence

'Neutral' flexor/extensor balance

An anterior pelvis/posterior thorax tends to flexor dominence

Fig 9.1 • Schematic sagittal view: altered pelvic position influences the body's neuromuscular response to the gravitational 'line of force'.

Roussouly et al.[12] comment 'the majority of degenerative disease occurs in spines that are well aligned in the coronal plane but exhibit highly variable morphology in the sagittal plane'. They performed a significant radiographic study examining the sagittal alignment of the lumbar spine in a cohort of 160 asymptomatic subjects. They found that 'normal' varied, and classified these variations into four groups. These subgroups resonate well with clinical impressions and so the features of each are described:

- *Type 1 lordosis.* The sacral slope is less than 35°; the apex of the lordosis is centered in the middle of the L5 body; the lower arc of lordosis is minimal decreasing toward zero as the sacral slope approaches horizontal; the inflection point (transition between the upper kyphosis and lumbar lordosis) is low and posterior creating a short lordosis with a negative lordosis tilt angle; the upper spine has a significant kyphosis of the thoracolumbar junction and thorax (Fig. 9.2).

- *Type 2 lordosis.* The sacral slope is less than 35°; the apex of the lordosis is located at the base of the L4 body; the lower arc of the lordosis is relatively flat; the inflection point is higher and more anterior decreasing the lordosis tilt angle but increasing the number of vertebral bodies included in the lordosis; the entire spine is relatively hypolordotic and hypokyphotic.

- *Type 3 lordosis.* The sacral slope is between 35° and 45°; the apex of the lumbar lordosis is in the centre of the L4 body; the *lower arc of the lordosis is more prominent*; the inflection point is at the thoracolumbar junction and the lordosis tilt angle is nearly zero; an average of four vertebrae constitutes the arc of the lordosis. *The spine is well balanced.*

- *Type 4 lordosis.* The sacral slope is greater than 45°; the apex of the lordosis is located at the base of the L3 vertebra *or higher*; the lower arc of the lordosis is prominent and the lordosis tilt angle is zero or positive; the number of vertebrae in lordotic orientation is greater than 5; a state of segmental hyperextension exists.

While demonstrating that sagittal alignment 'normally' varies significantly, the authors found the least common was Type 2 and the most common was Type 3 (construed as normal); where the apex of the lordosis was located on average in the centre of the L4 body. They also confirmed that the characteristics of the lumbar lordosis are most

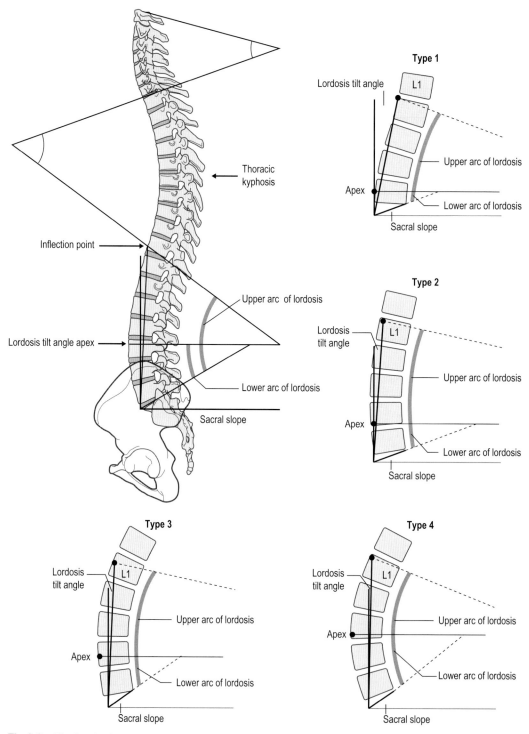

Fig 9.2 • The four lordosis types according to Roussouly et al. 2005. Change in the sacral slope effects reciprocal change in the lordosis.

dependent on the orientation of the sacral slope and the pelvis. They comment that there appears to be an association between loss of lordosis and an anterior shift of the vertical axis and the development of symptomatic back pain. Further, they comment that they have noticed that patients with symptomatic disc herniations are most commonly classified as Type 1 or 2; patients with spinal stenosis are most commonly classified as type 4 and that they rarely see patients with significant complaints who are classified as Type 3! A further study[13] compared the native sagittal alignment of patients with spondylolysis and low grade spondylolisthesis against a control group. They found increased lumbar lordosis, but less segmental extension between L5 and S1 than in the normal population. Reporting a later related study[14] in patients with lumbar degenerative diseases, they commented that previous data suggested that patients demonstrated less distal lordosis, more proximal lordosis and a more vertical sacrum; while that particular study found the loss of lordosis and a decreased sacral slope were significant. Their findings are important in corroborating the clinical impressions which underpin the pelvic crossed syndromes. Of particular significance are Type 1 with a reduced lordosis and Type 4 with an increased, albeit more cephalad or high lordosis.

In addition, Smith et al.[15] reported a photographic study examining sagittal alignment in 235 adolescents and also identified four subgroups – neutral, hyperlordotic, flat and sway. A higher proportion of the adolescent group that had never had back pain was in the 'neutral' subgroup.

The Pelvic Crossed Syndromes

These paradigms have elaborated upon the model of the Pelvic Crossed Syndrome described by Professor Vladimir Janda.[16–18] Attempts to validate the relationship between The Pelvic Crossed Syndrome as described by Janda and back pain have not been successful.[19] While the Pelvic Crossed syndrome as he described it certainly applied to some of this author's patients, it did not completely fit the picture for many, or at all for others. It took some time for this author to recognize the other patterns.
• *Posterior Pelvic Crossed Syndrome (PPXS).*
This fairly much equates to Janda's original 'pelvic or lower crossed syndrome'. In its pure form it does not appear to be as prevalent as might be expected,

however it often underlies a Mixed Syndrome presentation (see Ch. 10). It resembles a 'kyphosis-lordosis posture.[1]
• *Anterior Pelvic Crossed Syndrome (APXS).*
This appears to be the more common presentation within this author's clinical practice population either as the pure form or underlying the mixed syndrome (see Ch. 10). It resembles a 'sway-back posture'.[1]

These two syndromes form the basis of a proposed clinical classification system.

It is important to appreciate that not all patients will demonstrate the pure pelvic and related picture. Some will show some tendency, and others will exhibit a variable mixture of the two with a dominant tendency. Understanding the features of each helps understand the patient in front of you – possibly a Mixed Syndrome (see Ch. 10).

Posterior Pelvic Crossed Syndrome (PPXS)

The pelvis is back

Here the neuromuscular system is generally more switched on but in an abnormal manner of relative systemic global muscle system (SGMS) 'overdrive', with a tendency for *axial extensor muscle system dominance*. However, this extensor hyperactivity is regionally patchy and associated and related under activity of the deep system (SLMS). In its purest form it may be more common in males. The patient 'looks up'– the 'pseudo warrior' although he is tense, unyielding, generally tight and stiff, with poor selective control of movement within the torso (Figs 9.3–9.6).

Sagittal alignment characterized by:

• *Pelvis* is posteriorly shifted with increased anterior sagittal rotation or tilt. This appears to result from both psoas and erector spinae hyperactivity.
• *Trunk* – anterior translation of the thorax via thoracolumbar 'shunt' from increased thoracolumbar (T/L) extensor muscle activity creates a forward loaded trunk and associated compensatory anterior pelvic rotation. The line of gravity passes behind the thoracolumbar junction and the posterior wall of the body cylinder is shortened. An important normative study by

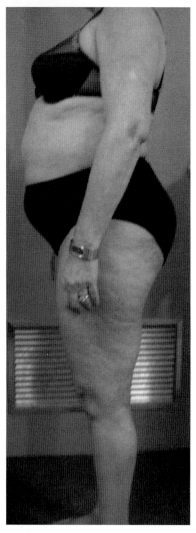

Fig 9.3 • PPXS: lateral view.

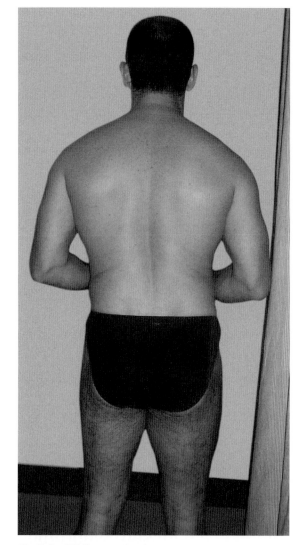

Fig 9.4 • PPXS: posterior view.

Harrison et al.[20] showed that trunk muscle activity can also influence pelvic position. Anteriorly translating the thorax at the level of T12 without restraining the pelvis resulted in it anteriorly tilting (and shifting posteriorly as shown, though not commented upon). The sacral base angle increased, the T12/L1 and L1/2 segments extended on average a total of 5° from the neutral position while L4/5 and L5/S1 flexed by a combined total of 6°. The flexing of the lower lumbars and the extension in the upper lumbars around the lumbar curve apex at L4 is interesting. In a later study,[21] they calculated that the increased thoracolumbar

extensor muscle activity associated with an anterior thoracic posture significantly increased the disc loads and stresses for all levels below T9. The IVD compressive and shear loads and the corresponding stresses were most marked at L5/S1 and L3/4 level.

• *Hips* are in relative flexion in the pure form as Janda originally described it. However, in the mixed syndrome (see Ch. 10) it is also common to see some patients lock their knees, externally rotate the hips, 'butt grip'[22] and hang the torso forward off the pelvis by holding with sustained activity of the thoracolumbar extensors.

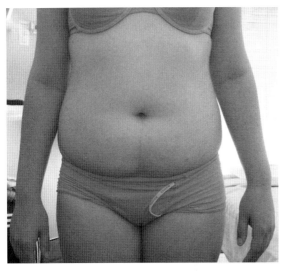

Fig 9.5 • PPXS: anterior view. The patient is 17 years old. Also see Figs 9.8 and 9.9.

• **Cursory glance** shows they look 'extended' with an increased lordosis. This is principally high lumbar and over the thoracolumbar junction. The Roussouly[12] Type 4 lordosis is extant. However, closer inspection generally reveals that the lower lumbar levels in fact show some relative flexion and are poorly controlled. The further findings reported by Roussouly et al.[13,14] and those of Harrison

et al.[20] with regard to reduced segmental extension of the lower levels in response to thorax position somewhat confirm this clinical impression. The chest is held more in the inspiratory position. Quick appraisal reveals a big belly, bottom and calves and bulky thoracolumbar extensor groups. Puffy superficial tissues and poor definition of the bony landmarks over the low lumbar levels and lumbosacral junction are usual.

• The altered length/tension relationships of the various muscles contributing towards this picture are shown in Table 9.1, Fig. 9.6.

As Janda[17] described the 'cross', there is an oblique relationship between the iliopsoas/hip flexors and erector spinae which are overactive/tight with poor

Table 9.1 Altered myofascial length/tension contributing to PPXS

Muscle hypoactivity/ lengthened	Muscle hyperactivity/ adaptive shortness
Lower pelvic unit synergy (LPU) in particular: • transversus and internal oblique • lumbosacral multifidus • iliacus in controlling intrapelvic movement and anterior pelvic rotation AT the lumbosacral junction • probably pelvic floor Entire abdominal wall +++ Glutei – medius + Inefficient diaphragm activity	Thoracolumbar erector spinae +++ Serratus posterior inferior+ Anterior hip flexor groups: • primarily psoas ++ • RF TFL Obturator group including piriformis? Hamstrings? ? hip internal rotators > external rotators? ?? lateral fibres of: • internal oblique and • latissimus dorsi

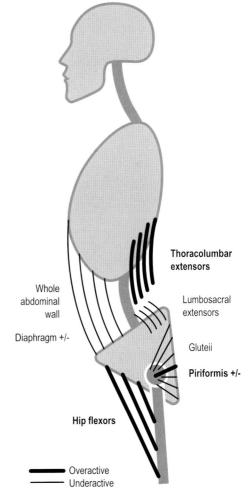

Fig 9.6 • Schematic view of PPXS.

control of eccentric lengthening. The spatially oblique gluteals and abdominals are weakened resulting in an anterior pelvic tilt, increased lordosis and a slightly flexed position of the hip (Fig. 9.3; Fig. 9.6). If the lordosis is deep and short the imbalance is principally located in the pelvic musculature. If it is shallower but longer extending into the thoracic area the imbalance is more marked in the trunk musculature.[17,23] Clinically, the latter appears more common and many also have quite bulky buttocks. Janda noted that those who stand with an opened lower thoracic aperture have a shortened diaphragm in association with underactive abdominals with decreased excursion in breathing.[23] Janda also noted that hamstrings could be tight in this syndrome either as a compensatory mechanism to lessen pelvic tilt or possibly as a functional compensation for the inhibited glutei.[17] He also noted that an imbalance can exist in the lateral pelvic muscles where a weak gluteus medius can be compensated for by over-activity and tightness in the ipsilateral quadratus lumborum and tensor fascia latae. An increased thoracic kyphosis and further compensatory increase in the cervical lordosis develop in efforts to balance the body and keep the head and eyes in the upright position.[17]

Toppenberg and Bullock[24] examined lumbopelvic muscle lengths and their interrelationships in healthy adolescent females and found significant positive correlations between shorter (by implication overactive) erector spinae and iliopsoas and rectus femoris with a tendency for longer abdominals (by implication weaker) in association with longer gluteals and shorter iliopsoas muscles. They concluded that the pattern of length relationships which constitute the pelvic crossed syndrome as described by Janda can be seen in normal pain free adolescent females. This study lends weight to the premise that movement dysfunction is present and observable before pain appears. A prospective study would be nice in determining which subjects went on to develop pain syndromes.

As a consequence we can expect or predict that in movement:

• **Patchy extensor synergies** tend to dominate in most movements – particularly T/L extensors. Inhibition of the overactive muscles can be difficult and they often can't let them go, e.g. in standing forward bending the T/L extensor muscle groups keep holding instead of eccentrically lengthening. This helps explain why some though not all patients with back pain demonstrate increased erector spinae EMG and a lack of flexion relation phenomenon[25–27] in forward bending.

• **Trunk extension is generally reduced** particularly through the thorax. In attempting extension, both poor spatial prepositioning of the pelvis and poor hip and intra-thoracic extension leads to further over activation of the extensor muscle groups over thoracolumbar junction (T/L/J) and upper lumbar levels.

• **Thoracolumbar region becomes hyperstabilized** by overactive erector spinae groups, serratus posterior inferior and psoas producing a 'Central Posterior Cinch' (CPC; Fig. 9.4). This reflex response begins to become the postural set that supports the ensuing movements. CPC hyperactivity over-anchors the lower thorax posteriorly, further reducing movement within the thorax and over the thoracolumbar junction to the upper lumbar spine. This then creates a tendency for a compensatory functional 'break' in the mid/low lumbar spine – these levels become relatively over stressed in movement with less intersegmental control. Examining the mechanics of lifting in a group of power lifters who clearly hyper develop their erector spinae, McGill reports a chance recording by video fluoroscopy of a segmental buckling/instability injury at L3/4[28] (later reported at L2/3[29,30]) (see Ch. 6, p. 134; and Ch. 13, p. 335). CPC activity can be so entrenched that it is even evident when recumbent (Fig. 9.7).

• **Poor control of the pelvis in space, on the lumbar spine and hips** in posture and movement because of inadequate control of the lower pelvic unit (LPU) and hence the fundamental pelvic

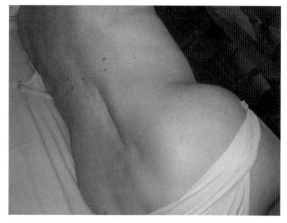

Fig 9.7 • Segmental irritation can further drive central posterior cinch behavior such that it is evident 'at rest'.

patterns. Instead, sagittal pelvic rotation control is indirectly attempted by an abnormal strategy which utilizes his CPC – anterior rotation primarily from the T/L extensors and the anterior pelvic femoral muscles – particularly psoas. The apparent anterior pelvic rotation is *not controlled* *at* the lumbosacral junction. This group has more difficulty shifting the pelvis anteriorly. When shifting it posteriorly, poor abdominal control to support anterior alignment in the body cylinder is evident.

• *Decreased hip extension range* because of tight/overactive psoas/anterior hip muscles and related underactive glutei (Fig. 9.8). Difficulty performing the 2nd fundamental pelvic pattern (FPP2) means shifting the pelvis anteriorly/posterior rotation and control of closed chain hip extension is deficient particularly in kneeling (see Fig. 11.8). Difficulty with the 1st fundamental pelvic pattern (FPP1) makes open chain hip extension control more difficult. Active hip extension movements are associated with increased CPC activity. The poor contribution and control of the lumbosacral region towards anterior pelvic rotation/low lumbar lordosis

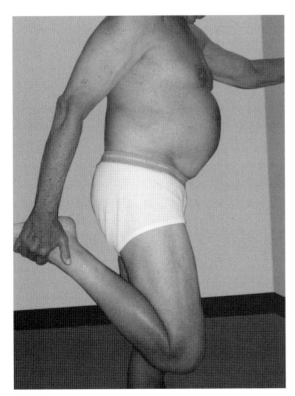

Fig 9.8 • Difficulty achieving closed chain hip extension is associated with disturbed patterns of axial alignment.

to support hip extension is interesting. Psoas is overactive in synergy with thoracolumbar extensors, and iliacus seemingly underactive in concert with the abdominals. The observed imbalance between psoas and iliacus activity in this group will hopefully interest future researchers.

• *The important standing forward bending pattern.* The pelvis is already posteriorly shifted and anteriorly rotated, and so a reasonable contribution of hip flexion is more often seen. The better developed buttocks seen in this group is evidence that they are using them somewhat! Poor control of the 'body cylinder' with imbalance between the underactive abdominals and the dominant posterior cinch patterns is the key deficient component with diminished dynamic adjustments in the legs. Reduced control of the FPP1 coupled with poor control of the anterior wall of the body cylinder is compensated by increased thoracolumbar extensor activity. This leads to…

• *Relatively increased intersegmental flexion over the mid/low lumbar levels* occurs during spinal flexion (and other movements) as the thoracolumbar contribution to movement is reduced from CPC hyperactivity. This becomes exacerbated by the frequent therapeutic misdirective to 'tuck the tail under' in a misguided attempt to decrease thoracolumbar extensor hyperactivity.

• *Sitting postures* will further stress the low lumbar levels into flexion if a collapsing strategy is adopted (see Ch. 8). Conversely they may 'sit up' by locking in with a CPC strategy and inadequate lumbopelvic contribution.

• *Abnormal axial rotation* – lack of general and rotary mobility in the thorax and over the thoracolumbar junction because of CPC activity and a 'dome' (Ch. 8) and diminished mobility and control in the hip–pelvic unit, means any rotation imposed on the system tends to occur abnormally in the mid/low lumbar spine.

• *Walking* further increases the altered loading patterns. Decreased hip extension and poor triplanar control pelvic rotation leads to further stress in the lumbar spine. Lateral weight shift (Ch. 6, Part B) is further compromised by the CPC fixing strategies holding the spine more centrally and limiting lateral shift of the thorax over the base – the lumbar spine becomes stressed in both the sagittal and frontal planes. When dysfunction is marked walking is characterized by a waddling gait as the mass of the thorax is heaved over the standing leg and the lumbar spine is observed to both side bend and rotate. The incidence of foot pain symptoms and the wearing of orthotics as well as chronic knee symptoms are common to see – both related to chronic somatic and autonomic influences resulting from compromised segmental dysfunction.

• *Dysfunctional breathing patterns* – Poor abdominal tone does not provide the stability for effective diaphragm activity which is further hampered by CPC strategies reducing posterior basal expansion. The thorax is frequently held in the (abnormal) inspiratory position[31–33] where its lower pole and the diaphragm assume a more oblique position. Liebenson[34] notes this position will inhibit the postural function of the diaphragm (Fig. 9.9).

In very general terms the prognosis for this group is perhaps more limited. Inhibiting the dominant CPC neuromuscular behavior can be really difficult and can represent a real therapeutic challenge. Chronicity is more likely and particularly so in those who have spinal surgery. Surgery may be more likely in this group.

Anterior Pelvic Crossed Syndrome (APXS)

The pelvis is forward!

Here, the neuromuscular system is more 'switched off' – both the deep SLMS and the superficial systems (SGMS). However, while less dominant, the superficial system is still abnormally used though more intermittently. Those with generally low muscle tone fall into this group and sensory system dysfunction seems more apparent. These people rely more on passive strategies for antigravity support – hanging on the iliofemoral ligaments, adopting a wide base of support, hyperextending the knees and generally limiting the opportunity for postural perturbations to influence the system (see Ch. 8).

In its purest form, it is probably more common in females. The patient appears somewhat collapsed and exhausted while 'up'. The tail bone is 'tucked under' and aspects of posturomovement patterns tend to reflect elements of 'psychological withdrawal' (Figs.9.10–9.13).

Sagittal alignment is characterized by:

• *Pelvis* is *anteriorly shifted with an increased posterior rotation or tilt.* Psoas is underactive

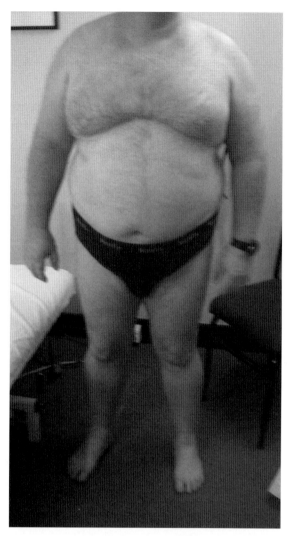

Fig 9.9 • The thorax appears to migrate more cephalad because of decreased inferior stability from the abdominals.

and they passively hang relying on their iliofemoral ligaments. This requires little postural demand in the LPU. The poor pelvic control is primary.

• *Trunk.* The thorax is *shifted more posteriorly* and the line of gravity passes anterior to the thoracolumbar junction. The axial posture is one of more general flexion, creating more loading stress on the anterior structures throughout the spine. The anterior wall of the body cylinder is shortened. There is loss of the lumbar lordosis and in some, lumbar kyphosis is apparent. This equates to the Roussouly[12] Type 1 lordosis (p. 219–220). Adaptive shortening and/or overactivity of the upper abdominals with underactivity in the lower region is evident.

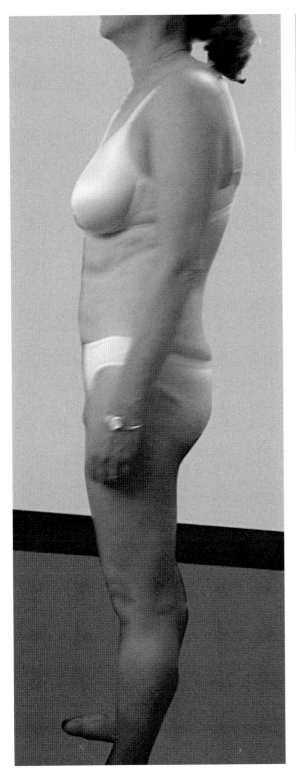

Fig 9.10 • APXS: lateral view. Her buttocks and calves are more developed than usual as she is a marathan runner!

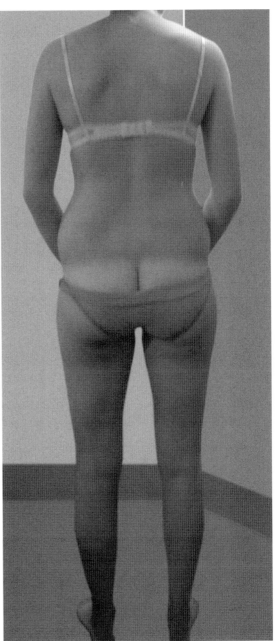

Fig 9.11 • APXS: posterior view.

• **Hips** are in extension with adaptively tight posterior hip structures. This can vary between reliance on the passive structures or active holding with the obturator group – the hips are externally rotated and the buttocks usually poorly developed. Active 'butt-gripping'[22] is more a feature of the mixed syndrome (see Ch. 10).

227

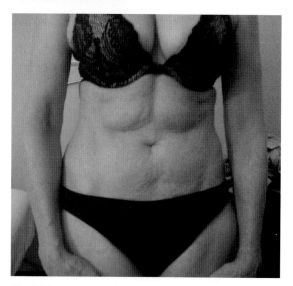

Fig 9.12 • APXS: anterior view.

Table 9.2 Altered myofascial length/tension contributing to APXS

Muscle hypoactivity/ lengthened	Hyperactivity/ adaptive shortness
Lower pelvic unit synergy: • Lower abdominal group • Lumbar multifidus – particularly over lower levels • Diaphragm – reduced excursion ++ • Iliacus and psoas + • ? weakness of anterior pelvic floor Glutei – reduced postural and movement demand and often adaptively shortened	Hamstrings +++ Obturator group including piriformis+++ Upper abdominal group including lateral internal oblique+ Hip external rotators ⟩ internal rotators +/− T/L erector spinae Posterior pelvic floor: anterior?

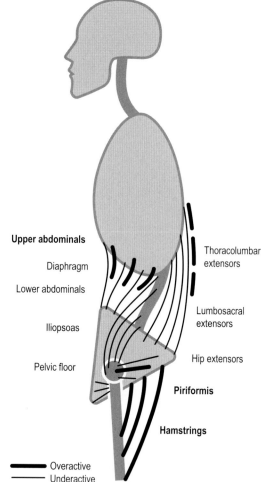

Fig 9.13 • Schematic view of APXS.

• *Quick appraisal* shows poorly developed buttocks; forward loaded head posture; thoracic kyphosis and the thorax is collapsed towards pelvis in the expiratory position. Calf development is poor.

The altered myofascial length/tension relationships observed in this picture of dysfunction are shown in Fig. 9.13 and Table 9.2.

In this presentation, the 'cross' consists of the oblique relationship between the hyperactive/tight upper abdominal group and the lower obturator/piriformis group with the posterior pelvic floor and hamstrings. The other 'diagonal' is under activity/weakness of the lower abdominal group, iliacus and psoas with lumbar multifidus. In standing this creates a posterior tilt of the pelvis, loss of the lumbar lordosis and hip extension. Active neuromuscular synergies for lumbopelvic support and control are in short supply.

As a consequence we can expect that in movement:

• *Patchy flexor synergies tend to dominate in posture and movement* – e.g. upper abdominals and pectorals coactivate in antigravity trunk

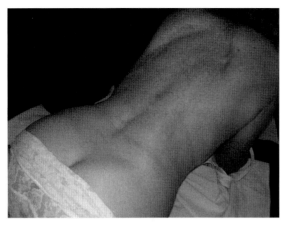

Fig 9.14 • General loss of extension is evident when prone on elbows.

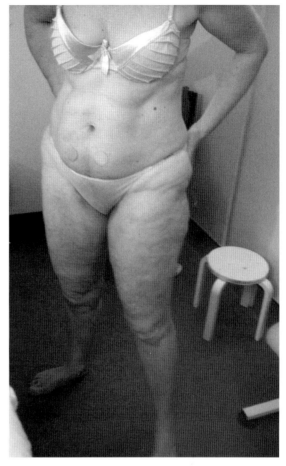

Fig 9.15 • Chronic CAC: the thorax is pulled down anteriorly; note the inactivity in the lower abdominal wall, anteriorly shifted pelvis and wide base of support.

flexion. Insufficient SLMS activity means the initiation and sustaining of appropriate postures to support movement is wanting.

• *Generalized loss of extension through the spine is marked* – both in the thorax and lumbar spine. Loss of lordosis is marked through the lumbar spine (Fig. 9.14). Most active extension is achieved by intermittent thoracolumbar extensor activity and/or further swaying pelvis forward and hyper extending the hips to compensate.

• *Thoracolumbar junction hyperstabilized in flexion.* Upper abdominal overactivity or 'cinch' creates a 'central anterior cinch' (CAC) which holds the anterior thorax down, inhibiting good descent of the diaphragm, increasing the thoracic kyphosis and 'dome' and further reducing the contribution of the thorax in axial movement. This reflex action invariably becomes the postural set adopted for axial stability to support limb movement. It can be acute (Fig. 4.9), or a chronic intrinsic problem (Fig. 9.15); or result from excessive 'training' (Fig. 9.16).

• *Poor spatial control of the pelvis, pelvis on the hips and lumbar spine.* When standing, particular underactivity in psoas/iliacus means the pelvis shifts forward and they passively hang off the iliofemoral ligaments. The patient utilizes the CAC with the hamstrings/obturators to bring the pelvis forward. Increased vertical loading stresses on the pelvic floor are more likely and Spitznagle suggests this risks stretch weakness of the PFM.[35] Clinically the posterior floor often appears tight. Delay, underactivity and imbalanced activity of the

LPU means poor spatial pre-positioning of the pelvis to provide support to the 'body cylinder' as well as for lower limb movement. The tendency to readily shunt the pelvis forward in movement means shifting it posteriorly is particularly disabled and 'unknown' (Fig. 8.29). A healthy study showed that if posterior shift of the pelvis was prevented when bending forward, inhibition of erector spinae occurred earlier in range than that normally given for the flexion–relation response.[36] The underactivity in psoas/iliacus is further reflected in difficulty in anteriorly rotating the pelvis, controlling sacral nutation and the low lumbar lordosis. The development of lumbopelvic girdle pain syndromes including the so called 'instability' syndromes of the lumbar spine and sacroiliac joint (SIJ) become a predictable eventuality. Incidentally, Mens et al.[37] note the possible

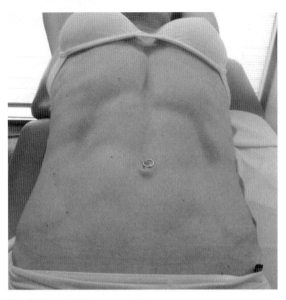

Fig 9.16 • CAC from overtraining.

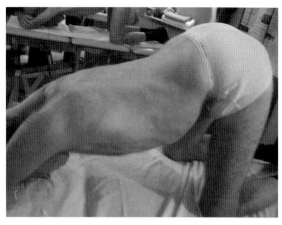

Fig 9.17 • The subject is attempting closed chain hip flexion in the 'Allah' stretch. Note the loss of axial alignment and poor anterior pelvic rotation.

increased risk of developing peripartum pelvic pain when delivery positions involved a flexed spine.

• **Decreased hip flexion** due to underactivity in iliacus-psoas and disordered LPU synergies with corresponding tight posterior pelvic and hip muscles which show poor eccentric lengthening – the obturator group including piriformis, posterior pelvic floor gluteus maximus and particularly hamstrings. Difficulty with FPP1 means anterior rotation of the pelvis and active control of closed chain hip flexion is particularly deficient and is compensated by further increased low lumbar flexion in movement (Figs 9.17 & 9.18). Hip extension becomes associated with posterior pelvic tilt. Poor control of the fundamental patterns means open chain hip movements particularly extension, are built on a poorly controlled pelvic base of support hence the movement is not well localized to the hip but is transferred to the lumbar spine. 'Hip stretches' invariably become stretches to the lumbar spine (Fig. 9.18) and may also create altered patterns of axial alignment higher up (Figs. 8.15 & 9.17) because of inadequate control of the LPU synergies.

• **The important pattern of forward bending in standing.** Instead of the sagittal axis of rotation being in the hips it becomes more the spine. Deficient control of the FPP1 & FPP2 is particularly evident in this action. The bending action is initiated more from relying on a

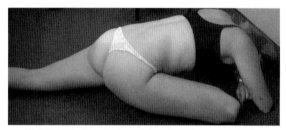

Fig 9.18 • Neurologically the patient is asleep. Passive collapse without directing the stretch from the ® ischium means the lumbar spine is the victim. The subject is the same as that in Figs 8.8, 8.26 and 11.4 who cannot initiate lateral weight shift through the pelvis in sitting.

combination of holding with the hamstrings while engaging the upper abdominals (CAC) and 'folding' forward in a pattern of generalized flexion (Figs. 9.19 & also 8.6 & 8.9) The spinal flexion–relaxation response is likely to occur early in range. In fact 'hanging off the hamstrings' allows one to rely more on the passive tissues and the hamstrings may not achieve flexion–relation at the end of flexion which is deemed to occur[38] (Fig. 9.20). This habitual initiation of forward bending by actively 'tucking the tail', creating posterior pelvic tilt and flexion of the spine has been alluded to as the 'click-clack phenomenon'[39] – an unfavorable loading state for the lumbosacral and sacroiliac structures. Poor control of FPP2 means the lifting/return phase is characterized by poor coactivation within the LPU and the 'body cylinder' with little contribution from gluteus maximus, the hamstrings being

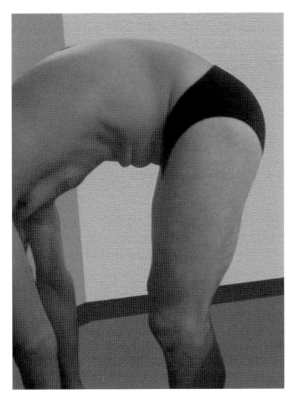

Fig 9.19 • Forward bend pattern with axial 'folding'.

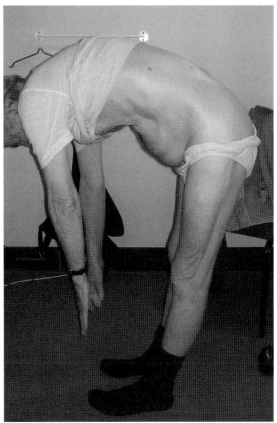

Fig 9.20 • Forward bend pattern relying upon 'hanging off the hamstrings' & the posterior axial 'passive system'.

dominant throughout the movement. The pelvis is hyperstabilized inferiorly thus held in posterior tilt through both phases and hyper flexion of lumbar segments occurs (Fig. 9.21). Adherence to the advice to 'bend the knees' generally results in more posterior pelvic rotation and lumbar flexion (Fig. 9.22) (see Ch. 6, Part B.). The key component is the lack of pelvic-hip control, and poor control of alignment in the 'body cylinder'. Lumbopelvic control suffers.

• *Relatively increased intersegmental flexion* over low lumbar levels occurs as a result of poor lumbopelvic control as well as compensation for associated posterior hip and pelvic tightness. (Fig. 9.23). Lumbar joints and intersegmental structures including the disc are used in untenable, more unstable and vulnerable end range flexion. Disc, facet and the plethora of other various 'diagnoses' are a predictable consequence over time.

• *Sitting generally involves passive collapse* (Ch. 8) with little initiation and control from the LPU, with minimal weight shifts and an inappropriate sacral position for 'axial column lift'

including control of the lumbar lordosis. Any attempts 'to sit up' are achieved by the adoption of a transient CPC in concert with their habitual CAC which serves to constrict the lower pole of the thorax in a 'central conical cinch' (CCC).

• *Abnormal axial rotation* – a general reduction in extension and rotation because of the dominant CAC patterns and thoracic 'dome', in addition to deficient lumbopelvic control and relative hypomobility in the hip and pelvic joints means any imposed rotation will abnormally occur in the lumbar spine.

• *Walking.* Gracovetsky[40] suggests that loss of control of psoas has a major effect upon locomotion as lordosis control is lost. Similarly, Rolf[41] considered that grace and efficiency in walking requires the psoas not the erector spinae as the primary antagonist of the rectus abdominus. Rather than walking with 'a spring in the step' and the easy oscillatory rhythm inherent in contralateral

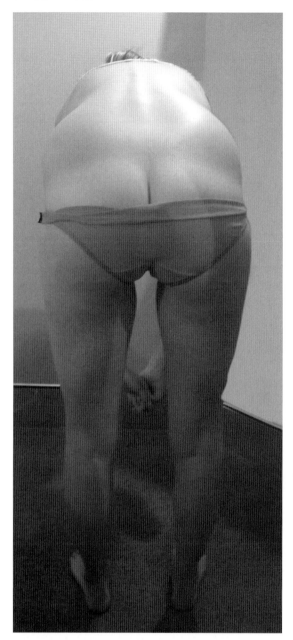

Fig 9.21 • Forward bend pattern from behind with poor eccentric lengthening in the postero-inferior pelvi-femoral muscles – "inferior tether".

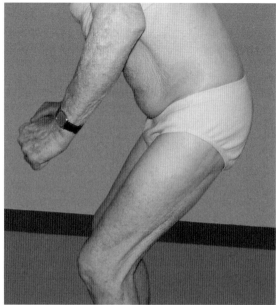

Fig 9.22 • Basic pattern tendencies are carried forward into other actions (Fig. 9.20). 'Bending the knees' in forward bending often results in increased posterior pelvic rotation.

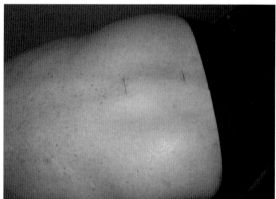

Fig 9.23 • Viewed from above. Segmental 'break' can occur in hyper-flexion of the lumbar spine.

pelvis–shoulder rotation, walking appears an effort and lacks vitality. Reduced range and control of rotation and weight shift through the kinetic system means that walking becomes more sagittal and two dimensional. Some 'pull themselves along' with their arms rather than push off well through the feet. Others appear to 'walk up to, but not past themselves', bringing the body to the weight bearing leg rather than over and past it where push off can be more effectively achieved through an extended hip in ipsilateral backward pelvic rotation.

• *Dysfunctional breathing patterns.* The thorax tends towards the more collapsed 'expiratory' position and becomes distorted by the effects of the hyperactive CAC responses and the more transient

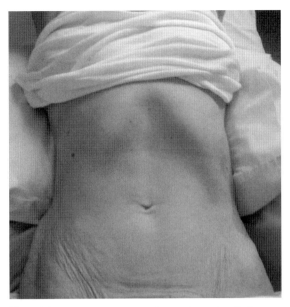

Fig 9.24 • General collapse and central anterior cinch diminishes adequate support function from the diaphragm.

CPC activity which serve to externally compress and reduce the dimensions of the inferior aperture (Fig. 9.24). This hampers diaphragmatic descent and the widening and opening out of the centre creating the internal support so important for axial stability and control (Ch. 6, Part A). When the diaphragm loses its dynamic function the action of transversus is also lost and the resting tone of the pelvic floor muscles is potentially reduced.[42] Diminished basal breathing is compensated by increased upper chest breathing with sympathetic dominance and related upper body tension. Cervical pain syndromes can also be expected to occur.

It is important to note that when attempting to be 'up', performing certain movements, trying too hard, or being over challenged, the tendency for this subgroup of patients is to flip to using a more primitive gross extensor synergy – principally utilizing the thoracolumbar extensors (CPC) in association with their retained upper abdominal 'central anterior cinch'(CAC) pattern. The lower thorax then becomes functionally converted to a cone shape. We have termed this a 'central conical cinch' (CCC) whereby the anterior, posterior and lateral thoracolumbar junction becomes hyperstabilized. Control of the pelvis is attempted from this habitual thoracolumbar strategy. The reflex reactive response becomes the postural set from which they move.

It is also important to recognize that during acute severe bouts of pain, marked muscle spasm can transform an APXS individual into one resembling a PPXS picture as their spine is held in extension with the pelvis more posteriorly placed. As joint irritability settles they revert to form.

Discussion: pelvic position and flexor or extensor proclivity

Altered pelvic shift and associated tilt has received almost no attention in the literature. Myers[43] mentions, 'the pelvis is commonly described as being anteriorly or posteriorly shifted relative to the malleoli with the understanding that "some tilts must occur along the way for that to happen".' A personal article by Schleip[44] describes 'The structural typology of Hans Flury'; however, this author found Flury's work difficult to locate. According to Schleip, Flury arrived at four combinations of pelvic tilt and shift. The two related to an anterior tilt he called 'internal'. This may be because clinically, the hip tends more to internal rotation in anterior pelvic tilt, although this is not stated. Similarly, those with a posterior tilt were termed 'external' – again not stated, but presumably because clinically, external hip rotation and posterior pelvic tilt certainly 'go together'. It appears Flury felt that an anterior and posterior tilt can occur in both an anterior and a posterior shift of the pelvis. However, at this stage, it is this author's clinical impression that posterior pelvic shift is coupled with anterior rotation and anterior shift with posterior rotation. Try it for yourself! Importantly, Schleip mentions that the two types with a posterior shift are considered to be 'tensional types' in which the fascial and muscular holding patterns are considered to be more apparent. This directly applies to the picture seen in the PPXS subgroup in the model presented here. Those with an anterior shift are considered 'compressional types' and this author interprets this as 'internal collapse' from inadequate SLMS activity – APXS as presented. Schleip hints that the emphasis for these names is in relation to the posterior trunk.

Brumagne et al.[45] recently found that persons with recurrent LBP showed a significant more forward inclination of their body when vision was occluded or in anticipation of postural instability. They noted however other studies have shown a tendency to more posterior inclination.

The important significance of the pelvic shifts and tilts is the real effect they have on the distribution of extensor and flexor muscle system activity throughout the torso:

- When the pelvis is anterior, flexor system dominance tends to prevail (APXS)
- When the pelvis is posterior extensor system dominance is more apparent (PPXS) (Fig. 9.1)
- When the pelvis is neutral balance between the flexors and extensors is likely.

Rock[42] defines the functionally normal neutral pelvic position as having a slight anterior tilt where the anterior superior iliac spines move slightly in front of the symphysis. In this position the reflex postural muscle chains are better activated and sacroiliac joint shear stress is minimized. This can be readily felt in standing.

Schleip[46] also offers a structural typology based on the effects of primary reflex behavior upon the functional relationship between the flexors and extensors (Ch. 7). This typology also shares many features in common with the crossed syndromes. Clinically, he notes a 'short extensor pattern' which equates to the PPXS and a 'short flexor pattern' – either contracted or collapsed, which equates to the APXS. Like this author, he has also been influenced by the work of Feldenkrais[47,48] and Hanna[49] and notes the associated psychological temperaments which tend to accompany each state. Feldenkrais saw that negative emotions and the 'the body pattern of anxiety' were flexor dominant. The APXS/flexor tendency group does appear more inclined to negative emotions, tension, depression, and anxiety, etc. The PPXS/extensor dominant individuals appear extroverted yet are stiff and rigid. Importantly his two typologies are not exclusive of one another, which is also the case in the crossed syndromes and further explored in the mixed syndrome in Chapter 10. However, Schleip believes the 'key indicator for the reflex patterns is not in the pelvis position in standing (like Flury's model), nor in the femur rotation (like in Sultan's), but the tonus balance between trunk-flexors and trunk-extensors specially (sic) around the rib cage'.[46]

The paradigm of the two crossed syndromes embraces the significant role that both the trunk and pelvis play and importantly, their ability to mutually influence one another. Essentially in the pure form, those with PPXS are axially hyperextended with relative hip flexion while those who are APXS are axially flexed with extended hips. Perhaps the pelvis is the primary dysfunction in APXS and the trunk is primary in PPXS. However, practically they are interdependent as trunk muscle activation patterns affect the pelvis and conversely pelvic activation patterns influence those in the trunk.

O'Sullivan described[6–8] five clinical patterns which are principally flexion or extension dominant, based upon pain behavior with movement. It appears that we are observing similar patterns of clinical presentation[6,50,51] namely:

- the APXS shares features in common with his flexion pattern which he thought was the more common underlying clinical presentation.[7,8,50]
- posterior pelvic crossed syndrome shares features in common with his extension pattern
- O'Sullivan's other directional patterns can be viewed as variations on these basic two patterns at differing stages of neuromusculoskeletal dysfunction.

Van Wingerden et al.[52,53] presented a study which lends support to the concept of the two pelvic crossed syndromes. They examined forward bending motion patterns of the lumbar spine and pelvis in two subgroups of patients with chronic pelvic girdle pain and chronic LBP against a control group. While they described the position of the trunk in standing as similar in all three groups, they found that those with pelvic girdle pain demonstrated a significantly increased posterior pelvic tilt and decreased lumbar lordosis in standing. When this group bent forward, lumbar flexion was significantly increased initially and through range while hip motion was significantly reduced (a common strategy adopted by those classified as APXS). Those with LBP initially maintained more lordosis when forward bending, but had more lumbar motion in the final stage of flexion i.e. they initially 'held' more with their thoracolumbar extensors and compensate at the end of range with increased motion probably over the lower levels. This group can clearly be sub-classified in the PPXS group. Predictably we can expect symptoms to differentially occur in both groups over time.

Other forward bending studies of subjects with CLBP have also shown early and increased lumbar movement with reduced hip movement,[54] especially when fatigued.[55] Porter and Wilkinson[56] found an overall reduction in the mean total range and mean maximum lumbar flexion in all symptomatic subjects with a subgroup showing a significant decrease in hip flexion. Sub classification as proposed would help explain the various findings.

If some show flexor dominance why work their abdominals so?

It has been exciting for this author to find resonance in the work of others who are describing similar clinical patterns with a certain common theme – some subjects show the influence of more dominant reflex flexor activity while for others it is extensor. This has important implications. The abdominal muscles receive a lot of attention in therapy and fitness programs in the pursuit of 'good core control'. However different presentations require different solutions.

In general those who are classified as APXS lack extension are flexor dominant and 'collapsed' when up. They generally show increased activity patterns in the upper abdominals and consistent underactivity of the lower abdominal region. The combination of reduced deep system activity and the adoption of the 'holding' and 'folding' strategies result in the axial spine becoming relatively *shortened*. The anterolateral abdominal wall bulges and they 'have a tummy'. Janda felt the lateral waist bulge was indicative of transversus hypoactivity. Unfortunately being told to 'hold their stomach in' has the effect of pulling them down into more flexion, shortening the torso increasing the 'dome' and further constricting function around the body's centre of gravity. These people need to develop control of their pelvis, the synergies for which require activation of the lower abdominals. Control of posterior pelvic tilt and achieving anterior tilt is difficult. Coactivation between the flexors and extensors for low load activities is also reduced, hindering control of alignment between the related segments in the kinetic chain. Consistently working them more into flexion compounds their problems and therapeutic misadventure is becoming a more common presentation in the clinic.

Those who are classified as PPXS *do* need to achieve better abdominal control, as they show underactivity in both the upper and lower regions. However, activation strategies also need to control the pelvis to prevent it punching into posterior tilt which is usual and serves to perpetuate the lumbo-pelvic dysfunction.

All abdominal activation strategies need to allow proper diaphragmatic breathing. Posterior tilting exercises have been a common therapeutic directive but this is hard to justify, when it is understood that the pelvis is usually found to readily tilt back but not forward. Posterior tilt places the lumbosacral junction in flexion[57] with well documented deleterious effects on the viscoelastic tissues and related neuromuscular responses.[58–60] Snook et al.[61] demonstrated significant reductions in pain intensity in CNSLBP when subjects completely avoided early morning lumbar flexion for the first two hours after rising. While not a particularly functional solution the benefits of reducing the flexion stress are shown.

While abdominal function *is* generally deficient in subjects with back pain, so are a lot of other things. Rather than muscle weakness, the problem is more usually inadequacy in the automatic reflex activity of groups of muscles cooperating in various synergies, to provide certain functionally important patterns of postural control and movement. The importance of this reflex behavior is attracting increasing research interest. There is recognition that attempting to consciously voluntarily alter trunk muscle coactivation might constitute a non optimal motor scheme and result in a drop in stability in demanding situations.[62] Reeves et al.[63] showed that increasing trunk muscle recruitment by 'bracing' degrades postural control. Brown and McGill[62] recently showed that the ability to increase spine stiffness by abdominal bracing is partially dependent upon trunk posture and it would appear reflex mechanisms. Normal subjects were placed in a set up which eliminated gravity and reflex responses and asked to voluntary brace the abdominals and trunk muscles while being slowly passively moved into different positions. In extension, spine stiffness increased with successive increases in voluntary muscle activation through range. However, in flexion and lateral bending, (the most commonly adopted trunk postures for ADL activities) spine stiffness increased between neutral and approximately 40% and 60% of maximum range respectively. After that, subjects became unaccountably less stiff despite maximal voluntary abdominal coactivation. The apparent 'yielding' phenomenon is being further researched.

Understanding the primary differences in presentation affords clearer insights into the specific movement problems of the presenting patient. This is further understood by examining the related clinical syndromes which ensue from these two primary patterns of movement dysfunction.

References

[1] Kendall FP, McCreary EK, Provance PG. Muscles: Testing and Function. 4th ed. Baltimore: Williams and Wilkins; 1993.

[2] Sahrmann S. Effects on muscle of repeated movements and sustained postures. In: Proc.1st International Conference on Movement Dysfunction. Edinburgh; 2001.

[3] Sahrmann SA. Diagnosis and Treatment of Movement Impairment Syndromes. St. Louis: Mosby; 2002.

[4] O'Sullivan PB. Diagnosis and classification of chronic low back pain disorders: Maladaptive movement and motor control impairments as an underlying mechanism. Man Ther 2005;10:242–55.

[5] O'Sullivan PB. Classification of lumbo-pelvic pain disorders – why it is essential for management. Man Ther 2006;11:169–70.

[6] Dankaerts W, et al. The inter-examiner reliability of a classification method for non specific chronic low back pain patients with motor control impairments. Man Ther 2006;11:28–39.

[7] O'Sullivan PB. Lumbar segmental 'instability': clinical presentation and specific stabilising exercise management. Man Ther 2000;5(1):2–12.

[8] O'Sullivan PB. 'Clinical instability' of the lumbar spine: its pathological basis, diagnosis and conservative management. In: Boyling JD, Jull GA, editors. Modern Manual Therapy. Edinburgh: Elsevier; 2004.

[9] Singer K, Malmivaara A. Pathoanatomical characteristics of the thoracolumbar junctional region. In: Giles LGF, Singer KP, editors. The clinical anatomy and Management series. Vol. 2: Clinical anatomy and management of thoracic spine pain. Oxford: Butterworth Heinemann; 2000.

[10] Kiefer A, Shirazi-Adl, Parnianpour M. Synergy of the human spine in neutral postures. Eur Spine J 1998;7:471–9.

[11] Neumann DA. Kinesiology of the musculoskeletal system: foundations for physical rehabilitation. St. Louis: Mosby; 2002.

[12] Roussouly P, et al. Classification of the normal variation in the sagittal alignment of the human lumbar spine and pelvis in the standing position. Spine 2005;30 (3):346–53.

[13] Roussouly P, et al. Sagittal alignment of the spine and pelvis in the presence of L5-S1 isthmic lysis and low grade spondylolisthesis. Spine 2006;31 (21):2484–90.

[14] Barrey C, et al. Sagittal balance of the pelvis spine complex and lumbar degenerative diseases. A comparative study about 85 cases. Eur Spine J 2007;16:1459–67.

[15] Smith A, O'Sullivan P, Straker L. Classification of sagittal thoraco-lumbo-pelvic alignment of the adolescent spine in standing using two dimensional photographic images and the association with back pain. In: Proc. 6th Interdisciplinary World Congress on Low Back and Pelvic Pain. Barcelona; 2007.

[16] Janda V. Muscles as a pathogenic factor in back pain. In: Proc. I.F.O.M.T. New Zealand; 1980.

[17] Janda V. Muscles and motor control in low back pain: assessment and management. In: Twomey L, editor. Physical Therapy of the Low Back. New York: Churchill Livinstone; 1987.

[18] Janda V, Frank C, Liebenson C. Evaluation of muscular imbalance. In: Liebenson C, editor. Rehabilitation of the spine: A practitioner's manual. 2nd ed. Philadelphia: Lippincott Williams & Wilkins; 2007.

[19] Nourbakhsh MR, Arabloo AM. The relationship between patterns of muscle imbalance and low back pain. In: Proc. 5th Interdisciplinary World Congress on Low Back and Pelvic Pain. Melbourne; 2004.

[20] Harrison DE, et al. How do anterior/posterior translations of the thoracic cage affect the sagittal lumbar spine, pelvic tilt, and thoracic kyphosis? Eur Spine J 2002;11:287–93.

[21] Harrison DE, et al. Anterior thoracic posture increases thoracolumbar disc loading. Eur Spine J 2005;14:234–42.

[22] Lee D. The pelvic girdle: An approach to the examination and treatment of the lumbo-pelvic-hip region. 3rd ed. Edinburgh: Churchill Livingstone; 2004.

[23] Janda V. Sydney: Course notes; 1989: 1984: 1985.

[24] Toppenberg R, Bullock M. Normal lumbo-pelvic muscle lengths and their interrelationships in adolescent females. Aust J Physiother 1990;36(2):105–9.

[25] Watson PJ, et al. Surface electromyography in the identification of chronic low back pain patients: the development of the flexion relaxation ratio. Clin Biomech 1997;12(3):165–71.

[26] Paquet N, Malouin F, Richards CL. Hip-spine movement interaction and muscle activation patterns during sagittal trunk movements in low back pain patients. Spine 1994;19 (5):596–603.

[27] Chiou W-K, Lee Y-H, Chen W-J. Use of surface EMG coactivational pattern for functional evaluation of trunk muscles in subjects with and without low back pain. Int J Industrial Ergonomics 1998;23 (1–2):51–6.

[28] McGill SM. Low back exercises: evidence for improving exercise regimens. Phys Ther 1998;78 (7):754–65.

[29] McGill SM. Low back disorders: evidence based prevention and rehabilitation. USA: Human Kinetics; 2002.

[30] McGill SM. Ultimate Back Fitness and Performance. Waterloo: Wabuno; 2004.

[31] Kolar P. Facilitation of agonist-antagonist co-activation by reflex stimulation methods. In:

Liebenson C, editor. Rehabilitation of the spine: A practitioner's manual. 2nd ed. Philadelphia: Lippincott Williams & Wilkins; 2007.

[32] Kolar P. Dynamic neuromuscular stabilisation: According to Kolar – an introduction presented by Safarova M. Courses (notes) conducted by CEA notes. Sydney; 2008.

[33] Cumpelik J. Breathing mechanics in postural stabilisation. Course (notes) conducted by CEA. Sydney; 2008.

[34] Liebenson C. Core training: the importance of the diaphragm. Dynamic Chiropractic 2007;13 (25):30–4.

[35] Spitznagle TM. Musculoskeletal chronic pelvic pain. In: Carrière B, Markel Feldt C, editors. The Pelvic Floor. Stuttgart: Thieme; 2006.

[36] Gupta A. Analyses of myo-electrical silence of erectors spinae. J Biomech 2001;34 (4):491–6.

[37] Mens JM, et al. Understanding peripartum pelvic pain: Implications of a patient survey. Spine 1996;21(11):1363–9.

[38] Sihvonen T. Flexion-relaxation of the hamstring muscles during lumbar-pelvic rhythm. Arch Phys Med Rehab 1997;78(5):486–90.

[39] Snijders CJ, et al. Effects of slouching and muscle contraction on the strain of the iliolumbar ligament. Man Ther 2008;13 (4):325–33.

[40] Gracovetsky S. The Spinal Engine. Austria: Springer-Verlag/ Wien; 1988.

[41] Rolf IP. Rolfing: The integration of human structures. New York: Harper and Row; 1977.

[42] Rock C-M. Reflex incontinence caused by underlying functional disorders. In: Carrière B, Markel Feldt C, editors. The Pelvic Floor. Stuttgart: Thieme; 2006.

[43] Myers TW. Anatomy Trains: myofascial meridians for manual and movement therapists.

Edinburgh: Churchill Livingstone; 2001.

[44] Schleip R. The structural typology of Hans Flury, Sourced: http://www.somatics.de/Flury. html.

[45] Brumagne S, et al. Altered postural control in anticipation of postural instability in persons with recurrent low back pain. Gait Posture 2008;28(4):657–62.

[46] Schleip R. Primary Reflexes and Structural Typology, Sourced: http://www.somatics.de/flex/ extens/primrefl.html.

[47] Feldenkrais M. Body and Mature Behaviour: A study of anxiety, sex, gravitation and learning. New York: International Universities Press Inc; 1949.

[48] Feldenkrais M. The Elusive Obvious or Basic Feldenkrais. Cupertino Ca: Meta Publications; 1981.

[49] Hanna T. Somatics: Reawakening the mind's control of movement. Cambridge: Da Capo Press; 1988.

[50] O'Sullivan PB, et al. The relationship between posture and back muscle endurance in industrial workers with flexion related low back pain. Man Ther 2006;11:264–71.

[51] Dankaerts, et al. Differences in sitting postures are associated with non specific chronic low back pain disorders when patients are subclassified. Spine 2006;31 (6):674–98.

[52] Van Wingerden JP, Vleeming A, Ronchetti I. Citation: physical compensation strategies in female patients with chronic low back pain and chronic pelvic girdle pain. In: Proc. 5th Interdisciplinary World Congress on Low Back and Pelvic Pain. Melbourne; 2004.

[53] Van Wingerden JP, Vleeming A, Ronchetti I. Differences in standing and forward bending in women with chronic low back or pelvic girdle pain: indications for physical compensation strategies. Spine 2008;33(11):E334–41.

[54] Esola M, et al. Analysis of lumbar spine and hip motion during forward bending in subjects with and without a history of low back pain. Spine 1996;21(1):71–8.

[55] Sparto PJ, et al. The effect of fatigue on multijoint kinematics and load sharing during a repetitive lifting task. Spine 1997;22(22):2647–54.

[56] Porter J, Wilkinson A. Lumbar-hip flexion motion: a comparative study between asymptomatic and symptomatic chronic low back pain patients in 18–36-year-old men. Spine 1997;22(13): 1508–13.

[57] Liebenson C. A modern approach to abdominal training. J of Bodywork and Movement Therapies 2007;11(3):194–8.

[58] Solomonow M, et al. Volvo Award Winner in Biomechanical Studies: Biomechanics of increased exposure to lumbar injury caused by cyclic loading: Part 1. Loss of reflexive muscular stabilisation. Spine 1999;24 (23):2426.

[59] Williams M, et al. Multifidus spasms elicited by prolonged flexion. Spine 2000;25 (22):2916–24.

[60] Solomonow M, et al. Biomechanics and electromyography of a common idiopathic low back disorder. Spine 2003;28(12):1235–48.

[61] Snook SH, et al. The reduction of chronic nonspecific low back pain through the control of early morning lumbar flexion: a randomized control trial. Spine 1998;23(23):2601–7.

[62] Brown SHM, McGill. How the inherent stiffness of the in vivo human trunk varies with changing magnitudes of muscular activation. Clin Biomech 2008;23 (1):15–22.

[63] Reeves NP, et al. The effects of trunk stiffness on postural control during unstable seated balance. Exp Brain Res 2006; 174:694–700.

Clinical posturomovement impairment syndromes

Changed muscle activation patterns produce altered alignment of the body segments against gravity. Observing the patient provides information about the more common patterns of posturomovement dysfunction. Chapter 9 dealt with the two primary pictures of torso dysfunction which underlie all the clinical syndromes. These provide a clinically useful classification system guiding assessment, diagnosis and therapeutic care. The presence of these syndromes result in altered stresses on the joints and soft tissues and the predictable development of various pain syndromes in time. Diagnosing the 'underlying mechanism driving the disorder'[1] rather than the often spurious diagnosis based upon pathology helps inform more rational treatment interventions.

Observing the subject in different planes affords different information. The clinical syndromes are listed and further explored below.

Sagittal view

The three pelvic syndromes and the common upper body posturomovement dysfunction:
- *The Posterior Pelvic Crossed Syndrome (PPXS)* (see Ch. 9)
- *The Anterior Pelvic Crossed Syndrome (APXS)* (see Ch. 9)
- *The Mixed Syndrome*: display features of both PPXS and APXS with a dominant tendency towards one or the other
- *The Shoulder Crossed Syndrome*. Described Janda,[2-4] this is also known as the upper crossed syndrome or the proximal crossed syndrome: it describes the common posturomovement dysfunction in the upper body and is usually always present albeit in varying degrees.

Coronal view

Layer or Stratification Syndrome. Described by Janda[3-5] this describes the commonly altered muscle activation patterns in the flexor and extensor systems.

Composite view

The Belted Torso Syndrome. This describes the observed dysfunction around the central torso and the body's centre of gravity which results from the combined influences of the pelvic crossed syndromes and the layer syndrome.

The 'pure' form of the pelvic crossed syndromes is not necessarily always present, yet the patient will generally display features which merit classification into one group or the other, and is then described for example as a 'mixed syndrome on a primary APXS picture'.

Mixed Syndrome (MS)

Clinically, this is perhaps the more common presentation. Appreciating each primary syndrome separately helps see the composite presentation and the relative underlying influence of one. The two basic pictures of dysfunction in the pelvic crossed syndromes are reflective of the developmental prowess or otherwise of the individual which not only includes the early developmental history but also subsequent influences. Psychological occupational and recreational factors all impact upon the primary picture of dysfunction and variously contribute to the development of the MS pictures in some patients. Unfortunately, poorly conceived therapeutic interventions and fitness industry programs appear to be responsible for the increasing prevalence and most flamboyant examples. The important role that the systemic local muscle system (SLMS) plays in the proper control of movement is generally not well understood. Instead, many myths abound and in particular with regard to 'core control' (see Ch. 6, Part B). In pursuit of this, many are entrenching central torso 'cinch patterns' and dysfunctional breathing patterns – a 'gym junkie syndrome' is becoming apparent (see Ch. 11, Sport and Recreation; Training and the fitness industry).

Regarding the mixed syndrome, it is useful to firstly reconsider the salient aspects of each of the two primary dysfunction pictures in order to more clearly see its genesis.

In general terms, the shared common dysfunction in the primary pictures consists of:

- Imbalanced activity between the SLMS and systemic global muscle system (SGMS) with general underactivity of the deep system
- Altered co-activation patterns between the axial flexors and extensors
- Poor lumbopelvic control providing inadequate support around the body's centre of gravity
- Increased SGMS activity occurs around the central and upper torso disturbing postural alignment and control including equilibrium, stability and breathing mechanisms.

However, within the common patterns above, variations occur in accordance with each primary syndrome and are summarized in Table 10.1.

'Central conical cinch' (CCC) behavior and 'butt-gripping'[6] are probably the most consistent distinguishing traits which unite the two primary pelvic syndromes in the MS. This results in a hyperstabilized central torso yet poorly stabilized lumbopelvic region with variable patterns of inferior pelvis/hip restriction.

These aspects are further explored.

Table 10.1 The cardinal features of altered function in the two primary pictures of dysfunction

	PPXS	APXS
Pelvis position re line of gravity	Posterior	Anterior
Thoracolumbar position re line of gravity	Anterior	Posterior
Flexor/extensor system tendency	Extensor	Flexor
Central cinch pattern	CPC	CAC → CCC
Suspected principal regional dysfunction	Thoracolumbar > pelvic?	Pelvic > thoracolumbar?
Pattern of hip/thigh muscle restrictions	Anterior > posterior	Posterior > anterior

Central cinch patterns (CCPs)

CCPs refer to the seemingly reflexive and somewhat obligatory *bilateral* neuromuscular responses which are observed to occur in posture and movement around the central torso. In most instances, their early activation means they become the postural set which initiate and support the ensuing movements. They hyperstabilize the central torso in one or more planes. They appear to be a response to reduced SLMS control and a compensation for inadequate proximal girdle control particularly in the pelvis. They are further magnified in the presence of a 'dome' (Ch. 8, Thoracic dysfunction). For whatever reason, the response is more dominant above the belt line than below. The patient finds it difficult to inhibit these responses and in essence only learns how to when better SLMS control is established, including control of the proximal limb girdles along with proper diaphragmatic breathing and better co-activation between the axial muscles.

Central posterior cinch (CPC)

CPC refers to the observed pattern of bilateral reflex overactivation of the superficial muscle groups which form a dense 'fan' which spans posteriorly from approximately the level of the mid/upper lumbar spine extending upwards to cover the lower pole of the thorax (Fig. 10.1). These work in synergy as a reflex 'mass response' with associated underactivity in the abdominals. Janda[7] considered that a clinically found muscle imbalance between different muscle groups is probably the result of a combination of both reflex and mechanical mechanisms. Regional extensor system hyperactivity may serve to inhibit the abdominals mediated by Sherrington's Law of reciprocal inhibition[2] or conversely, SLMS system dysfunction, abdominal underactivity and changed axial alignment creates the loading torque such that the CPC activity is necessarily facilitated. The presence of a 'dome' and generally reduced extension can mean that the CPC represents the region of 'active' extension. This can be readily observed when the patient simply lifts his head up in prone (see Fig. 8.18). The response is also a common compensation in forward bending when lumbopelvi-femoral control is decreased.

Clinically, the superficial posterior thoracolumbar muscle groups are usually but not always bulky, tender and tense with trigger points commonly found. Clinical impressions suggest they include (Fig. 10.2):

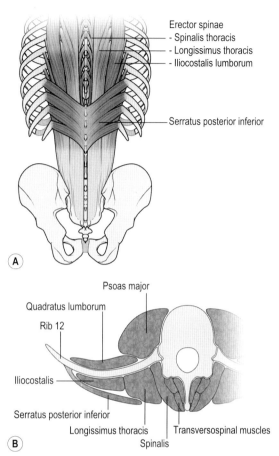

Fig 10.2 • Schematic conceptual view of the muscles involved in a central posterior cinch. Posterior view (A); cross-section around T12/L1 (B).

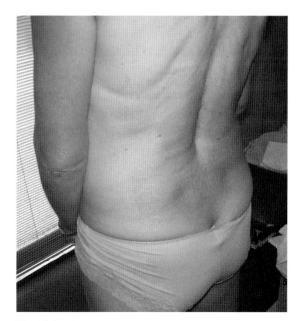

Fig 10.1 • Central posterior cinch: note the demarcation between the tension in the muscles above the waist and the atonic puffy, overworked tissues below.

- Those sections of the erector spinae which act over this region – the medially placed spinalis thoracis, longissimus thoracis pars thoracis and particularly the more lateral iliocostalis lumborum pars thoracis attaching to the angles of the lowest six or seven ribs.[8]
- Serratus posterior inferior extending from the spinous processes T11–L3 upwards and laterally to the posterior surfaces of ribs 9–12 lateral to their angles.[8]
- Psoas. Clinically one readily observes the activity of the superficial muscles but it is possible that the upper fascicles of psoas are also active in the response. Bogduk et al.,[9] suggest the upper fascicles tend to extend the upper lumbar spine while the lower fibres flex the lower lumbar levels. Penning[10] agrees and further considers psoas probably also functions as a stabilizer. Lateral weight shift requires eccentric contraction of one psoas and

concentric in the other but when bilaterally active the column becomes hyperstabilized centrally. In particular the thoracolumbar junction is pulled forward and 'fixed'.

• Similar involvement from the upper fibres of quadratus lumborum and lateral fibres of internal oblique and latissimus is also a probability. This tethers the lower pole of the thorax and limits elongation of the lateral wall of the body cylinder.

To a greater or lesser extent, practically all patients with spinal pain and related disorders can be observed to activate extensor dominant CPC patterns in posturomovement control. They are obligatory and particularly evident in the PPXS group, less so in the MS and intermittent in the APXS group. This is a reasonably constant response which the patient finds hard to inhibit. Eccentric lengthening is poor hence little adaptability/variability for postural control. The bilateral activation serves to 'fix' the lower pole of the thorax and the thoracolumbar spine in a 'central' position holding the region in a sagittal orientation and importantly, limits flexion, lateral and rotary movements and weight shifts through this region of the torso (Fig. 10.3). Neural irritability through segmental hypomobility further increases the tonus of the thoracolumbar extensors feeding into a vicious pattern generating cycle as the mid/low lumbar levels are further required to compensate.

Central anterior cinch (CAC)

CAC refers to the observed pattern of bilateral reflex overactivation of the anterolateral abdominal group above the level of the umbilicus. Given their superior attachments extend over the entire anterolateral surface of the inferior pole of the thorax; their overactivity has a significant influence. The bilateral activation creates a flexor torque, holding the central torso in a more flexed sagittal orientation thereby limiting extension, lateral and rotary weight shift and movements. Most significant is the narrowing of the inferior thoracic opening and limitation of the diaphragm's important functional role (Fig. 10.4). This 'reflex withdrawal' action is also initiated with anxiety, stressful states and fear (see Ch. 6, Part A). Janda[11] found that in healthy children and spastics with good postural development, unresisted and resisted knee extension in supine and sitting produced only slight or no

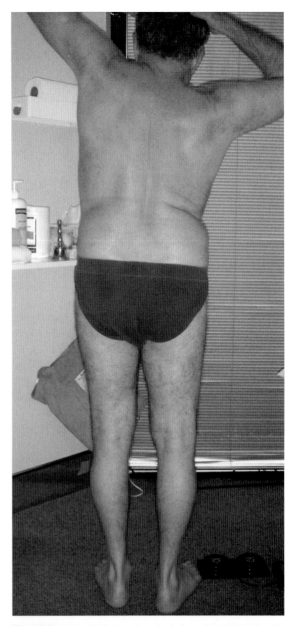

Fig 10.3 • A central posterior cinch fixes the spine centrally limiting lateral weight shift. The subject is attempting to 'grow one elbow to the ceiling (see Ch. 13). Note the lack of adaptive eccentric lengthening in the (L) erector spinae and probably psoas and the poor weight shift through the pelvis.

activity of the abdominal muscles. However, in those spastic children with a hypotonic trunk and bad posture, the activity of the abdominal muscles increased considerably in sitting during this test. Questioning whether this was the result of an altered reflex mechanism or due to possible mechanical stabilization

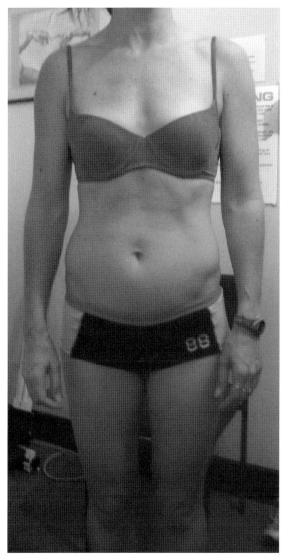

Fig 10.4 • Central anterior cinch: the anterior thorax is anchored inferiorly. Note the difference in abdominal tone above the umbilicus compared to that below.

dysfunction in these children, he examined healthy children with evident hypotonia of the trunk and also found a remarkable increase in their abdominal activity in sitting. The entire pattern of knee extension in this group was accompanied by a 'simultaneous backward tilt of the pelvis and a pronounced lumbar kyphosis and a curling movement of the whole trunk'. He surmised that altered reflex mechanisms were operant. It is interesting to note that low tone, postural collapse, CAC strategies and a tendency for 'total flexion patterns' (Ch. 8, p. 181) are all features observed in those classified as APXS. O'Sullivan

et al.[12] found that patients with CLBP had difficulty preferentially activating the deep abdominals with a tendency to higher levels of upper rectus abdominis activity. The CAC postural response is the obverse of that found in the normal state where the EMG onset of the upper region of transversus abdominus has been shown to occur later than that of the lower and middle regions in response to perturbation.[13]

CAC strategies are obligatory in 'pure' presentations in the APXS group and also predominant in those in the MS group but do not occur in the 'pure' PPXS group. See Figures 4.9, 8.28, 8.38, 9.12, 9.15.

Central conical cinch (CCC)

CCC refers to the combined activation of the CPC and CAC strategies and can subsequently develop in both primary pictures of dysfunction to create a MS. This simultaneous increased reflex activation serves to 'squeeze' the inferior region of the lower pole of the thorax and conceptually convert it into a conical shape. The lower pole of the thorax extending into the upper lumbar spine is hyperstabilized in all three planes. This is akin to a self inflicted functional 'straight jacket'. Rather than the 'body cylinder' (Ch. 6, p. 93) being open in the centre, it becomes constricted in posturomovement like squeezing a tube of toothpaste in the centre – the body cylinder now resembles an 'hourglass' (Figs. 10.5 & 8.38). This regional hyperstabilization coupled with inadequate and imbalanced lumbopelvic control renders the mid/low lumbar spine levels more vulnerable.

CCC strategies are seen intermittently in those classified as APXS and consistently in those in the MS based on either a primary underlying APXS (Fig. 10.6) or PPXS (Fig. 10.7).

Co-contraction of the superficial muscles was described by Radebold et al.[14] in 2000 and is being increasingly reported in the literature.[15,16] In an editorial on muscle function and dysfunction in the spine, Cholewicki et al.[17] note that while there is consensus that the muscle activation patterns exhibited by patients with low back pain are different to healthy subjects, the interpretations of such findings are divergent. Van Dieën et al.[18] analyzed the literature with respect to the changed activation of the lumbar extensor muscles derived from studies adopting the pain–spasm–pain model and the pain

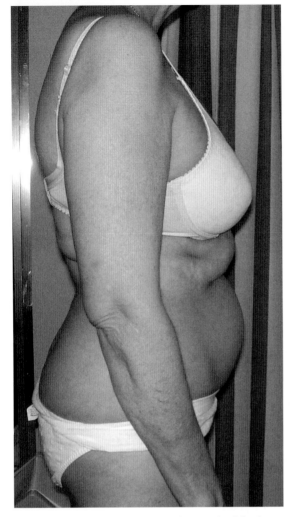

Fig 10.5 • Central conical cinch: the lower pole of the thorax is drawn in.

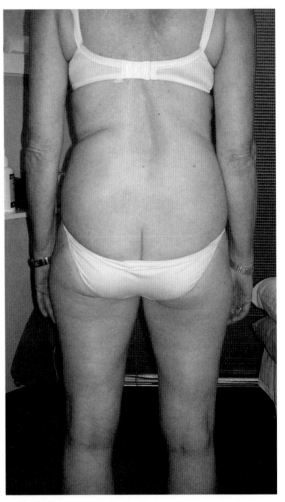

Fig 10.6 • Central conical cinch on a primary APXS picture. Note the asymmetry in the pelvis and the reaction around the thoracolumbar junction.

adaptation model. They found neither of the two models was unequivocally supported in the literature and proposed an alternate model which suggested that the altered trunk muscle recruitment is a *functional adaptation* to limit noxious tissues stress by limiting range and providing stabilization to the spine (Ch. 7 'Is the altered motor behavior observed in people...' p. 160) An appreciation of the central cinch patterns may help provide explanations for the diverse findings in the literature. They represent *evolving maladaptive responses which contribute to the development* of pain syndromes and which become further enhanced and entrenched in the presence of pain. Pain tends to facilitate activity in SGMS muscles and inhibit activity in SLMS muscles.

Overall effect of CCPs

The CCPs create significant impediments to healthy torso control as follows:

• The transmission of the segmental movement wave between the proximal limb girdles through the spine is variably impeded in three dimensions – flexion/extension, side bending and rotation.

• The small oscillating segmental shifts and adjustments necessary for equilibrium are blocked. Balance control begins to suffer.

• The bilateral activation hyperstabilizes the column 'centrally' compromising weight shift and thoracic aperture and inflation of the lung bases – particularly posterior basal. Many have absolutely no sense of diaphragmatic breathing. Postural support from the diaphragm and intra-abdominal pressure (IAP) is reduced. The breathing wave is damped thus the subtle segmental mobilizing effect of the breath is lost.

• Regional hyperstability sets the stage for segmental hypomobility and potential neural irritation (see Ch. 12). This is an interesting region neurologically in that all the lumbosacral nerve roots leave the cord in this region and the sympathetic thoracolumbar outflow extends to L2. This helps explain the common clinical finding of referred pelvic and leg pain when palpating the joints over the thoracolumbar junction. O'sullivan[19] notes the association between those patients who demonstrate abnormally high levels of muscle guarding and co-contraction, increased IAP and urge incontinence. Clinical observation also suggests that autonomic irritation from thoracolumbar segmental dysfunction may also contribute to this.

• The more 'fixed' one region of the spine becomes other regions and segments need to compensate creating a vicious pattern generating cycle.

'Butt-gripping' further affects function in ischial swing and pelvic floor myomechanics

The two primary pictures of dysfunction result in imbalanced control of pelvic tilt (Ch. 6, Part B) and the ability of the 'ischial swing' to adjust for weight shift in both the sagittal and frontal planes.

Clinically, in the APXS picture the pelvis predominantly shifts anteriorly and swings into posterior tilt reducing demand for postural activity of the gluteal group hence they are not well developed and show the signature 'saggy bum' or 'no bum' (Fig. 10.8).

In the primary PPXS picture the pelvis is more posterior and swings more into anterior tilt from more dominant erector spinae and psoas activity and poor abdominal activity. Although Janda described the glutei as 'weak' in his pelvic crossed syndrome,[3–5] clinically this is probably more the lateral glutei as most are observed to have well developed buttocks as could be expected in the necessity for an antigravity role in countering the

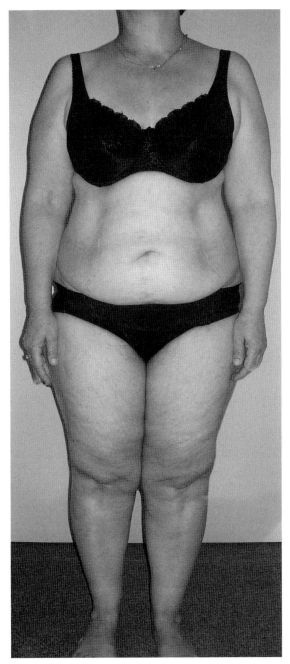

Fig 10.7 • Central conical cinch on a primary PPXS picture.

disallows adaptive lengthening of one side of the torso necessary in lateral weight transfer through the pelvis-legs.

• Poor stability for diaphragm descent in a CPC and CAC and the outer 'squeeze' in a CCC, limits diaphragm descent and expansion of the inferior

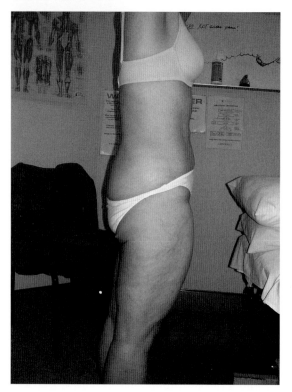

Fig 10.8 • The forward pelvis reduces postural demand in the buttocks with sometimes compensatory development of the anterior thigh muscles seen here.

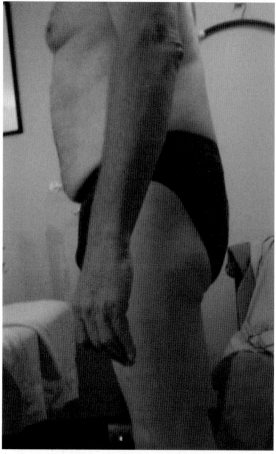

Fig 10.9 • Lateral view of mixed syndrome on a primary PPXS picture with 'butt grip' and dominant extensor activity in the trunk. Obturator activity is just discernable.

anterior pelvic tilt. Increased hamstring activity is also likely.[5]

Symptomatic of the MS is the adoption of more pronounced 'butt gripping' strategies in the PPXS group to help bring the pelvis forward and counter the activity of psoas. Described by Lee,[6] 'butt gripping' posteriorly tilts the pelvic girdle and flexes the L4/5 and L5/S1 joints and is associated with intra-pelvic postural change and narrowing of the inferior pelvis. Clenching the buttocks involves a synergy of gluteus maximus with the deep obturator group and the pelvic floor muscles (PFM) and hamstrings. The buttocks are more developed and the hips are externally rotated. Lewit[20] notes the synergistic relationship between the PFM and gluteus maximus in helping to control the anal sphincter.

Clenching the buttocks helps explain why those who appear to be extensor dominant and classified as PPXS show a proclivity for posterior tilt and flexion over the lower lumbar levels while still demonstrating dominant extensor activity in the trunk (Figs. 10.9 & 10.10). While bringing the pelvis more forward and neutralizing the hip flexion action of

psoas it probably shunts psoas' effect more into the spine, locking the thoracolumbar junction more forward in extension. Reduced eccentric lengthening of psoas during lateral weight transfer reduces postural adjustment through the thoracolumbar spine.

Increased buttock development and/or gripping in a MS from a primary APXS picture is more likely to result from habit, specific exercise endeavors and training effect (Fig. 4.4).

Clenching the buttocks is usually associated with hip external rotation and abduction with knee extension and there is little oscillatory postural activity in the lower kinetic chain. This directly influences pelvic floor myomechanics where the inferior bowl is mostly in the 'closed' shortened position and freedom in the ischial swing is reduced in both the sagittal and frontal plane.

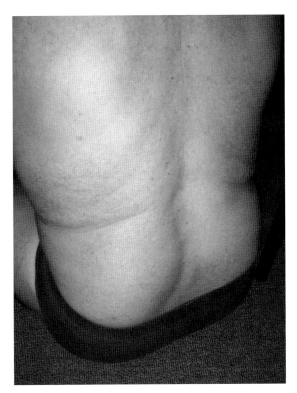

Fig 10.10 • Posterior view of mixed syndrome on a primary PPXS picture. Chronic 'butt gripping' and posterior pelvic rotation combined with dominant extensor activity in the trunk has resulted in an observable 'break' in the lumbar spine which is the predominant source of his symptoms.

The prevalence of MS and APXS syndromes point to an increasing incidence in the population where more and more of the pelvis assumes a position of more consistent posterior tilt, sacral counternutation and inferior bowl 'closure'. Stress urinary incontinence (SUI) has been associated with increased PFM and external oblique activity[21] (CAC) and altered recruitment, endurance and strength of the PFM.[22] Posturomovement wise the ability to close and in particular to open the inferior pelvic bowl is very important. Failure to re-educate eccentric PFM control in functional pelvic movement patterns may help explain why specific PFM training is commonly associated with improvement rather than cure and the benefits are not necessarily maintained long term.[23]

In the MS, the active 'holding patterns' around both the thoracolumbar junction and the hip/pelvis result in segmental dysfunction causing reactive facilitation in both the anterior and posterior hip/thigh muscle groups which show variable patterns of restriction.

Lateral shift or 'list' patterns of the trunk

These are generally an acute or subacute manifestation of a chronic problem and tend to reoccur in times of exacerbation. Left untreated, the neuromyoarticular patterns become further entrenched and more chronic (Fig. 10.11).

As explained, the development of the adaptive CCPs leads to varying forms of hyperstabilization around the thoracolumbar junction (T/L/J). Normal studies[24] have shown that lateral translations of the thorax relative to the pelvis are significant with most lateral flexion occurring at L1 but that segmental rotation angles for lateral flexion were largest at L3/4 (6.2°); L4/5 (5.7°); L2/3 (3.9°). When movement cannot occur though the T/L/J, the lower levels become more vulnerable to trivial provocations over time. In response to an acute segmental joint dysfunction, the associated muscles go into spasm and the trunk posture shifts or 'lists'. Lee[6] describes this as a multisegmental rotoscoliosis of the thoracolumbar spine coupled with a lateral shift of the thorax relative to the pelvis with associated intrapelvic torsion, internal rotation of one hip and external rotation of the other. O'sullivan[25,26] further

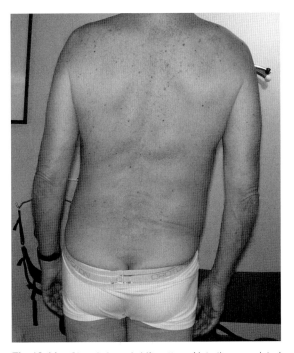

Fig 10.11 • Chronic lateral shift pattern. Note the associated buttock clenching and posterior cinch behavior.

describes it as usually unidirectional; with a loss of lumbar segmental lordosis and an associated lateral shift at the affected level; local multifidus atrophy and low tone on the contralateral side yet evident tone on the ipsilateral side; dominant thoracolumbar erector spinae activity; an inability to load the thoracolumbar spine directly over the pelvis when standing on one leg. During gait there is an observed tendency to weight transfer through the trunk and upper body rather than through the pelvis. Apart from an inability to satisfactorily co-activate SLMS synergies, movement tests demonstrate dominant activation of SGMS muscles including quadratus lumborum, lumbar erector spinae, and ipsilateral superficial multifidus associated with bracing of the abdominal wall and loss of breathing control.[25]

Psoas has been considered as one of the prime perpetrators in the development of adolescent idiopathic scoliosis.[27] Together with quadratus it is a sitting duck for being held primarily responsible for driving much of the lateral shift posture in the acute and subacute trunk list because of its activity in lateral trunk flexion and postural stability.[28] Clinically, unilateral segmental irritation of any level between T12 and L5 is capable of inducing unilateral psoas spasm and particularly so if the T12/L1; L1/2 segments are irritable. It has been proposed that when psoas contracts it produces extension of the upper lumbar levels and flexion of the lower,[9,10] and if only one psoas is facilitated, an ipsilateral side bending of the lumbar spine and rotation of the pelvis also occurs. The acute trunk list is consistent with the pain–spasm–pain response and represents a good example of an acute maladaptive response[1,29] superimposed upon a chronic evolving picture of dysfunction – the 'underlying mechanism driving the disorder'.[29] In a study of 50 patients with unilateral back pain, co-existing atrophy of psoas and multifidus was found at the symptomatic level on the side of pain; 48% occurred at L4/5 and 42% at L5/S1.[30] Effective treatment of the responsible joints should settle the acute muscle spasm and *then* movement re-education to redress the underlying dysfunction can commence.

Shoulder Crossed Syndrome (SXS) (refer to Ch. 6, Part C)

Common to all three pelvic syndromes is the variable coexistence of the shoulder crossed syndrome. Described by Janda,[2–4] this describes the typical changes in the postural alignment and movement function of the upper torso and shoulder girdle resulting from imbalanced myofascial activity. One diagonal of the 'cross' is formed by the overactive and tight obliquely opposite anterior chest muscles and the cervicothoracic extensors. The opposite underactive oblique pair consists of the deep neck flexors and lower scapular stabilizers (Figs 10.12–10.15).

The presence of the SXS substantially alters the regional biomechanical conditions[2] and clinically, in varying degree it underlies practically all cervicogenic syndromes[2] as well as many upper limb pain syndromes. The associated altered dynamic scapula control underlies 'shoulder impingement problems',[31] 'rotator cuff problems', 'frozen shoulder' and so on. Biomechanically, an evident SXS will also affect the alignment and related function in the lower torso, in particular around the thoracolumbar junction. Janda considered that the presence of this syndrome 'is just part of a general muscle imbalance involving the whole body'.[2] He saw his upper and lower crossed syndromes as 'key regions' where muscle imbalance starts to develop or where it is most pronounced. Wherever the imbalance starts

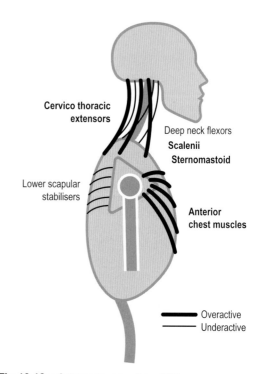

Fig 10.12 • Schematic view of the SXS.

Labels in figure:
Cervico thoracic extensors
Deep neck flexors
Scalenii
Sternomastoid
Lower scapular stabilisers
Anterior chest muscles
Overactive
Underactive

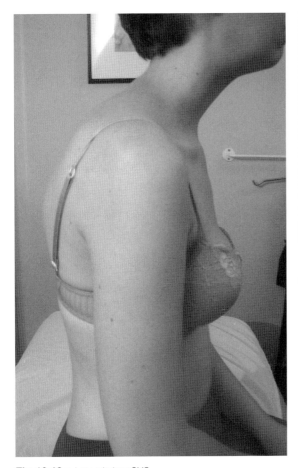

Fig 10.13 • Lateral view SXS.

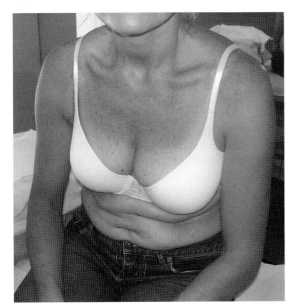

Fig 10.14 • Anterior view SXS.

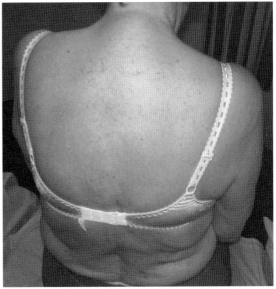

Fig 10.15 • Posterior view SXS.

it will tend to spread to involve the other region in time. The dysfunction in each region begins to affect that in the other.

In principle, the crossed syndromes describe the dysfunction in the two proximal limb girdles which not only affects control of the large ball and socket joints but importantly, also that of the cervical and lumbar spines and the spine as a whole.

SXS: characterized by altered sagittal alignment of upper pole of body

• *Head and neck*. The head is postured forward in relation to the thorax and the line of gravity (Fig. 10.13 & Fig. 10.16). Its balance on the occipital condyles is disturbed and the cervicocranial junction (CCJ) levels (C0/1/2) become stiffer in extension.[32] The cervicothoracic junction (CTJ) is held and becomes stiffer in flexion. The stress at the CTJ extends down to T4 provoking not only shoulder or cervical pain but even chest pain simulating angina pectoris.[32] Clinically, the forward head posture is usually associated with a dominant posteriorly tilted pelvis.

• *Thorax*. An increased thoracic kyphosis particularly of the upper dorsal segments[3] including a 'dome' (Ch. 8, Thoracic dysfunction) and probably a 'dowager's hump' over the

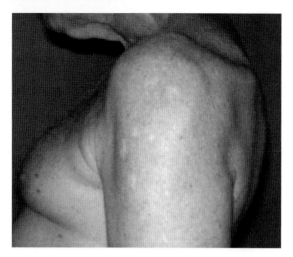

Fig 10.16 • The head is postured forward in relation to the thorax and the line of gravity. While a rather extreme example, the point is well illustrated.

Table 10.2 Patterns of changed myofascial activity seen in the SXS

Overactive/tight muscles	Underactive/weak muscles
Upper trapezius	Lower scapula stabilizers
Levator scapulae	• Middle and lower
Pectoralis major and minor	trapezius
Sternocleidomastoid	• Rhomboids
Masseter. temporalis digastric	• Serratus anterior
Suboccipital group: the recti and obliques[2,4]	Deep cervicocranial flexors; suprahyoid, mylohyoid2
Flexors of the upper limb[4]	Author also suggests:
Cervicothoracic erector spinae[4]	• Deep posterior intrinsic muscles extending from the
Author also suggests:	occiput down to the 'dome
• Serratus posterior superior	• Posterior region of
• *Lateral fibres* of latissimus dorsi	latissimus?
• Scalenes?	
• Serratus anterior?	

cervicothoracic junction is particularly significant. The thoracic kyphosis generally increases with age, often significantly,[33] and is probably most developed in females attributed to reduced physical activity and muscle tone.[34] In a radiographic study, Boyle et al.[33] found the mean location of the cervicothoracic curve inflection point moved from T3 towards C7/T1 with increasing age.

• **Shoulder girdle**. Posterior elevation and protraction of the shoulder girdle with 'round shoulders' and a variable degree of inferior winging of the scapulae which are also abducted and downwardly rotated.[2]

Overactivity and shortness of certain muscles and underactivity of others becomes evident. Those described by Janda[2,32] with some further additions are shown in Table 10.2.

Twenty years ago Janda wrote[2] 'controversy remains regarding the longus colli, longus capitis, rectus capitis anterior, the scaleni, subscapularis, supraspinatus and the rotator cuff'.... 'many concepts may well undergo change'. Janda considered serratus anterior and scalenes as 'phasic' muscles'[4] yet clinically their relative overactivity is often compelling. Janda did not include the spinal intrinsic muscles – multifidus, interspinales, rotators longus and brevis and levator costae brevis. Muscle activity over the posterior aspect of the upper pole of the thorax is often significantly diminished and

could even involve the more superficial muscles such as semispinalis and spinalis. Clinically, the interscapular region is frequently flattened with poor muscle bulk indicating deficient tone and activity. Commonly intersegmental movement through the region and medial scapular control is difficult.

Importance of shoulder girdle muscles in generating upper torso pain syndromes

The important relationship between the shoulder girdle musculature and the aetiology of cervical spine syndromes was well understood by Janda.[32] He stressed the following points:

• The neck–shoulder complex is strongly influenced by the limbic system,[2] impaired function of which leads to increased muscle tone which primarily affects this region. Hence when under stress, increased neck muscle activity readily occurs particularly in the upper trapezius (UT) and levator scapulae (LS). This activation is so common that their EMG activity is used as an objective measure in some psychological experiments.

• Fear activates the shoulder muscles in the 'defense reflexes' – to protect the head, we raise and elevate the shoulders. We protect the front of our body with our arms. Habitually folding the arms in front of our body is a common 'defensive' posture.

• Probably due to these reflexes above, we tend to simultaneously activate the shoulders girdle muscles and have a tendency for mirror movements with both arms which may explain the often seen irradiation of muscle activity to the contralateral side. Conversely we are in general, more accustomed to move the lower limbs alternatively. Janda[35,36] notes the similarity between the distribution of muscle tightness seen in postural defects and those occurring from cerebral lesions resulting in spasticity. In the upper body, the pectorals, upper trapezius and levator scapulae and the flexors of the upper limb are usually involved.

• The cervical muscles not only maintain and control the position of the head but also, all movements within the face as well as many other functions in the head area provoke cervical muscle activity. Any movement of the eyes immediately provokes activity in the neck muscles.

• The shoulder girdle and cervical muscles have a pronounced stabilizing function. There is practically no movement of the upper limb which does not involve their activation.

• In addition, the increasing incidence of sedentary work practices involving reading, writing and, in particular, computer use for long periods of time requires the majority of the 'muscle work' to come from within the upper pole of the body in sustained, relatively unphysiological postures.

Predominant patterns of shoulder girdle use create predictable patterns of muscle dysfunction

The extensive scope of the attachments of the large shoulder girdle muscles to the thorax and axial skeleton means that any alterations in their length/tension relationships exact a significant toll on axial alignment and control as well as disturbing scapular position and control and shoulder and upper limb function. Consider the more habitual patterns of modern man's upper limb use. Open chain upper extremity movements are generally bilateral, with the arms down in front of the body performing actions requiring eye/hand coordination. The head, upper spine and the upper limb are consistently

employed in variable degrees of a 'more total flexor pattern'. By comparison, arm movements up above the head or behind rarely occur. In general, the more consistent pattern of use predominantly involves the flexors, protractors and depressors of the shoulder girdle. Thus we tend to see shortening in the anterior chest muscles (ACMs) – the pectorals, serratus and lateral fibres of latissimus dorsi. The pattern of flexor dominance and tightness is carried into the upper limb muscles also. The girdle posturally hangs down and forward and in movement it is consistently pulled down and forward. This is related to an evident corresponding underactivity and 'stretch weakness'[37,38] in the muscles which stabilize the girdle posteroinferiorly – the lower scapular stabilizers – middle and lower trapezius (M&LT), rhomboids and the adjacent spinal muscles (see Fig 4.6). The orientation and position of the girdle changes. Inadequate inferior stability from M&LT allows the scapula to be pulled superiorly by dominant UT and LS activity and tip forward in the sagittal plane because of pectoral pull on the clavicle and coracoid.

The combined activity of the ACMs can also be likened to a 'cinch' becoming a common dysfunctional strategy for initiating and sustaining spinal postures, particularly if weight bearing through the upper limbs. When equilibrium is threatened or when moving from one body position to another, the observed habitual responses will generally involve this 'cinch' in the adoption of upper limb 'fixing' pulling, pushing or holding strategies to compensate for deficient support from SLMS activity, in particular from that around the pelvis. Try standing up from sitting yourself without using your arms!

This imbalance in the myomechanics of the girdle functionally fixes the upper pole of the thorax contributing to the development of a 'dome' and an increased kyphosis in general. The cervical and lumbar spines being more mobile compensate. The resultant increased stress on the neck disturbs segmental mechanics and can result in segmental irritation which further drives the overactivity in some muscles, e.g. irritation of the lower cervical segments contributes to hyperfacilitation of the pectorals creating a pattern generating cycle.

This anterior/inferior tethering of the girdle and the resultant increase and stiffening of the kyphosis together with reduced SLMS activity and poor pelvic control are probably the most important factors influencing the alignment and control of the entire spine.

Consequences of SXS

Changed alignment changes function through the junctions

The altered alignment means that gravitational and related forces impose eccentric loading stresses on the axial column with increased tensile and compressive stresses. The functional movement block within the CCJ and the CTJ means the mid cervical levels are forced to compensate, becoming relatively stressed and over mobile in posture and movement. Fairly predictable patterns of segmental joint hyper/hypomobility ensue (Ch. 8, 'Biomechanical changes...'). The altered alignment and 'fixing' of the CTJ and the upper thoracic spine further affects the position and control of the shoulder girdle. The lack of movement through the thorax and 'dome' means attempts to 'straighten up' result in CPC strategies over the thoracolumbar junction, serving to further hyperstabilize this region.

Head control suffers

Positioning of the head in space is regulated in a much finer way than any other motor function or body control mechanism.[2] The joints and muscles of the region also play an important role in equilibrium of the whole body. The upper cervical joints and muscles contain a large proportion of afferent fibres and are more sensitive to any alterations of proprioceptive input such as occurs with any joint restriction.

Altered alignment of the head causes/effects changes in the local neuromuscular posturomovement demand with shortening of the suboccipitals, dominance of sternocleidomastoid (SCM) and related weakness of the deep craniocervical flexors (CCF). Lifting the head in supine results in the chin leading the movement (Fig. 10.17). SCM can be so hyperactive/short that the muscle is still prominent when attempting to flex the occiput on the neck (Fig. 10.18). This dysfunction has attracted quite a lot of research interest. Delayed postural responses and reduced EMG activity in the CCF have been shown in subjects with chronic neck pain.[39,40] Similarly, objective weakness, reduced low load endurance and inaccuracy have also been shown.[41] The diminished flexor activity is associated with increased SGMS activity – in particular from the SCM, UT and LS. Specific *low load* exercise retraining of the CCF over 6 weeks has been shown

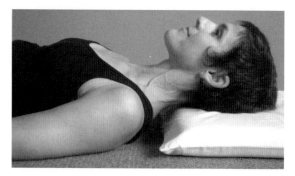

Fig 10.17 • When the deep neck flexors are underactive the sternomastoid is prominent and the chin leads the movement.

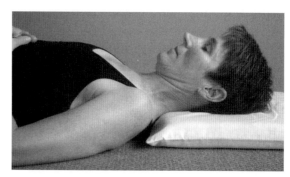

Fig 10.18 • When the deep neck flexors are engaged the chin drops and the back of the neck lengthens. Chronic overactivity and shortening in the sternocleidomastoid can mean inadequate lengthening in this action.

to decrease the EMG of the SCM and improve both the range of craniocervical flexion and the EMG of the CCF.[42] However, the reduction in SCM hyperactivity is not necessarily transferable to functional tasks.[43] Indeed SCM activity can be so entrenched, particularly in those with breathing pattern disorders (Ch. 8) that attempting to activate the CCF instead activates SCM. In a healthy study, Cagnie et al.[44] found that by asking for CCF on a slow expiration, SCM activity was less. A study monitoring activity of splenius capitis and sternomastoid during brief isometric cervical flexion and extension in chronic tension type headache suffers demonstrated greater coactivation of antagonist muscles.[45]

Sustained static loading of the head and neck in work related postures invariably tends to result in the head–neck moving forward at the CTJ [46] requiring sustained activity in LS and UT and causing associated neck and shoulder discomfort.[47] Increased activity levels in the cervical erector spinae and UT have been shown in children aged 4 – 17 when using a computer.[48] When these altered neck postures are adopted enough, the person begins to have an altered perception of what the correct alignment is.[49] The sustained forward loading into flexion at the CTJ means that over time, the joints stiffen in flexion. When looking up or extending the neck the mid cervical levels then bear the brunt. The forward head posture starts to become incorporated into movement. Plummer[50] notes that the great majority of people markedly protract and extend their head–neck when getting up and down from sitting. The dysfunction becomes self perpetuating.

Mutual dysfunction between the thorax and shoulder girdle

Thoracic joint dysfunction is often overlooked as many pain syndromes do not directly implicate it; however, segmental and rib dysfunction is implicated in a plethora of clinical symptoms, e.g. nausea and headache. The sympathetic outflow is confined to the thoracolumbar region between T1 and L3.[8] The thoracic sympathetic ganglia rest against the heads of the ribs.[8] Functionally 'there is the greatest possible integration between the autonomic and the somatic system'.[51] Increased activity and shortening in the ACMs and the lateral fibres of LD pulls the girdle forward if the hands are free or conversely flexes the thorax if the upper limbs are stable. Both ways the posterior structures in the upper pole become subjected to more repetitive postural and movement loading and the ability to extend the thorax decreases. Likewise free movements of the ribs under the girdle become lost.

Many shoulder and upper limb pain disorders are particularly associated with dysfunction in the levels within the upper pole of the thorax. The scapula becomes more tethered to the chest wall in a more elevated abducted and downwardly rotated position. Janda[2] points out that the angle of the glenoid fossa then alters becoming more vertical and affects the myofascial stability of the glenohumeral joint as the supraspinatus is required to constantly contract in order to stop 'head drop'. This helps explain why its tendon often shows so much attrition. The forward and abducted scapula position also induces more sustained abnormal postural holding from teres and infraspinatus which punches the head forward in the glenoid and limits abduction and elevation at the glenoid. Attempts at retracting the scapula invariably result in adducting the humerus, and instead activating teres/infraspinatus which

serve to further abduct the scapula. The reduced scapula and glenoid stability means that most free or stable upper limb postures and movements result in over activation of the ACMs antero/inferiorly and UT and LS postero/superiorly. The imbalanced myofascial activity results in stress on the neck and the shoulder and the thoracic spine.

Janda[2-5] considered serratus anterior a 'phasic' muscle and prone to weakness however clinically it is generally adaptively short, may be weak but is also often strong! Eccentric control is often defective particularly when working from a fixed upper limb. Clinically, serratus dysfunction is a common finding yet this author could only find one other reference to its overactivity and related overactivity of upper trapezius.[52] Serratus shortness holds the scapula more protracted and limits the ability to bring the thorax forward into extension when the girdle is fixed. Consequently, weight bearing through the upper limb then relies more upon anteriorly 'locking in' or 'cinching' with the ACMs and the thorax becomes hyperstabilized anteriorly and the dome perpetuated further affecting the cervical spine. True winging of the scapula is not that common clinically. What is often construed as 'winging' is more often the result of deficient activity in the lower scapular stabilizers not balancing increased pectoral, serratus and teres activity. The medial and inferior borders protrude (Fig. 10.19). The imbalanced activity between the LSS (MT: LT) and serratus also disrupts the force couple producing upward scapular rotation which is then further compensated by hyperactivity in LS and UT.

Tightness in the lateral fibres of latissimus further contributes to the problem. Frequently, the back pain patient cannot raise his arms because his shoulder structures are so tight! If he can, he has

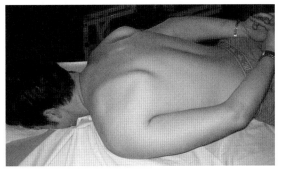

Fig 10.19 • The anterior chest muscles are winning here. The paucity of tone in the regional intrinsic extensors and the lower scapular stabilizers is obvious. Note also the active CPC.

difficulty sustaining the action. Attempts to do so result in compensatory movement in the cervical and thoracolumbar region (Fig. 10.20). Clinically, many LBP patients have coexisting shoulder problems and vice versa. The anteroinferior myofascial shoulder tightness acts like a functional 'tether' reducing the available range for lateral reaching rotary and extension movements of the upper body. The thorax is restricted in lateral elongation and opening necessary in weight shift and many unilateral limb activities.

The spatially altered scapula position influences its appropriate stabilization to support arm movements. A study of 53 junior elite tennis players found scapula dyskinesia in 43%, all of whom also showed a reduced passive and dynamic reduction of the subacromial space on ultrasound.[53] In a nice study observing the ability of healthy subjects to correctly orient their scapula to the neutral myofascial position, Mottram et al.[54] found the most consistent movements that the subjects needed to be taught were upward rotation in the frontal plane and posterior rotation in the sagittal plane. They found that all parts of trapezius demonstrated significant activity in maintaining the correct position while LD did not. Clinically it appears that more common pattern dysfunction in LD is probable underactivity of its posterior region in the synergy with MT and LT which provides dynamic postero/inferior stability to the scapula. Corresponding related shortness and increased activity in the lateral fibres of latissimus limiting movement at the glenohumeral joint is commonly found clinically.

Many therapeutic shoulder interventions rely upon stretching and strengthening the rotator cuff muscles. It is suggested that addressing the altered axiohumeral-scapular myofascial and related thoracic dysfunction will yield more promising results.

Further contributing factors

Variable combinations of the following also play into the dysfunction picture:

• Dysfunctional breathing patterns (Ch. 8) where the accessory muscles of respiration including the ACMs are activated during ordinary breathing

• Adverse training effect e.g. poorly conceived gym and exercise routines which over emphasize contemporary aesthetics over function – the desire

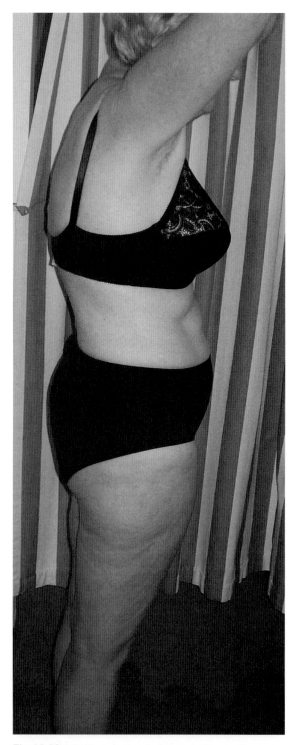

Fig 10.20 • Evident shortness anterior in the chest muscles contributes to a dome, limits freedom in the shoulder and creates compensatory movement in the cervical and lumbar spines.

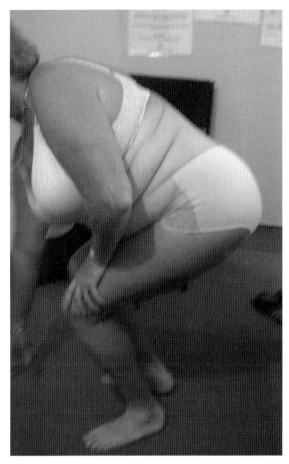

Fig 10.21 • Pushing down through the arms to come up is common when there is reduced dynamic control through the lower kinetic chain.

for 'good pecs' and 'a six pack' abdominals which further stiffen the thorax and reinforce the tendency to dominant upper body flexor synergies.

• Overuse of upper limb 'fixing strategies' (particularly in the elderly) to compensate for decreased lumbopelvic control and equilibrium reactions within the body (Fig. 10.21). Watch even young people in the train clinging and hanging off the bars instead of resolving the perturbations through the legs and trunk!

Stratification or Layer Syndrome (also see Ch. 8)

Described by Janda,[3–5] strata or 'layers' of muscle hyper and hypoactivity can be observed within the flexor and extensor muscle systems. When both the

pelvic and shoulder crossed syndromes are evident they are also expressed in this syndrome. Janda felt this was the most important of his 'syndromes',[55] its presence a sign of poor prognosis because the fixed patterns of muscle imbalance reflect severe and deeply fixed CNS dysregulation accompanied by very bad movement patterns.[3,4] However, he also says 'this syndrome is not rare. On the contrary it can be seen quite often in sportsmen who have trained heavily without precise check ups'.[3] Janda's genius is confirmed! Observing the posturomovement patterns of subjects with spinal pain disorders consistently reveals common patterns of response in the manner he described. The presence and related effects of this syndrome explains the frequent coexistence of cervical and lumbar and other pain syndromes in many patients.

The construct of the layer syndrome helps simplify and see at a glance the more common patterns of response and to predictably know what responses to expect when retraining posturomovement control. Viewing the patient's torso from the front and particularly from behind, we see layers or bands of overactive and hence bulky muscles alternating with regions of under active muscles with flattened contours. This provides clues to the probable habitual activation patterns of various muscle groups. Essentially there is 'emptiness' and poor contribution from the muscle groups over the posterior aspect of the proximal limb girdles and excessive yet variable central axial activity.

It is more easily observed in the ***posterior view*** (Figs. 10.22 & 10.23 and also Figs. 8.21 & 8.22).

In the ***anterior view*** Janda thought the most striking symptomatology was in the anterior abdominal wall where rectus abdominis and transversus show weak whereas the obliques are hyperactive.[3] This is seen as a groove on the lateral edge of the rectus (Fig. 10.24). Imbalance between the upper and lower abdominal wall is also apparent.

In the ***posterior layer syndrome*** there is poor muscular stability over the lumbopelvic and the mid dorsal/interscapular region and consistent hyperactivity in the cervicothoracic and particularly the thoracolumbar extensors. A normal study found that the lumbar fibres of longissimus thoracis and iliocostalis lumborum fatigued more than the thoracic fibres.[56] In the anterior Layer Syndrome there is poor muscular stability and support over the front of the cervical and lumbar regions.

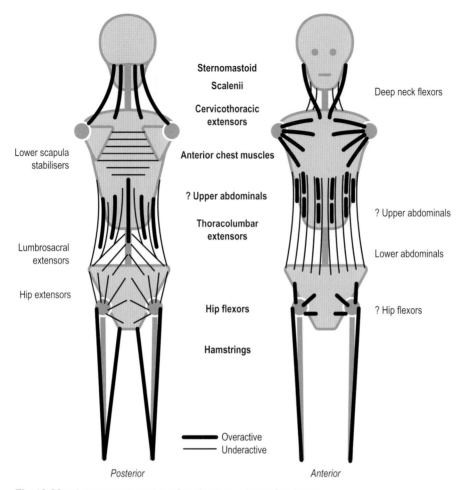

Sternomastoid

Scalenii

Cervicothoracic extensors

Deep neck flexors

Lower scapula stabilisers

Anterior chest muscles

? Upper abdominals

Thoracolumbar extensors

? Upper abdominals

Lumbrosacral extensors

Lower abdominals

Hip extensors

Hip flexors

? Hip flexors

Hamstrings

Overactive
Underactive

Posterior   *Anterior*

Fig 10.22 • Schematic view of the Stratification or Layer Syndrome.

It is important to appreciate that this pattern of trunk muscle activity *consistently plays out in all posturomovement's* e.g. reaching up, bending over, when on all fours and so on. Predictably, in time, this more obligatory pattern of muscle activity causes some regions of the axial skeleton to become hyperstabilized and stiff while other regions become undercontrolled and relatively mobile.

Appreciating this pattern of response in muscle activity presents a significant challenge to relearning effective therapeutic movement control. Attempts to facilitate activity of one hypoactive group will invariably risk early and over activation of the already dominant muscles, e.g. gaining activation of lumbar multifidus or lower scapular stabilizers without dominance of thoracolumbar extensors (CPC) and/or cervicothoracic extensors.

Belted Torso Syndrome (BTS)

This construct attempts to help further clarify torso dysfunction in a schematic composite which summarizes the more common patterns of muscle action as described in the pelvic crossed and layer or stratification syndromes. It is representative of more 'end stage' markedly entrenched neuromuscular dysfunction. This representation is a close up lens which helps to appreciate the dysfunction that occurs around the central torso and the body's centre of gravity in the pelvis. It just so happens that the conventional belt line at the waist seems to be a functional demarcation line! There appears to be a consistent difference in the muscle activation patterns above and below the belt in practically all our patients – variably hyperactive above the belt yet

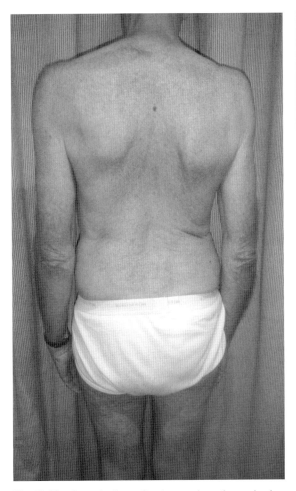

Fig 10.23 • Posterior Layer Syndrome where thoracolumbar extensors are prime.

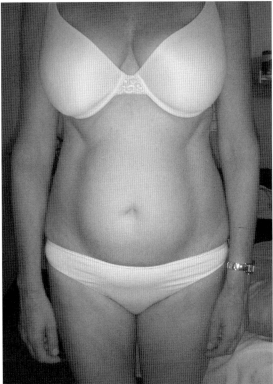

Fig 10.24 • The anterior Layer Syndrome is principally manifested by imbalance in the abdominal wall and increased activity in the anterior chest muscles.

consistently and appreciably hypoactive below. Defective spatial control of the pelvis is a universal observation it seems. The patient's presenting pattern will be a reflection of his primary pelvic dysfunction picture. This is represented in Figures 10.25–10.27 and Table 10.3.

The understanding of this consistently observed overactivation of muscles around the body's centre of gravity seen in our patients was greatly assisted by Hanna's[57] notion of the 'Reflexes of stress'. (Ch. 6) Stress is a response to both good things and bad and creates *unconscious, involuntary rapid reflex motor acts* which *primarily affect the muscles around the body's centre of gravity*. They are normal adaptive reflexes essential to our survival, which engage the entire nervous system and musculature. However, when repeatedly triggered in modern man, they *become habitual background neuromuscular activity*. The reflex response begins to become the postural set from which they move. The effects of emotional state on posture and consequent movement are becoming increasingly acknowledged.[58,59]

Disturbed central internal control

- The diaphragm ideally functions as a 'central piston' across the centre of the body. Imbalanced action between the two muscle systems and above and below the belt hampers its efficient action.
- Iliacus and psoas function 'at' the centre of gravity of the body; it appears:
  - psoas and iliacus both appear under active in APXS
  - show imbalanced activity between the two in PPXS (psoas over active; iliacus under active)
  - show variable findings in MS

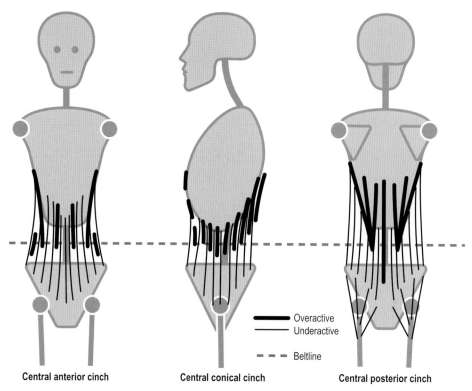

Overactive
Underactive
- - - Beltline

Central anterior cinch   Central conical cinch   Central posterior cinch

Fig 10.25 • Schematic view of the Belted Torso Syndrome.

- **PFM**. Imbalanced contribution to the LPU synergy either underactive or overactive with timing problems. Postural collapse in the APXS group reduces dynamic function of the diaphragm and transversus abdominus and because of their close functional synergy is also likely to reduce the resting tone of the PFM.[60] Poor activity in multifidus means balance in the force couple controlling the sacrum is disturbed and so it is generally counternutated with altered reciprocal PFM activity.[61] The obturator group hyperactivity also seen in this group and those classified as MS means that increased PFM tone is also likely. Lee and Vleeming[62] suggested probable imbalance in the floor with a tendency to under activation of the anterior floor and overactivation of the posterior floor. Clinically this is apparent. Dominance of hamstring and gluteal muscle activity is likely to be associated with posterior PFM shortening.[63] It is also common to find clinical relationships between PFM dysfunction syndromes such as SUI and the central 'cinch' muscle hyperactivation patterns which hyperstabilize the thoracolumbar region, creating segmental joint dysfunction and resultant altered autonomic effects.

In general, the emptiness is in the proximal limb girdles with poor initiation and balanced control of movement through them offset by reliance on the 'CCPs' instead. In addition to regional hyperactivity around the central torso there is in general an increased reliance upon upper limb use and in particular anterior shoulder girdle overactivity. Similar to the 'CCPs' we have termed this 'pectoral cinch' which disturbs balanced co-activation through the girdle.

Many axial patterns of movement are initiated from these 'cinch' strategies.

The 'inferior tethers'

When BTS is present, the dysfunctional patterns of muscle hyperactivity serve to 'tether' the proximal limb girdles and the centre of the body disturbing axial patterns of control (Fig. 10.28) as follows:

- The inferior pole of the thorax becomes more constricted by hyperactive superficial muscles, assuming a more conical shape at the base. Rather than resemble a 'cylinder' (Ch. 6, Part A),

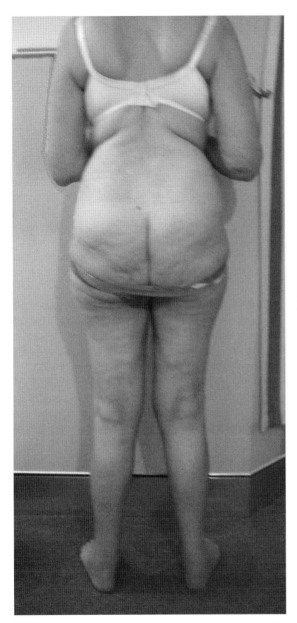

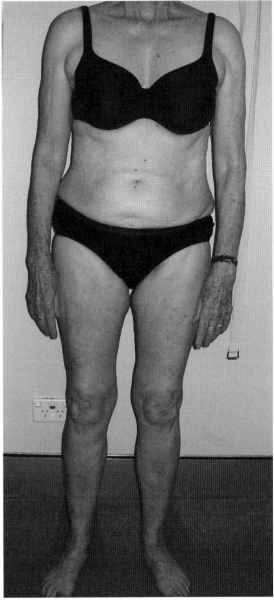

Fig 10.26 • Belted Torso Syndrome posterior view: note the inferiorly 'tethered' pelvis and thorax in both views.

Fig 10.27 • Belted torso syndrome anterior view: note the abducted legs and 'central fixing' in both views.

which is open in the centre, the body tends to be constricted in the centre, resembling an hour glass. This limits the expansive function of the thoracic diaphragm.

• Similarly the pelvic girdle is also constricted over its base resembling an inverted pyramid.[6] The lower pelvic bowl is more 'closed' while the upper is more 'open'. The pelvic diaphragm is compromised.

• The shoulder girdle is functionally 'tethered' antero-inferiorly disturbing shoulder girdle function and contributing to propagation of the 'dome' thereby affecting control patterns of the entire axial spine as well as feeding into syndromes in the upper pole of the 'body cylinder'.

In the BTS, the 'inferior tethers' thus restrict the pelvic and thoracic diaphragms disturbing the close

Table 10.3 Summary features of belted torso syndrome

Hyperactivity/over-stabilizing by the muscles acting above the belt

Posteriorly: a central posterior cinch in PPXS & MS; more intermittently in APXS
Anteriorly: as a central anterior cinch in APXS
Combination: in a central conical cinch in MS

Hypoactivity/defective posturomovement control below the belt

Anteriorly:
• Whole abdominal wall in PPXS
• Lower abdominal wall in APXS and MS
Posteriorly – lumbar multifidus is generally under active, particularly the deep fibres:
• Over the lower levels in PPXS, APXS and MS
• Also over higher levels in APXS

Disturbed internal function at the belt line creates a central disconnect

Centrally: altered co-activation patterns between the diaphragm, abdominals (particularly transversus) and psoas disturbs internal support provided by the breathing mechanism, IAP and psoas

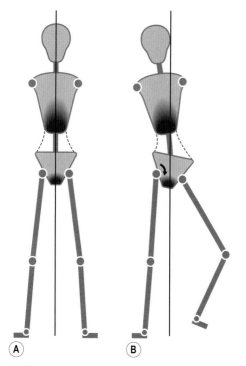

Fig 10.28 • Conceptual coronal plane view of the 'inferior tethers' acting over the lower pole of the thorax and pelvis change the shape and function of the 'body cylinder' (A). Note the effect during lateral weight transfer in (B) and compare with Figs. 6.24 & 6.36.

functional relationship between them. Greenman[64] suggests that the tentorium cerebelli can be viewed as the diaphragm of the craniosacral mechanism. In health the three diaphragms should function in a synchronous fashion. Upledger[65] regards the diaphragms as transverse support systems for the longitudinally oriented fascial lamina, being an integral part of the system and essential to its functional integrity. Disturbance in the diaphragms is thus likely to disturb the whole fascial system, modulation of the internal thoraco-abdominal internal pressure systems as well as influence the sucking action upon venous and lymphatic return. The functional importance of the respiratory diaphragm should not be underestimated.

The BTS helps us recognize that the most significant features common to all the other clinical syndromes are that antigravity support, breathing and the distribution of general body muscle activation patterns are conceptually somewhat 'upside down':
• The lower torso is underactive and poorly controlled on the legs. Deficient control of the pelvis in all its roles affects lumbopelvic function, effective control of the body on the legs and antigravity support as a result of what Bartenieff termed 'The Dead Seven Inches'.[66,67] Like frightened animals it is common for the tail bone to be tucked under. Significant challenge in weight

shift, limb loading and controlling antigravity hip flexion through range appears universal. Functionally, being 'dead on their legs' is prevalent.

• Altered function of the respiratory and pelvic diaphragms affects axial alignment and control. Inadequate diaphragm excursion and central expansion with an excess of accessory muscle respiration and upper body tension.

• Excess SGMS activity occurs in the upper body, as the patient attempts to 'hold himself up'. Increased role of the upper body in equilibrium and support.

The kinematic strategies adopted for forward bending will tend to reflect the basic primary patterns of dysfunctional control. Those who are more APXS dominant will tend to central axial folding because of poor pelvic hip control and tendency to flexor dominance. Those whose picture is more the picture PPXS will show more dominant axial holding because of poor hip–pelvis control and the tendency for extensor dominance. Both overly rely on 'hamstrings hang' and show poor axial co-activation (Fig. 10.29).

The BTS represents more end stage dysfunction when altered neuromyo-articular patterns of dysfunction are quite entrenched. Many 'diagnoses' such as 'spinal stenosis, 'instability' can be seen to display the common underlying patterns of neuro-myo-articular dysfunction seen in the BTS. Despite the radiological findings, appropriate treatment usually reverses the symptoms. However, this needs to be followed by appropriate motor relearning in a supervised class situation so that symptoms may remain at bay.

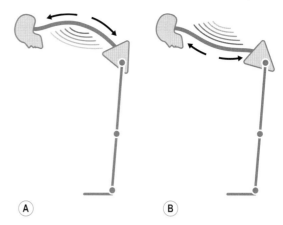

Fig 10.29 • Conceptual schematic view of the basic pattern tendency in the two primary pictures of dysfunction during forward bending. (A) Flexor dominance and 'folding' in primary APXS. (B) Extensor dominance and 'holding' in primary PPXS. Compare with Fig. 6.42.

The model presented suggests that the motor control changes *precede* pain onset and are responsible for its genesis. Understanding the patterns of neuromuscular dysfunction helps understand *why* the pain has developed. Once present, the pain will further result in either facilitation or inhibition of local and regional muscle responses. We can expect inhibition in SLMS muscles and facilitation of SGMS muscles. The recognition of the three pelvic syndromes and of the various CCPs and related underactivity in the SLMS dominant lumbopelvic muscles helps inform a different approach.

References

[1] O'Sullivan PB. Diagnosis and classification of chronic low back pain disorders: maladaptive movement and motor control impairments as an underlying mechanism. Man Ther 2005;10:242–55.

[2] Janda V. Muscles and Cervicogenic pain syndromes. In: Grant R, editor. Physical therapy of the thoracic spine. New York: Churchill Livingstone; 1988.

[3] Janda V. Muscles as a pathogenic factor in back pain. In: Proc. I.F. O.M.T. New Zealand; 1980.

[4] Janda V, Frank C, Liebenson C. Evaluation of muscular imbalance. In: Liebenson C, editor.

Rehabilitation of the spine: a practitioner's manual. Philadelphia: Lippincott Williams and Wilkins; 2007.

[5] Janda V. Muscles and motor control in low back pain: assessment and management. In: Twomey L, editor. Physical therapy of the low back. New York: Churchill Livingstone; 1987.

[6] Lee D. The pelvic girdle: an approach to the examination and treatment of the lumbo-pelvic-hip region. 3rd ed. Edinburgh: Churchill Livingstone; 2004.

[7] Janda V. Muscles, central nervous motor regulation and back problems. In: Korr IM, editor.

Neurobiologic Mechanisms in Manipulative Therapy. New York: Plenum Press; 1978.

[8] Williams PL, Warwick R. Gray's anatomy. 36th ed. Edinburgh: Churchill Livingstone; 1980.

[9] Bogduk N, Pearcy M, Hadfield G. Anatomy and biomechanics of the psoas major. Clin Biomech 1992;7:109–19.

[10] Penning L. Psoas muscle and lumbar stability: a concept uniting existing controversies. Eur Spine J 2000;9:577–85.

[11] Janda V, Stara V. Activity of abdominal muscles during knee extension in healthy and spastic children. In: Janda Compendium.

USA: Distributed in Australia by Body Control Systems for OPTP.

[12] O'Sullivan PB, et al. Altered patterns of abdominal muscle activation in patients with chronic low back pain. Aust J Physiother 1997;43(2):91–8.

[13] Urquhart D, Hodges PW, Story IH. Postural activity of the abdominal muscles varies between regions of these muscles and between body positions. Gait Posture 2005;22(4):295–301.

[14] Radebold A, et al. Muscle response pattern to sudden trunk loading in healthy individuals and patients with chronic low back pain. Spine 2000;25 (8):947–54.

[15] O'Sullivan PB, et al. Altered motor control strategies in subjects with sacroiliac joint pain during active straight leg raise test. Spine 2002;27(1):E1–8.

[16] Gregory DE, Brown SHM, Callaghan JP. Trunk muscle responses to suddenly applied loads: do individuals who develop discomfort during prolonged standing respond differently? J Electromyogr Kinesiol 2008; 18(3):495–502.

[17] Cholewicki J, van Dieën JH, Arsenault AB. Editorial: muscle function and dysfunction in the spine. J Electromyogr Kinesiol 2003;13:303–4.

[18] Van Dieën JH, Selen LPJ, Cholewicki J. Trunk muscle activation in low back pain patients, an analysis of the literature. J Electromyogr Kinesiol 2003;13:333–51.

[19] O'sullivan P. Motor control and pain disorders of the lumbo-pelvic region. In: Proc. 5th Interdisciplinary World Congress on Low Back and Pelvic Pain. Melbourne; 2004.

[20] Lewit K. Mobilisation of the fascia on the back in a caudal direction. In: Liebenson C, editor. Companion DVD for Rehabilitation of the spine: a practitioner's manual. Philadelphia: Lippincott Williams and Wilkins; 2007.

[21] Hodges PW. Women's Health Workshop. APA Conference Week. Cairns; 2007.

[22] Sapsford R. The pelvic floor: a clinical model for function and rehabilitation. Physiotherapy 2001;87(12):620–30.

[23] Bø, et al. Lower urinary tract symptoms and pelvic floor muscle exercise adherence after 15 years Obstet. Gynecol 2005;105:999–1005.

[24] Harrison DE, et al. Lumbar coupling during lateral translations of the thoracic cage relative to a fixed pelvis. Clin Biomech 1999;14:704–9.

[25] O'Sullivan PB. Lumbar 'segmental instability': clinical presentation and specific stabilising exercise management. Man Ther 2000; 5(1):2–12.

[26] O'Sullivan PB. Clinical instability' of the lumbar spine: its pathological basis, diagnosis and conservative management. In: Boyling JD, Jull GA, editors. Modern manual therapy. Edinburgh: Elsevier; 2004.

[27] Michele AA. Iliopsoas. Springfield, Illinois: Charles C Thomas; 1962.

[28] Andersson E, et al. The role of psoas and Iliacus muscles for stability and movement of the lumbar spine, pelvis and hip. Scand J Med Sci Sports 1995;5:10–6.

[29] O'Sullivan PB. Classification of lumbopelvic pain disorders – Why is it essential for management. Man Ther 2006;11:169–70.

[30] Barker K, Shamley DR, Jackson D. Changes in the cross sectional area of multifidus and psoas in patients with unilateral back pain: the relationship to pain and disability. Spine 2004;29 (22):E515–9.

[31] Mottram S. Dynamic stability of the scapula. Man Ther 1997;2 (3):123–31.

[32] Janda V. The relationship of shoulder girdle musculature to the aetiology of cervical pain syndromes. In: Proc: International Conference on Manipulative Therapy. Perth, Australia; 1983.

[33] Boyle JW, Milne N, Singer KP. Influence of age on cervicothoracic spinal posture: an ex vivo radiographic study. Clin Biomech 2002;17(5):361–7.

[34] Singer KP, Goh S. Anatomy of the thoracic spine. In: Giles LGF, Singer KP, editors. The clinical anatomy and management of back pain series: clinical anatomy and management of thoracic spine pain, vol. 11. Oxford: Butterworth Heinemann; 2000.

[35] Janda V. Comparison of spastic syndromes of cerebral origin with the distribution of muscular tightness in postural defects. International Symposium on Rehabilitation in Neurology. Rehabilitácia Suppl. 1977;14–5.

[36] Janda V. Pain in the locomotor system – a broad approach. In: Aspects of manipulative therapy. Melbourne: Churchill Livingstone; 1984.

[37] Kendall FP, McCreary EK, Provance PG. Muscles: testing and function. 4th ed. Baltimore: Williams andWilkins; 1993.

[38] Sahrmann SA. Diagnosis and treatment of movement impairment syndromes. Mosby: St Louis; 2002.

[39] Falla D, Jull G, Hodges PW. Feedforward activity of the cervical flexor muscles during voluntary arm movements is delayed in chronic neck pain. Exp Brain Res 2004;157:43–8.

[40] Falla D, Jull G, Hodges PW. Patients with neck pain demonstrate reduced EMG activity of the deep cervical flexor muscles during performance of the cranio-cervical flexion test. Spine 2004;29(19):2108–14.

[41] O'Leary S, et al. Cranio-cervical flexor muscle impairment at maximal, moderate and low loads is a feature of neck pain. Man Ther 2007;12(1):34–9.

[42] Jull, et al. Cervical flexor muscle re-training: physiological mechanisms of efficacy. In: Proc. 2nd International conference on movement dysfunction. Edinburgh, Scotland; 2005.

[43] Falla D, Jull G, Hodges P. Training the cervical muscles with prescribed motor tasks does not change muscle activation during a functional activity. Man Ther 2008;13(6):507–12.

[44] Cagnie B, et al. The influence on breathing type, expiration and cervical posture on the

performance of the cranio-cervical flexion test. Man Ther IN PRESS.

[45] Fernández-de-Las-Peñas, et al. Cervical muscle co-activation in isometric contractions is enhanced in chronic tension-type headache patients. Cephalalgia 2008; May 5 C.

[46] Szeto GPY, Straker LM, O'Sullivan PB. A comparison of symptomatic office workers performing monotonous keyboard work – 2. Neck and shoulder kinematics. Man Ther 2005;10 (4):281–91.

[47] Szeto GPY, Straker LM, O'sullivan PB. A comparison of symptomatic and asymptomatic office workers performing monotonous keyboard work – 1. Neck and shoulder muscle recruitment patterns. Man Ther 2005;10(4):270–80.

[48] Greig AM, Straker LM, Briggs AM. Cervical erector spinae and upper trapezius muscle activity in children using different information technologies. Physiotherapy 2005;91(2):119–26.

[49] Edmondston SJ, et al. Postural neck pain: An investigation of habitual sitting posture, perception of 'good' posture and cervicothoracic kinaesthesia. Man Ther 2007;12(4):363–71.

[50] An analysis of some exercise, therapies and techniques capable of correcting posture and muscle imbalance. In: Garlick D, editor.

Proprioception, posture and emotion. Sydney: Symposium UNSW; 1988.

[51] Grieve GP. Common vertebral joint problems. Edinburgh: Churchill Livingstone; 1981.

[52] Hruska R. Postural Restoration Institute: a setter's balanced attack requires a balanced back. www.posturalrestoration.com/.

[53] Silva RT, et al. Clinical and ultrasonic correlation between scapula dyskinesia and subacromial space measurement among junior elite tennis players. Br J Sports Med 2008; Apr 8.

[54] Mottram SL, Woledge RC, Morrissey D. Motion analysis study of scapular orientation exercise and subjects ability to learn the exercise. Man Ther IN PRESS.

[55] Janda V. Sydney: Course notes; 1984.

[56] Coorevits P, Danneels, et al. Fatigue related EMG median frequency characteristics of back and hip muscles during isometric back extensions. In: Proc 5th Interdisciplinary World Congress on Low Back and pelvic Pain. Melbourne; 2004.

[57] Hanna T. Somatics: reawakening the minds control of movement, flexibility and health. Cambridge MA: Da Capo Press; 1988.

[58] Vleeming A. Joint function: development of an integral model for diagnosis and treatment. In: Proc. I.F.O.M.T. Perth; 2000.

[59] Mosely GL. Psychosocial factors and altered motor control. In: Proc. 5th Interdisciplinary World Congress on Low Back and Pelvic Pain. Melbourne; 2004.

[60] Rock C-M. Reflex incontinence caused by underlying functional disorders. In: Carrière B, Markel Feldt C, editors. The Pelvic Floor. Stuttgart: Thieme; 2006.

[61] Snijders CJ, et al. Effects of slouching and muscle contraction on the strain of the iliolumbar ligament. Man Ther 2008;13 (4):325–33.

[62] Lee D, Vleeming A. Current concepts on pelvic impairment (workshop). In: Proc. IFOMPT. Perth; 2000.

[63] Spitznagle TM. Musculoskeletal chronic pelvic pain. In: Carrière B, Markel Feldt C, editors. The Pelvic Floor. Stuttgart: Thieme; 2006.

[64] Greenman PE. Principles of manual medicine. 2nd ed. Baltimore: Williams and Wilkins; 1996.

[65] Upledger JE, Vredevoogd JD. Craniosacral Therapy. Seattle: Eastland Press; 1983.

[66] Bartenieff I, Lewis D. Body movement: coping with the environment. Australia: Gordon and Breach; 2002.

[67] Hackney P. Making Connections: total body integration through bartenieff fundamentals. New York: Routledge; 2002.

Chapter Eleven

Examining probable contributions towards dysfunctional posture and movement

Backs complain when their movement diet becomes limited and repetitive. By and large, compared with the liberated curious child, the modern adult tends to use less variety and less expressive movement. The possible contributions to depleted posturomovement control are many and varied. In any one patient, the blend of these various influences contribute towards the presenting picture of changed motor function. The seemingly most pertinent are explored.

Neurodevelopmental aspects

The quality of our motor development is reflected in the manner in which we posture and move ourselves. It is possible that one never had very good motor control.

Mature motor behavior: what is 'normal'?

Sensorimotor development whilst progressing through common stages and patterns is nonetheless individual, adapting to various influences. Environment, opportunity, emotions, experience, cognitive and learning ability are some of the aspects that play a part in development. School and 'mental learning' mean we frequently sideline our sensorimotor learning. In some respects we 'stop developing' as our motor function deteriorates with the reduced demands and altered circumstances of sedentary lifestyles involved in education and work. For many of us, a certain untapped potential for developing

more highly refined sensorimotor function remains. Some however, attempt to further develop their motor potential in exploring various experiential awareness and somatic learning practices such as Feldenkrais, The Alexander Principle, yoga, dance the martial arts and so on. Alexander[1] drew attention to 'The use of the self' – *how* the person performs the ordinary movements involved during everyday activities can cause strain or otherwise on pain sensitive tissues.

More highly integrated sensorimotor development produces positive differences in the qualitative characteristics of the posture and movement responses. This begs the question – what is normal posture and movement? Just because a person does not have pain does not mean he moves 'normally' or well. Do 'pain free' and 'healthy controls' used in research design necessarily move in a well adapted way? Habitual behavior is common to us all – eating, drinking, smoking and the way we breathe and move. Changing any habit requires awareness of the problem, a desire to change it and application in doing so.

Abnormal early development: integrated versus more primitive control

Most of us develop the quantitative motor milestones – the ability to sit stand and walk and so on. However, we don't all do it in the same way as the quality of our eventual neuromusculoskeletal organization can demonstrate. *How* we posture and move may be less than ideal. How to discern what factors underlie this picture of 'soft dysfunction'?

Bartenieff[2] was concerned to identify innate constitutional factors that could be traced through childhood to adulthood which affected and reflected *how* the person was able to cope with his environment. Observing a series of films of the movement behavior between two 'normal' children at birth through to age 12, she was able to discern six core qualities which were significant in identifying to a greater or lesser extent, the adaptability of the child. The first three were observable in the first few weeks of life; the last three became evident as sitting posture and locomotion developed. All six features operate through childhood and are discernable in the adult. To quote her:

1. Differentiated vs less differentiated use of the limbs and their segments, head/trunk, and constellations of trunk and limb.

2. Dominance of asymmetrical vs symmetrical use of limbs. Asymmetric use stimulates greater mobility and develops selectivity and range in pattern.

3. Use of areas of reach space (personal kinesphere) around the body before full uprightness vs limited use of reach space.

4. Flexible vs fixed use of verticality.

5. Development of verticality and full use of kinesphere into a territorial space (locomotor space) vs limited use. This becomes visible in the sitting stage.

6. Organization of activity patterns into phrases – ordering, combining, alternating, and elaborating – vs short monotone flexion and extension actions

The differences in response were evident from birth in the Moro or Startle response. One infant demonstrated multi use of all limbs; emphasis on horizontal use of limbs; shifting the body from side to side and varying symmetrical and asymmetrical limb movements. The other showed less limb movements in predominant flexion/extension ranges; a rigid and fixed constellation of the limbs at the end of the response which was actually a postural reflex, with upper limbs flexed and lower limbs extended; a definite emphasis on symmetrical limb use. The qualities of the core parameters were carried through the developmental stages so that at the age of four, the child with the less ideal motor behavior displayed a collapsed posture and protective attitude of the arms reminiscent of her early startle response with flexed upper limbs and high tension extension of the lower. She moved within a limited kinesphere, lacked

variety in the movements she used and overall Bartenieff felt she showed a tendency towards rigid non-adaptability. Clearly some of us inherit a better neuromuscular apparatus than others. She believed that this small observational study revealed important insights for the movement therapist:

- the significance of core qualities which reflect interrelationships of movement behavior elements and
- the significance of pattern roots that appear in the early Startle behavior and are crystallized into later behavior patterns.

Inadequate integration during any stage of development creates the need for compensatory strategies which then become part of the person's movement repertoire, as they become learned and habitual. In time they more than likely become a patient.

Aspects of more primitive motor behavior are clinically evident in subjects with spinal pain disorders (Chs 7 & 8). Grieve[3] noted the awkward movements, poorly developed kinesthetic appreciation and 'physical illiteracy' of many of his patients making it difficult to teach them exercises.

Janda[4] knew the relationship between the inability to work out good movement patterns and the development of vertebrogenic conditions. In a group of back pain patients who had been 'therapeutic failures' he found symptoms attributable to 'minimal brain dysfunction' (MBD; see Ch. 7). He considered that about 10–15% of the child population suffers from at least some signs of this syndrome and about 80% of subjects with chronic pain fit the MBD category.[5]

'Acquired' aspects contributing to posturomovement dysfunction

While we may have enjoyed an exemplary early motor development, the continual influence of numerous ongoing intrinsic and extrinsic factors serves to modify our motor presentation as we adaptively respond to the prevailing conditions. The most apparent are discussed in brief.

Lifestyle

Chairs have a lot to answer for! Western industrial societies have progressively evolved towards the adoption of more sustained static sitting postures for education, work and leisure. Our heads are occupied with intellectual pursuits or otherwise distracted, yet the CNS is disadvantaged by the relative lack of sensory intelligence as a result of more limited body movement. Many never get down onto the ground and as Beach[6] observes, floor to standing transitions use deeply embedded archetypal musculoskeletal patterns that young children and premodern adults would use constantly during daily life. Sensory deprivation makes the system become rusty and leads to what Hanna[7] termed 'sensorimotor amnesia'. The posturomotor control system suffers and we develop changed antigravity responses when sitting and standing (Ch. 8). Repeated often enough they become habituated responses that start to 'feel normal'. Sitting with the spine flexed has been directly linked with back pain.[8,9] The desk worker then tries to become the 'weekend warrior' attempting the kinds of manual labor he is not well suited for, such as using the chain-saw. These activities inflict unreasonable kinematic demands upon an often struggling poorly organized posturomovement system.

The increasing incidence of obesity and associated inactivity is everywhere apparent within contemporary Western cultures and has been argued to predict back pain.[10] Maintaining activity levels and back muscle endurance may prevent it.[11]

In contrast, the subsistence farmer or hunter-gatherer 'uses his body' in a more physiological way as he walks daily for food and water, actively employing all his senses in hunting, manual work and possibly expressive dance and rituals. He is unlikely to have pain resulting from developing movement dysfunction.

Trauma

The influence of previous traumatic episodes is frequently overlooked yet can result in pernicious symptom development even many years later. If X-rays taken at the time were negative, the patient is usually told 'it's just soft tissue strain' and 'to rest'. Falls when skiing, off horses, out of trees etc. can be long forgotten, yet physical assessment can delineate the graveyards of old traumatic events. In particular, falls onto the bottom and knees and fractures of the coccyx can distort pelvic ring myomechanics and contribute to lumbopelvic symptoms.

Cultural trends

Volinn[12] reviewed the epidemiological literature and found rates of low back pain were 2–4 times higher in European general populations than in Nigerian and Asian farmers. Within the low income countries, rates were higher among urban than among rural populations. He concluded that hard physical labor itself is not necessarily related to low back pain and that its prevalence may be on the rise as urbanization and rapid industrialization proceed.

Probably the most significant posturomovement differences between those observed in the West and other cultures is in the manner of sitting, carrying and in fashion.

Sitting

Sitting in a chair and 'relaxing' invariably means collapsing (see Ch. 8).

Many in the world have never seen a chair and rest in either a cross-legged sitting or squatting position. Janda[13] relates that Fahrni had noticed that Orientals spend a large part of the day thus, which maintained the lumbar curve. He said that they manifest no increased incidence of disc degeneration with advanced age and have a very low incidence of back pain. He apparently had radiological data showing that the incidence of disc narrowing was 80% by age 55 amongst Swedish heavy workers, 35% in office workers of the same age, while in a jungle population in India the incidence was 9%.

Squatting also maintains good opening in the hips and pelvis. The base of support is active through the feet (or ischia in sitting) which serves to fire up the SLMS. In some cultures birthing could happen in the fields but now, in the West, more often than not it entails an operation. Most of us in the West have lost the art of squatting and cross legged sitting. Attempts to do so invariably result in hyperflexion over the lumbosacral spine and axial collapse because of limited range in the hip. Note the pandemic of hip replacement surgery – if you don't use them properly you need to replace them! As the saying goes – 'use it or lose it'.

It has also been argued that chair designers and users have generally been distracted by concerns for representing social status rather than the physiological and kinesthetic aspects which might contribute to physical wellbeing.[14]

Carrying

A significantly large proportion of the world carry loads on their heads - biomechanically sound as it loads the axial column providing much proprioceptive input and firing up the SLMS. The poorest untouchable in India can look more regal than a queen, such is her beautiful carriage. The effectiveness of head loading is demonstrated by a physiotherapeutic ruse for helping severely ataxic children to walk. Putting a weighted helmet on their head would immediately improve the antigravity response and stabilize them enough to be able to walk unaided! Head loading entails getting the arms up to place or balance the load, maintaining their elevatory function including thoracoscapula mechanics and basal breathing. The arms are free and can swing inducing the shoulder–pelvis counterrotation, minimizing the energy load of walking. In the west it is usual to carry the load in front with the arms. The body becomes eccentrically loaded and stress is imposed on the system. This occurs around the neck-shoulders and low back as we are pulled forward into a more general pattern of flexion. For many, struggling with the weekly shopping becomes a repetitive act which compounds patterns of improper muscle use. Contrast the serenity and relaxed demeanor of the African women despite coping with mixed spinal loading (Figs 11.1 & 11.2).

Balancing the head load ensures that the column is well aligned while also activating balanced antigravity responses.

Fashion

It is difficult to know why the concept of a small waist came to be. Tight belts, constrictive clothing and holding in the stomach all contribute to the development of dysfunctional breathing patterns.[15,16] The recent fashion for skin tight and low slung jeans means that the wearer cannot flex the hips properly without her buttocks popping out of her pants, thus she is impelled to sit in posterior pelvic tilt and excessively flex the lumbar spine.[17] Axial collapse of course ensues. Contemporary models frequently 'tuck the tail' and strike poses in lolling seductive, simpering postures which imply postural collapse is 'cool'.

The fad for 'trainers' and orthotics has to be one of the biggest marketing cons. The person is so trussed up with 'support' that they don't need and then can't find their own intrinsic support through

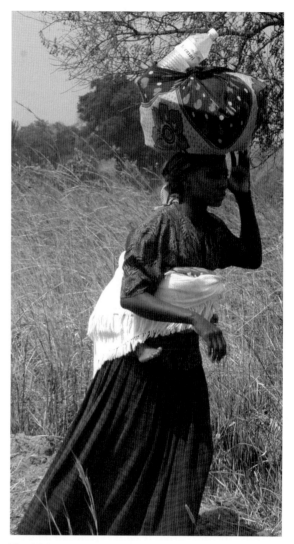

Fig 11.1 • Despite carrying two loads and hurrying she is graceful and relaxed!

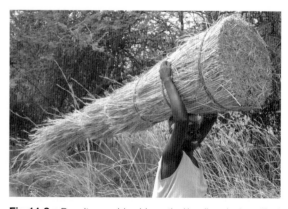

Fig 11.2 • Despite considerable vertical loading she is smiling!

active feet with a dynamic lower kinetic chain. Collapsed feet are indicative of poor systemic posturomovement control. Walking barefoot would be much better! Stand in any shopping centre and observe the waddling, plodding, loping and disjointed steps of many of those using this type of footwear. They are generally also obese.

Cultural expression and customs

Movement serves both function and expression. The religious act of frequent daily prostration has the added side benefit of maintaining fitness! Cultural practices and rituals involving meditating, chanting singing and wailing, effectively tune the breathing mechanism. Gestural body movements including clapping, tapping, stamping, dancing and so on in solo or group performances provide a lot of sensory input to the system as well as group interaction and entertainment. Reaching for the heavens in exultation leaps and shrieks are empowering. Conversely we in the West have become to rely on passive entertainment – magazines, TV, DVDs, computers, movies etc. – all while collapsing in sitting (again!) and often solo. Sadly the trend is spreading afar.

Psychosocial and emotional factors

Modern living has become stressful living. Many of us are in a constant state of hyper arousal and tension as we cope with a multitude of demands – the kids and the 'home front' while meeting deadlines, performance reviews, escalating mortgage payments, sick relatives and so on, while at the end of the day worrying whether we look good in bed! Stress is a potent potentiator in musculoskeletal pain syndromes.

Psychological factors play a great role in faulty central motor patterns. Lewit[18] considers that 'motor patterns *are* to a certain degree expressions of the state of mind: anxiety, depression and an inability to relax will greatly influence motor patterns. No less important is the subject's psychological attitude to pain'. In general, one never sees a depressed or very shy person who is 'up' and 'open'.

The 'human consciousness or human potential movement' evolved in the 1960s and 1970s and its many proponents included Ida Rolf, Alexander Lowen and Feldenkrais who variously explored disturbed somatic functioning and its relation to the psyche. Rolf[19] saw how each person's shape and

form constituted their personal history and suffering – genetics, trauma, habit and culture all contribute. Lowen[20] considered that neurosis and early psychologically traumatic events result in 'body armoring' where increased muscle tension limits motility and respiration. Feldenkrais[21] considered that 'to every emotional state corresponds a personal conditioned pattern of muscular contraction without which it has no existence'. He described 'The body pattern of anxiety' – a contraction of the flexor muscles especially in the abdominal region, and a halt in breathing soon followed by vasomotor changes as sweating and accelerated pulse and an increase in adrenalin. The head is lowered, we crouch and bend the knees and the arms come across the front of the body to protect the soft unprotected parts. He stressed that importantly 'the sensation of fear and anxiety due to the disturbance of the diaphragmatic and cardiac region *is actually abated by maintained general flexor contraction* and in particular that of the abdominal region'. He observed that introverts have some habitual reduction of their extensor tonus thus either the head or the hip joints are forward. The extrovert on the other hand has a more erect standing posture and gait.

Influenced by Feldenkrais, Hanna[7] described 'The reflexes of stress'. Fear avoidance behavior if repeated enough, becomes habitual (see Ch. 6., Part A and Ch 10). It is interesting to observe the very common postural habit of folding the arms in front of the chest in psychological protection and defense (see Fig. 3.3). Added to this, the adoption of further protective postures and splinting and guarding can ensue as a result of pain.

Breathing is the link between emotion and motion. Stress and anxiety alter the breathing patterns and hyperventilation syndromes[22,23] are common (Ch. 8.). Chaitow[24] remarks that breathing pattern disorders automatically increase levels of anxiety and apprehension which may be sufficient to alter motor control and to markedly influence balance control. A vicious pattern generating cycle is set in train.

Studies have certainly shown a clear relationship between low tolerance to stress and back pain.[4] Marras et al.[25] demonstrated that psychosocial stress produced statistically significant altered muscle coactivation patterns, increased spine loadings and kinematic responses. The erector spinae and the obliques generally exhibited greater mean activities. Different personality types responded to psychosocial stress differently. Most types increased their spinal compression stresses however introversion and intuition preferences were also associated with large increases in shear loading. In a prospective study, Mannion et al.[26] found that 'abnormal' scores from psychological questionnaires can precede back pain development.

Pain as a cause of altered motor control (see also Ch. 7)

It has been proposed that altered motor control eventually leads to pain. Pain itself causes further changes in movement. There are many possible mechanisms for this including changes in excitability in the motor pathway, changes in the sensory system, and factors associated with the attention demanding, stressful and fearful aspects of pain.[27,28] Pain can engender catastrophizing behavior and fear of movement and re-injury.[29,30] Predictable and unpredictable pain has been shown to increase CNS reaction times and anxiety about the impending pain further determines this effect.[31] Anticipation of pain can induce protective postural strategies[32] and the adoption of altered strategies which avoid or limit movement of the lumbar spine.[33] While the sensory perception of pain creates anticipatory and fear avoidance beliefs there are also usually significant objective findings such as strength deficits in the spinal muscles as shown by Al-Obaidi et al.[34]

Misinformed beliefs

A person's beliefs are strong drivers of any behavior. Many tabloid newspapers and women's magazines take pride in offering 'authoritative information' and advice on all manner of things including 'the best stretches' or 'losing that tummy' much of which can constitute little more than 'recycled garbage'. Believing the hype, various 'gismos to ease the pain' are peddled to the desperate and hopeful. Patients frequently present to the clinic proudly declaring that they 'exercise' and 'stretch' yet they cannot physiologically posture themselves against gravity. When these various exercises are assessed they can generally be held responsible for further contributing to the patient's symptoms. All kinds of misinformed beliefs

abound – 'don't let your back arch', 'touching your toes is good for you', 'sit-ups help your back', and so on. Rather, it is quality in control of physiological *patterns of movement* which need to be addressed in these people.

The belief that 'work caused the pain' is tricky territory to negotiate and made more so by the spectre of compensation and other forms of secondary gain.[35] Some clearly believe that their pain is 'serious' and can take to their bed or take time off work limiting their activity levels, yet rest in sitting (again and badly!) believing they are otherwise harming themselves. Correlations between activity level and pain intensity are poor.[36] It is more than likely that repetitive daily activities such as *the way he sits* and the kinematics of the movement pattern he adopts as he cleans his teeth that have more to do with aggravating his pain. Maluf et al.[37] suggest that daily repetitive posturomovements may result in preferential movement of the lumbar spine in a specific direction contributing to the development, persistence or recurrence of lower back pain (LBP). Some patients are loathe to accept responsibility for the manner in which they habitually posture and move as largely contributing to their pain, particularly where compensation is involved. Larsson and Nordholm[38] examined attitudes towards prevention, treatment and management of musculoskeletal disorders and the main associations found were that lower education, physical inactivity and sick leave for musculoskeletal disorders increased the odds of attributing responsibility externally to someone else. The best clinical practice is easily thwarted by the patient who is neither responsive to advice nor compliant with prescribed self help programs. Then there is the added problem of him doing it correctly: achieving the right pattern is difficult. In response to pain he may develop more fear avoidance motor behavior and these maladaptive and provocative responses[39,40] become superimposed on the poor habitual underlying patterns. He truly becomes a chronic back pain patient.

Intervention programs with a physical and behavioral therapy package aimed at altering lifestyle factors to help reduce current problems and prevent reinjury have shown favorable outcomes.[41] Return to work is often seen as an outcome measure yet this often underestimates functional impairment. Rather, objective kinematic functional performance measures are suggested as a more sensitive quantitative measure of outcome.[42]

Sport and recreation: 'stretching', 'Pilates' and yoga

While recreational sporting activities are a great way to work the body into the sorts of movement that the working week doesn't deliver, there must however be the underlying function to support the actions required. Inadequate organization and control of the forward bending pattern (Ch. 6, Part B) means that activities such as gardening produce 'gardener's back' instead of affording a positive 'physiological workout' for the body (Fig. 11.3).

The retired banker who takes up golf but has a stiff thorax and hips should not be surprised that he develops low back pain[43] – the rotation required in golf needs to come from somewhere! In pursuit of strength, the rower increases his time on the ergo machine yet the *kinematic pattern* he adopts may serve to shunt the movement stress to his low back. The tri-athlete needs to ensure he maintains good hip mobility and inner range extension and control of his lumbopelvic region in order to counteract the long periods of flexion on the bike. School sport often becomes a session supervised by the geography teacher. The type and method of stretching that some appear to have been taught would make your hair stand on end! Bad patterns learnt early become harder to change later.

'Stretching' has become the exercise mantra despite the fact that studies on stretching prior to exercise have shown little reduction in injury levels.[44] The reason so many want to do it is the fact that they *do 'feel stiff'*. One of the qualities of healthy physiological movement control includes *active elongation* of muscles as they variously contribute in the force couples that control posture and movement. One needs to stretch when movement control is poor. Imbalanced muscle action doesn't allow the spine to move properly. Axial collapse creates regions of segmental stiffness. Muscles innervated from irritated spinal segments become fired up – usually the large superficial muscles which when over-activated become tight (see Ch. 7 & Ch. 12). Added to this is the habitual overuse of the SGMS for posturomovement control which further compounds their tightness and influence. Unfortunately most of the stretching that is practiced is passive where the patient works against himself. Reduced SLMS control means little appreciation for the correct 'feel' and control of body segments, the pelvis in particular. 'Stupid stretches' result (Fig. 11.4) and become a potent precipitating and perpetuating factor in ongoing lumbopelvic pain syndromes.

Pilates has become a 'craze' which is now attracting increasing attention from the therapeutic community.[45] This is interesting as despite its popularity, little research supports the benefits of this form of exercise.[46,47]

Believing that civilization impairs physical fitness, Joseph Pilates designed a series of somewhat 'gymnastic' exercises he termed 'Contrology' which he

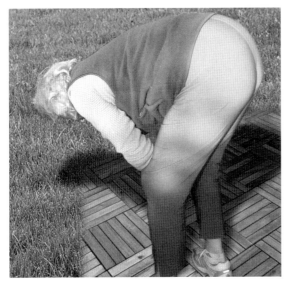

Fig 11.3 • Sprung! The subject 'thought she was bending properly'! There is inadequate release of the ischial swing from habitual holding (see Fig. 13.19). This is associated with poor axial co-activation.

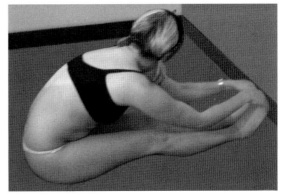

Fig 11.4 • Poor control of the pelvis and passivity in the stretch means that the low back is the structure receiving most of the stretch. It is the same subject in Fig. 8.26 who cannot weigh shift in sitting.

claimed 'develops the body uniformly, corrects wrong postures, restores physical vitality, invigorates the mind and elevates the spirit.'[48] Positive aspects of his approach include the 'mind's control over the muscles', awareness and concentration on the purpose of the exercises, patience and persistence and the importance of breathing during the exercises. The New York dance community found the approach beneficial to performance and it spread from there. It has become a marketer's dream – Polestar Pilates; Stott Pilates; Body Control Pilates; Clinical Pilates; Yogalates – you name it, everyone is having a go! The problem is the 'technique' is now so diverse it's hard to know what the client is receiving. Compounding this is its proponents, in general, lack a real understanding about 'function' and further, 'what's wrong' with movement in spinal pain patients.

Research has often been misappropriated to justify the approach – 'core strengthening' has served the industry well. Joseph Pilates stressed 'always keep the full length of the back pressed firmly against the floor'[48] and many of the exercises also involved movement and stretching the lumbar spine into hyper flexion. While he did counter these with strong 'extension exercises', it would appear that many contemporary approaches focus more on the flexion aspect. However, the big problem is that many with back pain already have a loss of lordosis and a tendency to more 'total flexor pattern' motor behavior (see Ch. 8) which becomes further reinforced by 'Pilates'. Those classified as an anterior pelvic crossed syndrome are particularly vulnerable (Ch. 9). Invariably patients work 'three stories too high'[2,49] entrenching central cinch behavior (see Ch. 10; Figs. 8.38, 9.12 & 10.4). Increasingly prevalent in the clinic are people presenting with neck pain and headaches with associated breathing pattern disorders and exacerbations of their low back problem that can be linked to their practice of Pilates.

Pilates' original routine would certainly help 'fitness' yet this is different to, and does not necessarily redress, movement dysfunction. It seems many therapeutic recommendations arise from not really knowing what else to do for the patient.

Yoga is now being offered on practically every street corner and one must question from where did all the teachers materialize given it takes many years to become a dedicated yoga teacher and those with integrity generally spend up to 5–6 hours a day refining their practice? In general, the potential

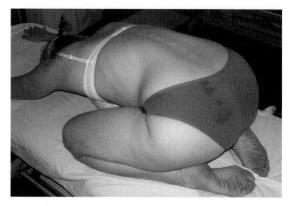

Fig 11.5 ● The subject is training to be a yoga teacher but not surprisingly is experiencing back pain. Note how she passively falls back into the pose without the necessary drive & support from the lower pelvic unit to open the postero-inferior pelvis and hips, hence the stretch is more in the low back.

problem is one of passive collapse and/or that 'postures' become fixed, 'held' and hard with little exploration within them (Fig. 11.5). Bartenieff[2] saw that 'the superficial appropriation of new materials can be observed in the frequently fragmented indiscriminate use of yoga' – 'attributable to casual teaching and studying that promotes misunderstanding and misuse of a valid discipline'. 'The misuse frequently results in diminished movement responses instead of full harmonious balance of action and non-action'. Aspects of all the six movement dysfunction syndromes described in Chapter 10 are readily apparent when observing participants in a yoga class. It takes great integrity of purpose and skill in the yoga teacher to guide subjects towards achieving higher level control rather than allowing them to merely further imprint their dysfunctional patterns. The 'adrenaline junkie' student approaches the practice of yoga as a work-out – a 'real challenge', employing ambition, end-gaining and effort which reliably increases SGMS activity and inhibits SLMS activity. Farhi[50] comments 'what they think they want and what they actually need are often two completely different things'. Weight bearing poses unfortunately generally demonstrate poor grounding through the base of support and so invariably show aspects of limb 'propping' and 'holding' in the torso, with disturbed breathing and excess tension in the upper body. Bartenieff[2] also described a 'preoccupation with pushing the body into the shape apparently desired by the teacher and a tendency to passivity particularly in initiating action and flow. Sloppily executed positions showed distortions in the tensions and countertensions inherent in them. Thus instead of balanced tensions that produce relaxation, the performer will experience abrasive exertions or muddy non-tension'.

A good teacher guiding the dedicated practice of 'proper' yoga which focuses upon inner awareness and mindfulness and 'soft control' is a wonderful way of improving SLMS function and inhibiting SGMS overactivity. The student is meaningfully relearning and further developing his sensorimotor potential.

'Training' and the fitness industry

There is a difference between cardiovascular 'fitness' and movement 'function'. Janda[51] notes 'the high incidence of functional impairment makes it extremely difficult to estimate the borders between the norm and evident pathology'. 'It is evident that a general dysfunction of the motor system occurs for years before a syndrome such as low back pain manifests itself by local pain. The altered function can be found predominantly in changed movement patterns, motor performance and muscle imbalances. Even the elite athlete who is 'fit' active and dedicated is often very dysfunctional in his movement patterning. Therefore more important than simply increasing muscle strength is the teaching of movement performance.[13] Gyms have become 'the definitive cultural icon' and a remarkably successful marketing exercise yet this author holds grave concerns about the veracity of their purpose. There is no doubt that inactivity and obesity are a contemporary problem and the gym seems an easy and appropriate option – a sort of playgroup for adults where the trainer actually does encourage some get up and go. Some go to the gym because 'everything aches' and the belief you 'need to keep it moving'. Many believe that unless they are 'busting a gut' 'nothing is really happening,' such is their woeful internal awareness.

However, clinicians increasingly have to contend with the 'Gym Junkie Syndrome': tense yet collapsed and exhausted bodies and the pumped up and grossly dysfunctional bodies which result from many 'training programs' which can be directly causally linked to the genesis of their pain. Just ask around your local gym and you may/not be surprised at the number of 'rotator cuff' and knee pain syndromes which are extant. Orthopedic surgeons are beginning to set up adjacent practices as the pickings are so good from these 'dysfunction factories'. I believe they have even coined the label 'knee – shoulder syndrome, as if you have one you will reliably get the other!

So what is so wrong you ask?
• The ethos in the fitness culture of the gyms and personal trainers is largely to 'get fit', develop strength, 'body sculpt' and look good (Fig. 11. 6). Many personal trainers possessed of limited understanding of pathology or dysfunctional control 'motivate' and push their charges to 'go for it'; 'work harder' with a 'no pain, no gain' approach based on notions of aesthetics with little regard for or understanding of their client's functional needs. Marketing and enthusiasm seem to win over integrity and quality control. The desire for 'strong abs' 'impressive pecs' etc. results in poorly conceived exercise programs being offered by many. When the personal trainers themselves are presenting with pain, there clearly is a problem.

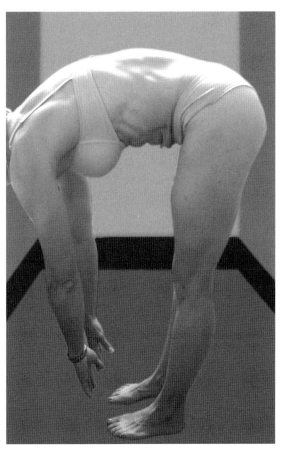

Fig 11.6 • All her hard work on 'body sculpting' has developed the SGMS but inhibited SLMS activity. Note the emptiness in transversus and the diaphragm in supporting the spine during the movement.

• The primary emphasis is on strength. Strong muscles are not necessarily healthy muscles. While many may be de-conditioned with reduced endurance which is a potential problem,[11] they are not necessarily 'weak'. They will, however, usually display muscle imbalance, some change in their ability to organize movement patterns and have difficulty sustaining certain postures at a low load level. This can even be the case in 'elite' sports people. Janda[52,53] said 'in athletes it is almost automatically assumed that the function of their musculoskeletal system is normal and the only target is to improve their otherwise normal status' – that all that needs to happen is to make them stronger. Impaired function, reflex changes and the patterning process[54] which can substantially influence the final result of a sportive effort are largely neglected.

Instead, *bad movement patterns are strengthened.* Strength training and the use of effort preferentially activates SGMS muscles and reinforces effort and tension patterns particularly if bilateral movements are used (Ch. 5). These have a tendency to be over active and dominant in our movement patterns as it is, and particularly in those who are symptomatic. Overactivity in the SGMS tends to have an inhibitory effect on the deep system (Fig. 11.7). Muscle imbalance and imperfect motor patterns do not allow perfectly adjusted movement.[52]

Similarly, McGill[55] sees that athletes are generally unhealthy from a musculoskeletal point of view and training should be for health where working smarter rather than harder is the goal. Requiring a different philosophy, 'it emphasizes muscle endurance, motor control perfection, and the maintenance of sufficient spine stability in all expected tasks. While strength is not a targeted goal, strength gains do result'.

• Most strength building maneuvers are practiced in sitting or lying with little focus on correct alignment. Pulling the highest weight is more important than the quality of movement and manner of breathing. It is unphysiological to sit at a machine and exercise. There is no active base of support and so little if anything is asked of SLMS control.

• Most resisted limb work is bilateral and in the sagittal plane further encouraging sagittal dominance of movement behavior (Ch. 8). In the upper body this further imprints already established patterns of dysfunction (Ch. 10). The important parameters to establish in the lower body are the control of weight shift on a dynamic unilateral support and usually this is not addressed. The stress encountered when 'pulling weights' is more often than not directed instead to the lumbar and cervical spines. Creative and expressive movements are not symmetrical.

• The hyper development of the SGMS limb muscles renders them tighter and accordingly they need to keep stretching them. Poorly devised and supervised stretching protocols invariably result in regions of the spine being further stretched, adding to the dysbalance.

• The training of a limited repertoire of certain bilateral patterns of movement associated with effort reinforces poor patterns of movement and creates conditioned responses such as the 'central cinch patterns' (Ch. 10) which are then applied in other situations. Managing to help these people inhibit these entrained responses can be really difficult.

Weight bearing exercise has been advised for osteoporosis which is very different from 'doing weights'.

McGill[56] draws attention to the Russian philosophy of training which encompasses briefly: awareness: all-round development; systematic increments in challenge; pacing; repetition; visualization; specialization; individualization and structure.

Therapeutic misadventure

The skill of appropriate therapeutic exercise prescription is a clinical art backed up by science.

Historically, 'back exercises' have been seen as flexion and/or extension exercises. The debate over many years was whether William's flexion exercises or McKenzie's extension exercises were the best

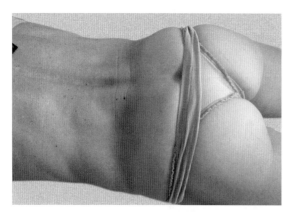

Fig 11.7 • Weight training has developed the superficial muscles but note the empty hollow from poverty in the transversus and diaphragm as she attempts to anteriorly rotate her pelvis.

for back pain! Inappropriate exercise prescription occurs when therapists have an inadequate understanding of healthy movement function, including biomechanically sound and functional kinematic patterns of movement. Secondly, without a comprehensive understanding of each patient's functional movement *needs*, therapists risk reinforcing their client's dysfunction. When they send their patients to Pilates it is hard to believe they are clear about what to do for their patient. Many poor patients have also been subjected to such a lot of stupid and poor advice such as 'don't let your back arch' or 'tuck your tail under'.

Pertinent also, is that the therapist is in touch with the status of their own musculoskeletal shortcomings. Just because they are 'the therapist' does not mean they necessarily function particularly well. The adage 'it takes one to know one' is apt and helps the therapist understand *how* function is altered and how to approach assisting others in effectively changing theirs. Which responses need to be inhibited or modified and which do we want to encourage, and *why*.

McGill[55] suggests inappropriate exercise prescription also probably results when the therapist does not understand the tissue loading that results in various tasks. Many exercises replicate injury mechanisms. Unfortunately there has also been a tendency for a one size fits all, 'recipe' approach which amounts to therapeutic 'hand me downs' for want of knowing better. The recommending of posterior pelvic tilting as an exercise is a good example. Some poorly conceived 'research' even advocates it.[57] Many patients perform this exercise despite the fact that this creates lumbar flexion[58], a pattern most have too much of, and which is probably contributing to their pain state. Another common example is what McGill[55] terms are 'silly stretches': toe touching and pulling the knees to the chest in supine first thing in the morning which not only hyper flex the lumbar spine but as he says, can cause instability. One never encounters the advice to teach anterior pelvic tilt, a pattern most can't control and which is basic to being able to properly move from and 'stretch' the hips.

Less experienced therapists may risk misinterpreting research outcomes.[5] Hodges and his colleagues have done a lot of nice research on transversus abdominus and have always stressed that functionally it is co-active with others in the synergy such as the diaphragm and pelvic floor.[59,60] However, as McGill[56] opines, despite the studies being fairly

reported by the authors, too many in the clinical community have tended to over focus on this one muscle and are creating very dysfunctional spines as the unfortunate patients become paralyzed by their own hyper-analysis of what transversus is doing. The pelvic floor has similarly suffered. Rather the need is to establish a muscle's synergistic role in various functional patterns – in McGill's[55,56] terms, 'establishing grooved motion/motor patterns'.

Post surgery outcomes are often modest because the underlying movement dysfunction with causal relations to the 'problem' has not been addressed.

Last but not least is referring the compensation patient with LBP to the gym for 'work hardening programs'. This needs to be criticized as this *reinforces and fixes bad movement patterns*.[61] It is as though the treating therapist doesn't know what else to do with the patient. For all the reasons mentioned this has to be the height of insanity – no wonder the patient is not getting better and is depressed!

Post script: epidemiological surveys among children and adolescents for low back pain

Generally, back pain in children is infrequently considered; however, clinically there may be an increasing trend for pain syndromes to present in younger age groups. This little girl (Fig. 11.8) does gymnastics and developed back pain. As we see, she tends to be extensor dominant posterior pelvic crossed syndrome (PPXS) and she had developed a bad habit of arching her back. However, she quickly learnt better control: the neuromyo-articular system is very flexible at this age (Fig. 11.9). Keeping it this way will be the challenge.

Kolar[62] maintains that in almost 30% of the child population, there is some degree of faulty posture caused by dysfunction in the muscle system. A study by Gunzburg et al.[63] found, a high prevalence of LBP in a cohort of 392 mostly 9-year-old primary school children; 36% reported suffering at least one episode and of these, 64% said that at least one of their parents complained of LBP. There was also significantly more LBP in those who played video games for more than 2 hours a day. In 1999, Balagué et al.[64] undertook a review of the literature published since 1992 on non specific LBP in children and adolescents. Prevalence in the various studies varied between 30% and 51%. They state that the role of certain factors remains

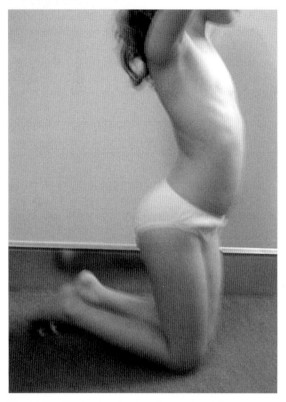

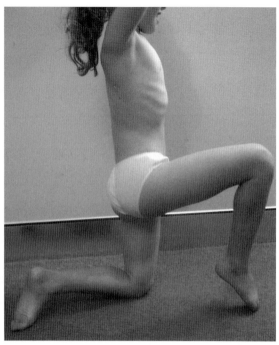

Fig 11.9 • The options for change are usually there if the motivation is there.

Fig 11.8 • The tendencies are often apparent from childhood.

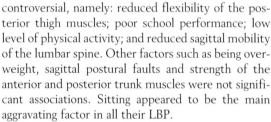

controversial, namely: reduced flexibility of the posterior thigh muscles; poor school performance; low level of physical activity; and reduced sagittal mobility of the lumbar spine. Other factors such as being overweight, sagittal postural faults and strength of the anterior and posterior trunk muscles were not significant associations. Sitting appeared to be the main aggravating factor in all their LBP.

In a South African cohort of mixed racial groups, Jordaan et al.[65] described an incidence of 52% prevalence of LBP with significant risk factors being: white racial group; high level of sport participation; high levels of sedentary activity; incontinence; decreased

neural dynamics and indifferent emotions towards life. A study on prolonged LBP in young athletes concludes that the reasons for the pain are usually established by imaging studies demonstrating cumulative stress changes, the most common of which can be classified as posterior vertebral arch stress injuries to the disc-vertebral end plate complex.[66]

In overview, LBP in children and adolescents appears to be associated with certain functionally meaningful trends namely: a significant prevalence by age 9 increasing with age; the association between postural collapse and sedentary activities and conversely the increased incidence in those with a high level of physical activity. The case for considering altered patterns of posturomovement control as a significant element in the genesis of these states appears overwhelming.

References

[1] Barlow W. The Alexander Principle. Victor Gollancz; 1990.

[2] Bartenieff I. Body movement: coping with the environment. New York: Routledge; 2002.

[3] Grieve GP. Common vertebral joint problems. Edinburgh: Churchill Livingstone; 1981.

[4] Janda V. Muscles, central nervous motor regulation and back

problems. In: Korr IM, editor. Neurobiologic Mechanisms in Manipulative Therapy. New York: Plenum Press; 1978.

[5] Janda V. Sydney: Course notes; 1984; 1985; 1989.

[6] Beach P. The contractile field: a new model of human movement – Part 2. J of Bodywork and Movement Therapies 2008;12 (1):77–85.

[7] Hanna T. Somatics: Reawakening the mind's control of movement, flexibility and health. Cambridge MA: Da Capo Press; 1988.

[8] O'Sullivan P, et al. The relationship between spinal posture and physical characteristics in an industrial low back pain population. In: Proc. 5th Interdisciplinary World Congress on Low Back and Pelvic Pain. Melbourne; 2004.

[9] O'sullivan PB, et al. The relationship between posture and back muscle endurance in industrial workers with flexion-related low back pain. Man Ther 2006;11:264–71.

[10] Ryan CG, et al. Activity levels in individuals with chronic low back pain and asymptomatic matched controls. In: Proc. 6th Interdisciplinary World Congress on Low Back and Pelvic Pain. Barcelona; 2007.

[11] Biering-Sorenson F. Physical measurements as risk indicators for low back trouble over a one year period. Spine 1984;9 (2):106–19.

[12] Volinn E. The epidemiology of low back pain in the rest of the world: a review of surveys in low and middle income countries. Spine 1997;22(15):1747–54.

[13] Janda V. Low back pain: trends, controversies, community-based rehabilitation approach. In: Proc. Consultation on Disability Prevention & Rehabilitation. Turku Finland; 1984.

[14] Galen C. The Alexander technique in the world of design: posture and the common chair Part 1: the chair as a health hazard. J of Bodywork and Movement Therapies 2000;4 (2):90–8.

[15] Clifton-Smith T. Breathe to Succeed. New Zealand: Penguin; 1999.

[16] Farhi D. The breathing book: good health and vitality through essential breath work. New York: Henry Holt and Company; 1996.

[17] Carrière B. Interdependence of posture and the pelvic floor. In: Carrière B, Markel Feldt C, editors. The pelvic floor. Stuttgart: Thieme; 2006.

[18] Lewit K. Manipulative therapy in rehabilitation of the motor system. London: Butterworths; 1985.

[19] Rolf I. Rolfing: The integration of human structures. New York: Harper and Rowe; 1977.

[20] Lowen A. The language of the body. New York: Collier Macmillan Publishers; 1958.

[21] Feldenkrais M. The elusive obvious or basic Feldenkrais. Ca: Meta Publications; 1981.

[22] Bradley D. Hyperventilation syndrome: breathing pattern disorders. New Zealand: Tandem Press; 1998.

[23] Chaitow L, Bradley D, Gilbert C. Multidisciplinary approaches to breathing pattern disorders. Edinburgh: Churchill Livingstone; 2002.

[24] Chaitow L. Breathing pattern disorders (BPD), motor control and low back pain. In: Proc. 5th Interdisciplinary World Congress on Low Back and Pelvic Pain. Melbourne; 2004.

[25] Marras W, et al. The influence of psychosocial stress, gender, and personality on mechanical loading of the lumbar spine. Spine 2000;25(23):3045–54.

[26] Mannion A, Dolan P, Adams M. Psychological questionnaires: do "abnormal" scores precede or follow first time low back pain? Spine 1996;21(22):2603–11.

[27] Hodges PW, Moseley GL. Pain and motor control of the lumbopelvic region: effect and possible mechanisms. J Electromyogr Kinesiol 2003;13 (4):361–70.

[28] Moseley GL, Hodges PW. Are the changes in postural control associated with low back pain caused by pain interference? Clin J Pain 2005;21(4):323–9.

[29] Vlaeyen JW, et al. Fear of movement/(re)injury in chronic low back pain and its relation to behavioural performance. Pain 1995;62(3):363–72.

[30] Crombez G, et al. Pain-related fear is more disabling than pain itself: evidence on the role of pain-related fear in chronic back disability. Pain 1999;80 (1–2):329–39.

[31] Moseley GL, et al. The threat of predictable and unpredictable pain: differential effects on central nervous system processing? Aust J Physiother 2003;49(4):263–7.

[32] Moseley GL, Michael N, Hodges PW. Does anticipation of back pain predispose to back trouble? Brain 2004;127 (10):2339–47.

[33] Thomas JS, France CR. Pain-related fear is associated with avoidance of spinal motion during recovery from low back pain. Spine 2007;32(16):E460–6.

[34] Al-Obaidi SM, et al. The role of anticipation and fear of pain in the persistence of avoidance behaviour in patients with chronic low back pain. Spine 2000;25 (9):1126–31.

[35] Moseley L. Does compo make it hurt more? In: Proc. 5th Interdisciplinary World Congress on Low Back and Pelvic Pain. Melbourne; 2004.

[36] Linton SJ. The relationship between activity and chronic back pain. Pain 1985;21 (3):289–94.

[37] Maluf KS, Sahrmann SA, van Dillen LR. Use of a classification system to guide nonsurgical management of a patient with chronic low back pain. Phys Ther 2000;80(11):1097–111.

[38] Larsson MEH, Nordholm L. Responsibility for prevention, treatment and management of musculoskeletal disorders – a matter for the medical professionals, employers or individuals? In: Proc. 6th Interdisciplinary World Congress on Low Back and Pelvic Pain. Barcelona; 2007.

[39] O'Sullivan PB. Diagnosis and classification of chronic low back pain disorders: maladaptive movement and motor control impairments as an underlying mechanism. Man Ther 2005;10:242–55.

[40] O'Sullivan PB. Classification of lumbopelvic pain disorders – why is it essential for management. Man Ther 2006;11:169–70.

[41] Linton SJ, et al. The secondary prevention of low back pain: a controlled study with follow up. Pain 1989;36(2):197–207.

[42] Ferguson SA, Marras WS, Gupta P. Longitudinal quantitative measures of the natural course of low back pain recovery. Spine 2000;25 (15):1950–6.

[43] Van Dillen LR, Sahrmann S, et al. Trunk rotation-related impairments in people with low back pain who participate in rotational sports activities. In: Proc. 5th Interdisciplinary World Congress on Low Back and Pelvic Pain. Melbourne; 2004.

[44] Herbert RD, Gabriel M. Effects of stretching before and after exercising on muscle soreness and risk of injury: systematic review. Br Med J 31 Aug. 2002;325:1–5.

[45] Chaitow L. Editorial. J Bodywork and Movement Therapies 2008;12(4):293–4.

[46] Shedden MS, Kravitz L. Pilates exercise: a research –based review. J of Dance Medicine and Science 2006;10(3&4): 111–16.

[47] Bernardo LM, Nagle EF. Does pilates training benefit dancers? An appraisal of Pilates research literature. J of Dance Medicine and Science 2006;10 (1&2):46–50.

[48] Pilates J, Miller WJ. Pilates' return to life through Contrology.

USA: Presentation Dynamics Inc; 1998.

[49] Hackney P. Making Connections; total body integration through Bartenieff Fundamentals. New York: Routledge; 2002.

[50] Farhi D. Personal communication. January 2007.

[51] Janda V. Introduction to functional pathology of the motor system. In: Proc. V11 Commonwealth and International Conference on Sport, Physical Education, Recreation and Dance, vol. 3. 1982.

[52] Janda V. Sport exercise and back pain. In: Proc. 1Vth European Congress of Sports Medicine Prague 1985. Prague: VICENUM Czechoslovak Medical Press; 1986. p. 231–5.

[53] Janda V. Postural and phasic muscles in the pathogenesis of back pain. In: Proc. X1th Congress ISRD. Dublin; 1968. p. 553–4.

[54] Janda V. Muscles as a pathogenic factor in back pain. In: Proc. I.F.O.M.T. New Zealand; 1980.

[55] McGill S. Low back disorders: evidenced based prevention and rehabilitation. Champaign IL: Human Kinetics; 2002.

[56] McGill S. Ultimate back fitness and performance. Waterloo: Wabuno Publishers; 2004.

[57] Shields RK, Heiss DG. An electromyographic comparison of abdominal muscle synergies during curl and double d straight leg lowering exercises with control of pelvic position. Spine 1997;22(16):1873–9.

[58] Liebenson C. A modern approach to abdominal training. J Bodywork and Movement Therapies 2007;11(3):194–8.

[59] Hodges PW. Is there a role for transversus abdominis in lumbo-pelvic stability? Man Ther 1999;4 (2):74–86.

[60] Richardson C, Hodges P, Hides J. Therapeutic exercise for lumbopelvic stabilisation: A motor control approach for the treatment and prevention of low back pain. 2nd ed. Edinburgh: Churchill Livingstone; 2004.

[61] Janda V. Sydney: Course notes; Feb 1995.

[62] Kolar P. Facilitation of agonist-antagonist co-activation by reflex stimulation methods. In: Liebenson C, editor. Rehabilitation of the spine: a practitioner's manual. 2nd ed. Philadelphia: Lippincott Williams and Wilkins; 2007.

[63] Gunzburg R, et al. Low back pain in a population of school children. Eur Spine J 1999;8:439–43.

[64] Balagué F, Troussier, Salminen JJ. Non-specific low back pain in children and adolescents: risk factors. Eur Spine J 1999;8:429–38.

[65] Jordaan R, et al. Prevention of low back pain: a new perspective. In: Proc. 6th Interdisciplinary World Congress on Low Back and Pelvic Pain. Barcelona; 2007.

[66] Kujala UM, et al. Prolonged low back pain in young athletes: a prospective case series study of findings and prognosis. Eur Spine J 1999;8:480–4.

Chapter Twelve

A 'functional pathology of the motor system'[1] involves a pattern generating mechanism underlying most spinal pain disorders

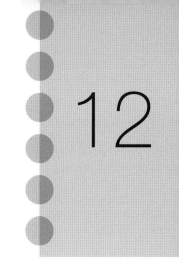

12

Janda[2] said: 'the biological function of pain is that it signals bad or harmful function; it is the motor system's way of protecting itself when overstressed. Pain will sooner or later force us to change our motor behavior. Pain may be considered as the major and most frequent sign of *impaired function of the motor system*. It is not a 'disease' as Western medicine chooses to see it. The patient's pain can help us unravel his functional problems and can also act as the incentive for him to change the bad movement habits that have generally created it.

Lewit'[1,3] adopted the term 'functional pathology of the motor system' to encompass the most important functional changes together with the *reflex changes* they produce. The impaired function may be reflected anywhere in the motor system; however, roughly speaking, there are three basic yet functionally interdependent levels where it is seen:[2] the central nervous system (CNS) corticosubcortical motor regulatory centers; the muscles; and finally the joints. Altered afference produces altered motor output and the muscular level represents perhaps the most exposed part of the system'[2] (see Ch. 7). Neuromuscular control of the spine is complex and involves the interaction of all levels of the motor system.

Whilst a clinically useful and compelling paradigm, it is only more recently that there has been more interest and emerging evidence which in principle supports aspects of the functional approach proposed by Janda and Lewit.[4–8]

Altered loading stresses through the functional spinal unit (FSU) affects local, regional and general neuromuscular responses

The segmented spinal column houses the main nerve trunks between the brain and the periphery. Its functional wellbeing ensures the health of the entire nervous system. The nervous system is a continuous tissue tract which continually glides, slides and stretches as it adapts to the movements it orchestrates.[9,10] When the activity level between the two muscle systems is out of balance, postural and kinematic patterns of movement alter and the whole spine suffers as the compression and tension loading stresses across it change. Altered neuromuscular control is reflected in essentially four ways:

Altered postural responses within the column

Altered alignment and loading patterns in one part of the spine will affect those in adjacent and more removed segments. While *resulting from* changed neuromuscular control they also *result in* the need for further postural compensations being brought to bear in the system. An example is poor spatial control of the pelvis alters the alignment and control of the lumbar lordosis and necessitates muscular 'holding' patterns higher up the torso in order to support the column and head upright. The ability for the pelvis to contribute to postural control is reduced.[11] Some segments and regions are loaded in more tension, others in compression. Reduced ability in finely adjusting and controlling intersegmental movement means individual segments become further compromised. Every spinal segment is susceptible and symptoms arise depending upon the individual circumstances. However, the discussion here will focus on the lumbar spine as most of the literature pertains to this region.

Habitual provocative posturomovement strategies

Neurologically we get used to firing some muscles repeatedly and forget to use others as we repeat various less ideal movement patterns again and again. A good example is when bending forward the action principally occurs by locking the knees and relying on the hamstrings and obturator group with poor contribution from the antagonists in the controlling pelvic force couple – the transversus, iliacus and psoas and other LPU muscles. The hamstring hyperactivity limits posterior pelvic shift and further defacilitates the antagonistic contribution (Fig. 12.1). The habit of crossing the arms in front

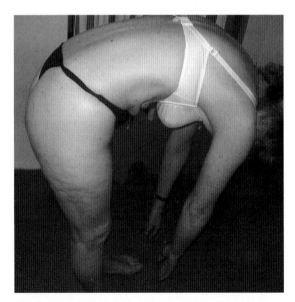

Fig 12.1 • Habitual forward patterns such as this where there is little spatial pre-adjustment of the pelvis to support the movement result in poor patterns of coactivation in the torso.

of the chest fires up the pectorals and serratus contributing to 'dome' development and disturbing cervical and shoulder girdle myomechanics.

Altered segmental muscle function

The passive viscoelastic structures within each FSU (Ch. 6, Part A) enjoy a rich sensory and autonomic innervation enabling them to transmit proprioceptive and nociceptive information.[12] The reflexive feedback control of local muscular contraction consists of afferents in the ligaments, disc and facet joint capsules, spinal interneurons and selected trunk muscles.[13] Altered alignment and movement stresses through the segment can induce progressive creep and hysteresis in the ligaments, the development of joint laxity reduced joint stability and the risk of injury.[14] Feline studies have shown that the induced creep in the viscoelastic tissues also desensitizes the mechanoreceptors and results in a dramatic loss of reflexive muscular activity and stabilization.[15] The induced laxity only showed partial recovery with rest periods twice as long as the loading duration and recovery of reflexive muscular activity follows the recovery of laxity in the viscoelastic structures.[16] More prolonged static loading in lumbar flexion (20 minutes) produced the initial sharp decrease in multifidus activity followed by spasms.[17] Full recovery of reflexive multifidus activity and viscoelastic tension did not occur for up to 24 hours. Static constant loading in flexion not only results in a complex neuromuscular disorder[18] but also importantly the time dependent development of local inflammation.[19,20] Repetitive static loading into flexion increases the likelihood of a cumulative neuromuscular disorder.[21] Injecting porcine facet joints with saline reduced paraspinal muscle activity.[22] Beith[23] showed delay in the short latency stretch reflex in multifidus but not in rectus abdominus or internal oblique in subjects with CLBP. In a porcine study, Hodges et al.[24] found rapid atrophy in multifidus 3 days after experimentally inducing an acute disc injury at L3/4 or an L3 nerve root injury. The changes after the disc lesion produced single segment atrophy and they concluded this may be due to disuse following reflex inhibitory mechanisms. Nerve root injury reduced the cross sectional area over three segments.

Thus depending upon the stage of disorder and tissue irritability, segmental dysfunction involves inhibition/wasting or weakness or conversely spasm of local muscles and segmental control further suffers.

Altered multisegmental muscle function

Local segmental irritation can either decrease or more usually increase activity in SGMS muscles which receive innervation from that segment(s). These large muscles span numerous segments and being large torque producers with domineering behavior, can act as 'yankers' further disturbing axial control (see Ch. 5) This may involve muscles within the torso such as the erector spinae or more peripheral muscles such as the hamstrings which then further influence pelvic control. Eccentric contractions and lengthening behavior in patterns of movement appear to be more difficult in these muscles.

Clinically increased tension in the hamstrings in association with back pain is well appreciated; however, the fact that the same mechanism can effect changes in other peripheral muscles is nor so well known. Upledger[25] suggests mobilizing the upper lumbar spine levels can relax spasm in iliacus. A statistically significant relationship between evident trigger points in the upper trapezius and cervical dysfunction at C3&4 has been reported.[26] Dishman and Bulbulian[27] demonstrated spinal mobilization and manipulation produced a profound yet transient attenuation of reflex excitability in the gastrocnemius. Sacroiliac and spinal manipulative therapy (SMT) has been shown to generate reflex activation of upper and lower limb muscles[28] and to decrease quadriceps inhibition in patients with anterior knee pain.[29] SMT to L4/5 has also been shown to change superficial abdominal muscle recruitment in postural activity in people with low back pain but not in controls.[30]

The potent influence of spinal segmental irritation as the driver of much limb muscle 'tightness' seems little appreciated in the clinical community. It is suggested that 'central axial drive' of peripheral muscle tightness or hyperactivity largely contributes to the pattern generating mechanism responsible for symptom development seen in many 'fitness industry' participants and particularly so in most functional spinal pain disorders (see 'The hamstrings/hip conundrum' p. 286).

Whether a muscle is under-firing or over-firing will thus variably depend on CNS influences, local segmental reflex influences as well as the habitual strategies chose in everyday posturomovement activity. Further, disrupted sensory feedback appears to have a greater effect upon eccentric control than concentric control.[31]

Altered loading stresses of any joint in the body will generally result in reactive inflammatory changes. It is important to recognize that a stiff spinal joint readily becomes an inflamed joint as does a joint that is relatively over mobile. Arguably, in the clinical realm, stiff joints appear to cause more abrasive neurally related symptoms than over-mobile joints. A joint can be stiff in all or some of its available ranges. A joint which is over stressed into flexion with probable creep/hysteresis will generally be stiff into extension and related movements particularly those through the junctional regions. The middle lumbar and cervical segments risk becoming overstressed into both flexion and extension, potentially developing a structural or 'functional instability'. Any inflammatory change within the FSU is liable to create neural irritation to some degree which in the early stages will be sub-clinical, manifesting as altered facilitation or inhibition of muscles which derive their innervation wholly or partly from that segment. The influence of segmental movements on muscle activity can be appreciated in a normal study which showed that moderate central pressures applied to L3 when the subject was prone produced statistically significant reductions in erector spinae EMG.[32] Janda[33] notes that when the intraarticular pressures change, the irritability of the muscles in the vicinity changes. Traction or separation of the joint surfaces facilitates the flexor groups, whereas compression of the articular surfaces in the joint's longitudinal axis facilitates the extensors.

The altered local and multisegmental muscle function results in altered afference to the CNS which in turn results in changed motor output from the CNS. 'This two way traffic of cause/effect/cause'[34] further adds to the pattern generating process in the developing neuromusculoskeletal dysfunctional disorder.

Altered loading stress through the FSU creates the conditions for neural irritation creating local and referred pain and other epiphenomena

The radiculopathic model for the genesis of many chronic pain syndromes is well understood by experienced clinicians. Irritation or damage to a peripheral nerve invariably at the spinal nerve root leads to muscle shortening, autonomic changes and some-times pain in the dermatomal, myotomal and scler-otomal target tissues supplied by that segmental nerve.[35] Simple inflammation rather than structural changes are more often the cause –'biologically or ergonomically triggered neurogenic inflammation.'[36]

The region around and within each FSU is richly endowed with nerves thus a brief review of some clinically relevant aspects of anatomy is useful.

Each FSU intimately encases and contributes to the protection of the spinal cord and the spinal nerve root as it exits through the intervertebral foramen (IVF). The nerves are numbered according to the vertebra beneath which they lie. Thus, the L1 spinal nerve lies below the L1 vertebra in the L1/2 IVF:[12] Centrally each spinal nerve is connected to the spinal cord by a dorsal and ventral root (Fig. 12.2).

The dorsal root of each spinal nerve transmits sensory fibres from the spinal nerve to the cord. The ventral root largely transmits motor fibres from the cord to the spinal nerve but may transmit some sensory fibres.[12] The ventral roots of L1 and L2 spinal nerves additionally transmit preganglionic, sympathetic, efferent fibres.[12] The spinal cord ter-minates in the central vertebral canal opposite L1/2 but this can be as high as T12/L1 or as low as L2/3. The lower lumbar, sacral and coccygeal roots are all enclosed together within the dural sac and descend together as the cauda equina.[12] (Fig. 12.3).

The dorsal root ganglion contains the cell bodies of the sensory fibres in the dorsal root and lies immediately proximal to its junction with the spinal

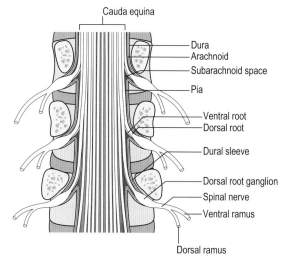

Cauda equina

Dura
Arachnoid
Subarachnoid space
Pia

Ventral root
Dorsal root

Dural sleeve

Dorsal root ganglion
Spinal nerve
Ventral ramus

Dorsal ramus

Fig 12.2 • Lumbar spinal nerve and its relations in the central and lateral canal after Bogduk 1987[12].

nerve within the intervertebral foramen. The spinal nerve root sleeve is surrounded by circumferential layers of connective tissue which indirectly bind the nerve to the margins of the IVF but importantly, *mainly to the capsule of the facet joint dorsally.*[12] This helps explain how clinically, a swollen or thickened facet joint can cause radicular symptoms.

Peripherally, *just outside* the IVF, each spinal nerve divides into a larger ventral ramus and a smal-ler dorsal ramus.[12]

• The **dorsal rami** divide into a medial and lateral branch as they approach the transverse processes
  • The lateral branches are principally distributed to iliocostalis but those from L1, L2 & L3 also become cutaneous and innervate the skin of the buttock over an area extending from the iliac crest to the greater trochanter.[12] This helps explain many clinical patterns – in particular why pain in this region should not necessarily be seen as primary pelvic girdle pain.
  • The medial branches are of paramount importance as they supply the two facet joints, the interspinous muscle and ligament and the multifidus.[12] Each medial branch also supplies the facet joint above and below. Each facet joint also receives additional innervation ventrally from the dorsal ramus in front of the joint.[12] The capsules of the facet joints are thus richly innervated with the appropriate sensory apparatus to transmit both proprioceptive and nociceptive information.[12] The muscular innervation is very specific at each segmental level – each medial branch supplies only those muscles that arise from the vertebra with the same segmental number as the nerve. *The Principal muscles that move a particular segment are innervated by the nerve of that segment.*[12]

• The **ventral rami** lie within the substance of the psoas muscle.[12] The L1–4 ventral rami form the lumbar plexus and the L4–5 ventral rami form the join to form the lumbosacral trunk which enters the lumbosacral plexus. The principal clinical importance of the ventral rami is their communication with the sympathetic nervous system via the grey rami communicantes and the innervation of the disc.

The **autonomic nervous system** must adapt to body movements if it is to function properly. Full utilization of bodily movement ensures its flexibility and health. The sympathetic trunk lies anterior to the whole column and in the thorax it is also attached to

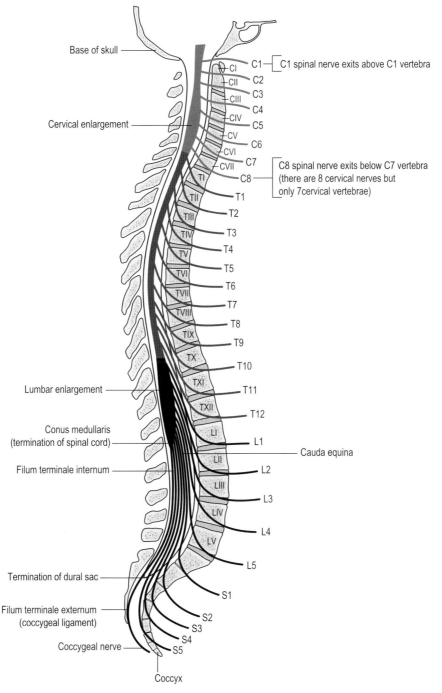

Fig 12.3 • The spinal nerves in relation to the vertebrae. Note the conus is adjacent to the thoracolumbar junction. Irritation of these levels potentially influences a number of nerves.

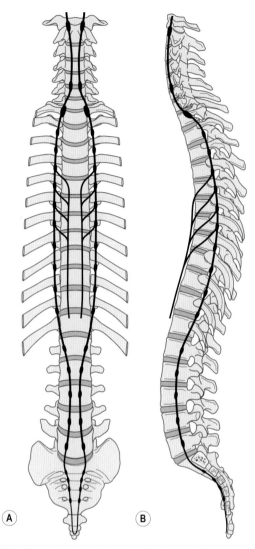

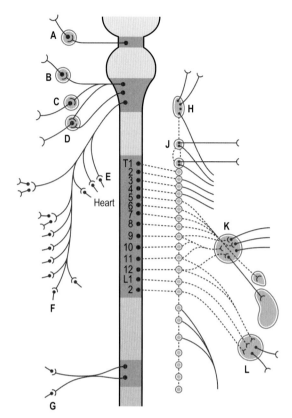

Fig 12.4 • Anterior view (A) and lateral view (B) of the sympathetic chain and its bony relations.

Fig 12.5 • General plan of autonomic nervous system. *On the left:* Cranial and sacral autonomic parasympathetic system. Thick lines from III, VII, IX, X and S2, 3 are preganglionic (connector) fibres. A, ciliary ganglion; B, sphenopalatine ganglion; C, submaxillary and sublingual ganglia. D, otic ganglion; E, vagus ganglion cells in nodes of heart; F, vagus ganglion cells in wall of bowel; G, sacral autonomic ganglion cells in pelvis; thin lines beyond = postganglionic (excitor) fibres to organs.
On the right: Sympathetic nervous system. Dotted lines from T1-12, L1, 2 are preganglionic fibres; H, superior cervical ganglion; J, middle and inferior cervical ganglia (the latter fused with the 1st thoracic ganglion to form the stellate ganglion); K, celiac and other abdominal ganglia (note other preganglionioc fibres directly supplying the adrenal medulla); L, lower abdominal and pelvic sympathetic ganglia; continuous lines beyond = postganglionic fibres. Reproduced with legend from Grieve 1981 with permission Churchill Livingstone.

the head of the ribs[9] (Fig. 12.4). In the lumbar spine the trunks lie next to the attachment of psoas.[12] Note in Figure 12.5 that the 'sympathetic outflow' extends from T1–L2 via the thoraco/lumbar somatic nerves; while the parasympathetic system utilizes the cranial nerves III, VII, IX, X and sacral somatic nerves S234 for its pathways – known as the 'craniosacral outflow'. Both the sympathetics and parasympathetics transmit pain; however, concerning pain in the lower body, the sympathetics will refer to dermatomes associated with the lower sympathetic trunk (T10–L2),[34] while parasympathetics refer to dermatomes associated with S2, and S3 (and S4) segments.[37] In the upper body, the

afferent sympathetic pathways to the head and neck travel with the segmental nerves T1–5, and those to the upper limb, T2–10.[34]

An unhealthy posture of increased thoracic and lumbar kyphosis and cervical extension is likely to place altered tension on the sympathetic trunk.[9] Mobilization to L4/5 has demonstrated significant changes in peripheral sympathetic activity in skin conductance.[38] Impairment of the sympathetic system could be an etiologic cause or perpetuating consequence for the development of active trigger points.[39]

Local and referred pain

Grieve[34] states 'in all pain states, the somatic and autonomic nervous systems are activated in a variety of manifestations and degree. Considerations of spinal pain and referred pain in spinal conditions should include attention to visceral reflex phenomena also'. Similarly, Lewit[1] notes that 'any localized painful stimulation will act in the segment to which the stimulated structure belongs. In this structure there is usually a hyperalgesic zone in the skin, muscle spasm, painful periosteal points, movement restriction of the spinal segment and (perhaps) some dysfunction of the visceral organ. One of the structures may be the source of the pain while others may show more intense reflex changes. However these reflex changes are not confined to a single segment but may affect distant segments constituting a 'chain reaction'.[1]

The somatic response mainly consists of muscle spasm or inhibition and changed motor patterns at the CNS level. The motor pattern may also change to spare the painful structure. The autonomic response is much more varied and can include hyperalgesic zones, pain spots, and vasomotor reaction and at the central level may affect respiration, the cardiovascular and digestive systems.[1]

Referred pain is 'pain perceived in a region topographically displaced from the region of the source of the pain'.[12] It can be referred via the sclerotome or myotome[34] known as 'somatic referral' or by the dermatome known as 'radicular referral'.[12] Dermatome, sclerotome and myotome charts are shown in Figures 12.6–12.8 as they can help towards exploring and localizing the principal joint problem. Pain in any region may arise directly from underlying tissues or be referred to the region from the spine.

When the subjective history implies referred pain, one is never relieved of the obligation to palpate the tissues both centrally and locally to discriminate the pain source. 'Finding the level' is ultimately determined by the 'feel' and response of the joint and related tissues to testing. As Grieve-[34] points out, clinical referral is not always neatly confined to the particular segment as the spinal joints themselves receive articular nerves derived from the segments above and below. Dermatomes are

not anatomical entities but neurophysiological entities whose boundaries may fluctuate according to the prevailing levels of cord segment facilitation. Virtually any source of local lumbar or lumbosacral pain is also capable of producing somatic referral into the limb; the mechanism for which according to Bogduk[12] must lie in the CNS. The quality of somatic referred pain is generally more deep and aching and hard to localize while 'radicular pain' is more superficial, sharp and lancinating. Bogduk[12] points out that compression of a peripheral nerve is not painful but causes changes in conductivity such as weakness and numbness. However, it appears that compression of the *dorsal root ganglia* does trigger nociceptive responses and pain.[12] Experimental compression of a lumbar nerve root demonstrated Wallerian degeneration not only at the site of compression but also at the synapses of spinal cord dorsal horns.[40] Back pain is somatic pain and emanates from local segmental irritation and/or is referred from adjacent of more removed segments e.g. low lumbar pain can emanate from joints in the upper lumbar spine or higher in the thorax.

Diagnosis based upon pathology is not necessarily relevant. Dysfunction in the FSU variably yet mutually involves the facet joint, disc, ligaments, nerves and local muscle control – it is never 'just the disc' etc. At best it is presumptuous guess work, not clinically reliable or particularly useful in delineating effective treatment. The mechanisms involved in neuromyo-articular dysfunction in spinal pain and related limb pain disorders are complex. Schäfer et al.[41] suggest a clinical classification for low back-related leg pain based upon identifying the underlying predominant pathomechanisms involved. They describe four subgroups: central sensitization; denervation; peripheral nerve sensitization and somatic referred pain. It is suggested that, clinically, this approach risks over complication and less effective clinical interventions as these categories largely represent different stages of disorder of an underlying problem and can be expected if the continued noxious input is not addressed.

Arguably there is one fundamental underlying mechanism *common to all* presentations which is *disturbed function* of spinal segments, some of which in Sahrmann's[42] terms, are the 'criminals' while others are the 'victims'. Assessment determines what is what. Examination of both local and regional joint and neuromuscular *function* will delineate *how* the altered function is more than likely to be affecting a number of structures and mechanisms, any and all

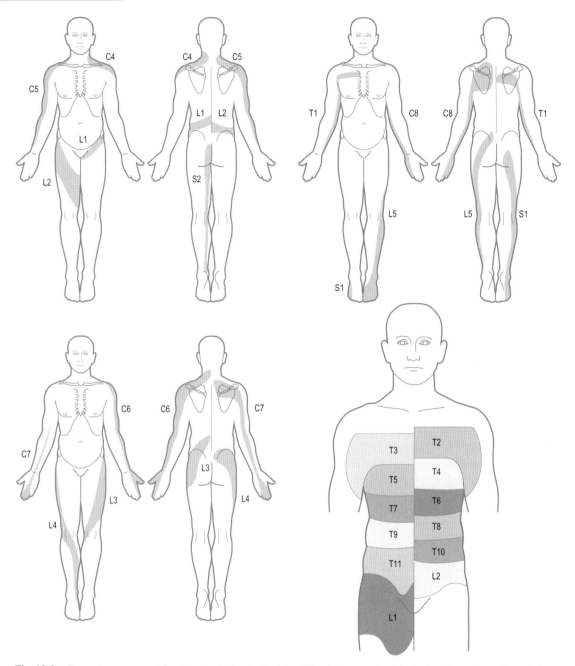

Fig 12.6 • Dermatomes are not fixed anatomical or territorial entities, but *neurophysiological* entities, whose boundaries fluctuate according to the prevailing levels of cord segment facilitation. The areas delineated above are those corresponding to body regions in which pain and other symptoms may often be partly or wholly distributed from joint problems in the general neighbourhood of associated vertebral segments. Reproduced from Grieve 1981[34].

of which can be variously contributing to the pain. Restoring function in the FSU and the adjacent functional regions generally ameliorates the pain and symptoms and helps normalize neuromuscular activation thus providing better and longer lasting clinical outcomes. Frequently overlooked is the potent ability of the facet joint to be the causal driver of most spinal and related pain syndromes. Mooney and Robertson[43] injected the region of the lumbar facet joints and reproduced both back and posterior thigh

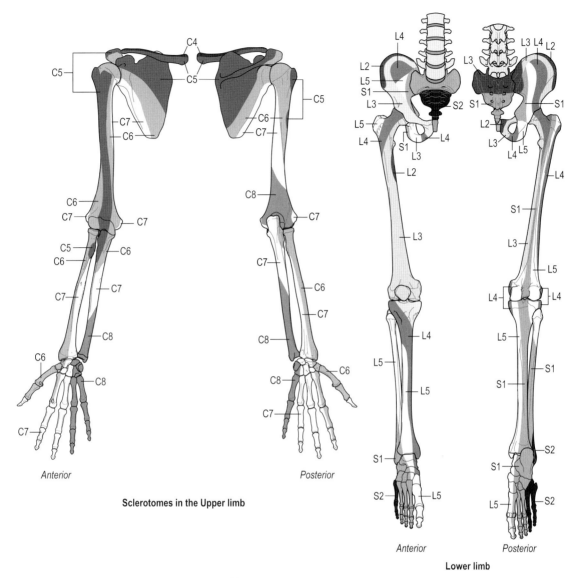

Anterior

Posterior

Sclerotomes in the Upper limb

Anterior

Posterior

Lower limb

Fig 12.7 • Sclerotome charts reproduced from[34] (Grieve 1981).

pain and painful reduction in the SLR. Facet joint dysfunction not only triggers local and somatic referred pain and related syndromes but when the joint is thickened and enlarged as is common, it has the common propensity along with the disc to act as a space-occupying lesion in the IVF engendering radicular symptoms. Nerve root compression has only occurred when the limb pain is accompanied by numbness, weakness or paresthesia.[12]

Segmental neural irritation may not necessarily involve much back pain but can certainly refer symptoms peripherally either somatic or radicular or a combination of both. Wong et al.[44] report a significant correlation between recurrent trochanteric bursitis and lumbar degenerative disease. It is a great mistake to disregard the coexistence of seemingly subtle spinal symptoms of 'stiffness' or 'discomfort' as of no consequence. Most patients have probably had this for years and see it as 'normal' and/or part of 'getting old', yet it can represent a potent potential source of referred symptoms. The semantics of the questioning are important as the term 'pain' can mean agony for some or 'just a niggle' for others. A patient will

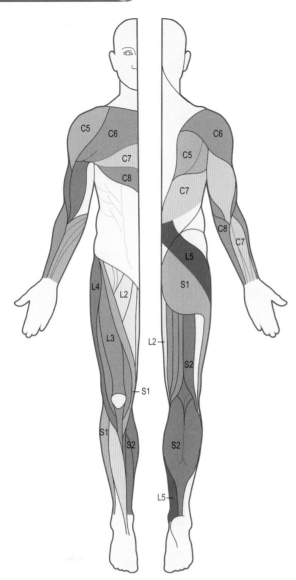

Fig 12.8 • Myotome chart. Reproduced from[91] (Martland 1977)

often deny back pain, yet an enquiring, gentle, palpatory joint and related tissue assessment can have the subject squirm. A similar mistake is to dismiss the spine as a potential cause of peripheral pain when active spinal movements don't reproduce the peripheral symptoms – they infrequently do. Nerve root compression represents and end stage dysfunction disorder yet despite this is it is usually amenable to appropriate conservative treatment. Butler[9] used the terms 'double crush' or 'multiple crush' to describe the co-existence of central and peripheral neurogenic symptoms and their mutual influence upon one another.

The complexity of clinical presentations and the reflex changes brought about by skilled spinal manipulative therapy is exemplified in a case report by Connell[45] in which manual treatment applied to locally symptomatic thoracolumbar and lumbosacral segments produced an immediate improvement in knee range and pain in a subject with anterior knee pain. In restoring neuromyo-articular function over these important junctional regions, the mid lumbar levels are reflexley and 'functionally de-loaded'. Further case reports describe relief of gluteal pain from treatment directed to thoracolumbar levels.[46] Similarly other peripheral syndromes such as tennis elbow are increasingly being reported as functionally associated with spinal dysfunction.[47]

'The hamstrings/posterior hip muscle conundrum'

Tight hamstrings are a common finding in many people and particularly so in those with low back pain. Various authors have attempted to understand this relationship including a possible causal link between tight hamstrings and the development of low back pain.[48–51] 'Problems with the hamstrings' are probably the largest bête noire in the sporting world and recurrent injury is common[52] particularly in the running and kicking sports where they are required to reach extreme lengths in combined hip flexion and knee extension.[53] They apparently accounted for 51% of all lower limb injuries at the 1996 Olympics.[54] The possibility of multifactorial etiology and a continuum of symptoms have been suggested including deficient lumbopelvic dysfunction[52,55], changed biomechanics and motor patterns.[56] These aspects will be further explored.

Their classification within the SGMS renders the more likely behavior of the hamstrings as hyperactive and dominating in movement patterns (Ch. 5). Studies on stretching the hamstrings demonstrate poor and non consistent length gains[57] and stretching in general has not been shown to reduce exercise related injuries.[58–60] Athletes with less range of motion in the standing toe touch test have shown stiffer hamstrings and a lower stretch tolerance than controls.[61]

Studies examining the relationship between the vertical static lumbopelvic posture and tight hamstrings have shown little association.[62–64] Kendall et al.[65] maintain that 'shortness of hamstrings *does* not cause (sic) a posterior pelvic tilt, but a posterior pelvic tilt and a flattening of the lumbar spine are often seen in subjects who have hamstring shortness'. Sahrmann[66] notes that those liable to persistent strain of their hamstrings have a sway back posture with posterior pelvic tilt and poorly developed gluteals (APXS!). However, Stewart et al.[67] applied functional electrical stimulation to the hamstrings in standing and showed that the hamstrings act strongly to retrovert the pelvis and extend the hip in all postures while their action at the knee changes from flexing to extending as crouch increases. Stokes and Abery[68] observed that if the hamstrings were tight, seated postures which involved partial extension of the knees produced pronounced flattening or reversal of the lumbar lordosis. In children with cerebral palsy, McCarthy and Betz[69] found a statistically significant correlation between hamstring tightness and lack of lumbar lordosis in sitting but this correlation was less significant in standing.

Forward bending has been clearly implicated as a risk factor for developing low back pain (LBP). Examination of the dynamic patterns of motion during forward bending in subjects with and without a history of LBP has shown different kinematic patterns. Those with a history of LBP had tighter hamstrings and moved more in the lumbar spine in the early part of the movement.[48,70] Similarly, when rising from bending the LBP group demonstrated greater lumbar motion and velocity in the initial phase of extension and had significantly tighter hamstrings yet hamstring length was not correlated with any kinematic variables.[48] Other studies have shown an overall decrease in range and a significant decrease in hip flexion.[71] Fatigue in forward bending has been shown to alter multi-joint kinematics with decreased knee and hip motion and increased lumbar flexion[72]. Sihvonen[73] found that the flexion-relaxation phenomenon (FRP) when forward bending is also apparent in the hamstrings but occurs later in range after the back extensors relax. However McGorry et al.[74] found this hamstring FRP was less consistent. The different results may be due to their research design which allowed both free standing and restrained standing with the knees held in some flexion. However, their restraint device did not allow the pelvis to posteriorly shift. A fundamental flaw in research design occurs when subjects are instructed to 'keep the knees straight' when bending forward.[48,62,70,71,75] This misunderstands the hamstring's role acting over two large joints as kinematically, full knee extension disallows the pelvis to posteriorly shift and anteriorly rotate, which is necessary to manage the body's center of mass within the base of support (Ch. 4). Kendall notes that when the hamstrings are tight and the knee is extended there will be restriction of hip flexion. Examining the effect of tight hamstrings on gait, Whitehead et al.[76] simulated hamstrings shortening in normal subjects and noted increased effort in walking with decreased speed, stride and step length; decreased hip flexion and increased knee flexion in stance; increased posterior pelvic tilt, decreased pelvic obliquity and rotation.

Neurally, it seems that the hamstrings appear to become readily super charged. Hungerford et al.[77,78] found early timing onset in hamstrings EMG activity in ipsilateral weight bearing in subjects with SIJ pain. A pilot study also reported dominant ipsilateral activity of biceps femoris and underactivity of gluteus maximus in a subject with SIJ pain when walking.[79] In states of heightened mechanosensitivity in the nervous system defensive hamstring hyperactivity can be obser-ved prior to pain onset during the passive SLR test.[80] Mooney and Robertson injected the L4/5 and L5/S1 facet joints with hypertonic saline and in 15 seconds increased EMG activity was apparent in the hamstrings with a reduced SLR. Schleip[81] describes an interesting study he found which showed that stretching the suboccipital muscles resulted in nearly twice as much increase in the SLR test as stretching the hamstrings themselves indicating complex functional reflex relationships between tonic neck reflexes, antigravity control and the hamstrings as part of the extensor system response. Clinically acute lumbar 'discogenic' presentations often appear to be a combination of spasm of the hamstrings posteriorly rotating the pelvis with abnormal co-activity of psoas.

The hamstrings are not the only supercharged posterior hip muscles

While hamstrings hyperactivity is more readily apparent, also pernicious in limiting anterior pelvic rotation/hip flexion on a stationary femur is tightness of the one joint hip extensor –gluteus maximus and those muscles that help control the sagittal movements of the pelvis on the femur – the obturator group and piriformis. When overactive and tight there is static and dynamic restriction of hip flexion, internal rotation and adduction. So why are they so often tight?

Why are the posterior hip and thigh muscles so commonly overactive and tight?

Based on clinical impressions, the following causal sequence of events is suggested to help illustrate the self inflicted, self sustaining dysfunction loop in which so many patients become enmeshed. This cycle serves to not only precipitate but also perpetuate his various symptoms through mutual reinforcement.

1. Habitually adopted *collapsed sitting* postures = repeated posterior pelvic rotation and hyper-flexion of the lumbosacral junction levels.[82] Habitual 'tail bone tuck' postural sets become the basis of subsequent movements which then do not ask for physiological hamstring lengthening in everyday function.

2. Habitual patterns of forward bending principally rely upon dominant hamstring and posterior inferior pelvi-femoral 'holding' where 'hanging from the hamstrings' is associated with back extensor activity and/or Reliance upon the passive tissues with associated poor LPU activity and antagonist coactivation and (Fig. 12.9) →

3. Altered loading stress on lower lumbar segments creates irritation and inflammation within the FSU causing inhibition of local segmental muscles and hyper-facilitation of muscles innervated by the spinal nerves emanating from these levels, i.e.→

- Dysfunction of the L4 root can affect changes in the facilitation/inhibition of quadriceps, tensor fascia lata, the adductors and obturator externus.[83]
- Similarly, the L5, S1 & 2 roots innervate[83] the obturator group (except for obturator externus supplied by L3 & 4); piriformis; hamstrings; glutei.[83]
- The S2, 3, 4 roots innervate the urogenital diaphragm.[83]
- S4 & 5 innervates the pelvic diaphragm (levator ani, coccygeus).[83]

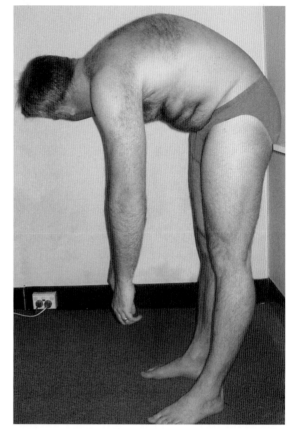

Fig 12.9 • Relying upon 'hanging from the hamstrings' & locking the 'ischial swing' in forward bending. This subject had been diagnosed as 'having a disc'. Intrathecal injections produced no ease. Observing 'his exercises' showed that he was reinforcing his problem (see Fig. 12.10).

4. Movement quality becomes further affected with *decreased hip flexion and anterior pelvic rotation* because of poor antagonistic coactivation and more overactivity, tightness and reduced eccentric control in these posterior pelvic-hip muscles particularly during the forward bending pattern (FBP) repeatedly involved in many ADL activities.

5. FBP thus involves more compensatory *excess low lumbar flexion* and further irritation of lumbar segments and related changes in the muscles; → beginning of a pattern generating mechanism as the more distal muscles become further facilitated.

6. The over-facilitated posterior pelvic–hip muscles serve to functionally hold the pelvis in posterior sagittal rotation, the sacrum in counternutation hyperstabilizing the inferior pelvic bowl during all other posturomovements. Conjunctly, the superior pelvic bowl and SIJ are held in the more open and hypostabilized 'unlocked' position with **reduced or asymmetrical 'distorsion'** and so physiological movement control of the legs and lumbopelvic control is jeopardised during all functional activities.

Hungerford et al.[77,78] speculated that the early onset of biceps femoris in unilateral weight bearing in subjects with sacro-iliac joint (SIJ) pain was compensatory for delayed gluteus maximus activity and/or to augment force closure across the SIJ. The authors do not appear to have considered the influence of segmental and SIJ dysfunction upon the facilitation/inhibition of more distal muscles such as the hamstrings. It is suggested that hyperactivity of hamstrings results both from their habitual over engagement in posturomovement strategies plus their neural overdrive resulting from related segmental spinal and sacroiliac joint dysfunction. Hamstring overactivity will tug the innominate into more posterior rotation carrying the sacrum and 'opening' the ipsilateral lumbosacral junction segments, further aggravating segmental SIJ function. A pernicious pattern generating cycle is operant.

7. Because the buttocks and hamstrings feel tight and sore and the subject is inclined to **stretch** them ⟶

8. However related reduced SLMS activity means segmental and LPU control is poor and so 'posterior hip stretches' are usually 'passive' and instead become lumbar stretches into more flexion further aggravating the segments and **further perpetuating the cycle** (Figs. 12.10–12.12).

9. **The changed patterns of neuromuscular activity can be overt or covert** in general function however, when the hamstrings are hyper-facilitated, increased and sudden demand especially in activities and sports requiring sudden explosive actions such as sprinting and kicking and those entailing bending at the hips, will more easily lead to symptoms such as 'tears'. Most muscle strain injuries are deemed to occur when the muscles are eccentrically contracting.[59]

10. It is suggested that *reduced eccentric activity and active lengthening* (Ch. 4) in these posterior pelvic–hip muscle groups, related *poor coactivation in the LPU* activity and *poor lumbopelvic control* represents the **underlying mechanism driving many lower limb disorders**. The L5–S3 nerves supply the lower limb muscles including the foot

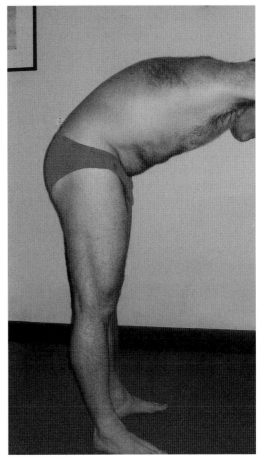

Fig 12.10 • Rather than lengthen, note how active the hamstrings are here! The knee hyperextension and external rotation in the hips effectively lock the 'pelvic swing' so the trunk is required to further flex instead.

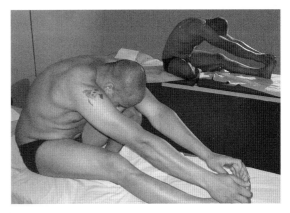

Fig 12.11 • There is no activity from the LPU in controlling the pelvis hence the hamstrings continue to win and the whole back continues to be victimized. Note again how much the arms are involved in the stretch further reinforcing the 'dome'.

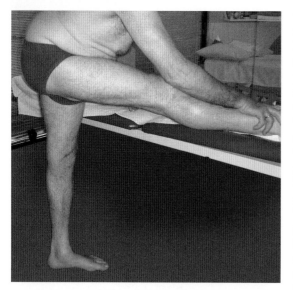

Fig 12.12 • Again note how the tail bone is tucked under and the pelvis is posteriorly rotated with flexion of the lumbopelvic region and poor coactivation in the trunk. This is the same patient as in Fig. 10.10. He has created this ghastly problem in his back through ill informed exercising including this. He practiced 'yoga' for many years.

intrinsics. Clinically, 'diagnoses' such as shin splints, achilles tendonitis, plantar fasciitis and even foot cramps can all have a neurogenic basis and represent 'double crush'[9] insults. The same applies for many 'developmental' hip and knee pain syndromes which occur with no readily apparent reason.

Recurrent hamstring tears in the dancer or sports person can occasion prolonged recovery time. In subjects with a previous posterior thigh injury, Sole et al.[84] reported significantly earlier EMG onsets in the hamstrings on the injured side when preparing for single leg stance. In a prospective study of 30 patients with hamstring strains, Askling et al.[53] found 47% had decided to end their sports activity because of the injury. In the remaining group the median time for return to sport was 31 weeks (range 9–104). It is suggested that specifically addressing the passive and active neuromyo-articular movement dysfunction of lumbopelvic-hip region will reward much shorter return to sport with less reoccurrences (see Ch. 13). There is some evidence that active dynamic stretching seems to be more effective.[85] When hamstring 'stretching' occurs as *active lengthening in controlled patterns of movement* the neuromuscular pathways are 'grooved'[86] and when better established, the opportunity to incorporate them automatically into functional movements becomes more likely. Movement and posture modification may produce the same length gains as 'active inhibitory restabilization'.[87] Increased hamstring length has been shown after muscle energy technique[88] suggesting that when lengthening involves neural control, bigger length gains are achieved and stretch tolerance will improve. However, if the pelvis is not well controlled during active lengthening, no significant length gains are achieved.[89] Maintaining the pelvis in anterior tilt preserves the lordosis, protects the joints and will achieve greater gains in flexibility.[90]

References

[1] Lewit K. Manipulative therapy in rehabilitation of the motor system. London: Butterworths; 1985.

[2] Janda V. Introduction to functional pathology of the motor system.

[3] Lewit K. Managing common syndromes and finding the key link. In: Rehabilitation of the spine: a practitioner's manual. 2nd ed. Philadelphia: Lippincott Williams and Wilkins; 2007.

[4] Vicenzino B, Collins D, Wright A. The initial effects of a cervical spine manipulative physiotherapy treatment on pain and dysfunction of the lateral epicondylalgia. Pain 1996;68:69–74.

[5] Schmid A, et al. Paradigm shift in manual therapy? Evidence for a central nervous system component in the response to passive cervical joint mobilisation. Man Ther 2008;13(5):387–96.

[6] McGuiness J, Vicenzino B, Wright A. Influence of cervical mobilisation technique on respiratory and cardiovascular function. Man Ther 1997;2(4):216–20.

[7] Vicenzino B, et al. An investigation of the interrelationship between manipulative therapy-induced hyperalgesia and sympathoexcitation. J Manipulative Physiol Ther 1998;21(7):448–53.

[8] Berglund KM, Persson BH, Denison E. Prevalence of pain and dysfunction in the cervical and thoracic spine in persons with and without lateral elbow pain. Man Ther 2008;13(4):295–9.

[9] Butler DS. Mobilisation of the nervous system. Melbourne: Churchill Livingstone; 1991.

[10] Butler DS. The sensitive nervous system. Adelaide: Noigroup Publications; 2000.

[11] Mok NW, Brauer SG, Hodges PW. Hip strategy for

balance control in quiet standing is reduced in people with low back pain. Spine 2004;29(6): E107–12.

[12] Bogduk N, Twomey LT. Clinical anatomy of the lumbar spine. Melbourne: Churchill Livingstone; 1987.

[13] Solomonow M, et al. Neuromuscular neutral zones associated with viscoelastic hysteresis during cyclic lumbar flexion. Spine 2001;26(14): E314–24.

[14] Solomonow M. Ligaments: a source of musculoskeletal disorders. J Bodywork and Movement Therapies. IN PRESS.

[15] Solomonow M, et al. Volvo Award Winner in Biomechanical Studies: Biomechanics of increased exposure to lumbar injury caused by cyclic loading: Part 1. Loss of reflexive muscular stabilization 1999.

[16] Gedalia U, et al. Biomechanics of increased exposure to lumbar injury caused by cyclic loading: Part 2. Recovery of reflexive muscular stability with rest. Spine 1999;24(23):2461.

[17] Jackson McL, et al. Multifidus EMG and tension-relaxation recovery after prolonged static lumbar flexion. Spine 2001;26 (7):715–23.

[18] Solomonow M, et al. Biomechanics and electromyography of common idiopathic low back disorder. Spine 2003;28(12):1235–48.

[19] Solomonow M, et al. Muscular dysfunction elicited by creep of lumbar viscoelastic tissues. J Electromyogr Kinesiol 2003;13 (4):381–96.

[20] Le P, et al. Cyclic load magnitude is a risk factor for a cumulative lower back disorder. J Occup Environ Med 2007;49(4):375–87.

[21] Sbriccoli P, et al. Static load repetition is a risk factor in the development of lumbar cumulative musculoskeletal disorder. Spine 2004;29 (23):2643–53.

[22] Indahl MD, et al. Interaction between the porcine lumbar intervertebral disc, zygapophysial joints and paraspinal muscles. Spine 1997;22(24):2834–40.

[23] Beith ID. Short latency stretch reflexes are delayed in lumbar multifidus but not in the abdominal muscles in chronic low back pain, In: Proc. 6th Interdisciplinary Congress on Low Back and Pelvic Pain. Barcelona; 2007.

[24] Hodges PW, et al. Rapid atrophy of the lumbar multifidus follows experimental disc or nerve root injury. Spine 2006;31 (25):2926–33.

[25] Upledger JE, Vredevoogd JD. Craniosacral therapy. Seattle: Eastland Press; 1983.

[26] Fernández-de-Las-Peñas C, Miangolarra JC. Musculoskeletal disorders in mechanical neck pain: myofascial trigger points versus cervical joint dysfunctions. A clinical study. J Musculoskeletal Pain 2005;13 (1):27–35.

[27] Dishman JD, Bulbulian R. Spinal reflex attenuation associated with spinal manipulation. Spine 2000;25(19):2519–25.

[28] Herzog W, Scheele D, Conway P. Electromyographic responses of back and limb muscles associated with spinal manipulative therapy. Spine 1999;24(2):146–52.

[29] Suter E, et al. Decrease in quadriceps inhibition after sacroiliac joint manipulation in patients with anterior knee pain. J Manipulative Physiol Ther 1999;22(3):149–53.

[30] Ferreira ML, Ferreira PH, Hodges PW. Changes in postural activity of the trunk muscles following spinal manipulative therapy. Man Ther 2007;12 (3):240–8.

[31] Enoka RM. Neuromechanics of Human Movement. 3rd ed. USA: Human Kinetics; 2002.

[32] Krekoukias G, Petty N, Cheek L. Comparison of surface electromyographic activity of erector spinae before and after the application of central posteroanterior mobilisation on the lumbar spine. J Electromyogr Kinesiol IN PRESS.

[33] Janda V. Muscle and Joint Correlations, In: Proc. IVth Congress FIMM Prague Rehabilitacia Suppl. 1975;10/11:154–8.

[34] Grieve GP. Common vertebral joint problems. Edinburgh: Churchill Livingstone; 1981.

[35] Gunn CC. The Gunn approach to the treatment of chronic pain: intramuscular stimulation for myofascial pain of radiculopathic origin. 2nd ed. New York: Churchill Livingstone; 1996.

[36] Zusman M. Irritability. Man Ther 1998;3(4):195–202.

[37] Briggs C. Functional anatomy of the pelvis, In: Proc. Aust Physiotherapy Assn. NSW Branch Conference; 1997.

[38] Perry J, Green A. An investigation into the effects of a unilaterally applied lumbar mobilisation technique on peripheral sympathetic nervous system activity in the lower limbs. Man Ther 2008;13 (6):492–9.

[39] Fernández-de-Las Peñas. Neural and joint afferences as etiologic or perpetuating factors of myofascial spinal trigger points, In: Proc. 6th Interdisciplinary Congress on Low Back and Pelvic Pain. Barcelona; 2007.

[40] Kobayashi S, et al. Synapse involvement of the dorsal horn in experimental lumbar nerve root compression: a light and electron microscopic study. Spine 2008;33 (7):716–23.

[41] Schäfer A, Hall T, Briffa K. Classification of low back-related leg pain – A proposed patho-mechanism based approach. Man Ther IN PRESS.

[42] Sahrmann SA. Sydney: Course notes; 1996.

[43] Mooney V, Robertson J. The facet syndrome. Clin Orthop Relat Res 1976;115:149.

[44] Wong L, et al. Is recurrent trochanteric bursitis due to lumbar degenerative disease? In: Proc. 6th Interdisciplinary Congress on Low Back and Pelvic Pain. Barcelona; 2007.

[45] Connell AT. Concepts for assessment and treatment of anterior knee pain related to altered spinal and pelvic biomechanics: a case report. Man Ther 2008;13(6):560–3.

[46] Sebastian D. Thoracolumbar junction syndrome. Physiother Theory Pract 2006;22(1):53–60.

[47] Berglund KM, Persson BH, Denison E. Prevalence of pain and dysfunction in the cervical and thoracic spine in persons with and without lateral elbow pain. Man Ther 2008;13(4):295–9.

[48] McClure PW, et al. Kinematic analysis of lumbar and hip motion while rising from a forward flexed position in patients with and without a history of low back pain. Spine 1997;22(5):552–8.

[49] Rebain R, et al. A systematic review of passive straight leg raising test as a diagnostic aid for low back pain (1989 to 2000). Spine 2002;27(1&):E388–95.

[50] Feldman DE, et al. Risk factors for the development of low back pain in adolescence. Am J Epidemiol 2001;154(1):30–6.

[51] Zhu Q, et al. Adolescent lumbar disc herniations and hamstring tightness: review of 16 cases. Spine 2006;31(16):1810–4.

[52] Wallden M, Walters N. Does lumbopelvic dysfunction predispose to hamstring strain in professional soccer players? J Bodywork and Movement Therapies 2005;9:99–108.

[53] Askling CM, et al. Proximal hamstring strains of stretching type in different sports: injury situations, clinical and magnetic resonance imaging characteristics and return to sport. Am J Sports Med 2008; Apr 30.

[54] Nannini L, et al. The centennial olympic games and massage therapy: the first official team. J Bodywork and Movement Therapies 1997;1(3):130–3.

[55] Devlin L. Recurrent posterior thigh symptoms detrimental to performance in Rugby Union: Predisposing factors. Sports Med 2000;29(4):273–87.

[56] Croisier J-L. Factors associated with recurrent hamstring injury. Sports Med 2004;34(10):681–95.

[57] Magnusson SP. Passive properties of human skeletal muscle during stretch maneuvers. A review. Scand J Med Sci Sports 1998;8(2):65–77.

[58] Herbert RD, Gabriel M. Effects of stretching before and after exercising on muscle soreness and risk of injury: systematic review. Br Med J 31 Aug. 2002;325:1–5.

[59] Weldon SM, Hill RH. The efficacy of stretching for prevention of exercise-related injury: a systematic review of the literature. Man Ther 2003;8 (3):141–50.

[60] Pope R. Muscle stretching for the athlete: friend or foe? Aust Physiotherapy Association Sportslink 2002; Sept:4–5.

[61] Magnusson SP, et al. Determinants of musculoskeletal flexibility: viscoelastic properties, cross sectional area, EMG and stretch tolerance. Scand J Med Sci Sports 1997;7(4):195–202.

[62] Li Y, McClure P, Pratt N. The effect of hamstring muscle stretching on standing posture and on lumbar and hip motions during forward bending. Phys Ther 1996;76(8):836–49.

[63] Toppenberg RM, Bullock MI. The interrelation of spinal curves, pelvic tilt and muscle lengths in the adolescent female. Aust J Physiother 1986;32(1):6–12.

[64] Gajdosik RL, Hatcher CK, Whitsell S. Influence of short hamstring muscles on the pelvis and lumbar spine in standing and during the toe touch test. Clin Biomech 1992;7(1):38–42.

[65] Kendall FP, McCreary EK, Provance PG. International edition: muscles testing and function. 4th ed. Baltimore: Williams and Baltimore; 1993.

[66] Sahrmann SA. Diagnosis and treatment of movement impairment syndromes. St. Louis: Mosby; 2002.

[67] Stewart C, et al. An investigation of the action of the hamstring muscles during standing in crouch using functional electrical stimulation. Gait Posture 2008;28(3):372–7.

[68] Stokes IA, Abery JM. Influence of hamstring muscles on lumbar spine curvature in sitting. Spine 1980;5(6):525–8.

[69] McCarthy JJ, Betz RR. The relationship between tight hamstrings and lumbar hypolordosis in children with cerebral palsy. Spine 2000;25(2):211.

[70] Esola MA, et al. Analysis of lumbar spine and hip motion during forward bending in subjects with and without a history of low back pain. Spine 1996;21(1):71–8.

[71] Porter JL, Wilkinson A. Lumbar-hip flexion motion: a comparative study between asymptomatic and chronic low back pain in 18- to 36-year-old men. Spine 1997;22 (13):1508–13.

[72] Sparto PJ, et al. The effect of fatigue on multijoint kinematics and load sharing during a repetitive lifting test. Spine 1997;22(22):2647–54.

[73] Sihvonen T. Flexion relaxation of the hamstring muscles during lumbar-pelvic rhythm. Arch Phys Med Rehab 1997;78(5):487–90.

[74] McGorry RW, et al. Timing of activation of the erector spinae and hamstrings during a trunk flexion and extension task. Spine 2001;26(4):418–25.

[75] Norris CM, Matthews M. Correlation between hamstring muscle length and pelvic tilt range during forward bending in healthy individuals: an initial evaluation.

[76] Whitehead CL, et al. The effect of simulated hamstring shortening on gait in normal subjects. Gait Posture 2007;26(1):90–6.

[77] Hungerford B, Gilleard W, Hodges P. Evidence of altered lumbopelvic muscle recruitment in the presence of sacroiliac joint pain. Spine 2003;28(14):1593–600.

[78] Hungerford B, et al. Altered lumbo-pelvic muscle recruitment occurs in the presence of sacroiliac joint pain, In: Proc. 5th Interdisciplinary World Congress on Low Back and Pelvic Pain. Melbourne; 2004.

[79] Hossain M, Nokes LDM. A biomechanical model of sacroiliac instability resulting in low back pain, In: Proc. 6th Interdisciplinary World Congress on Low Back and Pelvic Pain. Barcelona; 2007.

[80] Hall T, Zusman M, Elvey R. Manually detected impediments during the straight leg raise test. In: Proc. 9th Biennial Conference. MPAA; 1995. p. 48–53.

[81] Schleip R. How upper neck muscles influence hamstring length. Sourced. http://www.somatics.de/NeckAndHams.html

[82] O'Sullivan PB, et al. The relationship between posture and back muscle endurance in industrial workers with flexion-related low back pain. Man Ther 2006;11:264–71.

[83] Williams PL, Warwick R. Gray's Anatomy. 36th ed. Edinburgh: Churchill Livingstone.

[84] Sole G, et al. Altered muscle activation of hamstring muscles following posterior thigh injury. In: Proc. 6th Interdisciplinary Congress on Low Back and Pelvic Pain. Barcelona; 2007.

[85] Wiemann K, Hahn K. Influences of strength, stretching and circulatory exercises on flexibility parameters of the human hamstrings. Int J Sports Med 1997;18:340–6.

[86] McGill S. Low back disorders: evidence-based prevention and rehabilitation. Champaign Il: Human Kinetics.

[87] De Vito G, et al. Comparison of two stretching techniques on hamstrings flexibility. In: Proc. 6th Interdisciplinary World Congress on Low Back and Pelvic Pain. Barcelona; 2007.

[88] Ballantyne F, Fryer NDG, McLaughlin P. The effect of muscle energy technique on hamstring extensibility: the mechanism of altered flexibility.

J Osteopathic Medicine 2003;6 (2):59–63.

[89] James M, et al. The effects of a Feldenkrais program and relaxation procedures on hamstring length. Aust J Physiother 44(1):49–54.

[90] Sullivan MK, Dejulia JJ, Worrell TW. Effect of pelvic position and stretching method on hamstring muscle flexibility. Med Sci Sports Exerc 1992;24 (12):1383–9.

[91] Maitland GD. Vertebral Manipulation 4th Ed. Butterworths: London; 1977.

Therapeutic approach

Pain can result from overt traumatic incidents or where altered posturomotor control over some time creates repetitive micro trauma, setting the scene for an often trivial incident becoming the 'tipping point' for symptom development. When looked for, other associated sub-clinical symptoms have usually also been apparent as part of the dysfunction picture.

The treatment rationale is determined by assessing the patients neuromyo-articular *function*, and redressing the specific neuromyo-articular dysfunction found as the actual or likely cause and perpetuator of the pain picture in that particular patient. When the pain and the reasons for it can be effectively dealt with in the early stages there is less likelihood of secondary problems developing such as chronic pain and central pain hypersensitivity, fear of movement, passive coping, depression, catastrophizing etc.

The *diagnosis is based on movement dysfunction*, not structural pathology. Restoring improved function will generally ease the pain while structural pathology such as 'a bulging disc' remains the same. The structural pathology generally represents the point of tissue distress resulting from altered posturomovement function over time.

Simply looking at the patient tells us a lot about him. Appreciating the model presented – the salient aspects of normal function (Ch. 6); the common features of dysfunction (Ch. 8); and the clinical patterns (Chs 9 & 10) provides a helpful framework through which to assess the patient. Which joints do we expect to be symptomatic: stiff or overstressed? Knowing what to look for helps decide the test movements and in particular, when

passive joint testing, refine the direction of enquiry for possible joint restriction. Assessment confirms or otherwise our predictions and hunches. 'The model' hopefully helps the therapist discern 'the wood from the trees' and 'see' the problem more clearly and find and understand the pain source. Assessment will ideally delineate which are the 'key elements' to address, indicate the level of dysfunction and stage of the disorder.

Centrally important is the recognition of the interdependence between spinal joint and muscle function. Symptomatic spinal joints emanate from altered posturomovement control but in turn when irritable, further adversely affect neuromuscular function. Improved muscle function cannot be expected while the joints are symptomatic and vice versa. Ideally, manual and exercise therapy complement and mutually reinforce one another.

Therapeutic algorithm

Altered control of the spine not only results in various spinal pain syndromes but because it houses much of the nervous system, a plethora of related symptoms seemingly in other organ 'systems' or in the head and limbs are possible. The therapeutic approach considered here will principally focus upon 'spinal pain' and related proximal girdle disorders with more emphasis on the pelvic girdle. However, it is very important to appreciate that dysfunction in the upper pole of the body also affects function in the lower pole and vice versa, affecting spinal function as a whole. In this respect the upper pole *is* considered within the therapeutic algorithm and the exercise and movement control approach. Ideal motor function relies on integrated control between the spine, head, both proximal limb girdles and their large ball and socket joints.

The therapeutic algorithm can be distilled into the following main components (summarized in Table 13.1). The irritability of the patient's condition will dictate how many of the movement tests are performed. The art of the clinician is to gauge the stage of disorder and only test what he/

Table 13.1 The therapeutic algorithm: assessment and management

1. Assessment

- Subjective: dealt with in summary form only
- Objective comprehensive treatise as follows:

A) Observation:

- General
- Clinical syndromes
- Muscle contours
- Soft tissue clues

B) Movement testing

- **Patterns** of active movement in:
- *Standing:* (*=sufficient in more acute presentations where assessment is limited because of irritability)
  - *Forward bend pattern
  - *Spinal extension, side bending, rotation
  - *Sit to stand to sit
  - Bilateral arm elevation
  - Pelvic translation
  - Standing on one leg
  - Grow one elbow with hands on head
  - Hitch one hip
  - Squat pattern
  - Single leg semi-squat
- *Sitting feet supported:*
  - *Achieving a neutral pelvis
  - *Breathing pattern
  - Sagittal and lateral pelvic weight shifts
  - Neutral pelvis with hip flex; knee ext.
  - Pattern of hip int. rotation/adduction
  - One hip external rotation
- *Supine crook lying:*
  - *Breathing pattern
  - *Three fundamental pelvic patterns
  - Loading for bridge
  - Limb load challenge
    - Bent knee fallout
    - Hip flexion from ilio-psoas
    - Hip, knee & ankle flexion 90°
    - Active straight leg raise?
  - Coordination IAP, breathing and axial stabilization
  - Supine low f/ab/er test
  - Supine high f/ab/er test
- Supine f/ad/ir test
- Posterior pelvi-femoral opening
- Modified Thomas position screening
- Craniocervical flexion (CCF)
- Bilateral arm elevation
- *Prone:*
  - *Breathing pattern
  - *Habitual leg posture
  - *Fundamental Pelvic Patterns
  - Prone on elbows
  - Prone knee bend (PKB)
  - Length/tension balance in hip rotators
  - Prone f/ab/er test
  - Backward pelvic rotation pattern
  - Prone limb load and pattern of hip extension:
    i) in PKB
    ii) with knee extension
  - Prone push up/passive extension in lying
  - Posterior-inferior opening of the pelvis and hip

C) Passive testing/treatment of joints and myofascia with reference to the junctional regions:

- Lumbosacral junction
- Thoracolumbar junction
- The 'dome'
- Cervicothoracic junction
- Cervicocranial junction

2. Therapeutic approach

- Manual: the 'key' positive assessment findings become the focus of manual treatment aimed at clearing pain and related symptoms
- Modify the symptom producing habitual postural behavior
- Simple adjustments to common daily activities
- Therapeutic exercise: should complement manual treatment, be problem specific and redress the general features of dysfunction as described
- Home exercise program: practicality and pitfalls
- Exercise therapy and spinal pain:
  - Review of literature −ve and +ve
  - The case for therapeutic exercise and movement classes

It is important to establish fundamental patterns of movement required in ADL activities she needs to in order to discern the reason for the patient's pain. For someone in severe pain, simple observation and gentle manual exploration might be the only measures the patient can comfortably tolerate. As pain settles, more detailed movement testing can ensue. Motor performance will be markedly compromised if the patient has marked pain.

Assessment

The committed and experienced practitioner has learned to understand and see the often subtle nuances inherent in 'normal' posturomovement function and the significance of seemingly small differences seen in the dysfunctional state (see Ch. 4). The competent therapist is deft at ferreting out the information needed to help delineate the presenting picture of dysfunction.

Subjective examination

Relevant aspects to explore include the exact area, extent and description of *all* symptoms; this includes the presence of other pains and symptoms which may not seem related. Is there an apparent reason for their sudden or gradual onset; symptom frequency and whether worsening or stable and the stage of the disorder; symptom irritability and sleep patterns; behavior of symptoms in relation to postures and activities; past history of trauma; occupational posturomovement demands; past and present exercise and leisure activities; previous treatment and demonstration of any exercises prescribed; general health status, medications and results of investigations; patient beliefs as to the source of symptoms; compensable status? Screening for any 'red flags' or 'yellow flags',[32] also begins during the subjective examination.

Objective examination (see Ch. 4)

A) Observation

1. *General*. Many valuable insights are gleaned during the subjective examination when the patient's habitual posturomovement behavior can be observed without him realizing. This includes his sitting and standing postures; breathing patterns; willingness and manner of moving as he undresses and psychomotor aspects.

2. *Clinical Syndromes*. The standing observation looks for any asymmetry and the relative influence of the clinical syndromes – the Pelvic Crossed Syndromes (PXS; Chs 9 & 10), the Shoulder Crossed Syndrome (SXS), the Layer Syndrome and the Belted Torso Syndrome (Ch. 10). Notice the habitual posturing of the legs and the quality of the feet in being likely to offer dynamic support (Ch. 8, p. 207). The pelvic position, muscle contours and symmetry help decide the Clinical Syndromes and individual patterns within these.

3. *Muscle contours*. The following descriptions have largely been influenced by Janda.[1,3,4,5]

Posterior view

- Careful attention should be paid to the back muscles. A healthy back has a healthy distribution of muscle tone. Unhealthy backs have too little and look 'empty' (Fig. 13.1) or too much and look 'straightjacketed' (Fig. 13.2). The **erector spinae** bulk should be compared from side to side as well as from the lumbar to the thoracolumbar regions. According to Janda there should be no difference between sides or regions and 'prevalence of the thoracolumbar portions of erector spinae is a poor sign in relation to prognosis'.[2–4] This is common in the PPXS and MS.

- The inter scapular area should be observed for loss of bulk of the **inter-scapular muscles**. If so, in addition the distance between the thoracic spinous processes and the medial border of the scapula is increased and the scapulae are rotated, with their inferior angles improperly fixed to the rib cage such that apparent winging occurs[5] (Fig. 13.3). If present there is probably a corresponding tightness in the levator scapulae and upper trapezius muscles which is associated with neck pain. If so the neck/shoulder line is changed such that the person displays 'Gothic shoulders'[4] – all indicative of the SXS.

- Imbalanced **rotation in the hip joint**. Janda confounded this author in claiming a patient had a right sacroiliac joint problem when he had just walked into the room! This pronouncement was predicated upon the marked external rotation evident in the right hip indicating hyperactivity and shortening of piriformis.

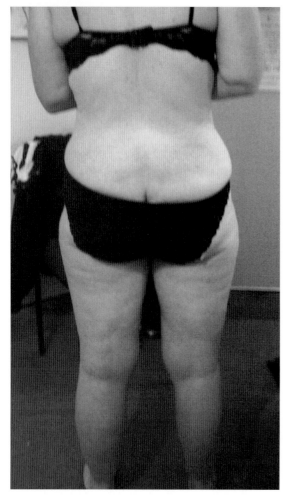

Fig 13.1 • A back with too little tone looks doughy and lifeless.

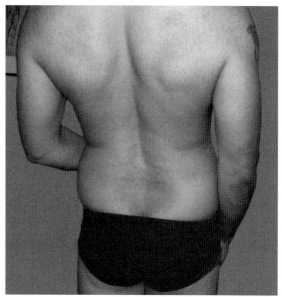

Fig 13.2 • A back with a lot of superficial muscle activity is not necessarily healthy.

- An ***abducted position of the legs*** indicates possible shortness of the abductors – gluteus medius and minimus and tensor, with 'long' adductors. Indicative of all PXS and reduced active support from the systemic local muscle system (SLMS)
- The ***glutei*** should be symmetrical and rounded. If weak or inhibited the muscle tends to 'hang' loosely[3] – common in APXS. Asymmetry may indicate problems in the lumbar spine, sacro-iliac joint or hip.
- The ***hamstrings*** are usually well developed but it is important to look at their bulk relative to the glutei as when these are inhibited the hamstrings become predominant[3] and knee hyperextension is

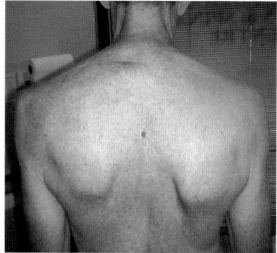

Fig 13.3 • Emptiness in the interscapular region.

common. Commonly found in all PXS. Their activity can markedly increase in forward bending if dysfunctional.
- Tightness of the ***short hip adductors*** is seen as a distinct bulk of muscle in the upper third of the thigh.

- A normal calf has a spindle form.[6] Tightness of the **gastrocnemius-soleus (**GS) is characterized by an apparent broader tendo-achilles.[4] If the soleus is tighter there is increased bulk on the medial side of the TA tendon[6] and the lower leg becomes more cylindrical.[4] The normal heel shape has a quadratic form and if more pointed this can indicate that the GS is tighter, which shifts the center of gravity forward.[6] More common in PPXS.

Anterior view

- The **abdominal wall** should be flat. A sagging protruding abdomen reflects a generalized weakness of the abdominals. There may be imbalanced activity between the different abdominal muscles. When the obliques are dominant, a distinct groove will be seen on the lateral side of the recti, indicating that there may be a decrease in the stabilizing function of the recti in the anteroposterior direction, an important factor in stabilization of the spine.[3,4] (Fig. 10.24). When the transversus is underactive a lateral bulge in the waistline is apparent.[6] This can even be obvious in someone who has 'worked out' at a gym where the emphasis has been upon the superficial abdominals while there is little 'inner support' (Fig. 13.4). Conversely, the abdominals as a group can be over activated and so over developed that they overly fix the lower pole of the thorax and equally compromise axial control (Fig. 13.5). There may be imbalance between the upper and lower regions with fullness of the lower abdominal wall - common in APXS (Fig. 13.6).

- The **pectorals**. The tighter and stronger these are, the more prominent is the muscle belly. Typical imbalance will lead to rounded and protracted shoulders and slight medial rotation of the arms.[5] This is particularly common, especially in people who use weights at the gym. The nipple is shifted laterally and superiorly and if pectoralis minor is tighter there is increased bulk above it. The anterior axilliary fold is thickened if major is tight.[6] However, appearances can be deceptive as tightness can also occur without bulk through adaptive shortening (Fig. 13.7).

- The **sternocleidomastoid** in normal states is just visible. If the insertion, particularly the clavicular insertion, is prominent it is a sign of

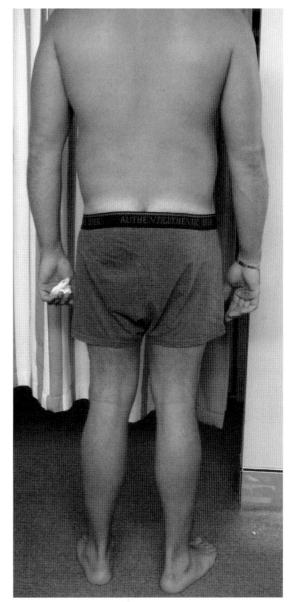

Fig 13.4 • Despite 'working out', many 'gym junkies' display this lateral bulge.

tightness. If so there is usually related weakness of the deep neck flexors[5] (see Fig. 10.14).

- Normally the bulk of the **tensor fascia lata** (TFL) should not be distinct. If it is and there is also a groove on the lateral side of the thigh the muscle is being overused and both it and the iliotibial may be tight (Fig. 13.8). When the **rectus femoris** is tight

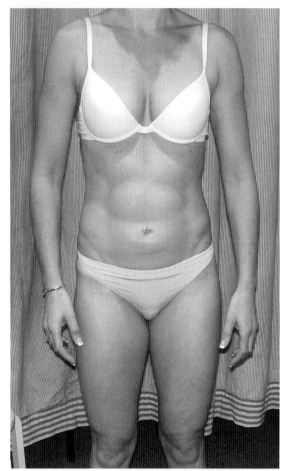

Fig 13.5 • Overdeveloped abdominals can act like a tight 'bib' anteriorly restricting freedom of the lower pole of the thorax.

the position of the patella moves slightly upwards and also laterally if there is concurrent tightness in the iliotibial band.[6]

4. _Soft tissue signs_ can also reveal valuable clues. A segmental 'divot' or reactive bony prominence may be apparent in the spine hinting at altered function. A soft tissue 'bubble' is often apparent over L3/4 or L4/5 when marked 'hinging' stresses have been occurring over these levels and the local soft tissues begin to resemble over stretched elastic (Fig. 13.9). Segmental and long muscle spasm is reliably indicative of segmental dysfunction when later confirmed by palpatory examination.

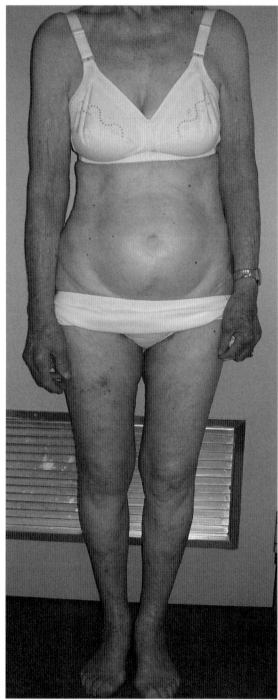

Fig 13.6 • Evident imbalance in the tone between the 'upper' and 'lower' abdominals is common and indicative of poor spatial and intrapelvic control.

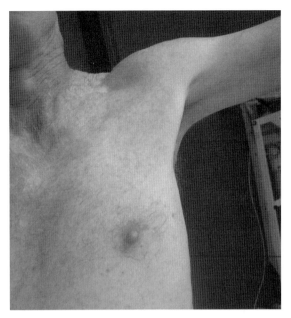

Fig 13.7 • Tight pectorals are not necessarily bulky.

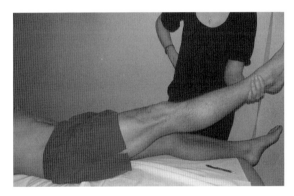

Fig 13.8 • Evident tight TFL.

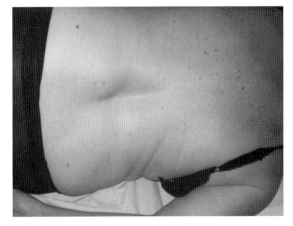

Fig 13.9 • Soft tissue 'bubble' relating to marked 'hinging' stresses in function.

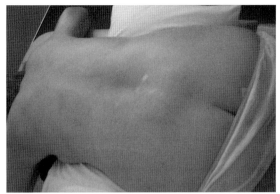

Fig 13.10 • Puffy superficial tissues and poorly delineated bony landmarks over the lumbosacral junction.

Segmental wasting may also be apparent over attenuated levels. Poor muscle bulk, puffy and reactive superficial tissues and poorly defined bony prominences are often apparent over the lumbosacral junction and indicative of the region sustaining a lot of abnormal loading stress (Fig. 13.10). When the skin is mottled and discoloured (livedoreticularis) it is a sure sign the person has been going to bed with a hot-water bottle to ease the pain over some time. The soft tissues feel very tough and inelastic and expect that accurate joint testing can be more difficult.

B) <u>Movement testing</u> (refer to Ch. 4)

Imbalanced activity between the deep (SLMS) and superficial systemic global muscle system (SGMS) muscle systems is reflected in *altered kinematic motion patterns* resulting from imbalanced length/tension relationships of muscles contributing to the *control of force couples in movement*. Examination of patterns of movement begins to indicate the abnormal loading patterns that various joints may have been subjected to. Uneven segmental motion with segmental or regional 'hinges' and/or 'blocks' may be apparent and symptom producing (Fig. 13.11). Further testing of joint function confirms or otherwise these impressions.

Patterns of active movement

While possible combinations of movement testing are endless and will depend upon the region of pain and stage of disorder, at the initial assessment those which appear to yield the more significant information are mentioned. One is not compelled to perform

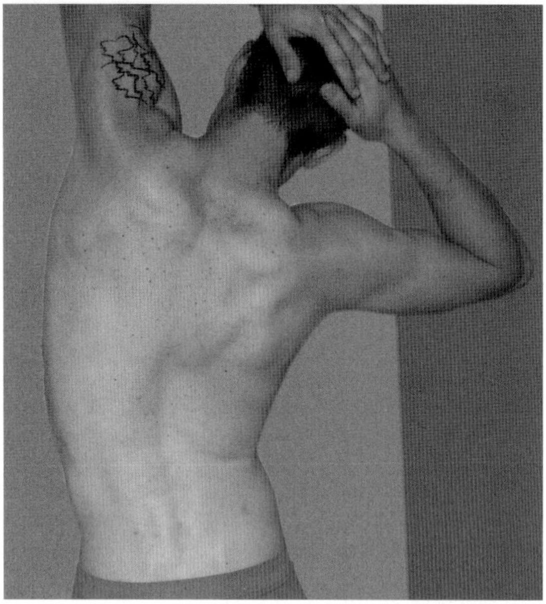

Fig 13.11 • Apparent segmental 'block' around the 'dome'.

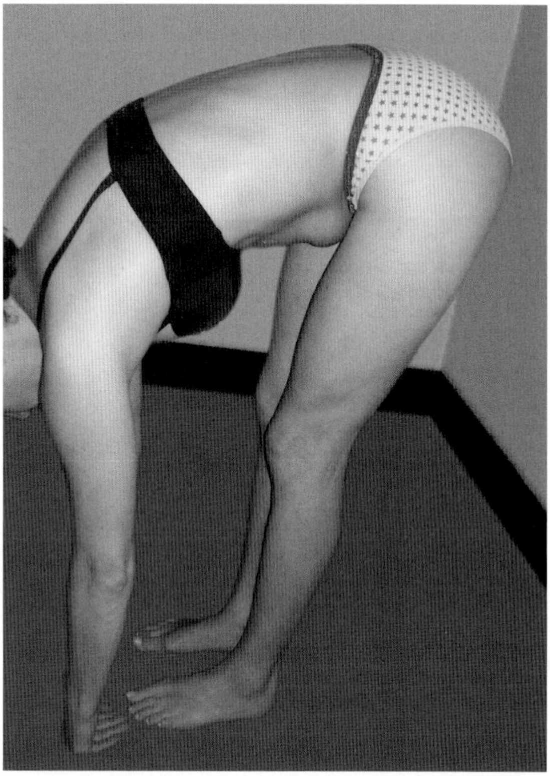

Fig 13.12 • This is a better forward bend than most. However, ideally one would like to see better anterior pelvic rotation and co-activation in the abdominal wall (see Fig.13.116).

all those tests listed and clearly in an acute presentation, only a few of the basic tests (marked *) are examined. However, one may need to chase symptoms in say an elite athlete and many if not all may be performed. We are most interested in the ability and quality of the movement patterns the alteration of which can limit or increase range in different regions of the spine and explain symptom development. Altered length/tension relationships in various pelvi-femoral muscles affect pelvic myomechanics and control. Some, none or all of these movements may reproduce the pain or a symptom which is informative however, symptom reproduction is not the primary goal. It is important that the therapist does not over-challenge the patient beyond his abilities as otherwise he will use what he can draw upon and 'knows'– invariably dominant SGMS activity in predictably provocative kinematic patterns and thus risk exacerbating symptoms. Poor performance of any test indicates avenues for treatment.

In standing:

- *__*Forward bending pattern and return*__: the patient's habitual preferred strategy tells a lot about his motor function in general. The axis of movement, pattern of pelvic control and intersegmental movement through the whole spine are observed (Fig. 13.12). Repeat while palpating the inferior aspect of the posterior inferior iliac spines (PSIS) and noting if the movement is symmetrical. A torsion or 'twist' indicates altered intrapelvic movement and/or stiffness in one hip or altered hamstring tension. Importantly, also note to what degree the whole pelvis posteriorly shifts and anteriorly tilts on the femoral heads and is this sufficient that the sacrum nutates and the coccyx and ischial tuberosities lift through the movement? Is there co-activation between the flexors and extensors or does he simply rely on the extensor system and/or the passive tissues and 'hanging off the hamstrings'?
- *__*Spinal extension, lateral flexion and rotation*__ observing for 'hinges' and 'blocks' in segmental movement throughout the spine as well as range and symmetry and importantly the amount of pelvic shift and tilt to provide the axis and support for the sagittal and coronal movement. In extension does the pelvis shift anteriorly and tilt posteriorly so that the axis of movement is in the hip (Fig. 13.13)? In lateral flexion does it shift contralaterally and tilt on the femoral heads and what of segmental movement

in the spine? (Fig. 13.14). In rotation is there ipsilateral backward pelvic rotation and relative hip internal rotation? Repeat while palpating the PSIS during the movements which should be symmetrical in extension but asymmetrical in side bending and rotation to reflect flexible 'distorsion'. When the pelvis is mobile Lee[7] notes that in side bending the contralateral innominate posteriorly rotates thus, ipso facto the ipsilateral lumbosacral

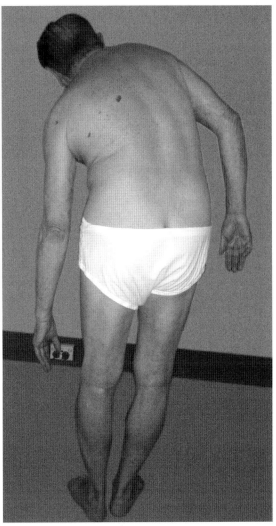

Fig 13.14 • While the pelvis has shifted there is reduced freedom in 'distorsion' and dissociation within the joints of the hip–pelvis and lumbosacral junction complex with poor intersegmental movement through the lumbar spine.

junction can move into a 'closing' pattern. Similarly, in axial pelvic rotation the contralateral innominate anteriorly rotates and the sacrum rotates ipsilaterally[7] initiating axial rotation through the spine. Altered length/tension in the hip rotators influences intrapelvic motion and that of the pelvis on the femoral heads (Fig. 13. 16).

Standing to sitting and return to standing: observing the quality of sagittal weight shift in the pelvis and trunk, axial alignment including head control, lower limb kinematics and the ability to come up to stand without pushing down through the arms (Fig. 13.15).

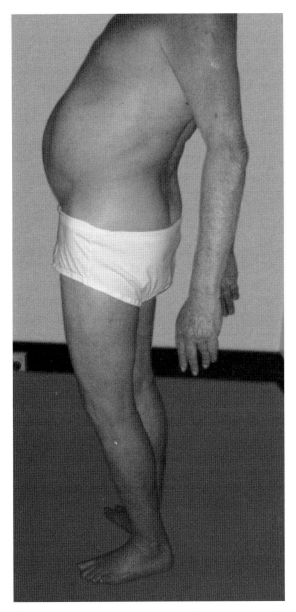

Fig 13.13 • Notice the poor anterior shift of the pelvis and opening in the hips coupled with poor support from the abdominal wall.

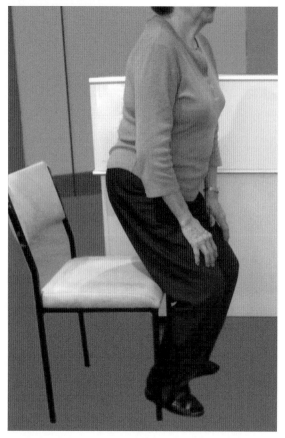

Fig 13.15 • It is unusual for 'patients' to stand up without pushing down with their arms particularly when the base of support and control of sagittal weight shift is poor.

• ***Bilateral arm elevation:*** looking for quality of shoulder girdle support for the movement and whether there is adjustment through the thorax or overcompensation in the lumbar spine and neck.

• ***Pelvic translation*** in the sagittal frontal and horizontal planes: the ability to *initiate movement from* the pelvis and the sequencing of intersegmental movement from the lumbosacral junction through the spine, its symmetry and any symptom response (Fig. 13.16).

• ***Standing on one leg.*** Observing the adaptability of the lower kinetic chain for unilateral flexible support; the quality of pelvic control both on the supporting leg and also as the base of support for the torso; and also the balance strategies adopted. The pelvis as a whole should not tilt anteriorly, posteriorly, laterally or rotate on the standing leg. Frequently the patient maintains a level pelvis in the

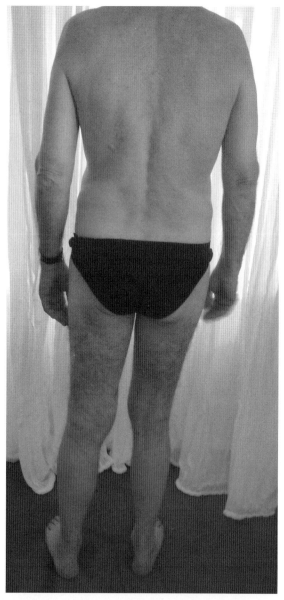

Fig 13.16 • The patient was asked to shift his pelvis to the right. There is reduced intrapelvic/hip dissociation extending into the spine and he experiences pain.

frontal plane although it is posteriorly tilted with loss of lordosis and poor 'distorsion' When 'distorsion' is defective the movement is shunted into the lumbar spine with holding strategies higher up the spine (Figs 6.22, 8.7 & 13.17). If a more physically competent patient, repeat while palpating both PSIS while flexing, extending and abducting one leg. Here one is further testing 'distorsion' available in the pelvis to support the open chain hip

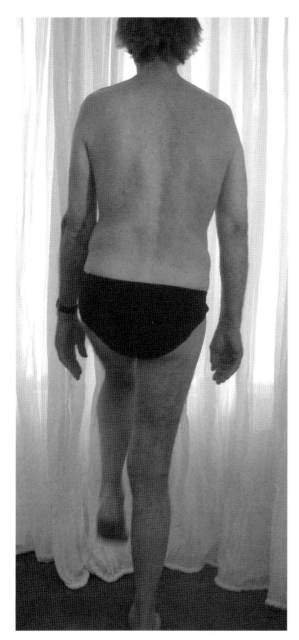

Fig 13.17 • The same patient as in Fig. 13.16 experiences pain and finds balance difficult. Note the response in the left limbs to aid stability.

movement while also maintaining lumbopelvic alignment on the standing leg. The PSIS on the weight bearing standing leg should remain reasonably still and the lumbar lordosis should be preserved. The PSIS on the moving leg should posteriorly rotate around mid hip flexion; anteriorly rotate in hip extension.

• *Growing one elbow* to the ceiling with hands on the head: provides clues about the quality of lateral weight shift through the pelvis and 'body half' support with postural adjustment through the thorax and thoracolumbar junction. Central cinch pattern (CCP) behavior in response to inadequate pelvic control reduce the ability for elongation one side of the torso necessary in lateral weight shift and elevating one arm (Figs 13.18,13.19 & 8.27).

• *Hitching one hip* with 'straight' legs provides further information about 'distorsion' and the quality of ipsilateral 'closing' patterns over the lumbosacral junction and may produce symptoms. Commonly the movement is 'taken' over levels higher up (Figs 13.20,13.21).

• *Squat pattern*. Observe the preparedness to load the lower kinetic chain into antigravity flexion patterns – the ability to control closed chain hip flexion and spinal and lower limb alignment on dynamically adjusting legs. Commonly there is poor posterior shift and the pelvis rolls into posterior tilt (Fig. 13.22) & (Fig. 13.24).

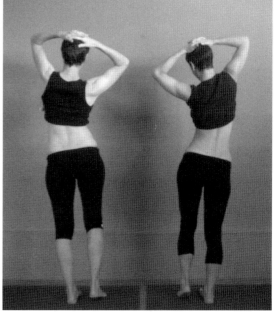

Fig 13.18 • More ideal organization for growing one elbow to the ceiling. The individual responses show a common pattern of ipsilateral weight shift and lengthening in the torso. Note the obliquity of the pelvis through its rotation in the frontal plane on the femoral heads.

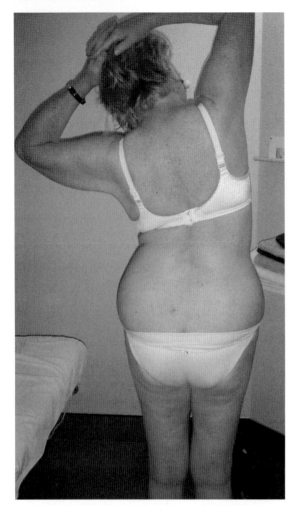

Fig 13.19 • Inadequate organization for growing one elbow to the ceiling. Note the buttock clenching and consequent lack of spatial pelvic shift and frontal plane rotation on the ipsilateral femoral head. Central posterior cinch behavior holds the spine centrally limiting adaptive response and weight shift through the torso to bring the body weight over the standing leg.

- **Single leg semi squat**. Provided the patient has good control of the previous tests, the ability for lateral weight shift and closed chain pelvic control during antigravity lower kinetic chain flexion is tested here. With the weight mostly on one leg and the other acting as a balance prop behind, the patient is asked to 'semi-squat' onto one leg. Observe the ability to align the knee in relation to the foot, control of rotation at the hip as well as triplanar control of the pelvis. Does the pelvis posteriorly shift and anteriorly rotate on the femur? Observe patterns of muscle activity in the trunk (Fig. 13.23).

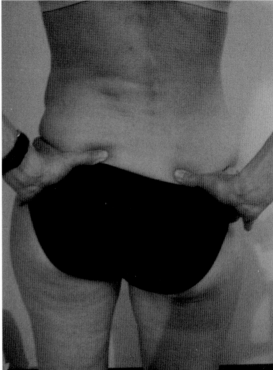

Fig 13.20 • Hitching one hip. Note the initiation in the pelvis and the left 'lumbosacral closing'. Incidentally note the "Block" around the thoracolumbar junction.

In sitting with feet supported:
- *The ability to assume a **neutral pelvic posture** with active lift *from* the ischial base of support, a corresponding neutral axial posture and head position (Figs 13.25 & 13.26) without torso holding patterns while breathing from the diaphragm assesses active control in the deep system.[8-10]
- ***The breathing pattern:** the ability to *widen* the lower pole of the thorax on inspiration from primary diaphragm activity.[11-13] Breathing should not involve any superior movement of the chest[12] and/or protraction of the shoulder girdle[13] (Figs 8.30 & 8.31).
- **Sagittal and lateral weight shifts through the pelvis:** the ability to *initiate from* the 'sitz bones' with postural adjustment through the whole spine and no 'central fixing' strategies (Figs 13.27, 13.28, 13.29 & 13.30 see also Figs 6.25, 6.26 & 8.26).
- The ability to **control the neutral position of the pelvis** while extending one leg or flexing one hip (Fig. 13.31).

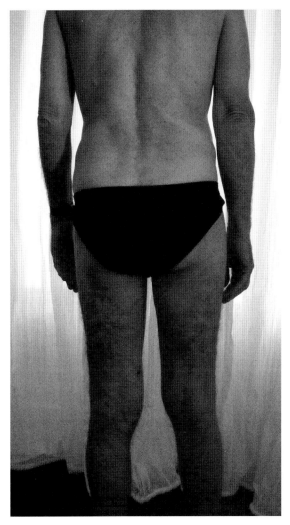

Fig 13.21 • Incompetent hitching the right hip with poor right 'lumbosacral closing' and the movement axis becomes higher up.

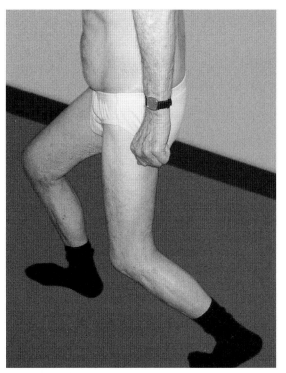

Fig 13.22 • This patient has had a hip replacement and 'rehab' and this is how he has been taught to 'squat'! He drops his body mass down 'between' both legs and does not shift the pelvis posteriorly. Consequently the action is hard on the right knee.

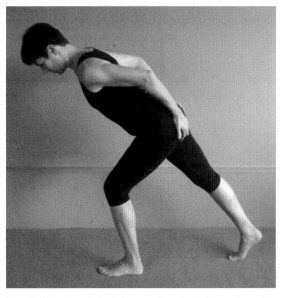

Fig 13.23 • Good single leg squat controlled from the pelvis which orients the torso.

• The ability to **adduct and internally rotate one or two hips** in sitting observing patterns of axial and pelvic alignment and control.

• The ability to **externally rotate one hip** at a time while controlling pelvic position.

In **supine crook lying** ('standing' on the feet with hips and knees flexed) with support under the head

• *Breathing pattern*: observing for abdominal and lower lateral costal breathing which should predominate.[11] There should be no elevation of the thorax on inspiration or tension in the scalenii and sternocleidomastoid.[11,12] Is this different to being upright? Is the patient able to maintain an expiratory position of the thorax after you have

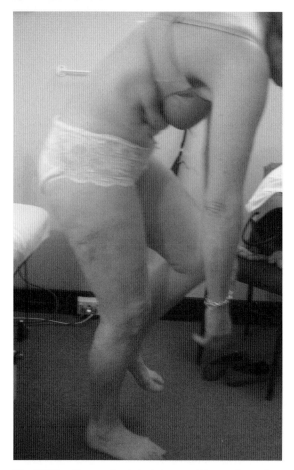

Fig 13.24 • Disorganized single leg squat in a pattern of 'more total flexion'.

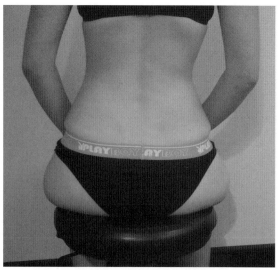

Fig 13.25 • Good base of support for sitting; note the width through the base of the pelvis and nice even tone in the back muscles.

brought him into it (Fig. 13.32)?[13] Can he widen the lower pole of the thorax on inspiration? Many can't.

• *The ability to **perform the three fundamental pelvic patterns** (Ch. 6, Part B; Ch. 8). Proponents of a motor control approach[14,105,108,114] which focuses upon the deep muscle 'canister'[14] of the lumbar spine, advocate initial specific and independent activation of the individual muscles before co-activation of the local synergy. However, the back pain population seen in the clinic are in general more akin to 'sensorimotor morons' and some find independent activation frustrating or nigh impossible. Even so called 'healthy' subjects have had to be excluded from research studies because they could not activate transversus in isolation.[15] The fundamental patterns provide a clinically expedient and practical solution to achieving activation of the muscles in the lower pelvic unit

(LPU; Ch. 6, Part B) in physiological, functionally relevant synergistic patterns of modulated movement. As the focus of the axis of movement is low within the pelvis there is less tendency for hyper-activation of SGMS torso muscles which has generally been the patient's habitual response and which is hard for him to inhibit.

The fundamental patterns involve the ability to *initiate movement from* the tail bone and sitz-bones through the LPU while the subject is in crook lying.

• **FPP1.** Place one hand at the posterolateral or if possible under the *lower* lumbar spine and the other medial to one anterior superior iliac spine (ASIS) and just north of the symphysis to monitor LPU activity and ask 'can you gently roll your back off my hand?' When LPU control is deficient, anterior pelvic rotation with a low lumbar lordosis is poor and attempted from a central posterior cinch (CPC; Fig. 8.3). The pattern of muscle activation should ideally be felt anteriorly, posteriorly and within the pelvis 'below the belt' while diaphragmatic descent expands the lower pole of the thorax above the belt during regular breathing. Placing a thumb and fingers over the subject's ischial tuberosities can assist the action by asking for and emphasizing *widening* the sitz bones, which facilitates a better LPU response and helps lessen the tendency to CPC behavior (Fig. 13.33). When the action is correct the groins deepen, the lower abdominals are

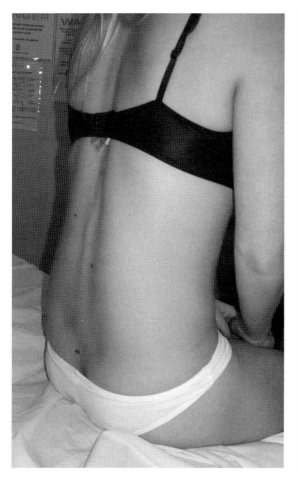

Fig 13.26 • Poor pelvic base to support sitting; notice the necessary flexion over the lumbosacral junction and holding higher up in order to get the column upright.

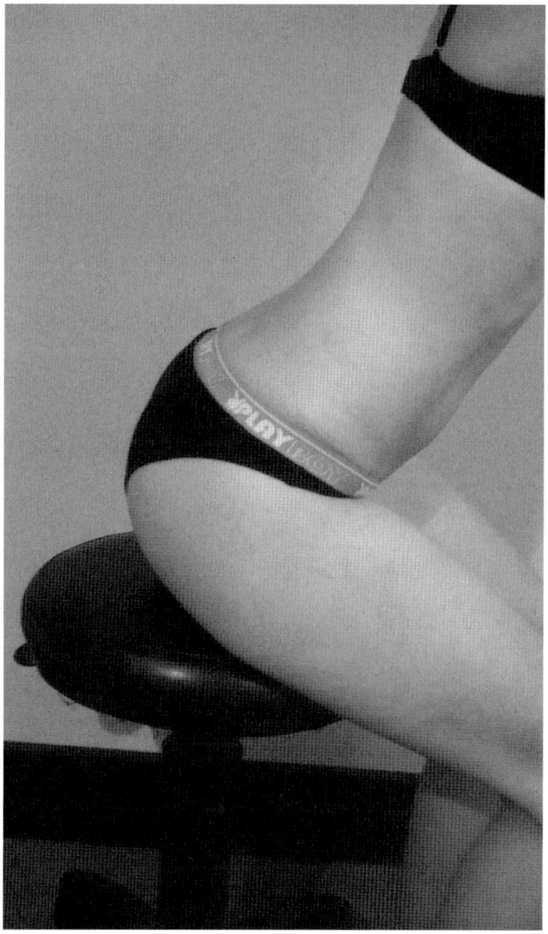

Fig 13.27 • Good sagittal anterior pelvic rotation; note the nice co-activation in the trunk.

more active than the upper, the spine elongates and the chin drops and breathing is unobstructed (Fig. 13.34). If the patient cannot inhibit CPC activity, a full inspiration and holding it (without tension) while attempting the LPU activation can help. If the patient is really struggling with the idea of the movement, the therapist can help provide the *sensation* of the correct movement by placing her hands on the patients anterior thigh and 'distracting' them caudad (Fig. 13.35).

• *FPP2.* While palpating the sitz bones and the other hand palpating medial to the ASIS, ask 'can you gently flatten your back onto the bed' by drawing your sitz bones together. Generally this action is 'easy'; however, when LPU control is poor pushing through the heels with hamstrings and gluteus maximus and upper abdominal hyperactivity

are dominant (Figs 13.36 & 6.30). When coming from the LPU the lower abdominals should be more active (Fig. 13.37).

• *FPP3.* Place a hand on each ASIS and ask 'can you grow one knee long and away' and monitor the amount of 'distorsion' and symmetry between sides (Fig. 13.38). When control is poor lateral flexion of the lumbar spine occurs rather than 'distorsion' (Fig. 13.39). Seemingly subtle it is an important action for the patient to feel.

The fundamental patterns can be taught from day one in side lying, supine and prone and help reduce local muscle spasm and holding patterns as well as 'milking' swollen joints and initiating motor relearning. In the acute scenario, movement is only to just short of any pain, whereas in the subacute or chronic, movement is into stiffness – particularly

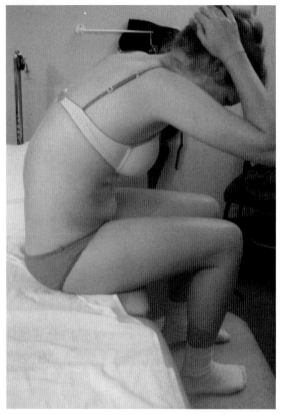

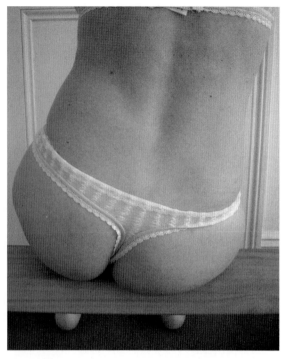

Fig 13.29 • Good frontal plane weight shift through the pelvis. Note the adaptive lengthening in the ipsilateral extensor system and lateral body wall. Stronger activity in the LPU would show more definition in multifidus over the lower levels.

Fig 13.28 • Poor initiation of sagittal anterior pelvic rotation and forward weight shift in sitting. The patient is 15.

FPP1 and FPP3. *Their establishment is fundamental for properly developing all other functional patterns of pelvic control.*

• *Loading for bridge*. Further tests able performance of FPP1 in two steps. The ability to bring the pelvis into slight anterior rotation via the LPU and *maintain the position* while:

1. 'Grounding' the feet and taking the lower body weight through them while breathing normally. The pelvis does not move. If able to do this:

2. Slightly unweighting the pelvis, maintaining the lordosis and *sustaining the action while breathing normally* (Fig. 13.40). Commonly this is difficult and the patient attempts the movement by coming up high into the bridge in posterior tilt where he can lock in with dominant hamstrings, gluteus maximus and obturator group action and, possibly, reliance upon CPC behavior (Fig. 13.41). This probably explains the findings of Stevens et al.[15] where

stabilizing exercises administered to a healthy population produced higher activity in the abdominal muscles but not the local back muscles despite the subjects being asked to maintain the lumbar spine in a neutral position.

• *Limb load challenge* to lumbopelvic control where a triplanar neutral pelvis is maintained throughout each hip movement. Maintenance of the low lumbar lordosis is particularly important:

1. *Bent knee fallout*[16] (BKF). One leg is extended from the heel with neutral hip and pelvic rotation monitored by the patient palpating his anterior iliac crests; while the bent knee is moved laterally as far as possible and returned without the pelvis moving or any disruption in breathing. In the correct action, the LPU provides appropriate support so that the action derives *from the hip*.

2. The ability for *prime ilio-psoas activity in flexing the hip*. The position is as for

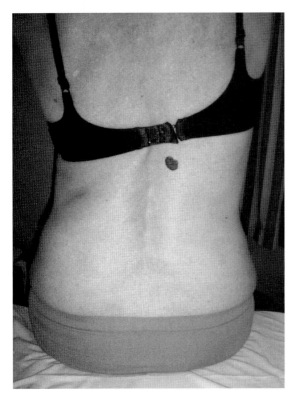

Fig 13.30 • Dysfunctional control of attempted lateral weight shift to the right. Note there is no initiation or shift through the pelvis and instead she tries to 'pull up' from above. The bilateral CPC behavior does not allow adaptive weight shift through the torso. See also Fig. 8.26.

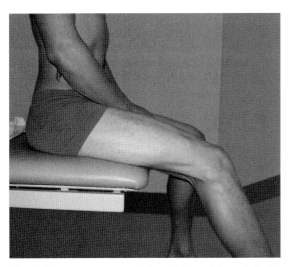

Fig 13.31 • When controlled, the pelvis provides stability for active lengthening in the hamstrings.

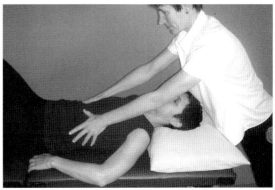

Fig 13.32 • The lower pole of the thorax is brought into the expiratory position and the patient asked to maintain the position while continuing to breathe with posterior lateral basal expansion.

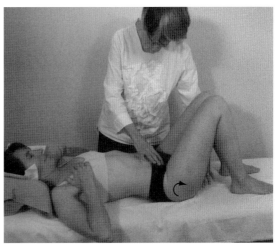

Fig 13.33 • FPP1 is facilitated by the therapist's hands over the lower belly and the ischia; lower abdominals are more active than the upper abdominals.

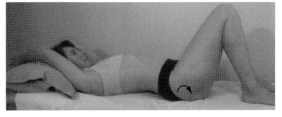

Fig 13.34 • In the correct action the movement is initiated from the pelvis, there is co-activation between the flexors and extensors, the groins deepen and the tail bone and chin drop down.

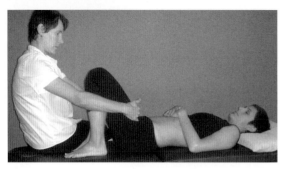

Fig 13.35 • Manual distraction provided by the therapist helps provide the sensation of the required movement.

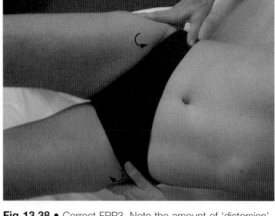

Fig 13.38 • Correct FPP3. Note the amount of 'distorsion' in the pelvis. This is best gauged by the relative distance between the thumbs on the ASIS resulting from the contra-rotation between the innominates. Note the deepening in one groin.

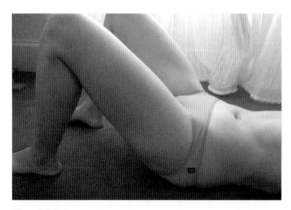

Fig 13.36 • Incorrectly actioned FPP2 shows more upper abdominal action over lower.

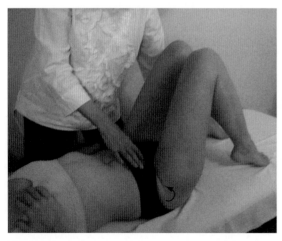

Fig 13.37 • Coming onto the toes helps inhibit gluteal and hamstring activity and facilitates the correct response in FPP2 from the LPU.

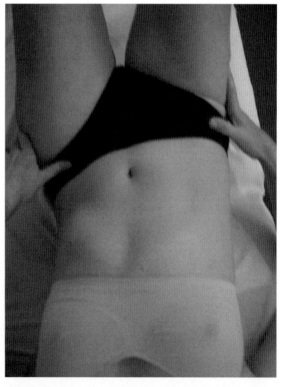

Fig 13.39 • Abnormal FPP3 rather than 'distorsion' in the pelvis there is more side bending in the waist; less 'twist' discernable between the thumbs; and the groin depth is more the same.

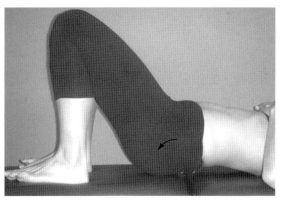

Fig 13.40 • Good loading for bridge maintains the anterior pelvic rotation and the lordosis.

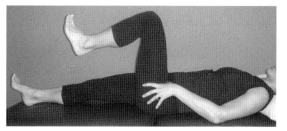

Fig 13.42 • Ideal hip, knee and ankle flexion to 90° involves iliacus-psoas and deepening of the groin without the ischia lifting.

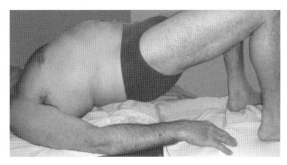

Fig 13.41 • Poor loading in bridge is actioned from predominant posterior tilt and hamstring activity and probably CPC holding.

(1) above and the patient slides the 'standing' foot away into hip extension and return. Placing one hand under the *lower* back and the other over the lower belly helps monitor control of the lordosis and frontal and transverse plane pelvic position and inhibition of CPC activity. In the correct action, palpation of the rectus femoris tendon of the moving groin helps determine whether psoas/iliacus with support from others in the LPU are primarily involved. The moving heel is aimed exactly towards the ipsilateral ischium and remains so through the movement.[17]

3. The ability to *flex the hip, knee and ankle to a right angle*. The position of the pelvis and extended leg is the same as for (1) and maintained with appropriate patterns of axial stabilization including breathing. From the 'standing' leg the patient activates the LPU and flexes the hip knee and ankle each to a right

angle while monitoring the lordosis as in (2). Again he palpates the rectus femoris musculotendon attempting to inhibit the 'jump' which occurs when LPU with prime action from psoas/iliacus[17] is deficient. This pattern is dependent upon the ability to perform FPP1. The groin should fold around the palpating finger and widening and reaching the ipsilateral ischium long and back helps facilitate this. The neck and shoulders should remain relaxed and breathing pattern rhythm unchanged (Fig. 13. 42). Should this be managed reasonably competently and irritability allows, test the active straight leg raise[18] (ASLR).

4. The ASLR test involves a significant limb load challenge to pelvic-axial control strategies for many with back pain (see Ch. 4) and should not be attempted in states of irritability. Modifications are suggested to stage the test as described by Mens et al.[18] as follows. The resting leg is in 'standing flexion' while the active leg is extended and then lifted up and lowered while observing the response. When well controlled, the pelvis and torso alignment is maintained with no disruption to the breathing or CPC activity and hip rotation is neutral through the movement. If this is managed, the leg is again lifted 5 cm above the couch and sustained for up to 10 seconds while subjective sensations and effort are monitored. The test is positive if the patient cannot achieve quality control as described above, uses a lot of effort or experiences a profound sense of weakness heaviness or pain.[18,19] A positive test does not necessarily mean sacro-iliac joint (SIJ) 'instability' (Fig. 13.43). If 'positive', the movement is

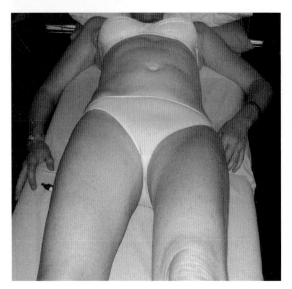

Fig 13.43 • With inadequate support from the LPU the pelvis has subtly rotated in the transverse plane.

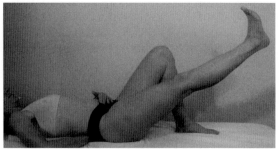

Fig 13.44 • Ideal control of the ASLR is achieved through LPU co-activation.

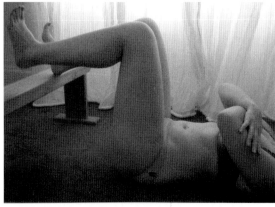

Fig 13.45 • 'Kolar' stage two with one foot supported.

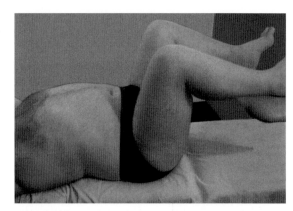

Fig 13.46 • This gentleman will need to keep working on improving his ability to bring the lower pole of the thorax back more in contact with the surface before we can think of asking him to attempt stage 2.

then retested not by manual external pressure over the lateral pelvis as has been described[7,18] but by facilitating improved activity in the LPU. To do this, one hand is placed under the low back and the other over the belly to monitor control of the LPU and pelvis while the action is initiated by elongating from the heel with an 'active foot' widening the sitz bones and reaching the tail bone to assist conscious engagement of the LPU prior to and through the lifting and lowering (Fig. 13.44). Competency in the fundamental pelvic patterns underlies quality control in this test. When managed well, extending the non moving leg while still monitoring control and breathing is a progression.

• **_Coordinating IAP, breathing and axial stabilization_**.[13] This is the ability to maintain the thorax in the expiratory position, achieve full contact of the lower pole of the thorax on the support surface while the flexed hips, knees and ankles are supported to a right angle; sustaining this 'posture' while _breathing normally_ (posterolateral basal) and keeping the neck and shoulders relaxed (Fig. 13.45). The head is supported. This stage 1 is difficult for most and particularly so for the PPXS group where attempting to bring the ribs back instead results in bringing the pelvis forward into posterior tilt. Inhibiting CPC behavior can be difficult (Fig. 13.46). A 6-month-old baby can easily

do this (Figs 3.13 & 3.14). Working for quality in the response is important and it may take time to master. The correct control requires synergistic co-operation between the abdominals, diaphragm

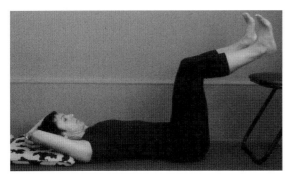

Fig 13.47 • When quality in the performance is achieved it can be progressed to stage three with both feet unsupported.

and psoas with the LPU. Widening the ischia and heels helps the LPU activation. When able to perform step 1 properly, it is progressed by unweighting one and then later two feet, maintaining the right angles, alignment and breathing (Fig. 13.47).

• *Supine low flexion/abduction/external rotation test.* This tests freedom of 'distorsion' in the pelvis and hip, length/tension in the adductors and internal rotators and may reproduce pain in the symphysis or posterior hip/pelvis. The non test leg is maintained in neutral hip rotation and extension and a neutral pelvis, while the test leg is in 'standing flexion' and passively abducted while the contralateral ASIS is stabilized. Overpressure to the test medial knee is applied noting the response. Next, active raising of the test knee is resisted commensurate with the patient's ability and the response noted (Fig. 13.48).

• *Supine high flexion/abduction/external rotation.* This also tests freedom of 'distorsion' in

the pelvis and hip movement and requires length in the lateral glutei and possibly the posterior adductor magnus. Stabilizing the other leg in neutral hip rotation and extension and ensuring triplanar neutral pelvic position helped by the patient's hands under the low lumbar spine; the tested leg is flexed fully *without posterior pelvic tilt* and then externally rotated. Extending the lower leg further tests hamstrings (Fig. 13.49).

• *Supine flexion/adduction/internal rotation test.* Also tests freedom of pelvic 'distorsion' and the hip. More specifically the ability for the deep hip external rotators and all glutei to lengthen with related opening of the postero-inferior pelvic bowl. The non test leg is stabilized in neutral rotation and extension. The test frequently causes an anterior 'impingement' pain in the hip/groin if the posterior-inferior myofascial hip structures are tight. This is also usually associated with increased posterior rotation of the ipsilateral innominate (Fig. 13.50).

• *Posterior hip and thigh flexibility.* Tests the ability for the hamstrings to actively elongate *while actively controlling the pelvis* (Fig. 13.51). Placing a hand under the low lumbar spine to *monitor the lordosis* the patient brings his thigh to the vertical and *sustains this* while actively extending the knee as much as he is able *without disturbing the vertical thigh or lumbopelvic position*. At the limit, further discrimination is afforded by dorsi- and plantar-flexing the foot, which also tests neural mobility and sensitivity.

• *Modified Thomas position pelvi-femoral screening test.* This one test position can divulge

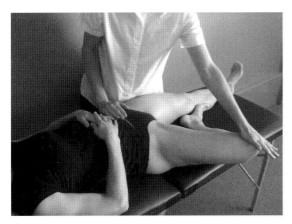

Fig 13.48 • Supine low F/AB/ER (combined flexion/abduction/external rotation).

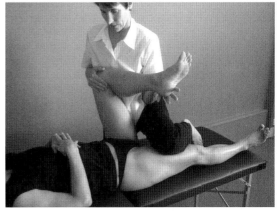

Fig 13.49 • High F/AB/ER (combined flexion/abduction/external rotation) test.

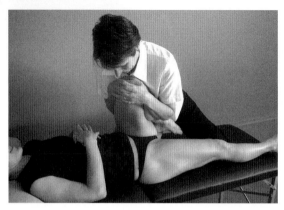

Fig 13.50 • F/AD/IR(combined flexion/adduction/ internal rotation) test supine.

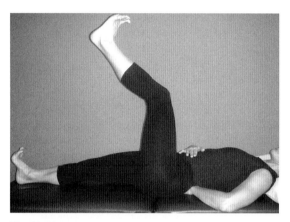

Fig 13.51 • 'Active elongation' of the hamstrings controlling lumbo/pelvic/ hip alignment.

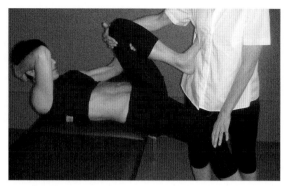

Fig 13.52 • Thomas testing position: there is some tightness of rectus femoris.

information about possible tightness of a number of large pelvi-femoral muscles as well as flexibility into more end range 'distorsion'. It should not be attempted if the patient's condition is irritable. The patient sits with his buttocks almost off the side of the bed and lies back as he is assisted to hold one hip in full flexion while his other hand supports his head. The operator's body stabilizes the flexed leg at the foot. It is important that the pelvis is not side bent. The position of the freely hanging leg is observed for muscle tightness patterns (Fig. 13.52):

- If the thigh hangs above the horizontal and/ or resists passive hyperextension of 10–15°, ilio-psoas is tight.[4] Compensatory knee extension will occur if rectus femoris is also tight.

- If the lower leg hangs in an oblique position and/or resists passive flexion of the knee to 100–105°, rectus femoris is tight.[4] Compensatory hip flexion may occur.

- If the thigh hangs into abduction and resists passive adduction to 15° or less while the ipsilateral lateral pelvis is stabilized, the tensor fascia lata and iliotibial band are tight.[4] A deepening of the groove on the lateral thigh may be evident if tight.

- If the thigh resists abduction to less than 25°, there is shortness of the joint hip adductor.[4] Compensatory hip flexion may also occur.

Patterns of muscle tightness may potentially implicate certain spinal levels e.g. a tighter ilio-psoas with dominant innervation from L1 and L2 roots[20] may implicate the L1/2 and/or 2/3 joints,[21] while a tighter rectus femoris with dominant innervation from the 3rd and 4th lumbar roots[20] could implicate the L3/4 or 4/5 joints. Assessing the joint confirms the relationship or otherwise.

- ***Craniocervical flexion test (CCF).*** The subject is asked to raise the head in the habitual way. If the chin juts forward there is over activity in the scalenii and sternocleidomastoid and inhibition/weakness in the deep neck flexors.[4] This may be associated with poor patterns of axial stabilization where the thorax moves cranially during the movement[13] and the shoulders protract (Fig. 10.17). The test is repeated by cueing the patient to gently widen the clavicles and sink the elbows into the support to activate the lower scapular stabilizers; drop the chin and look down at the chest and sustain this while *slightly unweighting* the head and breathing normally (Fig. 13.53). This determines if he can isolate flexion of the occiput on the neck[22] with the fulcrum around

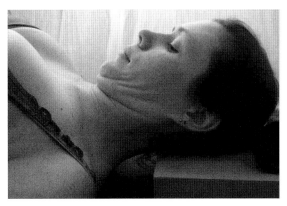

Fig 13.53 • Facilitating CCF with co-activation of the lower scapula stabilizers and FPP1. Ideally when overall spinal alignment is good a pillow is not necessary – most need one!

CO/1 as well as create a pattern of co-activation between the lower scapular stabilizers and the deep neck flexors necessary for good alignment of the upper pole of the body. Sustained pre-activation of FPP1 further facilitates the correct action.

• **Bilateral arm elevation**. The ability to extend straight arms above the head with a neutral cervical spine and thoracolumbar junction. This gives clues about shoulder girdle and thoracic mobility which will influence cervical and lumbopelvic movements. Shortness in latissimus dorsi and the anterior chest muscles contributes towards a 'dome' (Ch. 8) and poor stabilization of the lower pole of the thorax results in cephalad movement during the action[13] (Fig. 13.54).

In **prone**:

• The **breathing pattern:** the ability for posterior basal chest expansion; the presence of a respiratory wave and the quality of pelvic respiratory mechanics.

• The **habitual posturing of the legs** provides clues to the patterns of hip muscle activity or restriction and associated pelvic function. When extremely externally rotated with little gluteal bulk, expect woeful lumbopelvic-hip control (Fig. 13.55)

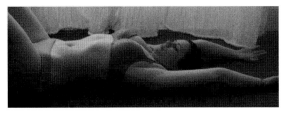

Fig 13.54 • Testing flexibility through the thorax and shoulder.

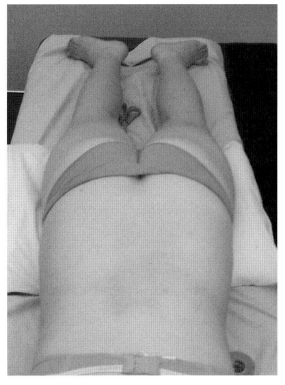

Fig 13.55 • The degree of external rotation in the hips implies heavy reliance upon the obturator group and hamstrings.

• The **three fundamental pelvic patterns** in prone involve the ability to *initiate movement from* the tail bone and sitz bones through the LPU:

   • FPP1 should produce isolated *lumbosacral* extension while the thoracolumbar extensors remain relaxed (Fig. 13.56).

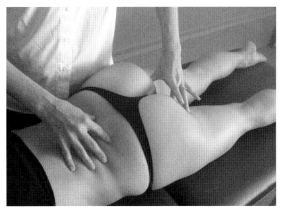

Fig 13.56 • Facilitating FPP1 in prone.

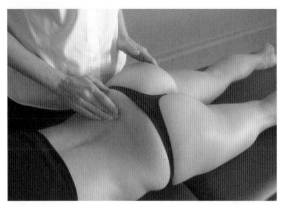

Fig 13.57 • FPP3 initiates backward pelvic rotation.

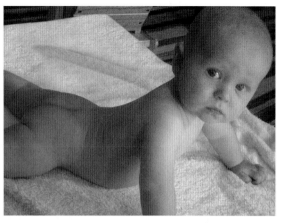

Fig 13.59 • Observe the lovely extension in the baby at around 6 months old.

- Does FPP2 come from the LPU or from dominant gluteal and hamstrings activity?
- With FPP3 only expect slight lift of one ischial tuberosity and slight contralateral weight shift with 'closing' of the ipsilateral lumbosacral junction. Palpate for L5/S1 joint movement and multifidus activity (Fig. 13.57).

• *Prone on elbows:* this passive test readily shows the degree to which extension is reduced through the spine (Fig. 13.58) and may indicate 'hinges' and 'blocks' in segmental flexibility (Fig. 8.40 & 8.41) as well as the quality of co-activation and support provided by the shoulder girdle. Commonly a 'pectoral cinch' fixes the thoracic 'dome' and the whole spine and pelvis show a disinclination to 'hang loose' except for the head which often overly does! Note the nice extension in the baby at around 6 months and how the head leads the movement (Fig. 13.59).

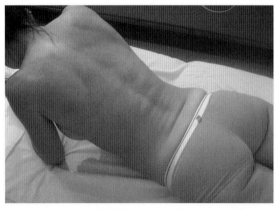

Fig 13.58 • Lack of extension becomes apparent. Note the prominent reactive segments over the thoracolumbar levels – the source of her symptoms.

• *Prone knee bend (PKB).* The ability to flex the knee to 90° tests length in the anterior hip and thigh structures while also controlling pelvic position and a neutral hip rotation.
• Testing *balanced length/tension relationships in the hip rotators* in PKB gives clues to the probable myomechanics of intrapelvic movements. When the hip external rotators are tighter and the internal rotators 'weaker' expect decreased anterior rotation of the innominate, nutation of the sacrum and tightness in the inferior syndesmosis. Tighter internal rotators reduce posterior rotation of the innominate. When all the rotators are tight, pelvic rotation in the sagittal and transverse planes is reduced and likely to lead to compensatory movement in the lumbar spine when walking etc. (Figs 13.60 & 13.61).
• *Prone flexion/abduction/external rotation test.* Tests 'distorsion' and length of hip adductors and internal rotators and anterior hip structures further into range and is a useful position in which to test and free up the sacrum as well as gain release in the tight muscles including trigger points (Fig. 13.62). Ideally the pelvis lies flat on the table and foot rests on the leg as shown but both are lifted when tighter.[23]
• The ability to perform *backward pelvic rotation* initiated from the coccyx/ischia via the LPU (Fig. 13.63) and not as a mid lumbar 'wind'. Note the lack of coactivation in Figure 13.64 with extensor dominance.
• *Prone limb load test* and *pattern of hip extension* with a flexed and extended knee. A flexed knee requires adequate length in rectus

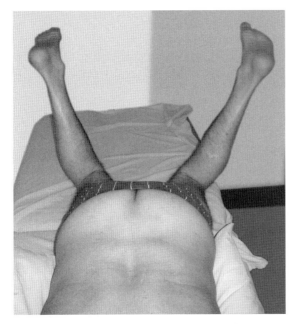

Fig 13.60 • The external rotators of the hip are tight. However this is not a reliable index on its own as range may appear better than it actually is when pelvic/hip myomechanics are more closely examined. Note here the asymmetry and puffiness over the low lumbar levels.

femoris and lessens hamstrings activity asking more dominant gluteus maximus action. Lifting with an extended knee requires more control of limb load torque in the torso and allows hamstrings to be more active. Given 'more total patterns of extension' can tend to predominate in the lower limbs; this is usually the preferred mode. Observe patterns of lumbopelvic control and the early use of central cinch strategies (Figs 10.1 & 10.3) and the sequence of muscle activation. Janda[4,6] considered early activation of the hamstrings and thoraco-lumbar erector spinae a dysfunctional pattern. Effective lumbopelvic control should involve a *neutral* pelvis at initiation of the movement which then moves into some ipsilateral anterior innominate rotation to support the leg action. Those who are APXS or who habitually 'buttock clench' attempt the movement from posterior pelvic tilt and hip hyperextension, while those with a pure PPXS picture initiate the movement from excess anterior tilt as a result of thoracolumbar extensor hyperactivity and related tightness in the anterior hip structures. Compare the nice action in Figures 13.65 and 6.23.

• **Prone push up/passive extension**. Tests for balanced control in the shoulder girdle and opening

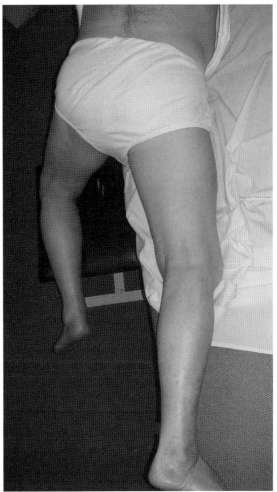

Fig 13.61 • Viewed from above one hip is flexed over the edge with the knee supported. This can quite dramatically reveal just how tight the rotators are as shown. It is a good position to release posturo-inferior pelvic hip tethering but great care must be taken to position the patient so that the lumbosacral spine is in the neutral position. For this patient, modified positions need to be used and more freedom gained before he can be safely treated in this position.

of the 'dome'. Commonly the patient will 'lock in' with the pectorals and a CPC strategy, hyper-extending his neck and fixing the thoracolumbar region with little opening through the thorax or he comes high and 'hangs' (Fig. 13.66).

• *Posterior inferior opening of the pelvis and hip (PIOPH.)* This tests the ability of the patient to open the posterior pelvis, pelvic floor and hip while simultaneously preserving a neutral spine, in particular the lumbar (Fig. 13.67 also see Fig. 3.24 – "Allah"). It is almost universally difficult for

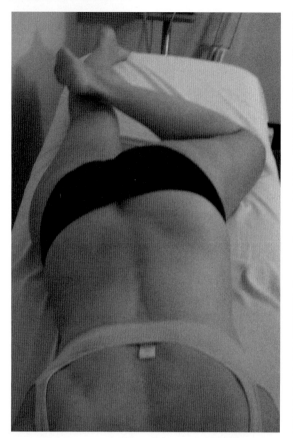

Fig 13.62 • Prone F/AB/ER position (combined flexion/abduction/external rotation).

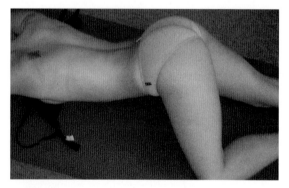

Fig 13.63 • Good backward pelvic rotation is initiated from the tailbone and ipsilateral ischium, the movement sequencing through the spine.

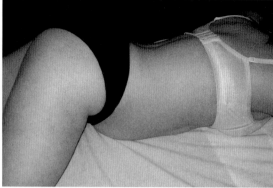

Fig 13.64 • Deficient backward pelvic rotation. Note the poor contribution from the LPU and lack of co-activation in the abdominal wall.

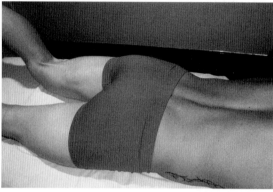

Fig 13.65 • Prone hip extension/limb load ideally involves even activation of the extensors as shown.

patients to do particularly those classified as APXS. The PPXS manage somewhat better though the tendency is to attempt this from CPC dominant strategies with poor abdominal co-activation (Figs 8.13, 8.17 & 9.17).When posterior opening is achieved the ischia widen, and lift up and back (Figs. 13.67 & 13.68). Note the reduced ability to achieve the correct action in Figure 13.69 which needs to be worked towards by specific drilling of FPP1 in various ways. 'Allah' is an exercise to target the correct action (Fig. 13.70). Note that this is very different from the commonly practised collapse in Figure 13.71 where *all prevailing patterns of lumbopelvic dysfunction are reinforced* including propagation of the 'dome'.

C) Passive testing of the joints and myofascial tissues

Passive joint and myofascial testing confirms or otherwise, impressions gleaned from the history, observation and movement testing. Sometimes these are unremarkable and the 'feel' of the tissues is all you have to go on. While Bogduk[24] said that 'virtually any source of local lumbar or lumbosacral pain is

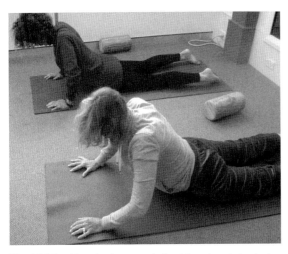

Fig 13.66 • Note the increase in the 'dome' and shortening in the neck with poor posterior girdle support in both subjects partly resulting from the poorly formed base of support in the hand, best seen in the subject closest.

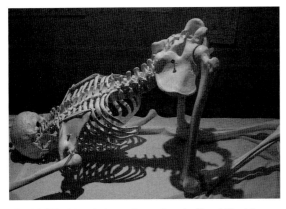

Fig 13.67 • The skeleton shows the significant lift of the ischia in relation to the femur in ideal 'Allah.'

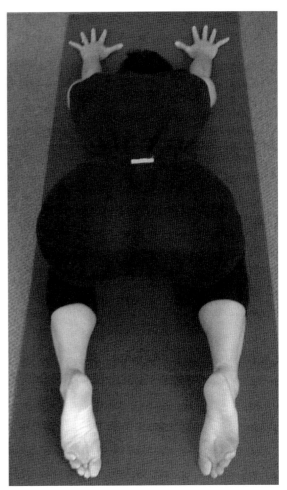

Fig 13.68 • Ideal 'Allah' involves opening the pelvic floor as shown. Also, note the good base support in the hands.

also capable of producing somatic referral into the limb, in this author's clinical experience it is the *joint dysfunction* which is the principal initial and sustaining pain driver of most spinal pain and related musculoskeletal disorders. Joint dysfunction emanates from muscle dysfunction and in turn further influences muscle function leading to either hypo or hyper activity. Bear in mind that when cranky, the joint irritability will also create secondary changes such as muscle spasm, trigger points, various autonomic symptoms, referred pain etc. Joint dysfunction also affects changes in other soft tissues such as fascia and ligaments as well as neural tissue (see Ch. 12). When local and or long spinal muscles are hyperactive it makes joint assessment

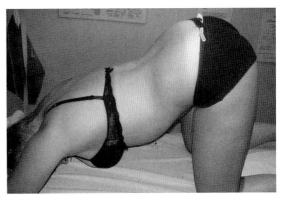

Fig 13.69 • Inadequacy of both coactivation and alignment in the torso and anterior pelvic rotation in 'Allah'.

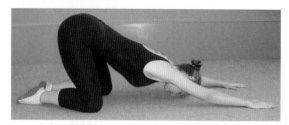

Fig 13.70 • 'Allah' as you like to see it! There is good elongation and alignment between the head and tail bone and the hands and knees are well grounded facilitating correct action in the pelvis and opening of the 'dome'.

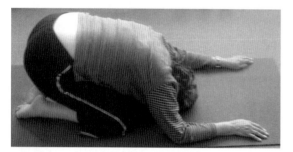

Fig 13.71 • Unfortunately many people collapse into this 'more total flexion' position which does nothing other than reinforce the prevailing dysfunctional posturomovement tendencies. The base of support is inactive.

more difficult possibly contributing towards a lot of the poor therapeutic outcomes. If sensing a symptomatic joint may be 'under there', the therapist may need to 'linger longer' and wait for neuromuscular abatement such that she can adequately access the joint.

Respect for irritability is important. Altered joint function creates local inflammatory changes and the chemical irritation can make the tissues 'irritable'[25] where even the mildest of mechanical stimuli can 'open Pandora's box' and markedly exacerbate symptoms. Reproducing 'the pain' may not be possible because of protective muscle spasm hence the need for proficient 'feel'. Joint dysfunction includes that in the functional spinal unit as well as that in the large joints such as the sacroiliac, hip and shoulder joints. It is, in general, stiffness dysfunction in these large joints and their proximal girdles which, in everyday function, adversely impacts on spinal myomechanics. Within the spine itself, stiff joints can stress levels above and below them.[7] Manual assessment is concerned to *find the level* which is principally producing the pain. This joint may be relatively mobile or stiff and either way can be

irritable. Manual testing will delineate the *pattern of altered joint function*. While we talk of 'finding the level' in clinical practice it is never just one joint but a family of dysfunctional joints and related neuromyofascial tissues which all feed into the picture of dysfunction. Similar to family pathology, each member plays their part in the general ailment. Specific joint assessment delineates which joints are the cause of the pain and which are the source of the pain[26] – the 'criminals' and the 'victims'. However, symptomatic joints don't necessarily allow themselves to be so easily found and it is here that the skill of the practitioner carries the day. Those joints that are the main offenders can be the most elusive and difficult to find, so encased are they in a reactive cocoon of muscle spasm. However, when found and you do the right thing with it, the symptoms will settle. When findings are apparent and understood, the assessment generally segues into treatment part of which always involves *constantly monitoring the response in the tissues* and the patient and adjusting the intervention as indicated.

Clues for successful manual examination and treatment

Space precludes a full treatise on possible manual assessment and treatment procedures in the spine. Various texts[7,11,27–36] provide descriptive accounts which the reader may like to consult as it is not intended to replicate those passive movement tests already described in the literature but to proffer some which more specifically apply to the approach offered herein. A few methods well applied far outweigh a 'bagful of techniques' shoddily actioned. Some principles help guide effective assessment and subsequent treatment of the spine.

The competent manual therapist is an artist

Upledger[37] wrote 25 years ago that 'palpation is an art which is grossly neglected in the health care professions'. Unfortunately, contemporary training institutions appear to offer less practical training and mentoring now than they did then. This is one of the central problems facing effective outcomes from manual therapy. While systematic reviews conclude that spinal 'manipulative therapy' offers no clinically worthwhile decreases in pain,[38] the patient 'knows' the worth of the therapist and simple cost/benefit principles usually apply.

It cannot be stressed enough that competency in manual therapy involves hard won skills which are achieved by application, dedication, determination and experience involving lifelong learning in their refinement with respect for the potential pitfalls. It is easy to miscalculate and underestimate the potent effects of spinal joint dysfunction and the need for sensitive artful interventions. For the novice, achieving treatment success can be frustrating and elusive but with guidance, care and commitment, understanding and competency evolve and grow.

This is one of the central problems in attempting to validate manual testing procedures and the benefit of manual treatment interventions in back pain as each therapist will bring their own stamp to the situation. This is a clinical reality and no amount of research studies will produce consistent and uniform clinical outcomes as there are so many different ingredients in the recipe of the patient's dysfunction picture let alone variability in the therapist's understanding, abilities, and clinical decision making.

Palpation involves three elements: the perception of motion, the perceived nature of tissue compliance and the reaction of the tissues to the applied manual stress, and the provocation of pain.[39] In a recent literature review[40] palpation for movement abnormality was found to have poor inter-examiner reliability while tests for pain provocation had more acceptable reliability. However the successful clinician simply *has* to also develop manual competency in detecting the subtle alterations in movement quality, tissue tension, reaction and tonus. For effective manual therapy of the spine, the ability to sense, or not, the small 'slides' of intersegmental movement at each FSU is paramount. Jull et al.[41] have shown that experienced and competent practitioners *can* identify 100% of symptomatic cervical segments cross referenced by diagnostic blocks. Similarly, Treleaven et al.[42] were able to successfully identify the most painful segments in subjects with post concussional headache. Reduced joint play is usually more significant than regional deformities or positional faults.

One could write an entire book on the salient aspects of therapeutic 'feel' – one of the most important tools in the entire therapeutic tool kit. It is the thing that the patient will most evaluate you on – they know whether you are 'getting the

spots' and whether as a pleasant versus an unpleasant experience. If they sense you are 'on the case' and symptoms change they will give you the chance to get them better. The patient is very adept at discerning the abilities and worth of a therapist, simply not returning if unimpressed. Proficiency involves the ability to sensitively examine tissue in a way that does not invoke defensive reactions; the care and the patience to be prepared to 'sink deep' and 'wait' while neuromuscular holding lets go such that one can access the joint and discover what it has to say; the ability to detect subtle nuances in tissue texture and the quality of the 'end feel' and the ability to sense when enough is enough. The artful practitioner works methodically and with their hands, head and heart. Again, pain reproduction should not necessarily be the goal, as it is neither reliable nor predictable[7] and can risk provocation. However, it is nice if you do and getting the 'sweet pain' reassures both therapist and patient that they are on the right track. Changed relationships, the quality of 'joint play' of 'give' and 'bind' and the 'feel' of the tissue response are much more informative. It can be surprising how seemingly relatively small differences in the quality of movement in a spinal joint can have such a marked influence on the surrounding neurology and hence pain and soft tissue function. Setting out to reproduce pain alone is likely to engender ham-fisted palpation by the less experienced practitioner. Hannon[43] suggests 'by using the least force necessary, we may increase the potential for perceiving more subtle sensory distinctions'. The therapist also needs to be mindful of not activating their own 'clench zones' and breathing 'properly'. 'God is in the detail' is an apt metaphor for effective manual therapy – small differences can mean a lot. The effective practitioner is able to resonate with the patient's inherent rhythms and oscillations such that her manual techniques also act as a somatic learning experience. For the interested reader, Hannon[44] has written nicely around this aspect; Chaitow offers interesting thoughts[45] and an excellent and comprehensive treatise on assessment and diagnosis through touch.[46] Lewit[47] and Upledger[37] also describe aspects of the art of palpation and soft tissue manipulation.

Importantly, the manual therapist needs to be moving and working from their own deep muscle system and possess a certain level of neuromuscular fitness. When effective SLMS activity provides effective 'grounding' and support, the therapist is better able to sense and gauge her manual intervention *according to what the tissue needs*. Unfortunately many manual treatments consist of imposing a 'technique' with little regard to the tissue response. Bad technique risks 'punching up tissues' and it is easy to 'trampoline' on hyper-facilitated tissue thereby increasing the neuromuscular defense. Instead the ideal tissue response is one of 'melting' and give. Most commonly the therapist either does not adequately 'get down to the joint' or conversely she suffocates it. Both result in poor outcomes. No matter what the intensity of the manual force there should always be enough sensitivity that the therapist can sense the patient's response.[48] Comprehensive examination will reveal many 'findings' and the art of the practitioner is to discern those most significant. Masterly 'feel' is the ultimate guide and effective treatment tool.

Expect joint restrictions according to observational findings

Observing the patient's posture and movement strategies and cognisance of the more common responses seen in spinal patients (Chs 8–10) helps delineate what to possibly expect when testing passive joint function e.g. the presence of hinges and blocks in movement means segmental examination will predictably test differently in different regions. Where there are regions of muscle hyperactivity, expect the underlying joints to be hyperstabilized, stiff, hard to get to although possibly irritable, thus perseverance is warranted for capable testing. Uneven intersegmental movement behooves one to fully explore all aspects of that joint's function and that of related segments. You may have impressions about the behavior of tissue but these can only be confirmed by actually testing it. It is easy to completely miss what is most important.

Mapping the territory

While appearing to be a truism, a good working knowledge of surface anatomy is necessary in order to find many of the structures needing to be assessed. Altered alignment and muscle activity can alter the bony landmarks quite surprisingly. It is not uncommon for quite experienced practitioners to mistake L5 for the sacrum or to completely exclude C1 from examination because of a lower hairline – problematic when they are such significant joints in spinal function. Because reactive

changes are common over the lumbosacral junction many even miss large landmarks such as the posterior superior iliac spine! In practice it is useful to map bony landmarks and when testing the joint, imagine oneself 'getting down to the bones'. However, where joints are most symptomatic in the spine, particularly where chronic muscle spasm and 'holding patterns' have prevailed, guarding and hypertrophy can be significant, making it even more difficult to locate the very problematic segment. The effective approach may need to come in through soft tissue work to 'get down there'. Slowly 'skiving' the articular gutters is helpful. Despite the handicaps often involved, it is important that the joint is not 'bothered' – seduction is preferable to rape. As Chaitow[49] suggests, the therapist is ideally offering the opportunity for change rather than obliging it. Sometimes you may not initially be quite sure what level you are on except that you have stumbled on a whole bolus of 'crud', the freeing up of which can release regional muscular holding sufficient to allow more refined assessment. The Catch-22 is that accessing and gently freeing the joint will bring about some letting go in the neuromuscular response and the more this occurs the better one can assess and help the joint to move. So called 'hypermobile' joints can be stiff in some movement directions. Radiology may show a spondylolisthesis at L5, yet clinically pain may only ease when the joint is mobilized into extension. The joint is telling you what to do by how it feels when you test it. It depends on whether you are listening.

Importance of breathing in manual therapy

Breathing is a connecting factor between the somatic and autonomic nervous systems.[50] It mirrors the status of the person. When relaxed, comfortable and trusting we breathe deeply and slowly through the diaphragm. If aroused and tense we are expectant and guarding ready for action. The therapist's touch must firstly reassure the patient to 'give themselves' to her. This facilitates the palpatory examination so the therapist can locate and do what is necessary in order to affect the pain. Observing the patient's breathing informs the therapist of the patient's experience of her touch – the spontaneous 'sigh' heralds a release – the therapist is on the right track. Conversely, holding the breath is 'defending against' the touch and can reinforce neuromuscular patterns of holding as well as 'stir things up'.

Shirley et al.[51] found that spinal stiffness changes throughout the respiratory cycle increasing with increased respiratory effort and being greatest during *maximum* expiration which involves the accessory muscles of expiration (Ch. 6). Breathing deeply (not maximally) should ideally involve movement of almost every vertebra in the spine and pelvis but this is generally reduced in people with spinal dysfunction. In general most patients have a very poor sense of diaphragmatic breathing with minimal basal expansion. This can be addressed from day one where physiological 'focused breathing' can be used in order to facilitate 'release' whereby the joint or myofascial tissue is specifically engaged and the patient asked to 'breathe into my hand' or 'gently push me away', while *expiration is passive*. Encouraging the breath mobilizes the joint on inspiration while on expiration the therapist sensitively takes up the tissue slack moving further into range. The 'inner expansion' from the breath also helps to inhibit and lengthen the superficial muscular 'outer holding', can deactivate trigger points as well as reduce segmental neuromuscular hyperactivity. When extensor spasm is marked it can really shroud the joint and even the gentlest enquiring palpation can engender a reactive sling of muscle guarding. In this case, sustained gentle though focused contact on any point on the vertebra and asking for 'try to expand back into me' and *not* following the joint further into range on expiration will usually result in the joint eventually 'floating up' towards your contact and allowing itself to be declared. The degree of tissue irritability will determine how many breaths this takes. The therapist's hands provide a valuable proprioceptive cue for the patient to direct the breath into hitherto unfamiliar regions. Initially, inspiratory expansion and the axial movement wave may be small and really need coaxing. It will however improve as the neuromyarticular irritability improves through the treatment and between treatments.

However, we can't necessarily assume that the patient can 'just do it'. 'Trying' to breathe deeply can engender central cinch behavior and paradoxical breathing. Entrenched muscle holding patterns and restricted myofascial and joint mobility (particularly in the APXS group) may require soft tissue and joint release around the lower pole of the thorax, deactivating any trigger points between the ribs and around the rim of the diaphragm to facilitate 'central' breathing. The use of strategies which reflexley activate the diaphragm help give him a sense of a relaxed and 'real diaphragmatic breath' e.g. extending the expiratory pause and/or activating postural reflex chains initiated from the limbs can assist this. It is also likely he is a hyper-ventilator, in which case further retraining on his breathing rate may be necessary. A Capnotrainer® or the Buteyko Breathing method is useful for this.

When retraining breathing or incorporating 'focused breathing' into manual treatment, care must be exercised not to 'hyperventilate' the patient (Ch. 8). The rate should not exceed 12 breaths/minute; the emphasis should be on a deep breath rather than a big breath and allow a ratio of 2:3:1 – as inspiration: expiration: pause.[52,53] The longer expiration not only improves the breathing pattern quality but also facilitates general and regional neuromuscular relaxation. 'Focused breathing' is particularly useful adjunct in treating thoracolumbar and lumbopelvic dysfunction.

Check the function in the junctions

This maxim is de rigueur in functional passive movement assessment of the spine as clinically *there is always associated disturbance in the functionally related junctional region*(s). Dysfunction here may be the symptom perpetrator or exert an altered biomechanical influence causing compensatory problems in functionally related and more vulnerable segments. Treating the more obvious 'painful level' alone can result in exacerbation of symptoms. A good example is a symptomatic L4/5, the genesis of which is usually always related to significant myo-articular restriction around the hip-sacroiliac joint and lumbosacral junction with further secondary problems higher up over the thoracolumbar junction. The adjacent and even removed 'stiff' levels are usually always exerting some neural influence on the local and regional neuromuscular responses (Ch. 12) as well as imposing a biomechanical block in the kinetic movement chain. Clinically, the vagaries of referred pain are such that leg pain in a presumed L4/5 distribution can be provoked from as high as T8 through all levels down to the coccyx.

Symptoms in the lower back, pelvis, hips and lower limbs deriving from a lumbar segment will always be associated with findings in the thoracolumbar and lumbosacral junctions although the significance of those in one junction will predominate over the other. Similarly, symptoms in the head, neck, shoulders and upper limbs emanating from a cervical segment will always be associated with findings in the cervicocranial and cervicothoracic junctions with the influence of one predominant. If the 'dome' is considered as a junctional region, its presence has some effect in all axial dysfunction syndromes.

The junctional regions can be tricky to assess well owing to the common occurrence of overlying reactive tissues including muscle hypertonicity. There is often more than meets the eye in terms of joint findings in these regions which need to be 'cleared' for effective function. Assessment and some treatment options for the more common 'junctional blocks' will be explored. These provide an example of the principles of an approach to treatment. Restoring movement in the junctional regions allows healthier movement not only within them but also in more vulnerable segments which may then only require a small amount of 'settling treatment' in order to render them asymptomatic.

Lumbosacral junction

The function of this junction is highly dependent upon that in the pelvic joints which in turn are also influenced by the hips hence these relationships are all examined. Sagittal pelvic rotation plays a significant role in the stiffness of the lumbar spine and particularly at L5.[54] Positioning the patient in side lying is best for those in acute pain and in all patients it yields lots of information about the possible state of his spine and habitual posturomovement habits (Fig. 13.72).

The sacrum-coccyx (S-C) is the largest member in the axial spine and while it plays a big role in supporting the superincumbent body load it also must be free to move. This allows proper kinematic function of both of the pelvic joints and L5/S1 in controlling forces and load transfer through the pelvis. Freeing the sacrum-coccyx also helps re-establish the initiation of posture and movements from the base of the spine – the coccyx. Otherwise compensatory movements need to occur and do – higher up – attested to in part by the commonality of degenerative findings more prevalent at L4/5 and higher.

The muscles with direct attachments to the (S-C) contribute to the movement force couples which control it, principally nutation and counternutation in the sagittal plane. The superiorly placed muscles – the iliacus ventrally and multifidus and erector spinae dorsally, contribute to sacral nutation and anterior pelvic rotation (APR) while the inferiorly placed

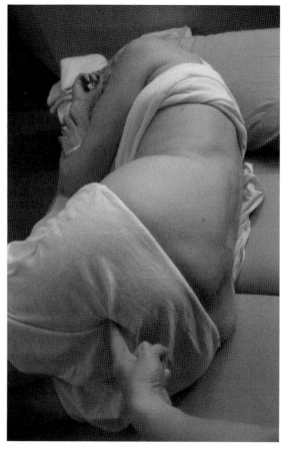

Fig 13.72 • The habitual side lying posture tells a lot. The operator's finger is palpating the ischium, revealing the extent of habitual tailbone tuck activity.

muscles – coccygeus and piriformis ventrally and gluteus maximus and levator ani dorsally, contribute to counternutation and posterior pelvic rotation (PPR). Imbalance in the force couple biases the posturomovement balance. Clinically, dysfunction of the sacrum-coccyx is more commonly one of postural counternutation[37]and PPR and reduced movement into nutation/APR. The lower force couple agents are adaptively or actively tighter serving to 'inferiorly tether' the S-C unit while the superiorly placed muscles counteracting this are underactive or show stretch weakness – iliacus, multifidus and lumbar erector spinae. The S-C hypomobility is linked to posterior restriction in the hips–pelvis and pelvic floor. Reinforcing this is the restriction between the femur and the innominate when either the iliacus-psoas or probably more commonly, the obturator group are also hyperactive or tight (Ch. 8).

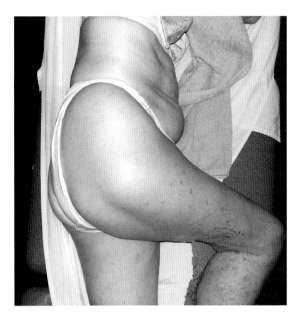

Fig 13.73 • Birdseye view with subject in side lying. Apparent divot and altered femoral position with obturator tightness.

Our patient population could be skewed and not represent a balanced spectrum of general presentations but most have a stiff sacrum and 'tucked tail' and we have still have yet to encounter a patient with a bias towards excess nutation and low lumbar extension. It would appear those sassy individuals with a pert bum and who 'stick out their tail' do not need our services!

The **side lying position** provides easy access to explore for probable 'inferior tethers' (Ch. 10) and associated patterns of joint restriction. When the femur is flexed to about 75°, if the posterior hip muscles are tight the pelvis lies in posterior rotation (Figs. 13.72 & 13.73) with an 'under-slung bum'. The femur resting position relative to the top and bottom of the innominate, informs about balance in the hip rotator 'fan' (Ch. 6, Part B). If the deep external rotators are tight the femur appears more caudad with a probable inferior recess or 'divot' over the muscles while superiorly, the gluteal space above the may appear 'long and 'empty' (Fig. 13.73). These external rotators are usually tense and stringy and really tender to palpate. If the internal rotators are hyper-facilitated, trigger point/tenderness and tension are also apparent.

Palpation of other soft tissues may reveal variable tenderness, fullness, tension and trigger points. While lying anterior to the sacrospinous ligament, the coccygeus is externally palpable at the level of the sacrococcygeal joint,[55] and the adjacent iliococcygeus part of the levator ani over the lowest two coccyx segments. Piriformis can be palpated just lateral to the greater sciatic foramen and through its length (Fig. 13.74). The position of the S-C is invariably counternutated and palpation of the L5/S1 reveals loss of nutation/extension. A number of maneuvers can be employed.

• *Freeing the sacrum/pelvis into nutation/APR*. Simply placing the heel of your hand over the sacrum and low lumbar joints immediately informs of their status. There is usually a poor breathing wave into the lower spine and pelvis. It is usual to feel thickened, pulpy, spongy and flaccid tissues over the lower lumbar levels with poor joint accessory movement and 'give' into an extension/side bending enquiry. Variously engaging the inferior PSIS; the sacral base centrally and/or laterally; L5 centrally or laterally and asking the patient to breathe into your pressure creates a counternutation torque. On expiration, the therapist carefully follows the APR/nutation/lumbosacral extension movement further into range while monitoring the response. This can be facilitated by asking the patient to 'widen the sitz bones' on the expiration (most need help knowing where they are and the request will seem to be 'out of the left field', so unused are they to this action!). This action is part of FPP1 and thus neuromuscular training also begins! Placing a hand towel or paper towel under one's carefully placed hand can help to 'collect' the bony prominence and so help to not slide off it. With the other hand the uppermost ischium can be facilitated into anterior innominate rotation which is synergistic to the action and helps with restoring the pattern for physiological lordosis. Freeing the joints assists soft tissue and trigger point release which further helps the joints. Posterior pressures through the lumbar spine are a nice way to gauge relative joint play and the status of the other lumbar joints. The L4/5 (and even L3/4) usually become the victim of restrictions through the lumbosacral junction either becoming hyper-flexed and sitting up like a 'knuckle' with reduced extension or, can feel relatively mobile and 'overworked' with an 'empty' end feel in one or more directions. This can be further exacerbated by a stiff 'plug' around L2/3 and related problems higher up. Each level reveals its plight and role in the story.

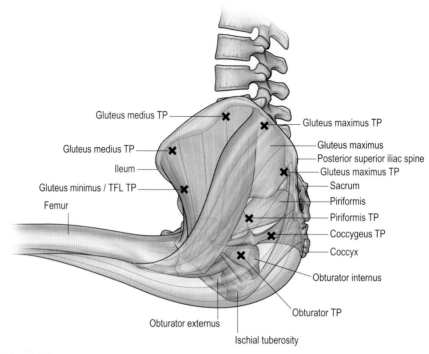

Gluteus medius TP

Gluteus medius TP

Ileum

Gluteus minimus / TFL TP

Femur

Gluteus maximus TP

Gluteus maximus
Posterior superior iliac spine
Gluteus maximus TP
Sacrum
Piriformis
Piriformis TP
Coccygeus TP
Coccyx
Obturator internus

Obturator TP

Obturator externus

Ischial tuberosity

Fig 13.74 • Palpation points for detecting potentially symptomatic pelvic myofascial structures.

• *Testing inflare of the ileum coupled with anterior rotation of the innominate*. This is stiff more often than reproducing pain. Similarly described by Grieve,[56] this involves approximation of the anterior superior iliac spines with pressure directed to the patient's opposite trochanter and importantly, the pressure is on the most anterior part of the ileum. This can be combined with therapist facilitated/active ipsilateral ischial outflare with or without 'active breathing' Activating the hip internal rotators and post isometric relaxation (PIR) of the external rotators can be employed to further improve hip and SIJ joint flexibility (Fig. 13.75). It is interesting that in cases with a positive ASLR test, the application of external compression of the ilia from a pelvic belt or the therapist's hands usually improves the test result.[7,18,57] It is suggested that improving the mobility and control of the test described herein will improve the patients control without the need for external compression. This test movement should not be confused with the pain provocation test usually described as the SIJ compression test.[7,35,58]

• *Palpating for trigger point tenderness in iliacus-psoas*. Baer's point is just medial to the

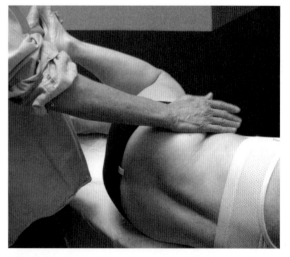

Fig 13.75 • 'Inflare' of the ileum while facilitating 'outflare' of the ischium through post isometric relaxation (PIR) of the hip.

ASIS. Gently sinking down into the medial wall of the ileum, palpable tension/tenderness can often be felt in iliacus.[56] Increased tension in psoas is felt slightly more cephalad through the abdominal wall, parallel to the spine[11] and anterior to the transverse processes (Fig. 13.76).

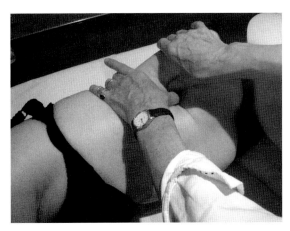

Fig 13.76 • Position for releasing both iliacus and psoas. Psoas is shown.

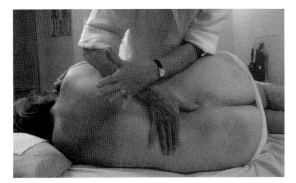

Fig 13.77 • Mobilizing both the ileum into 'inflare' and the lumbosacral junction into side bending.

• *Testing intersegmental movement.* The above maneuvers help to settle long muscle overactivity and facilitate further testing of the segmental joint play anywhere between the 'dome' and L5. The lower levels can be further addressed through combined medial mobilization of the innominate (Fig. 13.77) and/or PIR of the pelvic hip muscles (Fig. 13.75). Intersegmental movement can be assessed into rotation, side bending, flexion and extension noting where the reactive thickening and joint 'bind' is. Rotation maneuvers help inhibit bilateral superficial muscle spasm and 'holding patterns'. Soft tissues techniques which explore and 'skive' into the articular gutter help pick up further subtleties in joint and tissue texture and mobility. Asking for diaphragmatic inhalation which also affects intersegmental 'give' can also help to refine impressions.

Positioning the patient prone again confirms the lie of the pelvis at rest and is necessary to discern any a positional asymmetry and altered movement of the pelvic, hip and lumbar joints. Hypomobility is usual and seemingly small, subtle positional differences, asymmetry and reduced joint play can be significant. Exploiting the close functional relationship between the thoracic and pelvic diaphragms and utilizing respiratory lumbopelvic mechanics is helpful. Differences which may be found include:

• *Dissimilar level of the PSIS* indicating a fixed 'distorsion'. Also described as a 'so called subluxation of the sacroiliac joint….the common pattern is believed to be backward rotation of the innominate on the sacrum…and it is usually unilateral'.[20] The PSIS may appear level but display differences in 'give'. Placing the heel of the hands over each PSIS and feeling the quality and symmetry of innominate movement while the patient is asked to 'breathe into my hands' is confirmatory. Bringing the ipsilateral knee into flexion can reveal anterior thigh tightness which can be utilized to help mobilize the innominate into more anterior rotation if indicated (Fig. 13.78).

• *Sacral position and depth of the sacral sulcus.* When shallower, the sacrum is counternutated. If deeper on one side some torsion is present. This can be determined by sinking the thumb tips and 'skiving' along the sulcus while also noting any tenderness of the interosseous and long dorsal ligaments. Movement can be tested by placing one thumb along the sulcus over S1–3 to act as a 'chock' while the other hand overlies it. During inspiration the sacrum should rise up under your hand, while on expiration the pressure

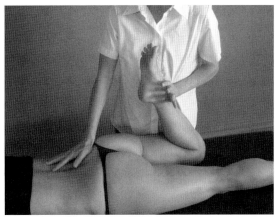

Fig 13.78 • Mobilizing the innominate into anterior pelvic rotation through prone knee bend (PKB).

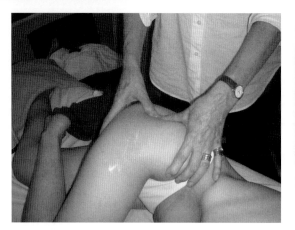

Fig 13.79 • Releasing trigger points in the piriformis.

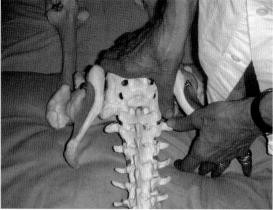

Fig 13.80 • Skiving the sulcus and locating L5/S1.

is gently increased to follow or coax the sacral base towards nutation. Active ischial outflare can embellish the expiratory response. Discern any asymmetry between sides. A deeper sulcus generally occurs on the side of the higher PSIS.

• *Deviation of the coccyx* to one side can occur if the ipsilateral pelvic floor[59] or synergist hip external rotators are tighter. This is usually associated with thickening and probable trigger points in coccygeus[12] and/or piriformis/gluteus maximus. Exploiting the functional relationship between the diaphragm and PFM, sustaining pressure on any trigger points in coccygeus, the obturator group, piriformis, and even the glutei while the patient 'breathes into' the pressure for 2–5 breaths can achieve a nice release (Fig. 13.79).

• The skiving exploration can extend both from the coccyx to the iliac crest to cover the attachments of coccygeus, piriformis and gluteus maximus (Fig. 13.74). Releasing the 'inferior tether' helps gain better physiological function of the sacroiliac joint and lumbosacral junction.

• *Prominence of one L5/S1 facet joint over the other*. When skiving the sacral sulcus, invariably at the top one encounters a thickened, woody or reactive L5/S1 joint which can be 'barnacle-like'. Continuing around and flush with the iliac crest, locate the 'wing nut' of the transverse process of L5. One or both L5 transverse processes may be flush with (or even posterior to!) the iliac crest if PPR and sacral counternutation has been excessive. Reactive soft tissues may make it difficult to delineate the transverse process from the iliac crest and persistence is warranted. If the sacrum is tilted back on the right, the right transverse process of L5

is more posterior, the L5/S1 joint will also be more prominent and 'stuck open' and segmental right closing movements will be less (Fig. 13.80).

• *Imbalanced length/tension between the internal and external hip rotators* and noting any asymmetry between sides. It is more common to find tightness of the external rotators and relative weakness of the internal rotators and this will be more apparent on the most painful side.[60]

• This will predictably reduce APR, sacral nutation and opening of the inferior pelvic bowl. Because of the pelvic attachments of the external rotators, this tightness can be exploited to help mobilize the pelvic, hip and lumbosacral joints by using PIR in the following ways:

  • Stabilizing either the coccyx, sacral base or L5 while activating the external rotators at 'the barrier' in a sustained 10s hold and then passively taking up the slack as the hip is moved into more internal rotation helps release and 'open' the posterior pelvic floor and pelvis/hip (Fig. 13.81).

  • Similarly, stabilizing one point e.g. S1/2 and/or L5 while the patient freely internally and externally rotates the hip and consciously breathes can help mobilize 'distorsion' patterns – the operator following the movement further into the more desired directions towards increasing range. Movements directed from the sitz bones and tail bone can be similarly employed.

  • The lumbosacral junction levels can also be mobilized in the position shown in Figure 13.61 either passively or combined with activation of the fundamental patterns (Fig. 13.82).

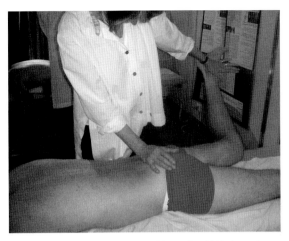

Fig 13.81 • Mobilizing the sacral base (and L5) through PIR of the hip rotators.

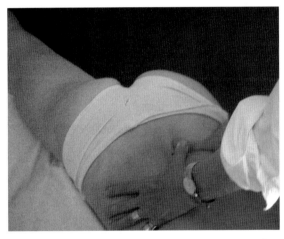

Fig 13.82 • Mobilizing the L5/S1 and related structures in prone with one hip flexed over with support under the knee (see Fig. 13.61).

Thoracolumbar junction

The significant contribution that dysfunction through this junction plays in many low back, pelvic pain and lower limb disorders is generally overlooked. In addition, those 'dirty backs' with gasping intense pain, breath holding and unpredictable behavior frequently involve prime input from the joints in this region. Altered loading stresses and neuromuscular patterns make T12 a site of frequent dysfunction.[31] The potential volatility of symptom behavior may be due in part to the influence of the sympathetic thoracolumbar outflow which extends down to L2.[20] Dysfunction here is always associated with reflex 'central cinch' neuromuscular behavior (Ch. 10), partly the cause of the dysfunction and further magnified when the underlying joints subsequently become irritable. This junction is thus generally hyper-stabilized in one or more planes. The function of the diaphragm is thus always compromised, reflected in poor expansion of the lower pole of the thorax and compromised IAP and stability mechanisms (Chs 6 & 8). Close attention to, and use of specifically directed 'focused breathing' as part of the treatment, particularly applies in this region. Commonly, sustained CPC behavior means that joint assessment is often really hampered by thick sausages of hyperactive muscle in the thoracolumbar 'fan' making it difficult to engage the bony prominences and it is easy to miss the real offenders. Importantly, graded soft tissue release in conjunction with 'focused breathing' helps gain access. When the diaphragm is 'empty' the posterior muscles may not appear so bulky yet the lower inferior pole of the thorax is recessed and pushed forward because their activity is not antagonistically matched by 'inner inflation' (Fig. 13.83). Gaining a diaphragmatic expansion can be really difficult as for many as it has been so underutilized in function and 'neurally forgotten'.

Initially the **side lying position** allows better approach to access target tissues. The therapist's hand acts as a proprioceptive breathing cue. Some possible treatment options are explored.

• **Assessing function of the diaphragm**. Simply place your open hand centrally over the thoracolumbar spine and ask the patient to 'breathe back into my hand'. Ideally, you would like to feel not only the expansion backwards and laterally but feel each vertebra slightly rise up under your hand in a slight flexion moment (Fig. 13.84). This requires a cooperative synergy between the psoas and abdominals to provide the stability for the crural fibres to act and at the same time, eccentric lengthening control from the extensors. There is a high correlation between erector spinae activity and increased segmental stiffness.[51] When their irritability is high they do not let go to allow the inflation synergy. Addressing the thoracolumbar joint and myofascial dysfunction begins to allow better facilitation of the diaphragm.

• **Assessing and releasing possible myo-fascial 'inferior tethers'** acting upon the lower pole of the thorax. This includes soft tissue exploration of the erector spinae (ES), serratus posterior inferior (SPI),

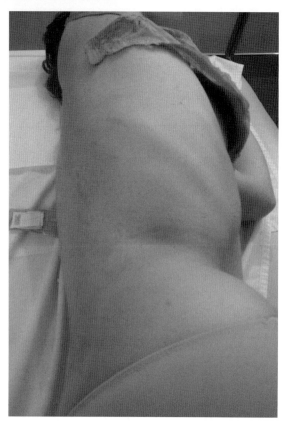

Fig 13.83 • The subject is lying on her left side. CPC behavior and 'empty' diaphragm and transversus activity appear to create a hollow as shown.

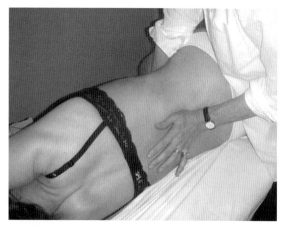

Fig 13.84 • 'Breathing back' into the operator's hand to assess diaphragm activity.

the intercostals and notably the diaphragm rim; psoas, quadratus lumborum and even the lateral fibres of internal oblique (IO) and latissimus dorsi (LD). This will involve covering territory from about T7 to L3 and the related thoracic cage including the circumference of the inferior rim. With the exception of latissimus, all those muscles over the lower posterolateral pole of the thorax mentioned above all derive their innervation from either the dorsal rami (erector spinae) or the ventral rami of the adjacent spinal nerves extending between T7 extending as low as L3.[20] In addition to its motor innervation from the phrenic nerve, the peripheral rim of the diaphragm also receives sensory fibres from the lower 6 or 7 intercostal nerves – themselves derived from the ventral rami of the adjacent thoracic spinal nerves.[20] Palpation of the diaphragm rim usually delineates local thickenings and trigger points affecting its function.

Hence dysfunction of any spinal segment from T7 to L3 can influence elements of CPC behavior. Again the 'Catch-22' is operant – mutual reinforcement between joint dysfunction driving the neuromuscular hyperactivity which drives the joint problem and so on. Asking for 'breathe back into my hand' can be really lamentable and generally needs to be worked for. When tense/tender tissues bands are found, the therapist carefully gauges the pressure and asks for 'breathing into it' and some release can generally be obtained, allowing further joint assessment and freeing and so on. It is important that the assessment clearly delineates and achieves dissociation between the lower four ribs and the transverse processes of L1 and L2. The assessment, soft tissue release and facilitated breathing and treatment of the joints segue into one another – as improvement in one allows further access in another and so on. Placing the patient's top arm above his head and asking for 'growing the arm long' as he inspires can aid further release (Fig. 13.85).

• *Assessing joint function in side lying.* When there is a lot of muscle spasm, careful and slowly applied central postero-anterior pressures[29] through the spinous process can help gauge joint play and gain slight movement enough to relax some of the neuromuscular hyperactivity and more clearly ascertain true joint status. However, when the spinal extensors are really hyper-facilitated, central posterior pressures can stimulate increased bilateral central cinch behavior hence the use of rotation is valuable to help inhibit this response.

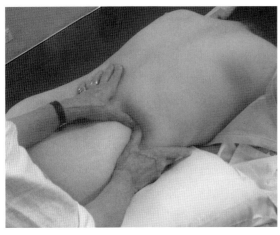

Fig 13.85 • Myofascial release of the 'lower golden triangle' gaining dissociation between the upper lumbar vertebrae and lower three ribs – with care!

Neuro therapies such as that of the Bobaths[61] advocate the use of 'reflex inhibiting postures', which adopt rotary components into postures and the facilitation of rotary movements to help inhibit the unwanted more primitive mass responses. Thus assessing rotation has the twofold benefit of banking down extensor hyperactivity as well as testing intersegmental movement into rotation which ideally is considerable yet usually markedly reduced in dysfunction of the lower pole of the thorax. While the therapist maintains her hold on a relevant bony prominence, the patient is asked to 'breath back' and 'fill out' the posterolateral thorax, 'think of' doing various *minimal movements* while myofascial release and mobilization are also incorporated to help free the joints (Fig. 13.86). The rotation can involve the top shoulder being rotated back or forward either as a position for treatment or as active movement.

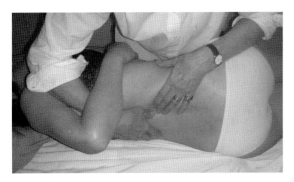

Fig 13.86 • Assessing segmental & myofascial rotary function through the thoracolumbar junction.

• The ***prone position*** affords the opportunity to better discern any asymmetry between sides at rest and when actively breathing. Placing two pillows under the lower pole of the thorax encourages more posterior basal expansion and superficial myofascial release during the treatment. CPC behavior (Ch. 10) fixes the region limiting segmental and cephalad rib movements needed for inflation as well as lateral weight shift. Trigger points in the involved muscles are common particularly in the ES, SPI and IO and their attachments with the diaphragm over the lower four ribs serve to 'tether' them. Placing the arms in as much elevation as is comfortable and supporting the shoulders is a preferred starting position and helps inhibit this neuromuscular response. Thoraco lumbar 'opening' can be further facilitated by lengthening one arm (Fig. 13.87) to help encourage patterns of lateral shift and lift through the lower pole of the thorax while also mobilizing the joints and soft tissues into this range. Care needs to be exercised if using leg lengthening if there is any concern about an 'unstable' level say at L4/5, as this can overwork the vulnerable level and exacerbate symptoms. Again the approach utilizes myofascial release, breath work and joint mobilization as indicated by the tissues. Positioning the patient in some rotation can also be used in the later stages of treatment to further improve the desired movement through the junction (Fig. 13.88). However this needs to be carefully

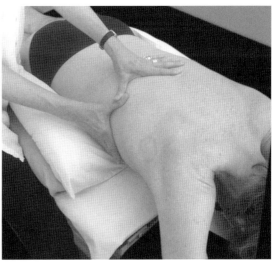

Fig 13.87 • Facilitating lengthening in the lateral body wall; releasing trigger points in serratus posterior inferior intercostals, lateral latissimus dorsi and asking for both diaphragmatic expansion and growing the ipsilateral arm.

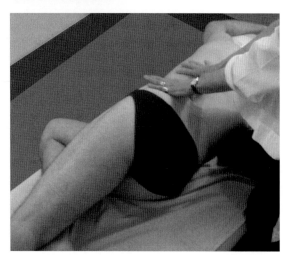

Fig 13.88 • Forward shoulder rotation positioning in side lying affords the opportunity for further nice release through the thoracolumbar junction.

gauged as if adopted before there is adequate freedom of movement through the lower pole of the thorax, aggravation of lumbar levels is possible.

• *Prone on elbows* can be used in later stage treatments to gain better segmental extension as well as regional and general extension. A pillow under the hips can further help this. As this position is usually stiff and unaccustomed, the patient will tend to tense, breath hold and 'pectoral fix' the thorax and 'dome' into flexion. This is particularly marked in those classified as APXS and prevalent central anterior cinch (CAC) activity where hypertonus in the upper abdominals can be really difficult to inhibit. The patient is encouraged to 'let go' these holding patterns, expand the center with the diaphragm and 'soften and lengthen'. *Gently* reassessing lateral, rotary postero-anterior movement at each segment from the 'dome' through to the sacrum will delineate where the 'blocks' are which still need more freeing.

• In the supine position any anterior myofascial tightness of the lower pole of the thorax due to CAC hyperactivity can be released. This narrows the infrasternal angle and limits lateral rib movement and 'lift' of the thorax. Diaphragm excursion becomes restricted. Myofascial tightness and trigger points around the anterolateral rim of the inferior thoracic aperture are common and will influence activity in both transversus abdominus and the diaphragm. These tight tissues are commonly very tender thus care needs to be

exercised to proceed with sensitivity in order to gain release rather than defensive holding (Fig. 13.89). Expansion usually visibly improves after this maneuver. At later stages, lying back over pillows or a bolster facilitates further opening (Fig. 13.101).

Is it possible that there is a 'basic lumbar pattern' of joint findings? Every patient with back pain requires individual assessment and treatment tailored to his particular deficits. However, common features can be observed (Ch. 8) with common patterns of presentation (Chs 9 & 10) This author is pondering the matter as to whether clinically, underlying each individual presentation a somewhat common underlying 'joint pattern' can be distilled which ensues from a combination of the skeletal/myofascial geometry (see Ch. 6, Part C) and the common patterns of altered posturomovement control. Tentatively proffered, and as much as one can generalize and I do so with caution, it would seem that the following *basic underlying pattern* of joint and soft tissue characteristics *may* be generally though variably observed, the extent of which further varies according to the stage of the presenting disorder:

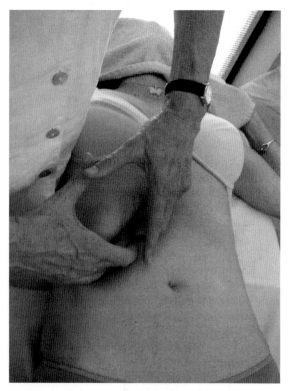

Fig 13.89 • Release of the diaphragm and transversus around the anterior/inferior thoracic rim.

- Variable neuromuscular hyper-activity of the muscle 'fan' over the thoracolumbar levels in a CPC creates joint hyper-stability. Brittle stiffness though potentially irritable joints. The tissues are generally more neurally 'hot' and 'alarmed'.

- Segmental and long muscle hypertonus/tightness frequently starts to become more apparent around L3 cephalad and can be particularly so around T12/L1. This is associated with 'different' increased segmental resistance to palpation. Does dysfunction of the diaphragm play a decisive role? Shirley et al.[51] demonstrated a greater stiffness at L2 than L4 during inspiratory efforts indicating a contributory spinal stabilizing role for the crural diaphragm. They also showed a high correlation between increased erector spinae activity during expiratory effort and increased segmental stiffness and ipso facto if more active in some regions these regions will be stiffer. When there is more hyper-activity in the erector spinae this may also involve psoas and more so if the abdominals are underactive (PPXS). Even when psoas and extensors are underactive (APXS) with increased upper abdominal activity there is intermittent CPC activity. Either way, when the co-activity between psoas, abdominals and extensors is altered the stability of the thoracolumbar spine alters and so affects the stability for the crural diaphragm attachments – L1-3. Clinically they consistently 'feel different'!

- Segments L3/4/5 tend to be more flexed and generally more 'empty' neuromuscularly with more developed reactive soft tissue changes. Probably more neurally 'burnt out' although frequent 'sprains' to these levels produce recurrent acute symptoms suggestive of 'instability' and similar presentations in some.

- Sacrum counternutated. L5/sacrum and the pelvic joints restricted particularly into the 'closing' movements with reactive myofascial changes.

- Variable patterns of hip restriction affect pelvic mechanics.

Consideration is ongoing!

The 'dome' (Ch. 8)

The 'dome' is the transitional area between the less mobile upper pole of the thorax and the more mobile lower pole – a local segmental kyphosis/restriction at the 'dorsal hinge' and part of a general increase in the thoracic kyphosis (Figs. 13.11 & 8.33). One of the contributors towards its genesis is imbalance in the myofascial fan attaching the shoulder girdle to the thorax (Ch. 6, Part C & Ch. 8). Tightness in the anterior chest/shoulder muscles act to flex the anterior thorax and pull the shoulder girdle forward becoming an 'antero-inferior tether', disturbing shoulder girdle function and limiting opening forward of the sternum with concurrent extension around the 'dorsal hinge'. The shape of the inferior pole of the thorax can become quite distorted (Fig. 8.35). A 'dome' is usually variably present in each of the pelvic crossed syndromes. Serratus anterior interdigitates with the external oblique and if both are short as in the APXS or the mixed syndrome (MS), the infra-sternal angle is more closed, and the whole thorax is more flexed. If the external obliques are underactive as in the PPXS, the lower pole of the thorax flares open anterolaterally and the person can 'look more extended'. However, a thoracic kyphosis and 'dome' are usually still evident in PPXS, the apparent extension occurring from compensatory hyperextension over the thoraco-lumbar junction. A 'dome' can thus drive a thoracolumbar problem and needs addressing in order to restore sequential movement transmission through the spine. The dome and related reactive intersegmental hypomobility risks chronic irritation of the sympathetic ganglia which rest against the rib heads. Apart from 'organ type symptoms' the sweat may have a metallic smell and the skin and superficial tissues may feel thickened, tense, congested and inelastic and may show changes such as 'peau d'orange'. Joint assessment can be further difficult. It need only take one symptomatic joint within the 'dome' and/or between it and the lumbar spine to fire up the whole thoracolumbar erector spinae mass making finding 'levels' even more difficult.

Examining the dome is indicated in all shoulder problems, primary cervicothoracic problems and also primary thoracolumbar junction problems. As its presence creates significant alterations to the transmission of segmental adjustments and movements throughout the axial spine one should even be prepared to examine this region in pain syndromes of the low back, pelvis and leg. Clinically, leg pain can be reproduced from as high as T7 and foot pains have been eradicated with treatment to symptomatic joints over this region when local treatment to the foot or lower spinal levels have made no change. Treatment is directed both at the symptomatic joints but in particular to the related

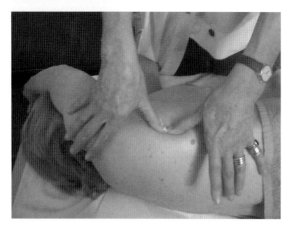

Fig 13.90 • Myofascial release of structures related to the 'dome' in side lying.

myofascial tightness and is best done in the side lying position. (Fig. 13.90). The principles are the same as described for the thoracolumbar junction.

Cervicothoracic junction

This junction serves an important crossroads marrying function between the cervical spine, thorax and shoulder and its examination should be undertaken for pain syndromes in any of these regions as well as any arm symptoms. It readily becomes the victim of postural collapse, a forward head posture and altered shoulder joint myomechanics which largely ensue from sitting and working – 'riting, reading and 'rithmetic' and the dreaded computer. Add the effects of stress and poor breathing habits and the recipe for symptom development is evident. The shoulder crossed syndrome is the expression of the altered spinal alignment and related myofascial imbalance (Ch. 10). Both the joint dysfunction and the neuromyofascial imbalance need to be concurrently examined and redressed in treatment. The *side lying position* affords the easiest initial access. Some approaches are explored.

• *Examining the 'upper ring'* (see Chs 6, Part C & 8). The scaleni collectively arise from all cervical segments and distally attach to the 1st and 2nd ribs[20] with segmental innervation variable but generally from the ventral rami C3-8;[20] hence, their hyperactivity can emanate from dysfunction in any cervical segment as well as from altered posturomovement and breathing habits. Their hyperactivity creates a tense web which acting like guy ropes, tends to 'lift' the 'upper ring' and more posteriorly. Postural collapse and coexistent overactivity of the subclavius and clavicular

pectoralis major, downwardly rotates the clavicle, dropping the 'upper ring' anteriorly while also pulling the clavicle 'down' on the 'upper ring'. Reactive changes occur at the sternoclavicular joint, the 1st and 2nd rib attachments front and back and the vertebral joints. The C7/T1/2 joints become stiff and reactive as they are relatively hyperstabilized in flexion, losing side bending, rotation and extension which further limits movement in the upper ring and adaptable postural setting for the shoulder and the head and neck (Fig. 13.91). This creates the 'dowager's hump' which when marked can be associated with overlying puffy soft tissues and a 'glassy' appearance of the skin. The hyperactivity in the scalenii, cervicothoracic extensors, upper trapezius and levator scapulae, make engaging the vertebrae for determining intersegmental movement very difficult and again a combined approach of myofascial release and joint mobilization is indicated – analogous to 'peeling the layers off an onion to get to the heart of the matter'. This junctional block also contributes towards the

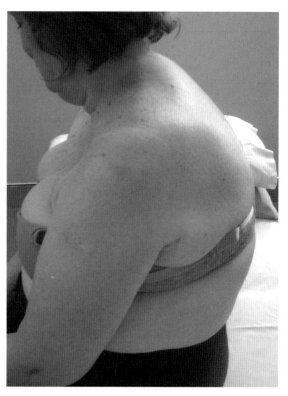

Fig 13.91 • Disturbed 'upper ring' function is apparent.

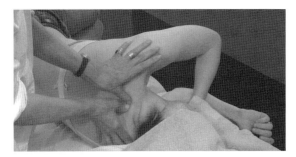

Fig 13.92 • Assessing postero-anterior intersegmental 'give' through the junction in side lying.

common findings of stiff yet reactive changes in C6 and associated variable signs of 'overwork' in the form of spasm, reactive change and altered kinematics between C3–5. Initially the patient's arm lies by his side but later when working further into range, can be variously positioned forward, above the head, etc. (Fig. 13.92).

• *Examining freedom in the claviscapular unit and related spinal function* (Chs 6, Part C. & 8). Dysfunction in the 'upper ring' is closely allied with claviscapula dysfunction. Hyperactivity of pectoralis minor tugs the coracoid down and forward and through the acromioclavicular joint attachment and pectoralis major hyperactivity, further contributes to the downward rotation of the clavicle. Posteriorly, the scapula is pulled superiorly, also considerably helped by increased activity in upper trapezius and levator scapulae. The cervicothoracic junction dysfunction becomes maintained through altered shoulder girdle myomechanics. Trigger points can abound in all the hyperactive muscles, seemingly resulting from both segmental hyper-facilitation and habitual overuse. Releasing these tight muscles is important in gaining a more centrated position of the upper ring and shoulder girdle (Fig. 13.93). Release of the pectorals assists in reinvigorating the lower scapular stabilizers and adjacent intersegmental extensors to lift the sternum and upper ring anteriorly. Pectoralis minor can create particularly pernicious effects including compression of the brachial plexus when it is tense and tight. It receives its innervation from C6,7 & 8[20] hence irritation of these spinal segments can further drive its overactivity creating a vicious cycle. Gaining active elongation through PIR and or free movements while stabilizing variously ribs 3–5 helps release while at the same time mobilizes the ribs. Upper thoracic segmental dysfunction arises from the altered kinematics and in turn further

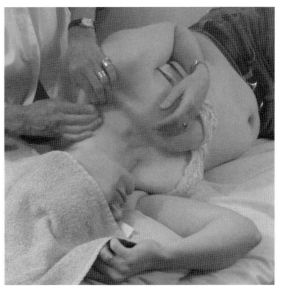

Fig 13.93 • Myofascial release of tight upper trapezius and levator scapulae.

contributes to hyperactivity in various myofascial tissues and many upper limb pain syndromes. There is often hypomobility/irritability between T2/3 and rib 2/3 where the divergent influences of the scalenii superiorly and pectoralis minor inferiorly play out. In addition when the claviscapula unit is out of balance, the upper fibres of serratus anterior appear to act like a syndesmosis where the superomedial scapula becomes 'bound' to the upper ribs – the 2nd and 3rd in particular, further influencing the problems here. The ribs thus become 'yanked' when the scapula moves and this is a frequent cause of many shoulder and so called 'rotator cuff' complaints. So called 'shoulder impingement' is often a rib 2–3 problem.[62] The 'handstand' position affords improved access for releasing the infra and supra clavicular fossae and nice mobility in the upper thoracic and junctional spinal joints and ribs can be also be gained by the therapist maintaining an appropriate contact point on the vertebra and the patient performing small multidirectional movements with the elbow – the claviscapula movements so produced, providing the mobilizing force to the vertebrae (Fig. 13.94). Fixing these ribs and asking the patient to slightly move the scapula is invariably really painful locally and can refer pain into the glenohumeral joint and also to the head. However when dissociation between the scapula and ribs improves so does the pain.

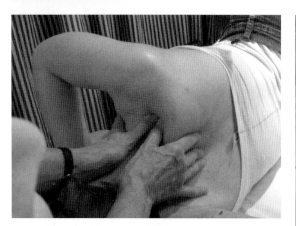

Fig 13.94 • The handstand position is nice for getting into the upper 'golden triangle' including testing upper rib mobility.

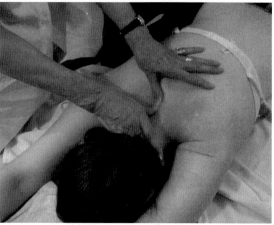

Fig 13.95 • If tolerated, bringing the arms up helps to present the segments for detailed testing.

• *Further examination of intersegmental movement in prone.* A marked forward head posture can lead to significant sagittal deformation through this junction and achieving a neutral spine when prone is not possible. Accordingly, placing a pillow or even 2 under the thorax initially accommodates the altered alignment until such time that it can be improved. Placing supports under the shoulders supports a more neutral position and stops them dragging the spine forward. All too frequently, joint problems are not picked up over this junction because of inadequate assessment. A focused persistence helps ensure getting down into the articular gutter and it is useful to 'skive' the gutter to delineate the finer differences between levels. Allodynia on palpation of the spinous process is a reliable sign that the joints of this vertebra are dysfunctional which should encourage more probing. Raising the arms into elevation, elbow extension and external rotation (Fig. 13.95) brings the junctional levels to more prominence making testing easier. However because of the frequent concurrence of shoulder problems with dysfunction here, a modified position with flexed elbows may need to be adopted and as improvement occurs can progress to the elbows extended.

Cervicocranial junction

The functional importance of this junction towards spinal function as a whole is in general not appreciated hence enquiring and competent assessment is unusual unless symptoms implicate its frank involvement such as headache and dizziness.[27,63] Given that nearly 50% of nodding and rotating the head occur through the joints in the upper cervical complex, any restriction in neck movements should invoke its examination.

Disturbed neuromyo-articular function in this region is likely to affect the essential afferent impulses arising from the receptor systems in the connective tissue structures and small muscles around and within the upper joints. These play an important role in the tonic neck reflexes and the mediation of postural tone throughout the body and limbs including equilibrium reactions.[27] Head posture thus largely influences postural control though the body. A forward head posture means that in order for the eyes to orient to the horizontal, the occiput is relatively extended on the neck. Weakness in the craniocervical flexors is common[3,4,5,22] with corresponding tightness in the suboccipital muscles. This is also associated with increased activity in the sternocleidomastoid, upper trapezius and levator scapulae[3-5] acting to further extend the occiput on the neck which means the occipital condyles are not free to disengage posteriorly from the articular surfaces of the atlas. All of the deep flexor and extensor suboccipital muscles receive innervation from C1-3; in particular the dorsal ramus of C1 plays a large role.[20] The altered alignment and muscle imbalance impair the complex and functionally important joint kinematics between C0/1/2 further influencing facilitation and inhibition of these deep muscles.

The 9th, 10th and 11th cranial nerves (respectively, the glossopharyngeal, vagus and accessory nerves) exit through the jugular foramen which is located just lateral to the occipital condyles[37] of the atlanto-occipital joint. Dysfunction of this joint creates local reactive tissue changes which can also extend to impair function in these cranial nerves potentially influencing far reaching function throughout the body. Difficulty swallowing and altered pharyngeal function implicates the 9th cranial nerve; the vagus nerve can be implicated in many vocal, digestive, respiratory cardiac disorders.[37] Importantly the accessory nerve innervates the sternocleidomastoid and the trapezius and if irritated can further add to their hypertonus, further compounding the upper cervical joint complex dysfunction as well as that in the neck and shoulder.

C0/1/2 dysfunction and the associated tissue change in the region of the jugular foramina is also reflected in dysfunction in the craniosacral system.[37] The close functional relationship between the head, neck and temporomandibular joint and proximity of the external auditory meatus mean that cervicocranial dysfunction is also often implicated in some ear and jaw symptoms.

Restricted movement in this joint complex will shunt movement further south to the mid cervical levels – C345, which frequently display variable soft tissue signs of overwork. It is particularly important that mobility is sufficient when expecting the patient to perform the craniocervical flexion test as an exercise (p. 316). Given that the nerves from the mid cervical levels provide the sole motor innervation to the diaphragm,[20] it is tempting to speculate further as to negative influences upon its function emanating from cervical dysfunction. Furthermore, the phrenic nerve also receives connections from the cervical sympathetic ganglia[20] in the neck and Rock[72] notes that the autonomic innervation of the diaphragm plays a key role in the automatic activation of the transversus abdominus and the pelvic floor. In similar vein, many shoulder muscles enjoy a mid cervical innervation.

Palpation and testing of this region is hampered by suboccipital myofascial thickening and tightness and tender superior attachment points of the long posterior hyperactive muscles. C1 can be elusive to engage and tenderness and fullness over the joints and articular processes can be marked hence a persistent yet sensitive approach is necessary. Many miss locating C1 as it is sometimes above the hairline. Some options are explored:

• **Assessing rotation at C1/2 and flexion/ extension at O/C1 in sitting.** The patient sits with a neutral pelvis and the therapist stands to the right and behind; adopting a soft pincer grip, the therapist places the pad of the left thumb and index finger on the transverse processes of C2. Imaging these to be the flanges of a wing nut is useful. This is often tender hence it is important not to 'poke' producing defensive responses. The other hand cradles the patient's head in neutral flexion/extension and side bending and the patient is asked to 'look' to the left. The eye movement creates a subtle tonus change in the suboccipital muscles and a discrete rotation at C2 which the operator carefully follows around and then gently 'fixes' the position of the vertebra at the barrier. Pressure of the thumb on the right transverse process of C2 is slightly increased to ensure it does not move back while the patient is then asked to 'look to the right' as much as they are prepared to do, as the therapist gauges the dissociation between C1 and C2. Rotation to the left is then repeated while the therapist gently brings the right transverse process slightly further forward and 'takes up the slack' within the limits of comfort. To gain effective release, generally about a 3–4/10 pain level needs to be experienced, however as the patient is in control, how much he 'moves' is up to him. (Fig. 13.96). The patient is asked to 'look with the eyes' rather than 'turn the head' as this usually results in a gross movement and far too much superficial

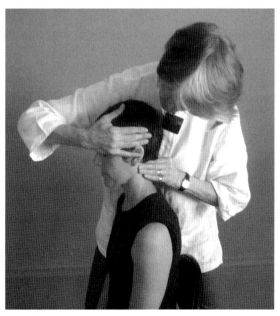

Fig 13.96 • Assessing freedom of the cervico/cranial joint complex in sitting.

muscle activity, negating accurate testing of the joint. The patient only moves within his comfort zone. As the joint becomes freer with a few repetitions, the local tenderness decreases and range increases. The same procedure is repeated to the other side noting any asymmetry. It is common for C2 to be rotated back on the right in right handed people with a related restriction in rotation to the left.

• In the same position as above, movement between the occiput and the atlas can also be gauged. The therapist slides her thumb and index finger slightly cephalad to rest over the arch of C1 which is stabilized while the patient 'looks up/down' as much as they are prepared to do while the therapist subtly applies counter-pressure further into range. Both these maneuvers can produce immediate improvements in active range of head and neck movement.

• *Freeing C1 and C2 in supine:*

  • The patient is supine and the therapist sits or stands at the head of the bed with the patient's head either resting on her stomach or supported in her relaxed hands. Her finger pads point vertically and sink and slide laterally into the suboccipital tissues providing deep pressure so that they eventually 'collect' C1. They act as the fulcrum for the head gently falling back more heavily into the therapist's palm and then rocking forward in a gentle oscillation. The suboccipital tissues are coaxed to relax by gently distracting the occiput during the flexion phase. Asking for 'imagine dropping or lifting your chin' can further facilitate the response. Look for any asymmetry of the skull on the atlas.

  • In the above position, slowly 'skiving' the suboccipital tissues transversely along the arch of C1 also assists release and helps break up fascial thickening. Distinguishing C1 from C2 is important as local thickening is frequently such that C1 feels like the occiput and can be missed. Both are usually stiff and tender but probably C1 is stiffer and C2 more tender. This can be segued into either fixing C1 and asking for 'think of looking up/down'; or fixing the 'peg' of C2 (the spinous process) as the patient is asked to 'think of looking' from side to side; or laterally flexing by 'imagine your ear being closer to your shoulder'. The therapist gently takes up the barrier through the maneuver as dissociation between C0/1/2 is sought.

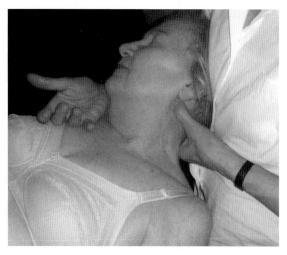

Fig 13.97 • Releasing C0/1 in supine rotation.

  • The patient's head is as above or on a pillow and slightly rotated to the left. Through gentle myofascial release the therapist explores around the occiput/C1 from posteriorly, around the lateral process of C1 continuing onto the anterior surface and under the jaw and around the superior attachment of the sternomastoid. This is usually all extremely tender and tense hence sensitivity and skill are necessary. As the tissues 'give' the release can begin to involve actual mobilizing the joint from behind, laterally or from the front (Fig. 13.97). The same is repeated on the other side addressing any asymmetry. In the neutral position, anterior pressure can be gently maintained on both lateral processes of C1 to 'fix' them while the patient is asked to gently 'look up and then down' – the patient will move as much as is comfortable. Again any asymmetry is noted.

• *Freeing C1 and C2 in prone*. The position is the same as for examining intersegmental movement in prone. C1 is palpated between the spinous process of C2 and the occiput and the movement continued laterally along the arch of C1 ensuring that C1 is actually engaged by directing the pressure up and under the occiput and towards the patient's eye. Transverse pressures on the 'peg' or spinous process of C2 help determine its rotary freedom as do unilateral pressures on the articular pillar in neutral or slight rotation. C3 (and probably C4) is frequently very sore with some guarding and overlying spasm when C1 and C2 are hypomobile.

Don't forget the rest

A case has been made for comprehensive assessment of the junctional regions because of the common propensity for their dysfunction, the significant biomechanical and neuromuscular effects that ensue and the general difficulty in assessing them well. Needless to mention, *all* segments in a symptom producing region are tested. For example, clinically, symptomatic C5/6/7 levels are always associated with cervicothoracic segmental and related myofascial dysfunction. A symptomatic 'plug' at L2/3 can be easy to miss and will usually be partly the result of thoracolumbar dysfunction and also relate to over-flexion and 'winding' at L3 and L4. Treating the junctional problem not only 'deloads' more highly symptomatic segments but also may reduce regional muscle hyperactivity such that finding the more potent segments is possible. Again, the process is akin to 'peeling the layers off the onion to get to the heart' of the problem!

Integrated therapeutic approach

In essence treatment, both manual and exercise/movement therapies, redresses the functional deficits found during the assessment – which joints and tissues are the pain source and why; which *patterns of movement* do we want to facilitate and gain improved control, and which are those that we need to modify or avoid?

Manual

The 'key' relevant assessment findings become the focus of manual treatment and some possible approaches were described. Manual treatment addresses the specific joint and soft tissue problems in order to change the pain and allow more normal neuromuscular function. Reassessment is ongoing and the choice and delivery of various techniques are accordingly adapted in response to the changes in tissue compliance.

Modify the symptom producing habitual postural behavior

Active

In order to 'stem the rot' explanation and an understanding of the role of faulty postural habits towards the development of symptoms is necessary. Be prepared to be very convincing as by and large, patients often expect that you are going to 'just fix them'. Some don't want to hear the message and can resist being actively involved in their own management. Paying for your services is a good incentive. Modifying provocative patient preferred alignments and movements can help decrease symptoms.[16,64] In the acute stages 'taping' the lumbopelvic region can help limit provocative movements and provides valuable proprioceptive feedback about more 'correct' alignment which has generally been relegated to the functional archive department (Fig. 13.98). There are good indications that neutral spinal postures facilitate spontaneous activity in the SLMS.[8–10,65–68]

Sitting is the most easily addressed in the early stages and should be covered even in a 'neck patient' due to the functional interrelationship between the head and tailbone. However it is not necessarily realistic to expect the patient to just simply 'sit up straight'. Combinations of a general or regional lack of spinal extension, reduced SLMS activity, and incompetent pelvic control with poor perceptuomotor appreciation of the neutral position make this difficult. He will invariably try and do this from increased SGMS activity around his mid torso which we do not want to further imprint. Thus it is important that 'correct sitting' is *built up* from:

• An effective base of support from the ischia or 'sitz-bones' appropriately positioned on a firm support with assistance from the feet (see Chs 6 & 8). Accomplishing FPP1 helps this (Fig. 13.25). Studies are beginning to show the importance of pelvic control in maintaining postural control in sitting.[69]

• The axial column is lifted from its base, the sacrum coccyx through inner support provided by

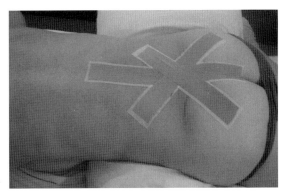

Fig 13.98 • Taping helps to control provocative postures in the early stages. Note the strap over the left innominate is deliberately tensioned to limit posterior rotation.

the SLMS and the LPU. This facilitates improved head control with more options and thus activity throughout the SLMS is further improved.

• This is further augmented by awareness of, and improvement in, diaphragmatic breathing by laterally expanding the lower pole of the thorax[70] against one's own hands adding proprioceptive input.

• In the early stages when improved SLMS activity is still wanting, it is helpful to supply the patient with a round or half round lumbar cushion along the lines of that proposed by McKenzie.[71] So that this is not entirely passive, the active base of support is still encouraged and breathing back into the support is also suggested.

Standing. This also needs to be built up from the base – the ground. Attending to:

• An active base of support through feet which are dynamic adjusters rather than stiff props (Fig. 13.99). Weight bearing through all four corners of the foot and particularly through the heel is necessary for 'grounding' the foot for antigravity 'push up' (Ch. 6, Part B).

• Avoiding hyperextended knees allows for flexibility of the lower limb kinetic chain and to spatially direct and control the pelvis.

• Avoiding a wide base of support and passive 'hanging' on one leg facilitates active support from the SLMS, particularly when the pelvis is slightly anteriorly tilted[72] and posteriorly shifted. As control improves, encouraging lateral weight shift more onto one leg *without collapse* further facilitates the LPU in a dynamic postural support role. Functionally it is so important to be able to come onto one leg with 'lift' in various permutations. When the upright postures are 'right' there is a lightness and freedom in being 'up'.

• Practice of the 'pelvic swing and shift patterns' (Ch. 6, Part B; Ch. 8; Figs. 6.42 & 6.43) helps provide competence in the forward bend pattern consistently repeated throughout the day in all functional activities e.g. gardening. 'Go back to come forward' when bending. The functional connection between the heel/sit-bone is important in driving this from the feet. (Fig. 13.100). The ischia lead the movement back and the knees must also be free to adjust. The hands are free to do whatever.

Passive

Most of our daily activities involve a predominance postures and patterns of movement into flexion.

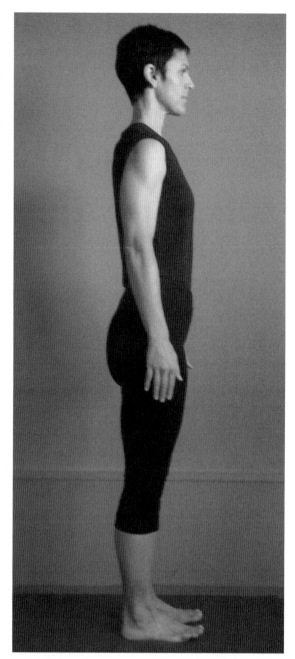

Fig 13.99 • Ideally uprightness should be effortless supported by 'inner lift' coming through an active base of support. The body segments are aligned and the 'center' is there.

Passive supported postures utilizing a 'bolster' help redress a number of deficient elements at once towards helping the patient achieve better 'active' postures. These include:

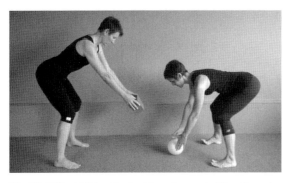

Fig 13.100 • Utilizing the 'pelvic swing and shift patterns' during ADL.

• Redressing stiffness providing passive extension and elongation of the whole spine and in particular the thorax while encouraging the physiological curves. This may also unload the functional spinal unit including the disc permitting rehydration.[73,74]

• Lengthening tight axioscapulohumeral muscles and pelvi femoral muscles, 'opening' stiff shoulders and hips.

• 'Opening the center' facilitating improved diaphragmatic excursion

• The opportunity for relaxation without collapse and 'letting go' superficial SGMS 'holding patterns'.

This can be done in numerous ways, e.g:

  • ***Bottom end over***. The patient sits on the floor and the bolster is brought in contact with the sacrum which is maintained while he lies back. If thoracic stiffness is marked, place a small pillow under the head to ensure a 'cervical/head neutral'. If lumbar extension is markedly reduced the patient may initially need to sit on a small pillow. The arm and leg positions can be varied as shown in Figure 13.101.

  • It is usual and in fact desirable to feel some 'stiff discomfort', the patient being

encouraged to breathe into this and progressively 'let go' the outer muscle 'straight jacket' during each expiration. Beware his tendency of 'holding against' any disease as protective responses are often very reflexley entrenched. It is important that any deficits are adequately supported and the positions modified so that he is not experiencing 'pain' and can properly focus upon breathing and 'release' e.g. placing a block under the thigh if hip opening is painful.

Simple adjustments to common daily activities

Taking time out 'to exercise' is often seen as a chore; however, just being mindful of simple shifts in the way we do ordinary things can often be much more effective than formal 'exercises' e.g. adopting a 'pelvic swing and shift pattern' when forward bending! Snook et al.[75] found reduced low back pain when patients avoided lumbar flexion in the early morning. Suni et al.[76] demonstrated that training in controlling the lumbar spine neutral zone during activities of daily living (ADL) and behavior modeling significantly reduced the intensity of low back pain. Similarly, when reading the newspaper, one can do so in the prone on elbows position (Fig. 13.102): also shown to be a useful position to

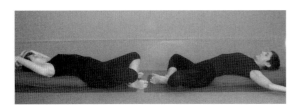

Fig 13.101 • Constructive rest positions supported by a bolster. The limbs can be placed in varying positions to facilitate 'opening'.

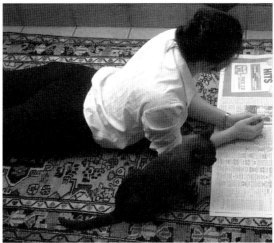

Fig 13.102 • Simply modifying usual activities helps gain functional mileage.

temporarily unload the spine after periods of sustained forward bending.[73] This facilitates a lot more extension, works the shoulder girdle in weight bearing and patterns of weight shift and rotation can be incorporated when turning the pages etc. However, for those with neck and shoulder problems this may be too challenging initially, in which case the more passive supine bolster poses can be used while further control is being attained. For those who work at a computer, encourage frequent weight shifts and movements which get the arms up, out and behind.

Therapeutic exercise

In principle, these should be problem specific and redress the local segmental motor control dysfunction as well as complement manual treatment e.g. if working to improve lumbosacral closing and mobility of the sacrum, unloaded patterns of movement are practised which functionally control this action such as FPP1 in prone, supine or side lying, or prone two knee bend, maintaining one leg neutral while moving the other leg into internal/external rotation. Establishing diaphragmatic breathing[77-79] and control of the simple deep muscle synergies such as the FPPs early in the treatment program is important in gaining control during primary ADL. The early stages are more difficult to teach and take longer to master. Key elements of a movement pattern are practised and mastered in order that competency of the whole pattern can be improved. Repetition 'grooves the motor patterns'[80] in the central nervous system (CNS). Quality control in the correct performance of a desirable component movement is the goal. Sustaining the action improves endurance and more so when done against gravity. Endurance and strength come when there is improved activation and coordination[81] in the SLMS. When patterns of movement are physiological, active lengthening is a natural feature of control and 'stretching' per se becomes less necessary.

Home exercise programs

The prescribing of 'home exercises' is expected and common therapeutic practice. However, what and how much a person does needs to be realistic and achievable. Given that the principal problem is *motor control impairment*[82] and the subject has a poor perceptual sense and control of more ideal

movements, the inevitable risk is that undesirable responses become further learnt and entrenched. For this reason the repertoire should be limited, reasonably straightforward and aimed at the most benefit for the least amount of input. It is easy for them to get the exercises wrong – they invariably do. Frequently, patients present who have been perpetuating their problem performing ill-advised 'stupid stretches' (see p. 291 and Ch. 11) and misdirected 'core' work. A few well mastered passive and active postural activities plus some fundamental motor control 'exercises' gain further mileage than a list of what often amounts to exercise nonsense in relation to the patient's actual functional needs. The 'Allah' stretch (Fig. 13.70) targets

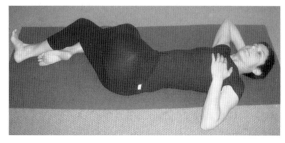

Fig 13.103 • The focus is upon distal initiation through gentle pressure from either the underside heel or elbow. This facilitates a postural reflex response of axial lift and opening including the diaphragm. The focus is on expansion in the center and 'letting go' on each expiration; **not** hardening the outer muscles and/or pulling oneself back.

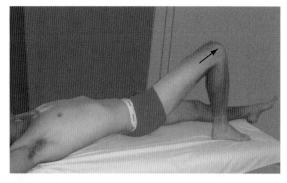

Fig 13.104 • Lying on the back with the hands behind the head and elbows relaxing back, the subject reaches the sitz bone of the standing leg 'long and away'. The action is initiated from the ischium/LPU and there should be co-activation in the torso while allowing weight shift and the movement to sequence through the torso. There is opening and no hardening in the center.

a number of desirable features. Two other examples are shown in Figures 13.103 & 13.104.

The dysfunction model described is complex and interrelated, and there are many aspects of dysfunction which need addressing. In order to achieve more positive therapeutic outcomes, a strong case exists for therapeutic exercises and movement classes where supervised motor control relearning can occur in small groups. Before examining this further it is instructive to look at the literature on therapeutic exercise for back pain

Therapeutic exercise and spinal pain

Overview of outcome studies

There are numerous studies examining the efficacy of exercise therapy in low back pain (LBP) yet it can be confusing for the clinician to make practical sense of the results given the differing etiological assumptions, seemingly random often inappropriate exercise protocols and the varying outcomes being measured. Reviewing trials up to 1990, Faas[83] concluded that 'in acute back pain, exercise therapy is ineffective whereas in subacute back pain exercises with a graded activity program, and in chronic pain, intensive exercising deserve attention'. Van Tulder et al.[84] found similar poor evidence for exercise efficacy in acute LBP with strong evidence for back schools and exercise therapy in chronic LBP. A further systematic review of 'all types of exercise therapy' for non-specific LBP[85] again found little evidence that specific exercises are effective in acute back pain while exercises may be helpful for chronic LBP to increase return to normal daily activities and work. In 2000, The International Paris Task Force on Back Pain[86] recommended that patients with chronic LBP should 'perform physical, therapeutic or recreational exercise keeping in mind that no specific active technique or method is superior to the other. Implementation of this recommendation should not be problematic, because it is current practice'!... No wonder there is a problem 'out there'!

'Exercise therapy' encompasses a broad spectrum of possible approaches and unless the patient's problem is more clearly defined, appropriate exercise prescription, relevant to the stage of disorder cannot occur. Common to many studies is that administered exercise protocols don't necessarily

redress the patient's actual movement function deficits. This is reflected in the title of Faas' paper, *Exercises: which ones are worth trying, for which patients and when?*[83]

The studies on exercise for LBP fall into several categories reflecting different approaches:

Strength and conditioning/functional restoration rehabilitation model

The belief that the major physical defect in patients with chronic low back pain was disuse- induced deconditioning led to programs which adopted a multimodal approach aimed at restoring spine mobility, muscular strength, endurance and cardiovascular fitness thus affording improved physical functional capacity.[87,88] The model has received a lot of attention and it is generally seen as superior to standard care for reducing work absence.[88] The Paris Report[86] will have further entrenched this approach. These programs have also exerted a significant influence within the general therapeutic, prophylactic and 'fitness' exercise spheres.

While more positive outcomes have been shown when adopting a more general active approach[81,87–90,93,94,91] the results are not necessarily as impressive as they seem, measuring different parameters and usually paying little heed to the patient's functional motor control status. The rationale for the exercise choice and delivery is seemingly based upon the general idea that 'any exercise' is beneficial with strength a prime goal. Descriptions of exercises applied in the studies include 'specific exercises'[87–89] (this is not defined); active therapy on strength, endurance, activation and fatigability of the back extensor muscles[81] – applied in three treatment groups as either: 'modern active physiotherapy'; muscle reconditioning on training devices; or 'low impact aerobics';[92] general aerobic exercises, exercises for strength and endurance of the back and abdominal muscles, mobility of the spine and hips;[93] intensive dynamic back exercises;[94] mobility, stretching and muscle strength exercises.[95]

The increased activity with a general lack of treatment specificity may as Mannion suggests[92,96] 'produce some 'central' effect, perhaps involving an adjustment of perception in relation to pain and disability.' However, the real danger is these results then become inflated as 'recommendations', e.g. 'the introduction of low impact aerobic exercise programs for patients with chronic LBP may reduce the enormous costs associated with its treatment.'[97]

In general, the poor attention to the quality of movement control and kinematic patterns and the emphasis on strength does little to change the patient's actual deficits and invariably further entrenches his neuromuscular dysfunction. This approach can hardly be called 'therapy' in the real sense of the word.

Furthermore, the waters become additionally muddied by studies which reflect a limited appreciation about functional spinal control, e.g. the effects of flexion versus extension exercises on pain[90] and 'evidence' which unfortunately advises the promotion of posterior pelvic tilt to gain more abdominal activation.[98]

Instability model for exercise prescription

The 'instability model' of low back pain proposed by Panjabi[99] has spawned the 'era of stabilization exercises'. Kavcic et al.[100] note that 'stabilization exercise' is a generic term which can be given to any exercise that challenges the stability of the spine. While these should ensure sufficient stability, if creating overly high levels of cocontraction, unnecessary compressive loading can occur on the tissues.[101] They quantified the amount of tissue loads versus stability of 'some commonly prescribed stabilization exercises' to help the practitioner determine the most appropriate exercise therapy. However, the danger here is that most chronic non-specific low back pain is assumed to be due to 'instability', and exercises with the 'highest measured stability index' are prescribed to all.[102] Further, the boundary between 'stability' and 'strengthening' has become confused and despite the widespread trend in rehabilitation for 'core strengthening' programs the research is meagre.[103] Performing many so called 'stability exercises' such as the 'abdominal curl', the 'side bridge' and 'bird-dog'[80,100] may well be far too challenging for the patient, encouraging and 'strengthening' further SGMS hyper-activity and does not necessarily restore motor control of the deep abdominals and other SLMS muscles.[104]

Treatment needs to match the disorder. Studies by Richardson and Hodges and their colleagues have improved our understanding of the deep muscle system function and led to a more specific approach to therapeutic exercise for lumbopelvic stabilization.[105] Specific stabilization exercises have been shown to produce favorable outcomes in pain reduction and reduced recurrence rates[106,107] and particularly when subjects are classified into clinical subgroups e.g. demonstrated instability[108] or pelvic girdle pain after pregnancy.[109]

However, it is important to appreciate that clinically patients can demonstrate *too much stability* in certain regions of the spine while other regions *are* less well controlled.

Unfortunately, exercise therapy approaches often reflect the latest fads and 'exercise recipes' which are applied willy nilly to all and sundry and positive outcomes become further remote. This is reflected in a small scale survey which recently investigated the current use of a range of exercise therapy approaches for LBP adopted by physiotherapists in acute hospital settings in Ireland. Specific spinal stabilization exercises were the '*most popular*' followed by the McKenzie approach and abdominal exercises. Do the practitioners understand what they are trying to 'fix'? Rightly the authors concluded there was lack of support from evidence based clinical guidelines for the exercise therapies used.[110]

The functional motor control model

There is increasing interest in the altered quality of motor control, posture and kinematic motion patterns in patients with LBP.[111–121] However, to date there are relatively few outcome studies on the effectiveness of exercise interventions of this kind in subgroups with LBP.

Magnusson[122] noted that preferred motion generated by physiologic submaximal effort may reveal details of motion that are masked by higher levels of effort. Range of motion and motion characteristics can be used to identify the source of dysfunction and assess the effect of rehabilitation While the goal of rehabilitation is return to work they argue that improved motion parameters including control and coordination could hasten return to work. While their administered rehabilitation program was 'non specific', they showed that functional rehabilitation significantly improved motion patterns and features in subjects with CLBP.

O'Sullivan[108] nicely demonstrated that a 'specific exercise' motor relearning treatment approach which trained coactivation of the *deep* abdominals and multifidus produced a statistically significant improvement in pain and functional disability levels in patients with spondylolysis and spondylolisthesis. Importantly, the muscle activation patterns were incorporated into previously aggravating static postures and functional tasks which explain the maintained improvements at 30-month follow up. Similarly, in a more recent study,[78] a specific motor learning intervention was conducted on nine subjects with a diagnosis of SIJ pain and a positive active straight leg raise test (ASLR). Improved diaphragm and pelvic floor kinematics and respiratory patterns during the ASLR test were associated with improvement in pain and disability scores.

Research by Hodges[114–16,123] has demonstrated that consistent delayed and reduced activity of transversus abdominus provides a marker of postural control dysfunction in people with recurrent LBP. In 22 subjects with recurrent LBP, Tsao and Hodges[124] demonstrated that a single session of training isolated voluntary activation of transversus abdominus can lead to automatic changes in feed-forward postural strategies, the magnitude of the effect being dependent upon the type and quality of motor training. In a further study,[125] nine subjects with CLBP received training in repeated voluntary transversus contractions over four visits (initial and at 2 and 4 weeks and 6 months) and subjects continued the training sessions twice a day at home. This specific exercise intervention lead to motor learning of automatic postural strategies during performance of untrained functional tasks and were maintained at 6 months follow-up. However, it is important to recognise that there was only a weak or non significant relationship between changes in pain VAS scores and the improved transversus onsets. Unfortunately, Hodges' important research findings are sometimes taken out of context in the clinical realm, and 'activating transversus' seen as an end in itself towards ameliorating pain. Based on the large outcome variability in their reported 2004 study,[109] Stuge et al.[126] performed a further study on the same population of women with and without longstanding post partum pelvic pain. They were interested to see if those who had continued pain differed in respect to their ability to activate transversus and internal oblique. They found no statistically significant difference between the two groups.

What can the clinician learn from these various outcome studies?

In summary, the systematic literature reviews conducted by Faas[83] and Van Tulder[84,85] and the Paris Report[86] found 'strong evidence' against exercise

therapy in acute back pain and in regard to chronic low back pain, the jury is still out. Included were studies reported between 1966 and 1999. Informed clinical practice assisted by subsequent studies has done much to increase our understanding since that time. Further review is useful:

• *Acute spinal pain syndromes*. While research has not yet delivered substantial evidence for exercise in acute back pain, effective clinical practice produces positive outcomes every day. The clinical priority is to ameliorate the source of pain with appropriate manual therapy and establish activation of specific muscles within the SLMS for local joint protection and support. These are *specific small actions and movements which ask for discrete control*. They can commence on day one of presentation. There is now good emerging evidence that 'appropriate, specific low load' exercise therapy is beneficial in the acute and subacute stages[106–109] for reducing pain intensity and disability. Establishing SLMS function is a prerequisite in any effective exercise therapy for addressing chronic spinal pain syndromes. Clinically, most acute pain episodes occur within a picture of chronic posturomovement dysfunction.

• *Chronic spinal pain syndromes.* Studies on the efficacy of exercise therapy in chronic spinal pain disorders show conflicting and inconsistent results. Returning to work, while a desired outcome, does not necessarily reflect the functional status of the worker who may still have some pain or experience recurrences of pain. Their kinematic movement patterns may be lamentable, the next 'bout' waiting to strike.

Some exercise therapy studies report clear negative outcomes and it is useful to explore the different features of these interventions and compare them with those reporting more positive outcomes including improved neuromotor function.

Negative outcomes

Mens et al.[127] studied women with peripartum pelvic pain. Subjects received a videotape with instructions for 'exercises which trained the diagonal trunk muscle systems for increased force'. These were hypothesized to increase stability of the pelvic girdle yet the ability of these superficial muscles to provide adequate support is questionable (Ch. 8). Patients received no supervision and not surprisingly, reported no change or increasing symptoms. 'A surprisingly large percentage of the experimental group (25%) had to cease training because of pain or fatigue'.[127]

Luoto et al.[128] found that after subjects with chronic LBP underwent a 'functional back restoration program' involving 'intensive physical training', one footed postural stability remained the same in the control and experimental groups but became significantly poorer in those subjects who reported increased pain and disability after the program.

Certain features were common to both these programs:

• Rather than based on the actual observed and found dysfunction, the exercise rationales demonstrate limited understanding of the real nature of the motor control problems seen in spinal pain patients and appear to be based upon hypotheses assuming 'weakness' as the principal physical deficit underlying the pain.

• Accordingly, both programs targeted increasing force and strength in the superficial SGMS which already show patchy dominance and are deemed a likely cause and perpetuator of spinal pain syndromes (Chs 5 & 7–10).

• The lack of adequate supervision[127] means that sensorimotor learning cannot occur. Instead the patient becomes more proficient in his already dysfunctional strategies.

• While standardized non individualized exercise protocols may well 'catch a few in the net' of improvement, many will suffer increased symptoms. No wonder pain related fear of movement/(re)injury and 'catastrophizing' behaviors ensue[129] further feeding into the complex picture of dysfunction which maintains the chronicity of the patient's pain.

Positive outcomes

Stuge et al.[130] addressed the apparent contradictory indications for 'stabilizing exercises' in the treatment of post partum pelvic pain which ensued as a result of the positive findings in their study[109] and the negative findings in the Mens study.[127] Pointing out the differences in the exercise interventions, Stuge argued for a more specific exercise approach which firstly targets the deep system muscles similar to the approach of Hides[106,107] and O'sullivan.[78,108] Common features contributing to the better results in these studies are apparent.

Common features of exercise therapy trials showing more positive outcomes

• The importance of individual assessment, customized prescription, supervision and correction of exercise therapy appropriate to the impairments linked to the patient's pain.

• Specific, accurate activation of local SLMS muscles, coactivation with other local muscles and sustained activation independent of the superficial SGMS muscles and breathing. This is more difficult than often realized and may take 4–5 weeks to master.[108] Activation is initially in positions with reduced gravitational loading is important in helping to change the known and entrenched habitual postural reflex responses.

• The exercises are 'low load' i.e. no more than 30% of the maximum voluntary contraction,[105] should not involve unnecessary effort and should not cause pain.

• Appropriate progression into antigravity positions and integration into functional patterns of posturomovement control. Building endurance and control in unsupported postures in the correct alignment.

• Patient cooperation, motivation, compliance and perceptual awareness in monitoring and adjusting less ideal responses.

• Repetition and practice of key elements of movement control which represent fundamental components of patterns of movement required in everyday function.

The case for therapeutic exercise and movement classes for more optimal relearning of motor control targeting the SLMS

Cholewicki[131] stated: 'clinical intervention does not make a spine more stable but provides a means for better control'. Research is increasingly suggesting that the 'kind of control' which spines lack is that provided by the SLMS

There is a saying 'you can't solve the problem with the same bad habits that created it'. The posturomovement dysfunction in those with spinal pain disorders extends throughout the torso, is interrelated, habitually entrenched and often considerable. For many, a few individual exercises will not appreciably change function even assuming they do them properly. Rolf[132] considered that in any individual at any age, the extrinsic muscles are more readily accessible to consciousness than the intrinsics. In the process of intrinsic motor relearning, 'getting it wrong' is easy. The manner in which they move is what they know and feels 'normal'. Changing the way we move involves motivation, application, dedication and particularly – *perceptual awareness*.

Once acute pain has settled and relearning control of the fundamental patterns, better alignment and breathing begun, the complexities of relearning further functional sensorimotor control are best addressed in small group classes with a maximum of eight people.

Moshe Feldenkrais[133] considered that because most of us lack a keenly developed perceptual awareness, we do not fully develop our abilities He was interested in our potential for organic learning, more so by 'doing' and he evolved a method of movement classes termed 'Awareness through movement' as a means of improving our biopsycho-social functioning. These classes are not 'problem oriented' but more concerned with perceptual experience and organizing new behaviors. 'Doing' these classes provided an interesting subjective learning experience of 'an easier, better posture' and helped me understand and better clarify the role of 'soft movement' in improving function in the SLMS. Regular participation in Iyengar yoga[134] classes has also provided similar insights and influence. A lot of therapeutic exercise has traditionally been 'hard exercise' addressing achievement and strength. The concept of therapeutic exercise classes which address motor control dysfunction and it is suggested, more specifically, function in the SLMS is reasonably novel.

The approach of this program is one of exploring movement within a context of therapeutic exercise. Appreciating the salient aspects of normal function (Ch. 6), the common deficiencies in function (Chs 7 & 8), and the more common clinical patterns of presentation (Ch. 9 & 10) allow us to construct series of safe and appropriate remedial exercises which specifically redress the more common motor impairments. The classes are 'themed' around various deficient yet functionally important aspects of movement. Which patterns do we want to encourage and which responses should be modified,

inhibited or avoided? Activation of desired muscle groups can be achieved by asking for movement in a way which involves their synergistic coactivation in controlling functional force couples and useful 'phrases' of movement. These 'phrases' are repeated in many different postural permutations and as they become more established, begin to form part of the subject's automatic repertoire of posturomovement control. Exercise interventions need to address the concurrent requirement for more mobility in some regions with the need for more control in others. Through an appreciation of the clinical syndromes such as the layer syndrome (Ch. 10), the therapist learns to expect certain predictable responses and counteract these by facilitating more desirable patterns. General principles which guide the facilitation of improved activity and control in the SLMS are incorporated.

The preceding content of this book endeavors to provide much of the understanding behind this approach. Without understanding 'what's wrong' you can't meaningfully help 'fix it'.

The guiding principles address the deficits while helping promote the SLMS.

General guiding principles for facilitating improved activity in the SLMS while addressing key aspects of control necessary for functional restoration

An inadequate understanding of function and the more common patterns of dysfunction mean that many exercise class situations be they therapeutic, yoga, Pilates etc., unfortunately resemble little more than a 'play group for adults' as the often young and dexterous instructor out in front plays a game of 'Simon says'. The participants struggle away trying to follow the often sloppy prompts for actions which may well beyond their capabilities. Over-challenging the patient only results in reinforcing bad habits with already dominant SGMS activity, as the patient calls on what he knows, and valiantly strives to oblige. Many 'exercises' seem to be 'hand me downs' with little applicability to what the patient actually needs.

If therapeutic exercise and movement classes are to offer meaningful motor control relearning, the prescription choice, staging and careful monitoring of the quality of the response is critical. The breaking up of movement into key components allows the practice and refinement of dysfunctional segments and their reintroduction into other patterns of movement.[135] We are aiming to change the habitual response. The aim is to repattern movement and the art is to do so without reinforcing old less ideal patterns.

Research to hand, the influence of certain talented practitioners and clinical practice have all contributed to the paradigm proposed in this body of work. Guiding principles have evolved which are offered to assist the practitioner redress the more common movement dysfunctions. These principles are functionally interrelated. They are not listed in order of importance. Of necessity they are presented in summary form:

• The approach incorporates the common features of those exercise trials demonstrating positive outcomes from a motor relearning approach targeting certain deep system muscles (p. 348).

• 'Boot camp for the brain'– tasking and training the brain to *organize and refine* better coordinated posturomovement solutions; we are not interested in strength per se but in getting the brain to solve the problems in the movement quality; while there is always a 'deconditioning' aspect, the primary problem is one of control; the senses change movement not strength; strength emanates from neural reorganization leading to effortless coordinated movement with multiple options, adaptability and flexibility. Endurance built upon this provides strength.

• Addressing the qualitative rather than the quantitative aspects of performance; altering habitual movement behavior through exploring potential rather than focusing on what is wrong;[133,143] we can't expect them to 'just do it' – re-introducing a forgotten movement vocabulary needs practice and repetition; to facilitate is to help make easier – providing the experience of moving with awareness and without effort; higher levels of effort disable the sensing of small discrete differences;[143] clarity of intent reinforces the movement; movement control is mostly automatic with cognitive override.

• The program is based upon a sensorimotor learning approach which recognizes the importance of the senses in movement control; maximizing proprioception[2,3,136–141] and exploiting the different aspects of the sensory system appropriate to the situation; focusing upon inner awareness and

the use of imagined movement;[142–144] the use of imagery to embellish, reinforce and integrate concepts of movement;[145,146] helping the person experience himself in a more sensory manner; bare feet are de rigueur in order to optimize sensory input through the feet.[136]

• The brain knows more about movement rather than about single muscles; co-activation of muscle synergies for axial and proximal limb girdle postural alignment; balanced activation in the muscle force couples controlling the proximal limb girdles; a tight/overactive muscle group may make its antagonists appear 'weak'; inhibiting muscles by activating the antagonists; muscle sequencing more important than strength in producing coordinated movement.[17]

• Posture and breathing are fundamental to movement hence need to be addressed in movement rehabilitation.

• The important postural and respiratory role of the diaphragm[70,149] is encouraged; coordinating breathing and moving – 'allowing the breath through' and 'opening the center'; allowing the breath to 'irrigate' a posture; using the breath both as a stabilizing and a mobilizing force.

• Correct breathing and control of the FPPs need to be established early and form the basis of 'core control' on which many other posturomovements are rebuilt.

• In general we are *facilitating and promoting* activation of the SLMS and *inhibiting or banking down* overactivity of the SGMS during functional patterns of posturomovement control; activating the 'inner' myofascial sleeve helps support and control internal forces and allows the 'outside holders' to let go; breaking up the more primitive habitual responses including 'holding patterns'; promoting better integrated responses to gravity[147] including feedforward responses;[135] other movement approaches facilitate 'inner support' and improved SLMS activity through conceptually 'activating support from the organs.'[77,164,165]

• Initial activation strategies are in gravity 'minimized' positions to free the CNS from habitual exteroceptive impulses through the feet, breaking the habitual antigravity response;[17,143] practicing control of 'key components' of a movement that are functionally necessary and useful; work towards increased gravity loading and endurance as patterns of control become better established.

• Certain key regions appear to play an important role in activating postural reflex chains; these responses may include related reflex postural activity of the diaphragm. Movements are variously *initiated from* each of these regions:

- • The feet and hands and indirectly the knees and elbows[148–150]
- • The pelvis: sitz-bones and tail bone; ASIS[149]
- • The head.[143,149,150]

• The importance of head orienting and control in spinal alignment and in initiating movement; movements involving 'looking' facilitate the head's role; all sensory experience is associated with movements of the head.[143]

• The concept of axial 'elongation' from the head and tail bone to facilitate co-activation in the deep system –'softening and lengthening'; the head–tail bone relationship in aligning the spine in posturomovement control.

• The concept of 'widening' through proximal limb girdles helps coactivation – nipples and sitz-bones are useful; 'lengthening' the limb aids proximal girdle co-activation; widening and opening through the center facilitates the diaphragm and helps inhibit central cinch behavior.

• *Initiating* movements *from* each of the '6 limbs' (hands, feet, head and tailbone) and the subsequent sequencing of closed chain movements through the spine; initiating movement from the proximal limb girdles and axial spine; specifically addressing movement transmission through the junctional regions.

• Building postures and movement from the 'inside' builds sensitivity in the tissue and better control; achieving a 'neutral spine' and maintaining alignment between the segments in posture and movement; creating, maintaining and adapting appropriate axial postural sets to support movement; the quality of the postural set determines the quality of ensuing movement; sustaining postural sets without superficial 'holding up' while breathing normally to build endurance yet flexible control.

• Coexistence of stability and mobility in postural control;[151] stabilizing and mobilizing elements continuously interact to produce effective movement;[17,152] adding even slight movement to

'postures' helps them to 'sensed' and hold the effect in the CNS.

• Moving slowly, sustaining and repeating the action gives time to process the sensory information and helps improve endurance in the SLMS and 'strength'; achieving even rhythm through the movement improves control; working for small discrete 'woosie' movements with selective points of initiation, e.g. interscapular region; functional co-activation is often an 'action' rather than a movement which may be miniscule.

• All functional movement patterns encompass elements of rotation and weight shift in varying degrees; both are important in sequencing movement through the spine; patterns of reach and rotation in the limbs to get more fully into the spine.

• Concept of active 'grounding' through the base of support in posturomovement; 'yield and push'[152] from the base of support to 'come up';[150] developing an adaptable base of support; encouraging weight shifts over the base of support – particularly initiated from the pelvis.

• When working for axial release – the value of 'yielding' the under surface of the body to the ground to aid 'opening' and movement in the upper surface; 'yielding' to the ground and/or the movement when 'stretching' without losing alignment or collapsing e.g. 'Allah stretch' (Fig. 13.71); waiting for the release and assisting with the breath.

• Controlling the alignment of the thorax on the lumbar spine; in particular posterior shift of the thorax on both a neutral and anteriorly rotated pelvis; a relaxed rib cage, elongated spine, horizontal respiration and centration of the thoracolumbar spine facilitates the SLMS and the LPU.[153]

• Soft versus hard exercise – 'growing the movement' slowly and the need to avoid effort; the importance of the quality of the response –'how' and 'where' the movement happens; holding tension cuts off the sensation.

• Strength comes when there is three-dimensional control and better endurance in the SLMS; strength is a function of reciprocal agonist, antagonist balance;[132] working with gravity as the teacher rather than repetitively pulling one dimensionally on a machine in recumbent positions.

• Taking movements out of a dominant sagittal orientation; asking for non habitual movements in three dimensions helps repatterning movement sequences and the nervous system and equips the patient with more options for response.

• Movement takes the path of least resistance; always incorporating axial alignment and control from the deep system while getting movement into the stiff regions and controlling the more mobile segments.

• 'Active elongation' versus stretching; reducing the use of SGMS strategies reduces the need to 'stretch'; active eccentric lengthening of short muscles in movement is assisted by activating the breath and the SLMS; the body's resistance should be respected for the useful feedback it provides.

• Addressing mobility and stability in the feet; aligning the feet in weight bearing; activating the feet: 'fanning' the toes; 'doming' the feet in weight bearing;[145] elongating the heel and 'grasping' in a free foot[150] (Fig. 13.105).

• The importance of establishing intrapelvic and three dimensional spatial control of the pelvis; control of the pelvis on the femora is all about initiating from the sitz-bones and tail bone; control of the lumbar lordosis is dependent upon this.

• Establishing good proximal girdle control supports the arms and legs in open and closed chain movements allowing more freedom in spinal control[150] and less reliance on central cinch strategies.

• Coactivation through the proximal limb girdles provides better control for limb weight bearing; building positive support reactions through the limb in weight bearing, helps avoid 'propping'; changing the addiction of the knees to lock.[166]

• The important functional relationship between the heel of the foot and the ischia; between the ball of the foot and the iliacus/psoas,[17,152] between the heel of the hand and the scapula in limb weight bearing.

• Establishing axial and proximal girdle rotary control and particularly through the thorax; using rotation to help break up tendency to total flexor/extensor pattern responses; the rotary element furnishes the third factor in three-dimensional movement.[17]

• Appreciating the reciprocal functional connection between the proximal limb girdles; in recumbent or all fours postures patterns of weight shift from one to the other establishes many axial patterns of control; opening the 'dome' is associated with anterior pelvic rotation in prone and supine all fours and needs to be worked for; closing the 'dome' is associated with posterior pelvic rotation and commonly easier to do.

• Working to improve eccentric control in posturomovement patterns; concentric/eccentric interplay underpins weight shift and postural adjustment; coordinated concentric/eccentric interplay imparts rhythm in movement.

• Gaining improved passive, active, selective and sustained control of extension; aided by supported passive poses e.g. a bolster or with self mobilizing activities such as the Spine Rolla©; activating the deep intrinsic extensors without increasing CPC behavior.

• Targeting the 'dome' and associated myofascial restriction in the shoulder girdle; establishing improved control of the shoulder girdle; initiating movement from the 'dome' while the lumbar and cervical spines are controlled; improving function through the 'dome' lessens the need for central cinching.

• Establishing movement *in* the large ball and socket joints – the hip and shoulder by addressing related tight myofascial structures while controlling axial alignment; balanced control and endurance about each axis; the axis of movement during active control is localized *in* the joint.

• 'Lengthening the sides' facilitates weight shift and opening the thorax and shoulders; 'body half' activities prepare for unilateral limb loading; therapeutic muscle activation while minimizing spine loads is achieved by unilateral activation of the spine muscle groups[154,155]; unilateral limb movements induce more unilateral low load spinal patterns.

• Task specific and functionally oriented training;[135] incorporating pelvic control patterns in practicing ADL actions: sitting, sitting to standing and reverse, standing, forward bending, reaching; learning to release the 'ischial swing'; ipsilateral/contralateral functional reach patterns.[156]

• Unilateral limb movements also help break up more primitive bilateral flexor and extensor patterns and encourage weight shift; incorporate contralateral movements; the use of diagonal and reach patterns sequencing through the torso from one proximal girdle to the other; muscles work best in diagonals or spiral patterns.[17,152]

• Encouraging disassociation between limbs; addressing tendency for total pattern responses between trunk and limbs; establish more competency in unilateral limb loading; encourage more flexor pattern loading in the lower limb and extensor in the upper limb; appropriate weight bearing challenge through all sections of the limbs.

• The ability to work the axial flexors and extensors without increasing more primitive 'total pattern' behavior or central cinch behavior; achieving balanced co-activation between the flexors and extensors; incorporating rotation, and side bending into flexion and extension movements.

• Movement should be painless; pain can indicate neuromyo-articular irritability and/or dysfunctional neuromuscular strategies and may require one on one manual treatment and revisiting specific basic exercises; accessing stiffness and myofascial tightness is necessary yet can be 'uncomfortable' and is assisted by 'breathing into it'.

• 'Challenging stability' should not mean 'throwing everything at it' as this risks 'fixing behavior' in the superficial system; instead we are training dynamic control of movement and less reliance on 'stiffening' strategies; labile surfaces such as 'physio balls' do not necessarily 'stabilize'[157] or increase target muscle activity,[158] and can foster more 'central fixing' strategies; they are not recommended unless optimal patterns of motor control are evident and maintained on them;[159,160]; the best devices for challenging stability are those with a firm surface to assist 'grounding', and better stimulating SLMS activity such as wobble boards and rocker boards;[136] the challenge should be achievable; the challenge is in the quality and organization of the response.

• Incorporating transitional posturomovements involving level change between the floor and standing;[161] inhibiting the compensatory tendency of the arms to 'push down' instead of the feet 'pushing down to come up' when getting up from the floor or from sitting; 'rooted' control in the pelvis allows the spine and upper limbs to reach out and 'fly'.[145]

• Moving with interest and curiosity rather than ambition and 'end-gaining'; 'playing the edges' and working with awareness of one's limitations; intention, attention and motivation all play an important role in movement.

• Avoid fatigue and cognitive overload; avoid inducing performance anxiety about 'getting it right' where tension patterns increase; healthy movement 'gives a sense of relief'[162] and feels pleasurable particularly if containing repeated rotary elements while the body is supported as in rolling.

• Rest periods in supported passive postures allow 'active reduction of somatic effort',[163] attention to residual sensations and focusing upon the 'inner'. A recalibration of self organization occurs allowing more freedom of choice when activating movement; supported postures help focus and access stiff regions.

• In essence we are building control from inside and below and reducing the habitual overdependence upon control strategies from the outside and above; to develop a balance between inner and outer and between movement initiated centrally and peripherally.[164]

Further practical aspects in functional control

There are literally thousands of 'exercises' that could contribute towards improved function. The guiding principles are offered as a reference framework to help direct the creativity and artfulness of the therapist in prescribing appropriate exercises. Some key aspects of this approach merit closer attention.

Effective 'grounding' through the base of support provides the stability for control

Ideal antigravity support comes from below and principally within. When 'grounding' is not well developed from the base of support (see Ch. 4), ineffectual and imbalanced control of the proximal limb girdles result, and the person develops compensatory 'holding patterns' around their center and 'core'.

When we 'yield' the base of support to the supporting surface, we 'ground' ourselves to the earth and proprioceptively 'connect' in order to 'push away', sensing our weight and gravity. Integration of the positive supporting reactions allows us to utilize the ground reaction force which provides the stable point from and through which we can 'push up', initiating a reflex chain of responses in the anti-gravity postural reflex mechanism.

Thus movements initiated from the periphery *from and through the base* sequence through the limb, proximal limb girdles and spine helping provide cross patterns of *inner support and control.* Weight shift is learnt between the girdles and between sides of the body through the basic homologous, homolateral and contralateral movement patterns (Ch. 3). Kinetic chains comprising groups of muscles are engaged either simultaneously or consecutively to produce either support or movement.[152] One part learns to provide a stable support while the other practices mobility.[152] Movement sequences from one girdle through the spine to the other providing the spine with the movement diet it likes.

The principle of 'grounding' and support preceding movement is basic to the work of Bainbridge- Cohen,[165] who influenced others.[164,152] The establishment of the 'yield and push patterns'[152] and 'grounding' supports the development of the 'reach and pull patterns'.[152,164,165] Many ADL activities involve these movement sequences. Hartley[164] notes that pushing must be supported and balanced by yielding mutually for effective grounding. 'Grounding' allows movement over the base of support necessary for weight shift and the development of all the transitions in movement. Being anchored to the ground by the legs and pelvis allows our spines to coil and uncoil elastically through space lending our arms power and range.[145]

However, while 'grounding' through the feet may seem an obvious feat when standing – you are on your feet after all – most are not *actively* 'on' them, attested to by the plethora of foot orthotics usage. 'Inactive' feet are generally associated with locked knees and standing becomes 'propping' instead of active control (Fig. 10.26). The same goes for weight

bearing through the hand. Focusing upon forming an *active base* through the heel and all four corners of the hand and the foot are important in gaining co-activation through the proximal girdles. 'Doming' engages the arches and 'fanning' the toes activates the feet base of support (Figs. 6.45 & 13.105). In 'yielding' to the support surface, we can more easily 'come up',[150] providing a buoyancy and lightness to upright postures. In fact 'the more you press into the ground the more it pushes you up'.[166]

An 'inactive' poorly 'grounded' base of support encourages the use of compensatory 'holding patterns' around the center or core limiting effective patterns of axial control and weight shift (Fig. 13.106). Establishing a proper base improves

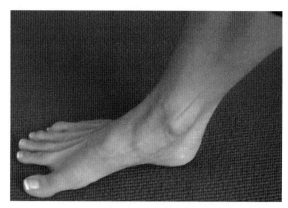

Fig 13.105 • An active foot combines elements of 'doming' for push off and support and 'fanning' the toes for stability.

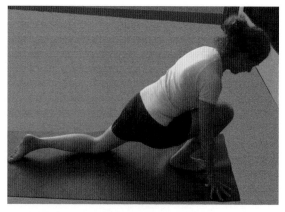

Fig 13.106 • Compensatory axial 'holding' is more likely with a poorly developed base of support. Note the right foot is not well grounded through the heel and there is evident CPC holding in the torso.

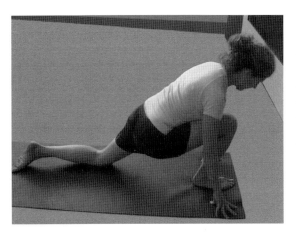

Fig 13.107 • When the foot is better grounded pelvic and axial control changes. She no longer needs to rely on as much CPC behavior.

control (Fig. 13.107). For this reason the popular use of exercise balls to establish 'core stability' needs some careful rethinking. In addition, cocontraction of the trunk flexors has been shown to decrease by up to 30% during trunk extension exercises over a ball.[157]

Activating the postural reflex responses from peripheral points provides the point of stability for patterns of closed chain movement sequencing which better facilitates SLMS control, allowing adaptable uprightness and movement in all planes while balancing and breathing. In a MRI study examining diaphragm movement, Cumpelik[150] was able to show that the diaphragm reacts to changes in the posture of the feet and head and movements initiated from the periphery. Establishing postural stability is basic to effective breathing. 'When the posture is right the breathing will come'.[150]

Tai Chi and similar Eastern practices are gaining more therapeutic interest[167,168] and represent various forms of 'soft exercise' in standing which facilitate activity in the SLMS. They afford the opportunity for practice in 'grounding' through the feet in whole body patterns involving 'yield and push' and 'reach and pull sequences' variously involving weight shift, with diagonal and rotary components. Evidence suggests that elderly subjects have a reduced ability to generate ground reaction force, relying on more central (i.e. more proximal than distal) and elevated cocontraction strategies.[169]

Building forward bending and squat patterns

Expecting the patient to suddenly change his habitual responses in ADL situations is unrealistic unless we 'exercise' key components of desired patterns of movement. McGill[80,155,170] recognizing frequent 'gluteal amnesia' in many back pain subjects advises building hip extensor and squat patterns. For many patients, control is so poor that they need help with component parts of the action. The major difficulty in forward bending is poor control of the pelvis (see Chs 6 & 8).

Controlling the pelvis is particularly difficult when it is loaded in anterior tilt and/or the hip is in flexion. Some will also have difficulty with extension loading. Loading pattern difficulties become even more apparent on one leg. Achieving control is dependent upon control of the FPPs. When basically established they can be further 'drilled' in various positions, three of which are examined to provide an example.

Bridging sequences

Preparatory loading for bridging was described previously (Fig. 13.40). The habitual non ideal response is to come up high in posterior pelvic tilt with the symphysis thrust forward with poor activity in the LPU. The other difficulty is adequate inhibition of CPC behavior and the ability to expand the diaphragm and breathe regularly. When the preparatory bridging sequences are mastered the action is sustained emphasizing the LPU, grounding through the feet and the heel sitz-bone connection while breathing normally. When proficient at this, all three FPPS can be drilled while the pelvis remains off the surface. The common difficulty is in achieving adequate APR from LPU control hence this really needs encouraging.

As quality control improves, appropriate progression towards various weight shift and unilateral loading activities while in the bridge can be explored:

• in the FPP1 unweighted position, lateral weight shift *through* the hip joint axis from the LPU without any twist or supra-pubic overactivity[17,152]

• working 'distortion' patterns by rotating the pelvis to place alternate sitz-bones on the ground.

- the sole of one foot can rest over the other kneecap while the fundamental patterns are repeated
- variously performing free one hip flexion thigh vertical; maintain thigh vertical and extend knee as able; or even free SLR if advanced.

Kneeling patterns can reveal a lot

Both the 2- and 4-point kneeling postures readily reveal the common problems and the basic tendencies towards APXS or PPXS often making clearer what the principle difficulty is. Review of Chapter 9 is instructive. Knowing what to expect helps direct the specific desired responses and 'downtrain'[7] the unwanted dominant SGMS activity. Kneeling sequences challenge the lower limb out of its habitual antigravity 'extensor prop'.

- **In all fours**. Difficulty with axial and proximal girdle 'neutral' because of poor LPU control and imbalanced co-activation of the deep system flexors and extensors. The tendency is to 'prop' like a table, keeping the center *between* all four limbs. Thus we can expect:

  - Difficulty achieving a neutral spine with good alignment between the head and tailbone. The basic tendencies to flexor or extensor dominance are apparent. The preference for initiating movements from the CCPs rather than control through the proximal limb girdles maintaining alignment between the segments is observable (see Figs 3.20 & 3.21). The commonly prescribed 'humping and hollowing' or 'cat/camel' further imprints this dysfunction.

  - The proximal limb girdles bear weight in more 'flexor patterns' – 'pectoral cinch', fixing the 'dome' and 'propping' in the upper (Fig. 8.14) and posterior pelvic tilt and forward shift in the lower (Fig. 8.32). Unless checked, this tendency increases in during weight shift: forward relies on more pectoral activity creating tension in the neck and more central fixing. Backward weight shift frequently results in collapse into end range lumbopelvic flexion (Figs 8.13 & 13.71).

  - These tendencies are further observed in single limb loading with a disinclination for weight shift in homologous, homolateral and contralateral patterns because of the reduced proximal girdle and axial control. Rather than

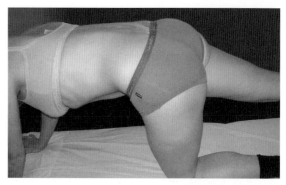

Fig 13.108 • Unilateral leg loading results in forward shift and posterior pelvic rotation. This is the same person in Fig.11.5 who is learning to teach yoga. Here she carries the same pattern into weight bearing.

control the pelvis on the femur in appropriate posterior shift / anterior rotation, they adopt a 'lock in' strategy of PPR and hip external rotation and tend to shift their weight more forward (Fig. 13.108) over relying on the arms for support.

- Initiating and controlling movement *from* the ischia and coccyx is really important in being able to control load transfer through a flexed or 'adaptable' hip (Fig. 13.109). Mastering this pattern is important for functional control of many patterns of movement in our ADL. As pelvic control improves it can be challenged with the center of gravity higher and moving outside the body. The focus is to *initiate and direct the movement back and up from the sitz-bones* while lengthening the tail bone. The possible 'moves' are innumerable once the basic dysfunction is understood and with a clarity of purpose in the rehabilitation of this. Open chain hip extension is further difficult because of difficulty controlling pelvic 'distortion' and generally results in further increased CPC activity.

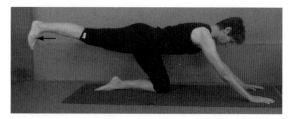

Fig 13.109 • Drilling dynamic unilateral weight bearing through the pelvis. In reaching the extended leg back, the principal focus is more upon the ischia of the weight bearing leg working up, back and wide.

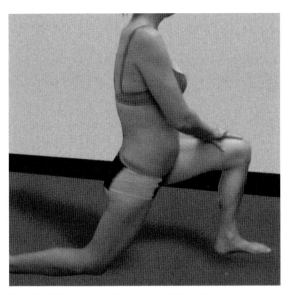

Fig 13.110 • Hanging the body weight halfway between the two limbs is more stable. This is the same patient as in Fig. 10.4. She is an APXS! Deficient LPU activity is reflected in the forward drift of the pelvis. Note how she relies upon her arms.

• **In upright kneeling**. Difficulty aligning the 'body cylinder' because of poor LPU activity and pelvic control and imbalanced co-activation between the axial flexors and extensors and imbalance in 'ischial swing' means we can expect:

- The thorax is forward in those with PPXS dominance. A tendency to tighter anterior hip structures and related difficulty with FPP2 and closed chain hip extension results in a further increase in CPC behavior and 'hanging the belly forward' (Figs 4.5 & 11.8).
- Inadequate 'grounding' through the base of support and control of the pelvis means lateral weight shift is hampered and associated with central cinch behavior (Fig. 13.111).
- There is reduced 'axial lift' with a tendency to 'hunker down' and 'grab' with the arms when perturbed. Poor axial adjustment and limited spatial reach patterns.
- All show some disinclination to 'unlock' PPR/ hip extension and posteriorly shift pelvis to weight bear in hip flexion needed for dynamic position changes of the trunk from vertical to horizontal. This is most marked in the APXS group (Fig. 13.112).

• *Half kneeling*. In general, the tendency is to 'hang the weight between the limbs' with a disinclination for posterior weight shift and

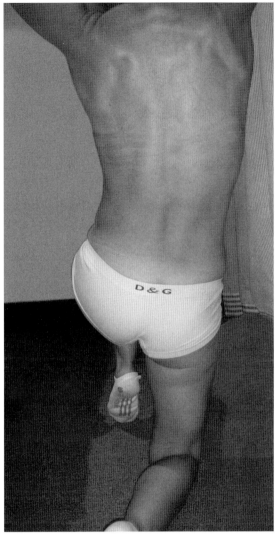

Fig 13.111 • Difficulty controlling lateral weight transfer onto one limb. Note the externally rotated hip and hamstrings activity from reduced LPU activity, and central cinch holding which limits lengthening the right waist to center the body over the leg.

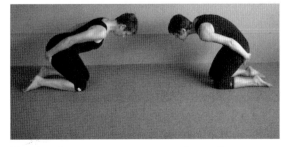

Fig 13.112 • The Key Alignment and Control Test. (L) Correct; (R) incorrect.

dynamically controlling the pelvic rotation from the LPU and balanced iliacus-psoas and hamstrings activity (Fig. 13.110). Related difficulty aligning the walls of the body cylinder is apparent.

Difficulties with lateral weight transfer are apparent in all forms of kneeing. In half kneeling, the usual compensation is to over rely on the forward leg and lose axial alignment because of difficulty directing the ischial swing and bringing the pelvis under the body (Fig. 13.111).

The Key Alignment and Control Test (KACT)

This functional test requires integrated control between the SLMS and SGMS in controlling axial alignment and in particular the pelvis under physiological sagittal loading conditions. It involves the ability of the *kneeling or standing* subject maintaining an axial neutral while executing dynamic position change of the trunk from the vertical towards the horizontal. Control of the 'pelvic swing and shift patterns' (Ch. 6, Part B) is obliged. From the neutral upright kneeling or standing position the subject's fingers locate the sitz bones to encourage widening in the two proximal girdles as the subject brings the pelvis *back* aiming to bring the spine more towards horizontal (Fig. 13.112). The quality of the response is monitored and corrections verbally prompted and manually adjusted if necessary. The action is repeated consistent with achievable challenge with the focus of the prompts being on the *correct pelvic action*, maintaining alignment and breathing. When the pattern is better established, the position is sustained as long as the subject can manage it with proper control. Doing so for 60 seconds is good. Initially it will be difficult for most to attain the proper position.

All of the inherent dysfunctional posturomovement tendencies will tend to come to the fore and need to be counteracted to help him gain control. These will be predictable in the subject depending upon which pelvic syndrome classification he fits and his stage of dysfunction. Prompts are offered as needed such as:

- 'Find the 'grounding' in your feet to support the weight and lift up of the pelvis'
- 'Widen and reach the sitz-bones up and back'
- 'Go long between the head and the tailbone'

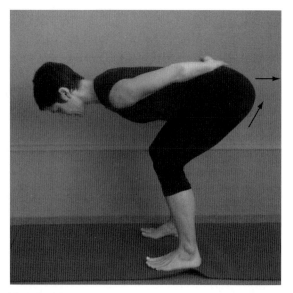

Fig 13.113 • Practising the KACT in standing improves endurance and helps imprint the relearned motor patterns. Note how the center of the body mass is balanced over the base of support.

- 'Widen the center and the shoulder girdle and expand the center with the breath'.

When the subject is aware of 'burn' in the buttocks they are actually using them! Practice in the 'test' provides further fuel for competent ADL patterns (Figs 13.100 & 13.113)

Stretching

The relative paucity of good SLMS function and the corresponding predominance of SGMS hyper-activity is reflected in just about everyone feeling stiff and needing to stretch. Stretching appears to be one of the most common interventions – but what about control? The problem is that by and large, most are perpetuating their dysfunction by the *way* they stretch. The tight muscles are generally those which relate to proximal girdle control, limiting hip and shoulder mobility while at the same time adversely affecting spinal alignment and control.

Some apparent general faults when stretching

- Loss of axial and proximal girdle alignment with axial collapse when and where possible!
- Stretching is 'passive' with little contribution from the SLMS. In fact the spine usually becomes the

victim of the stretch. The tight leg muscles win over adequate patterns of axial co-activation for control (Figs 8.8, 11.4, 12.10–12.12). 'Proper stretching' is a nice way to activate the SLMS.

• The tendency for lower limb stretches being actioned principally by the 'arms pulling' creating tension patterns in the upper body.

• The subject tenses against the discomfort, fighting himself as he disrupts his breathing and 'holds against it'.

• Lack of central and cortical intelligence in the procedure as neurologically the subject has learnt nothing, hence any lengthening is not sustained, probably accounting for the poor outcomes that stretching trials have shown.[171–173]

Features to consider in 'active elongation' or optimal stretching

This author prefers not to use the term 'stretching' as it might risk perpetuating the inherent problems listed above. Rather, *'active elongation'* signifies neuromuscular involvement where positive gains in sensorimotor experience and learning and SLMS system control are achieved at the same time. Whatever is being stretched, certain principles should be applied for optimal effects:

• Establish 'grounding' through the base of support so there is 'active lift' in the system.

• Establish axial alignment between the head and tail bone so the 'body cylinder' is balanced. In particular control the tendency to anterior rib shunt of the lower pole of the thorax.

• The stretch is *initiated from* the proximal limb girdles e.g. for the posterior hip muscles, directing the movement from the ischia which move 'back, up and wide' so that the posterior hip is asked to open. To do this effectively necessitates co-activation in the LPU and control of the FPPs with *eccentric lengthening* in the target muscles (Ch. 4; Fig. 13.114).

• Not hanging or 'propping' through the arms or conversely collapsing the whole body.

• 'Breathing into the center' and only going to the *point* where you can 'play the edges' of the discomfort, 'breathing into it' on inspiration and 'letting go' on expiration while 'softening and lengthening.

• 'Staying in it' and waiting for the release to come. If performed slowly with intent, the whole SGMS ideally begins to relax.

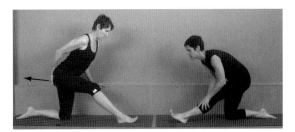

Fig 13.114 • 'Active elongation', directing the movement from the ischia and tail bone and maintaining alignment is apparent on the left. Collapse, propping, loss of alignment and stress to the low back and tension is apparent on the right.

The therapeutic use of rotation

Understanding and appreciating the importance of appropriate rotary control in optimal torso function is very often overlooked in most contemporary therapeutic approaches. The case for doing so is compelling:

• Normal movement patterns always contain an element of rotation and weight shift, even if slight (Ch. 3).

• Equilibrium and balance reactions depend on small rotary movements and postural shifts and adjustments.

• In situations of a lesion of the upper motor neuron such as cerebral palsy or stroke, reduced descending inhibitory control means movement patterns become more flexor/extensor with consequent difficulty rotating and shifting weight. Similar much more subtle tendencies are apparent in some people with back pain (Ch. 8). Neuro therapies such as that of the Bobaths advocate the use of rotary movements to both facilitate the activation of more normal movements and inhibit the unwanted more primitive responses.[174] Other therapies such as proprioceptive neuromuscular facilitation of Knott and Voss[175] also facilitate rotation in the diagonal patterns of movement they are helping to establish.

• In so called normal people, the use of patterns of rotary movement provide an increased movement repertoire and help break up habitual holding patterns. Hackney[152] notes that utilizing rotation in movements of the upper body can increase range and release habitual tension in the upper trapezius and levators which frequently become overused as a substitution for rotation when the arm reaches.

• The Feldenkrais method[133,144] of learning awareness through movement explores the non habitual three dimensional movements via gentle slow movements which utilize a lot of rotation in closed chain patterns – a marvelous way to activate the SLMS!

• The importance of rotation and weight shift in providing the added dimensions in movement control is also understood in the martial arts and many 'Eastern' movement approaches such as Tai Chi and similar practices. Their potential therapeutic benefits are attracting increased scientific interest.[167,168]

The importance of the senses in controlling movement

We have noted the interdependence between sensation and movement in motor development. Sensory information is richly supplied from proprioception, the vestibular apparatus, vision, and touch, interoception from internal organs, hearing taste, and smell. It is through the senses that we perceive our environment both internal and external. Movement occurs in response to perceived sensory information via feed forward mechanisms and is modified or adapted by it via feedback mechanisms. The quality of the motor response is largely dependent upon the quality and amount of sensory information that the central nervous system receives – 'garbage in becomes garbage out' rather like a computer or any programmed system of response. Ayres[176] recognized that defective sensory integration was reflected in less developed motor responses and learning difficulties

Bainbridge Cohen[165] discusses the dynamics of perception – 'how we filter, modify, distort, accept, reject and use that information is part of the act of perceiving. In order to perceive clearly, our attention concentration, motivation or desire must actively focus us on what it is we are to perceive'. She calls this 'active focusing'. This patterns our interpretation of sensory information, and without this active focusing, our perception remains poorly organized. Being able to come back to the inside and feel yourself provides life in the movement.[17,152] In a similar vein, Feldenkrais[133,143,144] maintains that if you are not aware of what and how you do something, you cannot change the way you do it. Even imagining a movement marshals the brain and helps

improve its execution. Hackney[152] draws attention to the important aspect of intention in movement control. 'Intent organizes the neuromuscular system. Clarity of intent enables the body to find the motor pattern to fill the intent'. Similarly, proponents of Ideokinesis and its related influence utilize mental imagery to help focus and refine the response.[142,145,146]

Most of us have developed inefficient and lazy movement habits. Changing movement requires perceptual acuity and many somatic education disciplines such as Laban/ Bartenieff, Feldenkrais, the Alexander Principle, yoga, and the martial arts focus on this aspect.

Stability and mobility are in constant relationship in movement

Feldenkrais[133] said 'Stability is nice. It also means difficulty to initiate movement as well as difficulty to be moved. Stability (when one is protected) increases the feeling of safety. Instability means risk but easy mobility. Both are biologically important. Becoming addicted to one of them makes one unsafe for lack of choice'.

In all movement, stability and mobility elements interact[17,152] – there is a continual shifting and gradation from one through to the other. Problems arise when there is too much or too little of either. 'Grounding' helps provide a stable support for movement. Effective weight shift onto one leg provides the stability for the other leg to move and so on.

In the spine, stability is achieved through control of mobility. Fundamental to this is active connection and control through the center of gravity at the pelvis – the 'core', to provide an inner adjustable base of support. There are continuous shifts in the body's center of gravity requiring simultaneous adaptive shifts and adjustments in the spine and proximal girdle joints. These movements also involve patterns of appropriate axial and proximal girdle pre-positioning and setting to support limb movements. Bartenieff[17] speaks of tensions and counter-tensions in movement. Counter-tensions help to create coactivation of the axial muscles. As the infant lifts his head (tension) he begins to push down on his arms and so creates a vertical counter-tension which leads to uprightness. As a limb moves away from the body it creates a spatial tension which becomes matched in the body by a counter-tension to balance the load. Many of these spinal countertensions are miniscule

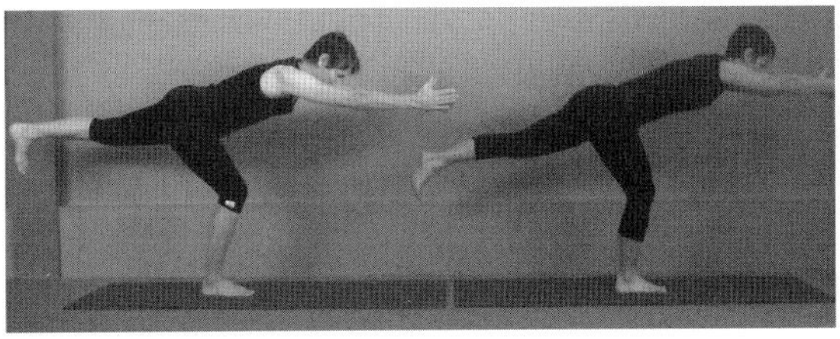

Fig 13.115 • Dynamic control of the lower kinetic chain allows innumerable movement options...

actions via deep muscle system activation. The more the limbs reach into space in three dimensions, and particularly in asymmetrical movements, the more the axial counter-tension response activates the patterns which provide spinal control. These movements should easily sequence up and down through the spine from side to side, rotationally and diagonally. Stability in the spine has been very misunderstood by many who have seen that the spine needs to be stabilized and not move! While it may be that some parts of the spine compensate with relatively too much movement, this is because other parts do not move enough.

Integrating movement through the whole spine and proximal girdles is the answer (Figs 13.115 & 13.116).

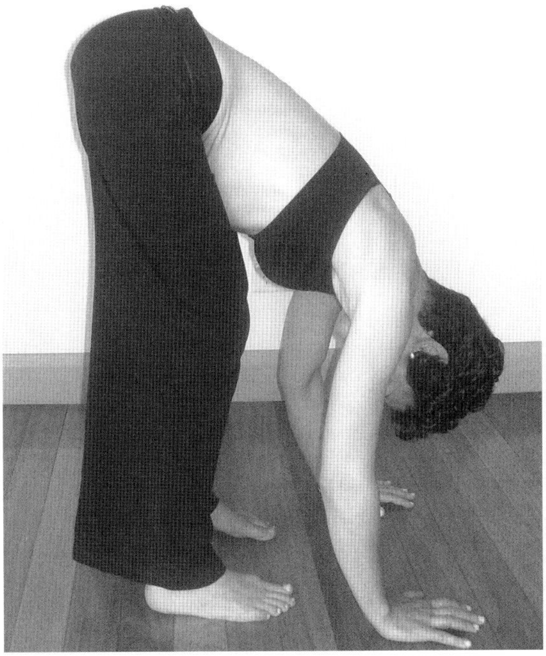

Fig 13.116 • ... including physiological forward bend without back pain. Well grounded feet are associated with good ischial lift and soft knees. In particular note the open front body in the pose.

References

[1] Janda V, Schmid HJA. Muscles as a pathogenic factor in back pain. In: *Proc.* International Federation of Manipulative Therapy. IFOMPT. New Zealand; 1980.

[2] Janda V. Motor Learning Impairment and Back Pain. J Manual Medicine 1984;22:74–8.

[3] Janda V. Muscles and motor control in low back pain: assessment and management. In: Twomey LT, editor. Physical Therapy of the low back. New York: Churchill Livingstone; 1987.

[4] Janda V, Frank C, Liebenson C. Evaluation of muscular imbalance. In: Liebenson C, editor. Rehabilitation of the Spine: a practitioner's manual. 2nd ed. Philadelphia: Lippincott Williams & Wilkins; 2007.

[5] Janda V. Muscles and Cervicogenic pain syndromes. In: Grant R, editor. Physical Therapy of the Cervical and Thoracic Spine. New York: Churchill Livingstone; 1988. p. 153–66.

[6] Janda V. Sydney: Course notes; 1984.

[7] Lee D. The pelvic girdle: an approach to the examination and treatment of the lumbopelvic-hip region. 3rd ed. Edinburgh: Churchill Livingstone; 2004.

[8] O'Sullivan PB, et al. The effect of different standing and sitting postures on trunk muscle activity in a pain free population. Spine 2002;27(11):1238–44.

[9] O'Sullivan PB, et al. Effect of different upright sitting postures on spinal-pelvic curvature and trunk muscle activation in a pain free population. Spine 2006;31 (19):E707–12.

[10] O'Sullivan PB, et al. Evaluation of the flexion relaxation phenomenon in the trunk muscles in sitting. Spine 2006;31 (17):2009–16.

[11] Lewit K. Manipulative therapy in rehabilitation of the motor system. London: Butterworths; 1985.

[12] Lewit K. Managing common syndromes and finding the key link. In: Rehabilitation of the spine: a practitioner's manual. 2nd ed. Philadelphia: Lippincott Williams and Wilkins; 2007.

[13] Kolar P. Dynamic Neuromuscular Stabilisation: According to Kolar-an introduction. Sydney: Course notes; 2008.

[14] Hodges PW. Is there a role for transversus abdominus in lumbo-pelvic stability? Man Ther 1999; 4(2):74–86.

[15] Stevens VK, et al. The influence of specific training on trunk muscle recruitment patterns in healthy subjects during stabilisation exercises. Man Ther 2007;12(3):271–9.

[16] Sahrmann SA. Diagnosis and treatment of movement

impairment syndromes. St. Louis: Mosby; 2002.

[17] Bartenieff I. Body Movement: Coping with the environment. Australia: Gordon and Breach Science Publishers; 2002.

[18] Mens JMA, et al. The active straight leg raising test and mobility of the pelvic joints. Eur Spine J 1999;8:468–73.

[19] De Groot M, et al. The active straight leg raise test (ASLR) in pregnant women: Differences in muscle activity and force between patients and healthy subjects. Man Ther 2008;13(1):68–74.

[20] Williams PL, Warwick R. Gray's Anatomy. 36th ed. Edinburgh: Churchill Livingstone.

[21] Bogduk N, Twomey LT. Clinical anatomy of the lumbar spine. Melbourne: Churchill Livingstone; 1987.

[22] O'Leary S, et al. Cranio-cervical flexor muscle impairment at maximal, moderate, and low loads is a feature of neck pain. Man Ther 2007;12(1):34–9.

[23] McConnell J. Recalcitrant chronic low back pain – a new theory and different approach to management. In: Beeton KS, editor. Manual Therapy Master Classes: The vertebral Column. Edinburgh: Churchill Livingstone; 2003.

[24] Bogduk N, Twomey LT. Clinical anatomy of the lumbar spine. Melbourne: Churchill Livingstone; 1987.

[25] Zusman M. Irritability. Man Ther 1999;3(4):195–202.

[26] Sahrmann S. Effects on muscle of repeated movements and sustained postures. In: *Proc.* 1st International Conference on Movement Dysfunction. Edinburgh; 2001.

[27] Grieve GP. Common Vertebral Joint Problems. Edinburgh; 2001.

[28] Grieve GP, editor. Modern Manual Therapy of the Vertebral Column. Edinburgh: Churchill Livingstone; 1986.

[29] Grieve GP. Mobilisation of the spine: A primary handbook of clinical method. 5th ed. Edinburgh: Churchill Livingstone; 1991.

[30] Maitland GD. Vertebral Manipulation. 4th ed. London: Butterworths; 1977.

[31] Greenman PE. Principles of Manual Medicine. 2nd ed. Baltimore: Williams and Wilkins.

[32] Liebenson C, editor. Rehabilitation of the spine: A practitioner's manual. 2nd ed. Philadelphia: Lippincott Williams and Wilkins; 2007.

[33] Bourdillon JF, Day EA. Spinal Manipulation. 4th ed. Norwalk: Heinemann Medical Books; 1987.

[34] Lee D. Manual Therapy for the thorax: a biomechanical approach. British Columbia: DOPC Delta; 1994.

[35] Laslett M. Pain provocation sacroiliac joint tests: reliability and prevalence. In: Vleeming A, et al., editor. Movement, stability and low back pain: the essential role of the pelvis. New York: Churchill Livingstone; 1997.

[36] Laslett M. Evidenced- based clinical testing of the lumbar spine and pelvis. In: Vleeming A, Mooney V, Stoeckart R, editors. Movement, Stability, & Lumbopelvic pain: integration of research and therapy. Edinburgh: Churchill Livingstone; 2007.

[37] Upledger JE, Vredevoogd JD. Craniosacral therapy. Seattle: Eastland Press; 1983.

[38] Ferreira ML, et al. Does spinal manipulative therapy help people with chronic low back pain? Aust J Physiother 2002;48:277–84.

[39] Jull G. Management of cervical headache. Man Ther 1997; 2(4):182–90.

[40] Murphy DR, Hurwitz EL, Nelson CF. A diagnosis based clinical decision rule for spinal pain: review of the literature. Chiropractic & Osteopathy 2008;16:7.

[41] Jull G, Bogduk N, Marsland A. The accuracy of manual diagnosis for cervical zygapophysial joint pain syndromes. Med J Aust 1988;148:233–6.

[42] Treleaven J, Jull G, Atkinson L. Cervical musculoskeletal dysfunction in post-concussional headache. Cephalalgia 1994;14:273–9.

[43] Hannon JC. The physics of Feldenkrais. Part 3: Stability. J of Bodywork and Movement Therapies 2000;4(4):261–72.

[44] Hannon JC. Wartenberg Part 3: Relaxation training, centration and skeletal opposition: a conceptual model. J of Bodywork and Movement Therapies 2006;10:179–96.

[45] Chaitow L. Are skilled manual practitioners and therapists artists or technicians, or both? Editorial. J Bodywork and Movement Therapies 1996;1(1):1.

[46] Chaitow L. Palpation and assessment skills: Assessment and diagnosis through touch. 2nd ed. Edinburgh: Churchill Livingstone; 1997.

[47] Lewit K, Kobesová A. Soft tissue manipulation. In: a Rehabilitation of the spine: a practitioner's manual. 2nd ed. Philadelphia: Lippincott Williams and Wilkins; 2007.

[48] Hannon JC. The man who mistook his patient for a chair: a speculation regarding sitting mechanical treatment of lower back pain. J Bodywork and Movement Therapies 1998;2(2):88–100.

[49] Chaitow L. Soft and hard evidence. Editorial. J Bodywork and Movement Therapies 2005;9:167–8.

[50] Carrière B. Interdependence of posture and the pelvic floor. In: Carrière B, Markel Feldt C, editors. The pelvic floor. Stuttgart: Thieme; 2006.

[51] Shirley D, et al. Spinal stiffness changes throughout the respiratory cycle. J Appl Physiol 2003;95:1467–75.

[52] Clifton-Smith T. Breathe to Succeed. New Zealand: Penguin; 1999.

[53] McLaughlin L, Goldsmith CH. Altered respiration in a case series of low back/pelvic pain patients. In: Proc. 6th Interdisciplinary World Congress on Low Back and Pelvic Pain. Barcelona; 2007.

[54] Chansirinukor W, Lee M. Latimer. Contribution of pelvic rotation to lumbar posteroanterior movement. Man Ther 2001;6(4):242–9.

[55] Travell JG, Simons DG. Myofascial pain and dysfunction: The trigger point manual: The lower extremities. Baltimore: Williams and Wilkins; 1992.

[56] Grieve GP. The sacro-iliac joint. Physiotherapy 1976;62(12): 384–400.

[57] Pool-Goudzwaard AL, et al. Insufficient lumbopelvic stability: a clinical, anatomical and biomechanical approach to 'a-specific' low back pain. Man Ther 1998;3(1):12–20.

[58] Laslett M, et al. Diagnosis of sacroiliac joint pain: Validity of individual provocation tests and composites of tests. Man Ther 2005;10(3):207–18.

[59] Bendová P, et al. MRI based registration of pelvic alignment affected by altered pelvic floor muscle characteristics. Clin Biomech 2007;22(9):980–7.

[60] Cibulka MT, et al. Unilateral hip rotation range of motion asymmetry in patients with sacroiliac joint regional pain. Spine 1998;23(9):1009–15.

[61] Bobath K. The motor deficit in patients with cerebral palsy. Clinics in Developmental Medicine No. 23 Spastics International Medical Publications in association with William Heinemann Medical Books Ltd; 1966.

[62] Boyle JJ. Is the pain and dysfunction of shoulder impingement lesion really second rib syndrome in disguise? Two case reports. Man Ther 1999; 4(1):44–8.

[63] Bogduk N. Cervical causes of headache and dizziness. In: Grieve GP, editor. Modern Manual Therapy of the Vertebral Column. Churchill Livingstone; 1986.

[64] Van Dillen LR, Sahrmann SA, et al. The effect of modifying patient-preferred spinal movement and alignment during symptom testing in patients with low back pain: a preliminary report. Arch Phys Med Rehabil 2003;84:313–22.

[65] Sapsford RR, et al. Coactivation of the abdominal and pelvic floor muscles during voluntary exercises. Neurology and Neurodynamics 2001;20:31–42.

[66] Sapsford R. The pelvic floor: a clinical model for function and rehabilitation. Physiotherapy 2001;87(12):620–30.

[67] Sapsford RR, Richardson CA, Stanton W. Sitting posture affects pelvic floor muscle activity in parous women: an observational study. Aust J Physiother 2006;52:219–22.

[68] Basler HD, Keller S, Herda C. Good postural habits: a pilot investigation using EMG scanning of the paraspinals. Appl Psychophysiol Biofeedback 1997;22(3):171–82.

[69] Kasahara S, et al. Lumbar-pelvic coordination in the sitting position. Gait posture 2008; 28(2):251–7.

[70] Kolar P. Facilitation of agonist-antagonist co-activation by reflex stimulation methods. In: Liebenson C, editor. Rehabilitation of the spine: a practitioner's manual. Philadelphia: Lippincott Williams & Wilkins; 2007.

[71] McKenzie RA. The lumbar spine: mechanical diagnosis and therapy. New Zealand: Spinal Publications; 1989.

[72] Rock C.-M.. Reflex incontinence caused by underlying functional disorders. In: Carrière B, Markel Feldt C, editors. The pelvic floor. Stuttgart: Thieme; 2006.

[73] Magnusson M, et al. Hyperextension and spine height changes. Spine 1996;21(22): 2670–5.

[74] Adams MA, et al. Effects of backward bending on lumbar intervertebral discs: Relevance to physical therapy treatments for low back pain. Spine 2000; 25(4):431–8.

[75] Snook SH, et al. The reduction of chronic non-specific low back pain through the control of early morning lumbar flexion: a randomised controlled trial. Spine 1998;23(23):2601–7.

[76] Suni J. Control of the lumbar neutral zone decreases low back pain and improves self-evaluated work ability: a 12-month randomized controlled study. Spine 2006;31(18):E611–20.

[77] Farhi D. The breathing book: Good health and vitality through essential breath work. New York: Henry Holt and Company; 1996.

[78] O'Sullivan PB, Beales DJ. Changes in pelvic floor and diaphragm kinematics and respiratory patterns in subjects with sacroiliac joint pain following a motor learning intervention. A case series. Man Ther 2007; 12(3):209–18.

[79] Liebenson C. Core training: the importance of the diaphragm. Dynamic Chiropractic 2007; 25(17).

[80] McGill SM. Lower Back Disorders: Evidence-based prevention and rehabilitation. Champaign Il: Human Kinetics; 2002.

[81] Mannion AF, et al. Active therapy for chronic low back pain. Part 1 Effects on back muscle activation, fatigability and strength. Spine 2001;26(7):909–19.

[82] Jull GA, Richardson CA. Motor control problems in patients with spinal pain: a new direction for therapeutic exercise. J Manipulative Physiol Ther 2000;23(2):115–7.

[83] Faas A. Exercises: which ones are worth trying, for which patients and when? Spine 1996;21(24): 2874–8.

[84] Van Tulder MW, Koes BW, Bouter LM. Conservative treatment of acute and chronic nonspecific low back pain: a systematic review of randomized controlled trials of the most common interventions. Spine 1997;22(18):2128–56.

[85] Van Tulder M, et al. Exercise therapy for low back pain: a systematic review within the framework of the Cochrane Collaboration Back Review Group. Spine 2000;25(21): 2784–96.

[86] Abenhaim L, et al. The role of activity in the therapeutic management of back pain: report of the International Paris Task Force on Back Pain. Spine 2000;25(45):1S–33S.

[87] Mayer TG, et al. Volvo award in clinical sciences: objective assessment of spine function following industrial injury:

a prospective study with comparison group and one year follow up. Spine 1985;10 (6):482–93.

[88] Rainville J, Kim RS, Katz JN. A review of 1985 Volvo Award Winner in Clinical Science: objective assessment of spine function following industrial injury: a prospective study with comparison group and 1-year follow up. Spine 2007; 32(18):2031–4.

[89] Frost H, et al. A fitness program for patients with chronic low back pain: 2-year follow-up of a randomised controlled trial Pain 1998;75(2–3):273–9.

[90] Elnaggar IM, et al. Effects of spinal flexion and extension exercises on low back pain and spinal mobility in chronic mechanical low back pain patients. Spine 1991; 16(8):967–72.

[91] Leggett S, et al. Restorative exercise for clinical low back pain: a prospective two-center study with a one year follow-up. Spine 1999;24(9):889.

[92] Mannion AF, et al. 1999 Volvo Award Winner in Clinical Studies: a randomized clinical trial of three active therapies for chronic low back pain. Spine 1999;24(23):2435.

[93] Dolan P, et al. Can exercise therapy improve the outcome of microdiscectomy. Spine 2000;25 (12):1523–32.

[94] Manniche C, et al. Intensive dynamic back exercises for chronic low back pain. A clinical trial. Pain 1991;47(1):53–63.

[95] Luoto S, et al. One footed and externally disturbed two-footed postural control in patients with chronic low back pain and healthy control subjects: a controlled study with follow up. Spine 1998;23(19):2081–9.

[96] Mannion AF, et al. Active therapy for chronic low back pain: Part 3. Factors influencing self-rated disability and its change following therapy. Spine 2001; 26(8):920–9.

[97] Mannion AF, et al. Comparison of three active therapies for chronic low back pain: results of a randomized clinical trial with one year follow up. Rheumatology 2001;40(7):772–8.

[98] Shields RK, Heiss DG. An electromyographic comparison of abdominal muscle synergies during curl and doubled straight leg lowering exercises with control of pelvic position. Spine 1997;22(16):1873–9.

[99] Panjabi MM. The stabilising system of the spine:1 Function, dysfunction, adaptation and enhancement. J Spinal Disord 1992;5:383–9.

[100] Kavcic N, Grenier S, McGill SM. Quantifying tissue loads and spine stability while performing commonly prescribed low back stabilisation exercises. Spine 2004;29(20): 2319–29.

[101] McGill SM. Low back stability: from formal description to issues for performance and rehabilitation. Exercise & Sport Sciences Reviews 2001; 29(1):26–31.

[102] Marshall P, Murphy B. Changes in the flexion relaxation response following an exercise intervention. Spine 2006; 31(23):E877–83.

[103] Akuthota SF. Core strengthening. Arch Phys Med Rehabil 2004;85(1):86–92.

[104] Hall L, et al. Immediate effects of co-contraction training on motor control of the trunk muscles in people with recurrent low back pain. J Electromyogr Kinesiol (IN PRESS).

[105] Richardson C, Hodges PW, Hides J. Therapeutic exercise for lumbopelvic stabilisation: a motor control approach for the treatment and prevention of low back pain. 2nd ed. Edinburgh: Churchill Livingstone; 2004.

[106] Hides JA, Richardson CA, Jull GA. Multifidus muscle recovery is not automatic following resolution of acute first episode low back pain. Spine 1996;21:2763–9.

[107] Hides JA, Jull GA, Richardson CA. Long term effects of specific stabilising exercises for first episode low back pain. Spine 2001; 26:E243–8.

[108] O'sullivan PB, Twomey L, Allison G. Evaluation of specific stabilising exercise in the treatment of chronic low back pain with radiologic diagnosis of spondylolysis or spondylolisthesis. Spine 1997; 22(24):2959–67.

[109] Stuge B, et al. The efficacy of a treatment program focusing on specific stabilising exercises for pelvic girdle pain after pregnancy. A randomized controlled trial. Spine 2004;29 (10):351–9.

[110] Byrne K, Doody C, Hurley DA. Exercise therapy for low back pain: a small-scale exploratory survey of current physiotherapy practice in the Republic of Ireland acute hospital setting. Man Ther 2006;11:272–8.

[111] Esola MA, et al. Analysis of lumbar spine and hip motion during forward bending in subjects with and without a history of low back pain. Spine 1996;21(1):71–8.

[112] McClure PW, et al. Kinematic analysis of lumbar and hip motion while rising from a forward, flexed position in patients with and without a history of low back pain. Spine 1997;22(5):552–8.

[113] Van Dieën JH, et al. Effects of repetitive lifting on kinematics: inadequate anticipatory control or adaptive changes. J Mot Behav 1998;30(1):20–32.

[114] Hodges PW, Richardson CA. Inefficient muscular stabilisation of the lumbar spine associated with low back pain: a motor control evaluation of transversus abdominis. Spine 1996; 21(22):2640–50.

[115] Hodges PW, Richardson CA. Altered trunk muscle recruitment in people with low back pain with upper limb movement at different speeds. Arch Phys Med Rehabil 1999; 80(9):1005–12.

[116] Hodges PW. Changes in motor planning of feedforward postural responses of the trunk muscles in low back pain. Exp Brain Res 2001;141(2):261–6.

[117] Mok NW, Brauer SG, Hodges PW. Hip strategy for

balance control in quiet standing is reduced in people with low back pain. Spine 2004;29(6):E107–12.

[118] Van Dieën JH, Cholewicki J, Radebold A. Trunk muscle recruitment patterns in patients with low back pain enhance the stability of the lumbar spine. Spine 2003;28(8):834–41.

[119] Moseley GL, Hodges PW. Reduced variability of postural strategy prevents normalization of motor changes induced by back pain: a risk factor for chronic trouble? Behav Neurosci 2006;120(2):474–6.

[120] O'Sullivan PB, et al. The relationship between posture and back muscle endurance in industrial workers with flexion related low back pain. Man Ther 2006;11:264–71.

[121] O'Sullivan PB, et al. Altered motor control strategies in subjects with sacroiliac joint pain during active straight-leg-raise test. Spine 2002;27(1):E1–8.

[122] Magnusson ML, et al. Range of motion and motion patterns in patients with low back pain before and after rehabilitation. Spine 1998;23(23):2631–9.

[123] Hodges PW, Richardson. Delayed postural contraction of transversus abdominis in low back pain associated with movement of the lower limb. J Spinal Disord 1998;11(1):46–56.

[124] Tsao H, Hodges PW. Immediate changes in feedforward postural adjustments following voluntary motor training. Exp Brain Res 2007;181(2):537.

[125] Tsao H, Hodges PW. Persistence of improvements in postural strategies following motor control training in people with recurrent low back pain. J Electromyogr Kinesiol 2008;18(4):559–67.

[126] Stuge B, et al. Abdominal and pelvic floor muscle function in women with and without long lasting pelvic girdle pain. Man Ther 2006;11:287–96.

[127] Mens JMA, Snijders CJ, Stam HJ. Diagonal trunk muscle exercises in peripartum pelvic pain: a randomized clinical trial. Phys Ther 2000;80(12):1164–73.

[128] Luoto S, et al. One-footed and externally disturbed two-footed postural control in patients with chronic low back pain and healthy control subjects: a controlled study with follow-up. Spine 1998;23(19):2081–9.

[129] Vlaeyen G, Crombez G. Fear of movement/(re)injury, avoidance and pain disability in chronic low back pain patients. Man Ther 1999;4(4):187–95.

[130] Stuge B, Holm I, Vøllestad N. To treat or not to treat postpartum pelvic pain with stabilising exercises? Man Ther 2006;11:337–43.

[131] Cholewicki J. Spine stability: the six blind men and the elephant. In: 6th Interdisciplinary World Congress on Low Back and Pelvic Pain. Barcelona; 2007.

[132] Rolf IP. Rolfing: The integration of human structures. New York: Harper and Row; 1977.

[133] Feldenkrais M. The Elusive Obvious or Basic Feldenkrais. California: Meta Publications; 1981.

[134] Iyengar BKS. Yoga: The path to holistic health. London: Dorling Kindersley; 2001.

[135] Van Vliet PM, Heneghan NR. Motor control and the management of musculoskeletal dysfunction. Man Ther 2006;11:208–13.

[136] Janda V, et al. Sensory motor stimulation. In: Liebenson C, editor. Rehabilitation of the spine: a practitioner's manual. Philadelphia: Lippincott Williams & Wilkins; 2007.

[137] Janda V. Rational therapeutic approach of chronic back pain syndromes. In: Symposium Chronic back pain, rehabilitation and self help. Proc 69-76. Finland; 1985.

[138] Janda V. Treatment of chronic back pain. Journal of Manual Medicine 1992;6:166–8.

[139] Brumagne S, et al. The role of the paraspinal muscle spindles in lumbosacral position sense in individuals with and without low back pain. Spine 2000;25(8):989–94.

[140] Bullock-Saxton JE, Janda V, Bullock MI. Reflex activation of gluteal muscles in walking: an approach to restoration of muscle function for patients with low back pain. Spine 1993;18(6):704–8.

[141] Page P. Sensori-motor training: a 'global' approach for balance training. J of Bodywork and Movement Therapies 2006;10:77–84.

[142] Sweigard LE. Human Movement Potential: Its Ideokinetic Facilitation. University Press of America; 1974.

[143] Feldenkrais M. Body and Mature Behaviour: a study of anxiety, sex, gravitation and learning. New York: International Universities Press Inc; 1949.

[144] Feldenkrais M. Awareness through movement: Health exercises for personal growth. San Francisco: Harper; 1990.

[145] Dowd I. Taking Root to Fly: articles on functional anatomy. 3rd ed. New York: Irene Dowd Publisher; 1995.

[146] Franklin E. Dynamic Alignment through Imagery. USA: Human Kinetics; 1996.

[147] Frank K. Tonic Function: A gravity response model for Rolfing Structural Movement Integration. Rolf Lines; March 1995.

[148] Pavlu D, Petak-Krueger S, Janda V. Brügger Methods for postural correction. In: Liebenson C, editor. Rehabilitation of the spine: a practitioner's manual. Philadelphia: Lippincott Williams & Wilkins; 2007.

[149] Kolar P, Safarova M. Dynamic Neuromuscular Stabilisation: According to Kolar – an introduction. Sydney: Course notes; February 2008.

[150] Cumpelik J. Breathing Mechanics in postural stabilisation. Sydney: Course; June 2008.

[151] Hodges PW, et al. Coexistence of stability and mobility in postural control: evidence from postural compensation for

respiration. Exp Brain Res 2002;144(3):293–302.

[152] Hackney P. Making Connections: total body integration through Bartenieff Fundamentals. New York: Routledge; 2002.

[153] Cumpelik J, Vele F. Yoga-based training for spinal stability. In: Liebenson C, editor. Rehabilitation of the spine: a practitioner's manual. Philadelphia: *Lippincott Williams & Wilkins*; 2007.

[154] McGill SM. Low Back Disorders: Evidence-based prevention and rehabilitation. USA: *Human Kinetics*; 2002.

[155] McGill SM. Ultimate back fitness and performance. Waterloo: Wabuno Publishers; 2004.

[156] Liebenson C. Functional fitness training: the functional reach. J of Bodywork and Movement Therapies 2006;10:159–62.

[157] Drake JDM, et al. Do exercise balls provide a training advantage for trunk extensor exercises. J Manipulative Physiol Ther 2006;29(5):354–62.

[158] Lehman GJ, Gilas D, Patel U. An unstable support surface does not increase scapulothoracic stabilising muscle activity during push and push up plus exercise. Man Ther 2008;13(6):500–6.

[159] Liebenson C. Functional training for performance enhancement Part 1: The basics. J of Bodywork and Movement Therapies 2006;10:154–8.

[160] Liebenson C. Functional training for performance enhancement – Part 2: Clinical application. J of Bodywork and Movement Therapies 2006;10:206–7.

[161] Beach P. The contractile field: a new model of human movement – Part 2. J of Bodywork and Movement Therapies 2008;12(1):76–85.

[162] Kagan B. Laban/Bartenieff post congress workshop. In: 5th Interdisciplinary World Congress on Low Back and Pelvic Pain. Melbourne; 2004.

[163] Batson G. Revisiting overuse injuries in dance in view of motor learning and somatic models of distributed practice. J of Dance Medicine and Science 2007;11(3):70–5.

[164] Hartley L. Wisdom of the Body Moving: an introduction to Body-Mind Centering. Berkeley: North Atlantic Books; 1995.

[165] Bainbridge Cohen B. Sensing, Feeling and Action: The Experiential Anatomy of Body-Mind Centering. Northampton: Contact Editions; 1993.

[166] Alon R. Sydney: Feldenkrais workshop; 2004.

[167] Wolf SL, Coogler C, Xu T. Exploring the basis for Tai Chi Chuan as a therapeutic exercise approach. Arch Phys Med Rehabil 1997;78(8):886–92.

[168] Gatts SK, Woollacott MH. How Tai Chi improves balance: biomechanics of recovery to a walking slip in impaired seniors.

Gait Posture 2007;25(2):199–214.

[169] Larsen AH, et al. Comparison of ground reaction forces and antagonist muscle coactivation during stair walking with aging. J Electromyogr Kinesiol 2008;18(4):568 79.

[170] McGill SM. Appropriate back exercise: from rehabilitation to high performance. In: Proc. 5th Interdisciplinary World Congress on Low Back and Pelvic Pain. Melbourne; 2004.

[171] Herbert RD, Gabriel M. Effects of stretching before and after exercising on muscle soreness and risk of injury: systematic review. Br Med J 2002;325 (Aug):1–5.

[172] Weldon SM, Hill RH. The efficacy of stretching for prevention of exercise-related injury: a systematic review of the literature. Man Ther 2003;8(3):141–50.

[173] Pope R. Muscle stretching for the athlete: Friend or foe? Aust Physiotherapy Association Sportslink 2002;Sept:4–5.

[174] Finnie N. Handling the Young Cerebral Palsied Child at Home. London: William Heinemann Books; 1974.

[175] Knott M, Voss DE. Proprioceptive Neuromuscular Facilitation: Patterns and Techniques. 2nd ed. New York: Harper & Row Publishers; 1968.

[176] Ayres J. Sensory Integration and Learning Disorders. Los Angeles: Western Psychological Services; 1972.

14

Inherent implications in this model

The back is the major highway of function in the body. A healthy spine ensures our general health and well being. When the spine loses its intrinsic support problems ensue. Being 'upright' involves a delicate balance in achieving effective control around the 'line' of gravitational force. One of the many challenges in our developmental progression is to strike the balance between too little and too much control. Compensations can begin early, are carried forward and are further built upon. And that goes for all of us.

Back pain appears to be a developmental problem in 'normal' 'healthy' people who don't move particularly well

The line between 'normal' and 'abnormal' is fuzzy. 'Dysfunction' is not necessarily overt but invariably involves subtle variations of what is usually considered 'normal'.

In general, seemingly subtle neuromuscular dysfunctions can be discerned in all of us, and have probably been present for a long while. Inefficient postural and movement responses exact their toll over time and by the stage of pain appearance, they are often well entrenched. The presence of pain further compounds the problems with movement control. Whether we 'succumb' or not will depend upon the quality of our intrinsic neuromotor blueprint and the further influence of various other factors which combine towards a 'tipping point' and so, various symptom development. Obese couch

potatoes get back pain but so do gymnasts and 'fit' secretaries.

The model presented attempts to assist the practitioner in 'seeing' what might be some of the more common *underlying altered patterns of neuromuscular function* which may underpin each individual patient presentation albeit with differing combinations of influential factors.

The movement dysfunction seen in patients with back pain is not a simple problem and there are no simple answers. Added to which for many, the neuromuscular 'changes' appear so subtle as to be considered insignificant. However the spine, like any column does not relish eccentric loading. Little changes can mean a lot where imbalance in its function is reflected in significant changes in the body's holistic function and wellbeing.

'Owning your problem' of back pain

The model presented argues that, in certain respects, the patient with back pain is 'caught in the loop' of a self inflicted, self sustaining cycle of posturomovement dysfunction. It is largely about habitual behavior. However, it is generally a case of 'Forgive them Father, for they know not what they do'. The job of the practitioner is to discern and effectively treat the reasons for the pain, and educate the patient about his role in its genesis. The patient needs to accept and see that the *way* he postures and moves contributes towards much of his problem through poor awareness and bad habits. He needs to be an active participant in his treatment program, and have a desire to get better, believing that change is possible. He needs to be prepared to make the necessary adaptations for change to ensue.

If nothing changes, nothing will change!

However, the degree to which change can be made will obviously vary according to the stage of the disorder, the degree of entrenched patterns of dysfunction, the magnitude of structural changes as well as psychosocial aspects. Therapeutic expectations need to be realistic and endeavors pragmatically directed to those who genuinely seek help. The 'helper' needs to possess an impressive 'armory' of clinical practice tools and abilities and above all, be altruistic.

The wider implications of the model

An understanding of the model presented invites its broader application into the rationales underlying most exercise and fitness programs, including the committed practice of yoga.

The model presents marked implications for both the medical and insurance industries in the manner in which they view and approach the treatment of back pain. The patient should not be the passive recipient. Frequently 'the fault' lies with the way the patient performs the simple everyday tasks rather than with 'someone or something else'. However, the patient really needs help in overcoming the pain that he has, in understanding why it is there and *appropriate and specific guidance* relevant to his problem and in learning new ways to counter the factors that have led to it.

There are also significant implications for research design in the hitherto use of 'healthy' and 'normal' controls. To date this has usually meant 'without pain'. The quality of a subject's kinematic patterns of movement may/not be less than ideal yet time and circumstance have been kind, with no pain episodes...to date. With a commitment to heal, simple observation, sensitivity, intuition and connection with one's own somatic intelligence, the practitioner can better appreciate the qualitative rather than the quantitative aspects of movement function. Herein it is suggested, lie the makings for a better understanding of 'back pain' and its management. This is more likely to lead to more functionally relevant therapeutic and research design and potentially better outcomes for all concerned.

ACMs	Anterior chest muscles		**I/Ts**	Ischial tuberosities
APA	Australian Physiotherapy Association		**IVD**	Intervertebral disc
APR	Anterior pelvic rotation		**IVF**	Intervertebral foramen
APXS	Anterior pelvic crossed syndrome		**LBP**	Lower back pain
ASIS	Anterior superior iliac spine		**LD**	Latissimus dorsi
ASLR	Active straight leg raise		**LOG**	Line of gravity
BOS	Base of support		**Logf**	Line of gravitational force
BPD	Breathing pattern disorders		**LPU**	Lower pelvic unit
BPR	Backward pelvic rotation		**LS**	Layer syndrome
BSR	Backward shoulder rotation		**LSJ**	Lumbosacral junction
BTS	Belted torso syndrome		**M & LT**	Middle and lower trapezius
CAC	Central anterior cinch		**MS**	Mixed Syndrome
CCC	Central conical cinch		**NPRM**	Normal postural reflex mechanism
CCJ	Cervico cranial junction		**PFM**	Pelvic floor muscles
CCPs	Central cinch patterns		**PIR**	Post isometric relaxation
CLBP	Chronic low back pain		**PKB**	Prone knee bend
CNSLBP	Chronic non specific low back pain		**PPPP**	Peri-partum pelvic pain
COG	Centre of gravity		**PPR**	Posterior pelvic rotation
COM	Centre of mass		**PPXS**	Posterior pelvic crossed syndrome
COP	Centre of pressure		**PSIS**	Posterior superior iliac spine
CPC	Central posterior cinch		**PXS**	Pelvic crossed syndromes
CTJ	Cervicothoracic junction		**RA**	Rectus abdominis
DBP	Dysfunctional breathing pattern		**S-C**	Sacrum-coccyx
EO	External oblique		**SCM**	Sternocleidomastoid
ERs	External rotators		**SGMS**	Systemic global muscle system
ES	Erector spinae		**SIJ**	Sacro iliac joint
FBP	Forward bend pattern		**SLMS**	Systemic local muscle system
FPPs	Fundamental pelvic patterns		**SPI**	Serratus posterior inferior
FPP1	1stFundamental Pelvic pattern		**STNR**	Symmetrical Tonic Neck Reflex
FPP2	2ndFundamental Pelvic pattern		**SXS**	Shoulder crossed syndrome
FPP3	3rdFundamental Pelvic pattern		**T/B**	Tail bone
FPR	Forward pelvic rotation		**T/L**	Thoraco-lumbar
FSR	Forward shoulder rotation		**TLJ**	Thoraco-lumbar junction
FSU	Functional spinal unit		**TLR**	Tonic Labyrinthine Reflex
HVS	Hyperventilation syndrome		**Tr A**	Transverse abdominis
IAP	Intra abdominal pressure		**UT**	Upper trapezius
IO	Internal oblique		**1°**	Primary
IRs	Internal rotators			

Index

M